Pulmonary Nursing Care

Patricia A. Dettenmeier, M.S.N., R.N., CCRN
Clinical Nurse Specialist
Division of Pulmonology and Pulmonary Occupational Medicine
Assistant Clinical Professor of Nursing
St. Louis University Medical Center
St. Louis, Missouri

150 illustrations

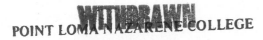

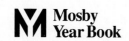
Mosby
Year Book

St. Louis Baltimore Boston Chicago London Philadelphia Sydney Toronto

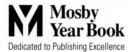

Mosby
Year Book
Dedicated to Publishing Excellence

Executive editor: Don Ladig
Managing editor: Robin Carter
Assistant editor: Linda Woodard
Project manager: M.S. Spann
Designer: Jeanne Wolfgeher

Printed in the United States of America

Mosby-Year Book, Inc.
11830 Westline Industrial Drive
St. Louis, Missouri 63146

ISBN 0-8016-5876-4

92 93 94 95 96 CL/DC 9 8 7 6 5 4 3 2 1

Consultants

Patricia Carroll, C.,C.E.N., R.R.T., M.S., R.N.
Owner, Educational Medical Consultants
Per Diem Staff Nurse
Emergency Department
Manchester Memorial Hospital
Manchester, Connecticut

Patti Coughlin Dalleske, M.S.N., CCRN, R.N.
Instructor
Youngstown State University
Youngstown, Ohio

Susan Donckers, Ed.D., R.N.
Associate Professor of Nursing
Radford University
Radford, Virginia

Margaret Eberts, M.S.N., CCRN, R.N.
Clinical Nurse Specialist
Ohio State University Hospitals
Columbus, Ohio

Clydia Frazier, M.S.N.
Clinical Specialist, Certified
Baltimore Veterans Administration Medical Center
Baltimore, Maryland

Cheri Howard, M.S.N., R.N.
Unit Director
Indiana University Hospital
Indianapolis, Indiana

Janet Larson, Ph.D., R.N.
Assistant Professor
College of Nursing
University of Illinois at Chicago
Chicago, Illinois

Colleen Mall, M.N.
Director
Nursing Education
Research Medical Center and Trinity
    Lutheran Hospital
Kansas City, Missouri

Edwina McConnell, Ph.D., R.N.
Independent Nurse Consultant
Madison, Wisconsin

Virginia L. Norman, M.A., M.S., R.N.
Associate Professor
College of Nursing
University of North Dakota
Grand Forks, North Dakota

Barbara Ogden, M.S.N., R.N.C.
College of Nursing
University of Florida/GVAMC
Gainesville, Florida

Tracy Riley, B.S.N., R.N.
Instructor
Aultman Hospital School of Nursing
Canton, Ohio

Carol M. Ruscin, B.S., R.N.
Level I Faculty
Baptist Medical System School of Nursing
Little Rock, Arkansas

Robert E. St. John, R.R.T., B.S.N., B.A., R.N.
Cardiopulmonary Nurse Clinician
Department of Nursing Administration
Jewish Hospital at the Washington University
    Medical Center
St. Louis, Missouri

Carol Thompson, Ph.D.
Assistant Professor
College of Nursing
University of Tennessee at Memphis
Memphis, Tennessee

Nancy Townsend, M.N., CCRN, C.S., R.N.
Program Director
Nursing Knowledge, Inc.
Metairie, Louisiana

Mary Wallace, R.N.C., M.S.N.
Assistant Professor
Northern Michigan University
Marquette, Michigan

Pamela Becker Weilitz, M.S.N.(R), R.N.
Pulmonary Clinical Nurse Specialist
Barnes Hospital at the Washington University
    Medical Center
St. Louis, Missouri

Preface

What do nurses and other health care professionals need to know in order to care for patients, primarily adults, with lung dysfunction? This is the objective of *Pulmonary Nursing Care* which is organized into 5 units based on clinically-functional components of the nursing process: assessment, diagnosis, and intervention.

Organization. To understand what happens in the patient (pathophysiology) and why treatments appropriate for one disorder are not appropriate for another, the nurse needs a foundation in what is normal. Therefore, Unit 1, Foundations of Pulmonary Nursing, includes the most important concepts of pulmonary anatomy and physiology, divided into 3 chapters.

Given this knowledge, the nurse is prepared to gather data. Unit 2, Methods of Assessing Pulmonary Function, is designed to provide the nurse with information about gathering and interpreting data specific to patients with lung dysfunction. This process begins with taking a history and performing a physical examination. Pertinent information about other body systems as they relate to the pulmonary system are also included. Other chapters in Unit 2 focus on analysis of arterial blood gases, chest x-rays, and pulmonary function tests. Components specific to critically ill patients are included throughout with additional specific concerns addressed in Chapter 9 Bedside Monitoring of Acutely Ill Patients. Some nurses might argue that they do not need to know how to interpret chest x-rays. Although it is true that a physician is ultimately responsible for "reading" a chest x-ray, it is important for nurses to understand abnormalities on chest x-rays to effectively direct nursing care. I have therefore included numerous examples of x-rays in this unit.

Unit 3, Diagnosis of Respiratory Dysfunction, discusses major lung diseases, of which there are basically two types: obstructive and restrictive. Some lung diseases, such as adult respiratory distress syndrome or chest trauma, traditionally cause acute respiratory failure and are discussed separately in Chapter 12 Respiratory Failure. In Chapter 12, I have tried to help the nurse separate basic ventilatory and oxygenation failure, which is critical for treatment.

Unit 4 Methods of Intervention discusses interventions applied in patients with respiratory dysfunction. Main interventions are classified into noninvasive and invasive, although noninvasive and invasive mechanical ventilation and weaning are covered in a subsequent chapter. Similarly, medications are discussed separately and not integrated into the treatment of diseases or with other interventions.

The final section—Unit 5, Home Care of Patients with Respiratory Dysfunction—is directed toward home discharge of patients with pulmonary dysfunction. This area has developed markedly in the past 2 decades. Patients are being sent home sooner, and with more technology for them to manage in the home. There is also a trend toward improving functional capabilities and quality of life in patients with chronic pulmonary diseases through rehabilitation. Unfortunately, reimbursement for pulmonary rehabilitation is not always optimal, and patients may need direction from the home health nurse.

A comprehensive patient education program, complete with reproducible patient education guides, is presented in Chapter 19 Pulmonary Rehabilitation.

Features. Each unit contains an introduction to focus the reader on important content. Each chapter begins with general learning objectives applicable to the student or practicing nurse to promote learning. This book is well illustrated—it includes over 100 illustrations to reinforce content visually. In addition, numerous tables and boxes are provided to help the nurse provide complete care for patients with pulmonary dysfunction.

Acknowledgements. I have many people to thank for their contributions over the years. First, there are the patients who helped me realize that I wanted to be a pulmonary nurse. Then, there are the nurses, therapists, social workers, and physicians who asked the questions that helped direct the content of this book. I am indebted to my colleagues, the pulmonologists and intensivists, who helped me to understand pulmonary medicine, which is critical for being an effective pulmonary nurse. I appreciate all the support and cooperation from family and friends. I also want to thank the staff at Mosby–Year Book, including Robin Carter, Don Ladig, Mark Spann, Jeanne Wolfgeher, and Linda Woodard. It is difficult to place a value on the advice I have received from a friend and colleague Anne Perry, who gave me my first opportunity to write in a major textbook. I am pleased that members of my COPD support group, the Breathers For Life, were able to demonstrate different types of oxygen devices. These people include John Cox, Daisy Dodson, Howard and Millie Jennings, Charles and Cedona Kendall, and Charles Peterson. I gratefully recognize Thomas M. Hyers for his thoughtful Foreword to this edition. Finally, I would like to thank you, the reader. I have tried to write an accurate, easy-to-understand book. I would appreciate any positive or negative comments you have. You can write to me at St. Louis University or through Mosby-Year Book.

Patricia Dettenmeier

For my boys
ROGER, DAVID, NICHOLAS, and MATTHEW
who charge my life and dreams

Foreword

It is a pleasure to write this Foreword to a new pulmonary book for nurses and other health care professionals. An understanding of lung function and lung diseases is increasingly important because these diseases continue to escalate in prevalence in western society; they now constitute the fourth leading cause of death in the United States. Although cigarette smoking has a great deal to do with this increase, other conditions, such as asthma and occupational health hazards, which are not directly related to cigarette smoking, also appear to be increasing. However, at a time when the prevalence of lung diseases is increasing, our understanding of them and our ability to intervene are also improving. Consequently, the pulmonary practitioner or student must constantly update knowledge and experience to care for these patients.

Diagnosis and treatment of lung diseases has increasingly become dependent on high technology. However, a basic understanding of anatomy and physiology must be coupled with a clear history and competent physical examination before high technology can be effectively applied. In my opinion, the three greatest advances in the diagnosis of lung disease in the last 20 years have been the widespread application of arterial blood gas technology, fiberoptic bronchoscopy, and computed tomographic scanning. These techniques have allowed for understanding of the pathophysiology of hypoxic-induced acute and chronic lung injury, and for widespread diagnostic approaches to the interior of the lung without resort to invasive surgical procedures. Each technology has already produced numerous spin-offs. Arterial blood gas measurements have lead to intravascular and cutaneous monitoring of oxyhemoglobin saturation. Fiberoptic bronchoscopy has led to a wealth of diagnostic and therapeutic techniques, which include transbronchial lung biopsy and needle aspiration and laser and brachytherapy for endobronchial neoplasms. Understanding the rationale and application of these techniques is essential in the approach to the modern day diagnosis of lung disease.

Similarly, in my opinion, the three greatest treatment advances in the last 20 years have been the widespread use of reliable mechanical ventilation in acute respiratory failure, the recognition that oxygen prolongs life in hypoxemic patients with chronic obstructive pulmonary disease, and the use of inhaled medications, particularly beta-2 adrenergic agonists and glucocorticoids, in the treatment of asthma. Again, to understand and apply these therapeutic advances, the student or practitioner must understand the basic pathophysiology of lung disease, the principles of gas exchange, and the mechanics of airway function.

Finally, the reader is reminded that the lung offers a much larger surface to the environment than does the skin. This gas exchange surface is constantly interacting with respirable environmental hazards. These hazards include dust, such as asbestos; noxious gases; and other particulates. The most important environmental hazard, however, remains a self-induced one. Cigarette smoke still accounts for the great majority of cases of lung disease, principally emphysema and lung cancer. In this regard, it is never too late to stop smoking. When a heavy smoker stops, the risk for lung cancer begins to decline immediately and returns to the risk of a non-smoker within 10 to 15 years. After smoking cessation, the accelerated rate of decline in airway function (decrease in FEV_1) in the emphysema patient rapidly returns to the rate associated with the non-smoking individual. Consequently, it is imperative that nurses and other healthcare givers understand and be able to explain to the patient the nature of lung diseases caused by cigarette smoking. Furthermore, the care-giver must be able to counsel individuals on the steps to smoking cessation. These steps are well outlined in the book and will prove useful in smoking intervention. This intervention is the most important therapy any care-giver can give a patient.

In summary, the book offers a basic summary of pulmonary interventions as appropriate for nurses and other care-givers. In addition to providing a physiological theoretical foundation, the book addresses assessment and treatment of the patient with lung diseases. Care-givers who understand the book and can apply its principles will render large benefits to their patients.

Thomas M. Hyers, M.D.
James and Ethel Miller Professor of Medicine
Director, Division of Pulmonology and Occupational Medicine
St. Louis University Medical Center

National Institutes of Health Clinical Trials Review Committee

Contents

Foundations of Pulmonary Nursing

In Chapter 1 anatomy and physiology are studied by monitoring air as it moves through the pulmonary system. Concepts follow the path of air from entry through the upper airway into the lower airway and finally into the bloodstream. With this understanding, the nurse is prepared to examine special properties of lung function in Chapter 2, titled "Ventilation/perfusion relationships." Ventilation depends on the compliance and resistance properties of the lung. Blood flow, or perfusion, in the lung is altered by many factors, including cardiac output and hypoxemia. The balance of ventilation and perfusion affects gas exchange. Understanding *ventilation/perfusion matching,* the final section in Chapter 2, is critical in recognizing gas exchange abnormalities common in respiratory dysfunction. Chapter 3 reviews the transport of oxygen and carbon dioxide across the alveolar-capillary membrane and discusses acid-base concepts. These concepts are a prelude to interpreting abnormalities in arterial blood gases and to applying appropriate interventions.

C H · A · P · T · E · R

1

Anatomy and Physiology

*O*bjectives:

- Identify upper airway structures on a diagram.
- State the functions of each upper airway structure.
- Identify lower airway structures on a diagram.
- State the functions of each lower airway structure.
- Discuss defense mechanisms of the upper and lower airways.
- Describe pulmonary circulation.
- Describe diaphragmatic function.

Respiration is the process of gas exchange in the lungs. Oxygen is diffused into the blood at the same time that carbon dioxide is removed from the blood. Air is directed to the gas-exchanging units through a complex system of upper and lower airways. These gas-exchanging units approximate in the pulmonary capillaries. This relationship allows for exchange of oxygen and carbon dioxide. Inhalation and exhalation of air are facilitated by the muscles of the thoracic cage. This chapter is designed to review fundamental concepts of the anatomy and physiology of respiration.

UPPER AIRWAY
Nose

The respiratory tract is divided into the upper airway and the lower airway. The upper airway is composed of the nose, pharynx, and larynx (Fig. 1-1). In the normal individual, air enters through the nares and passes into the nasal cavity. The nasal cavity is lined with a mucous membrane that contains serous glands and goblet cells. The serous glands and goblet cells secrete a thin layer of watery mucus over the mucous membrane. Also protruding from the mucous membrane are hairlike projections that beat in a waving motion to propel particulate matter for removal.

The primary respiratory functions of the nose are to warm, moisturize, and filter the inhaled air. Upon inhalation, air is warmed almost to body temperature by the time it reaches the trachea. This occurs because of the rich supply of blood vessels lying under the mucous membrane. Heat from these blood vessels warms incoming air.

Air is also moisturized by the nose as it is inhaled. The nose supplies mois-

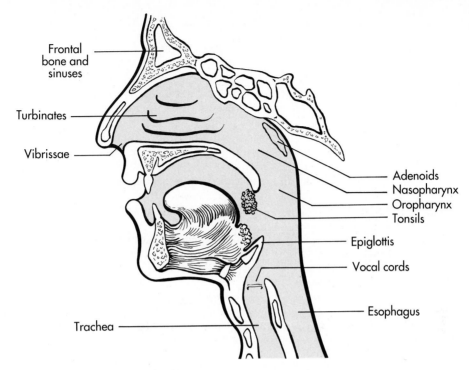

Fig. 1-1. Upper airway.

ture to inhaled air depending on the ambient temperature and humidity. When the temperature and humidity are elevated, as may occur in summer months, the nose supplies less moisture than when the temperature and humidity are lower, as may occur in winter months. The goal of 100% saturation of the air with water vapor is achieved by the time air reaches the alveoli. Most humidification of inhaled air occurs in the nose. To humidify inhaled air, the body loses approximately 250 ml of water in a 24-hour day.

Filtration of inhaled air is another very important function of the nose. Nasal hairs, or vibrissae, are responsible for filtering large particles of dust, germs, and other matter. Particles exceeding 10 μm are efficiently filtered by the vibrissae. This function can be appreciated on dusty days or days when particulate air-pollution levels are very high. For example, when the nose is blown, trapped dust or coal or hay particles are evident in the tissue. Smaller particulate matter is trapped by the mucus layer in the nasal cavity. Air flowing through the nasal cavity frequently changes direction, creating turbulent air flow, and causes impaction of particulate matter on the walls of the turbinate bones. The particulate matter lands on the mucus layer and is swept to the pharynx for expulsion. In some instances a sneeze will be generated to clear nasal passages.

Sinuses

Four sinuses surround and drain into the nasal cavity. They are the frontal, maxillary, ethmoid, and sphenoid sinuses. The ethmoid sinuses are associated closely with inspired air; they are also the smallest and most likely to be obstructed with mucus. Because of their posterior position, problems in the sphenoid sinuses are associated with vision impairment. The sinuses lighten the weight of the skull, produce mucus for the nasal cavity, and contribute to an individual's resonant voice characteristics.

Pharynx

After passing through the nose and nasal cavity, inhaled air reaches the pharynx, or throat. The pharynx has three anatomic divisions: the nasal pharynx, the oral pharynx, and the laryngeal pharynx. The nasal pharynx, also called the nasopharynx, is located posterior to the nose and above the soft palate at the rear of the mouth. The adenoids and eustachian tube openings are located in the nasal pharynx.

The oral pharynx, also called oropharynx, is located in the mouth. The boundaries of the oral pharynx are the soft palate superiorly, the base of the tongue inferiorly, and the palatine arches laterally. The tonsils are located in the oral pharynx.

The laryngeal pharynx, also called laryngopharynx or hypopharynx, is located posterior to the larynx from the hyoid bone to the esophagus. The epiglottis, arytenoid cartilages, piriform sinuses, and valleculae are located in the laryngeal pharynx.

The pharynx functions as a passageway for air into the lungs and for food into the esophagus. The pharynx, particularly the nasal pharynx, is also involved in filtering and humidifying the inhaled air.

Larynx

The larynx is the final portion of the upper airway. Another name commonly used to refer to the larynx is *voice box* because the vocal cords are located in the larynx. The larynx is located inferior to the pharynx and connects the pharynx to the trachea. The lower border of the larynx is about the level of the sixth cervical vertebrae. The glottis is the entrance to the larynx. During swallowing, the glottis is covered in a lidlike manner by the epiglottis. The thyroid, cricoid, and arytenoid cartilages are other essential components of the larynx.

The larynx has multiple functions, including separation of food and air, phonation, or voice production, and initiation of cough from the upper airway. The larynx is responsible for separating inhaled air from food that is being swallowed. Failure of the epiglottis to cover the larynx during swallowing results in aspiration of solid or liquid material into the lung. Because solids move through the larynx by propulsion instead of falling by gravity like liquids, they usually are aspirated less easily.

The vocal cords are located between the thyroid and arytenoid cartilages. They form the V-shaped opening of the glottis. Movement of the arytenoid cartilages by muscle contraction allows inhalation and exhalation of air and controls sound production. Sound is produced when the arytenoid cartilages pull together forcing exhaled air through a closed glottis and vibrating the vocal cords. Intubated patients cannot talk because of impaired vocal cord movement and because air does not pass over the vocal cords. Some patients with tracheostomy tubes can talk because vocal cord movement is not altered.

Cough from the upper airway is initiated by many irritants, including dust, smoke, pressure, chemicals, cold, and dry mucous membranes. Cough itself can initiate another cough. The physiology of cough is discussed as a lower airway defense mechanism later in this chapter.

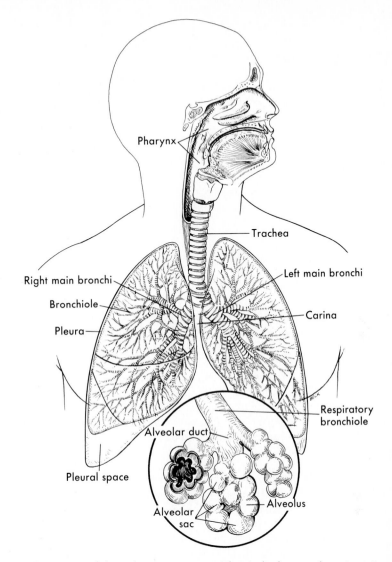

Fig. 1-2. Structures of the pulmonary system. The circle denotes the acinus, in which oxygen and carbon dioxide are exchanged. (From Thibodeau G: *Anthony's textbook of anatomy and physiology*, ed 13, St Louis, 1990, Mosby–Year Book).

LOWER AIRWAY

After inhaled air travels through the nose, pharynx, and larynx, it reaches the lower airway (Fig. 1-2). Structurally, the lower airway is composed of the trachea, carina, bronchi, bronchioles, and alveoli. Various cell types, including those that produce surfactant, are located in the lower airway.

Trachea

The trachea, also referred to as the windpipe, is a cylindrical tube 10 cm to 12 cm (5 inches) long and 1.5 cm to 2.5 cm (1 inch) wide located in the mid-

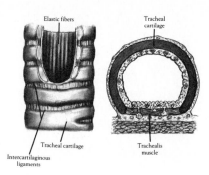

Elastic fibers

Tracheal cartilage

Tracheal cartilage

Trachealis muscle

Intercartilaginous ligaments

Fig. 1-3. The trachea (From McCance K, Huether S: *Pathophysiology*, ed 1, St Louis, 1990, Mosby–Year Book).

line of the neck. The trachea extends from the cricoid cartilage in the larynx to the bronchi in the thorax. The trachea is composed of smooth muscle with approximately 20 incomplete regularly spaced cartilaginous rings covered by a fibroelastic membrane. The posterior wall of the trachea is not supported by cartilage. Only the fibroelastic membrane separates the trachea from the esophagus posteriorly. A cross-sectional view of the trachea demonstrates the C-shaped cartilaginous rings and the flat posterior fibroelastic membrane, giving the trachea an overall appearance of being oval or D-shaped (Fig. 1-3). Mackenzie (1978) also reports elliptical and U-shaped tracheas in the adult.

Bronchial tree

The bronchial tree is often compared with a family tree, in which each generation is assigned a number. In the bronchial tree the first generation is the trachea. The trachea bifurcates into the two main stem, or second-generation, bronchi at the level of the carina. The carina is located at about the level of the second costal cartilage or fifth thoracic vertebrae. Many cough receptors are located at the carina.

The main stem bronchi are slightly different from each other. The chief differences are angulation, width, and length (Fig. 1-4). The left main stem bronchus is angled more sharply than the right main stem bronchus, which can impede both aspiration and sometimes expectoration of secretions or matter. Because the right main stem bronchus is angled less sharply and is more vertical than the left main stem bronchus, aspiration into the right lung and intubation of the right lung are more common. The left main stem bronchus is slightly narrower than the right main stem bronchus. Finally, the left main stem bronchus is longer, by approximately 5 cm, than the right main stem bronchus.

The left main stem bronchus divides into two lobar branches. One supplies the left upper lobe, and the other supplies the left lower lobe. The left upper lobe bronchus further subdivides into four smaller bronchi: apical posterior, anterior, superior lingular, and inferior lingular. The lower lobe bronchus

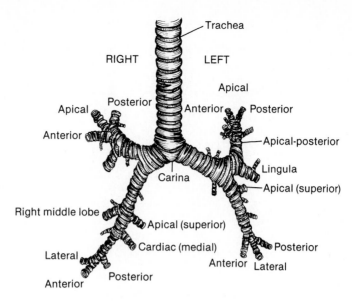

Fig. 1-4. Tracheobronchial tree (From Perry A, Potter P: *Clinical nursing skills and techniques,* ed 2, St Louis, 1990, Mosby–Year Book).

also subdivides into four smaller bronchi: superior, anterior medial basal, lateral basal, and posterior basal. These eight smaller bronchi, also called third generation bronchi, are termed *segments.* Each segment is named for its position in the lung.

The right main stem bronchus divides into three lobar branches. A branch supplies each of the three lobes of the right lung: upper lobe, middle lobe, and lower lobe. The right upper lobe bronchus divides into three segments: apical, posterior, and anterior. The middle lobe bronchus divides into two segments: lateral and medial. The lower lobe bronchus divides into five segments: superior, anterior basal, lateral basal, medial basal, and posterior basal. There are a total of 10 segments in the right lung.

The bronchi continue to subdivide 20 or more times into subsegmental bronchi, terminal bronchi, bronchioles, terminal bronchioles, and respiratory bronchioles. The respiratory bronchioles further subdivide into terminal respiratory bronchioles and ultimately into alveolar ducts, alveolar sacs, and alveoli.

The bronchi are supported by cartilage and muscle. Incomplete cartilaginous rings like those in the trachea are found in the main stem bronchi and lower lobe bronchi (Fig. 1-5). Less complete cartilage is present in the lobar and segmental bronchi. Bands of longitudinal and circular elastic connective tissue help to maintain the patency of the small bronchi and bronchioles. At the level of the smallest bronchi, i.e. bronchioles, there is no cartilage; only the property of elastic recoil of the smooth muscle is solely responsible for maintaining airway patency. Destruction of peripheral airways results in collapse of distal airways and alveoli.

The bronchi are lined with pseudostratified ciliated columnar epithelium (see Fig. 1-5). Goblet cells in the epithelium secrete mucus. The cilia and mucus together help to protect the lungs from dust, germs, and other particulate

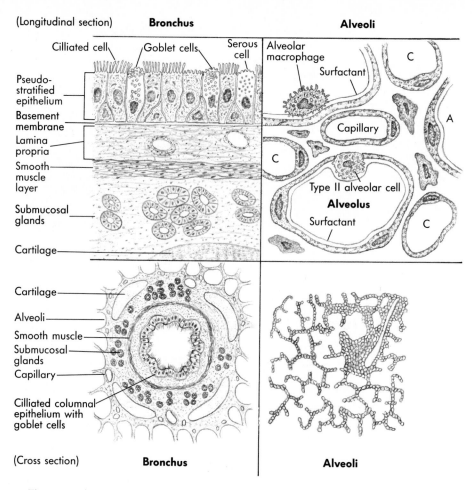

Fig. 1-5. Changes in the bronchial wall with progressive branching. (From McCance K, Huether S: *Pathophysiology*, ed 1, St. Louis, 1990, Mosby–Year Book).

matter. The epithelium of the bronchiole is a single layer. Epithelial cells are initially more cuboidal and then become flattened at the level of the bronchioles. In addition, at the level of the terminal bronchioles the cilia and most secretory gland cells are absent. Below the epithelium are two more layers, a basement membrane and the lamina propria. Blood vessels, lymphatic vessels, and nerve fibers are located in the lamina propria.

Mast cells lie just beneath the bronchial epithelium near the smooth muscle and blood vessels. The granular mast cell releases histamine in response to an antigen-antibody reaction or allergic response. Damage to the lungs, such as cardiopulmonary bypass or pulmonary embolism, can also cause the mast cell to release granules.

Blood is supplied to the bronchial tree down to the level of the terminal bronchioles by bronchial arteries, which branch off the aorta. At the level of the terminal bronchioles, the pulmonary circulation is responsible for supplying blood to the airways. Blood is drained from the bronchial tree via the pulmonary veins.

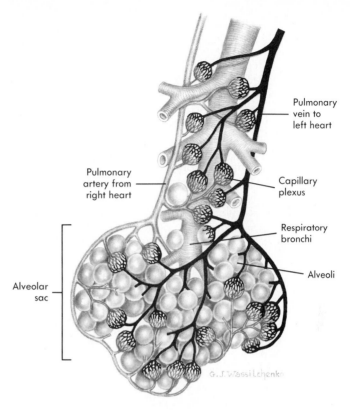

Fig. 1-6. Terminal respiratory units (From Thompson J et al: *Mosby's manual of clinical nursing,* ed 2, St Louis, 1989, Mosby—Year Book).

Gas-exchanging lung units

The gas-exchanging units of the lung collectively are called the acinus, or terminal respiratory unit (Fig. 1-6). The gas-exchanging units consist of the pulmonary structures distal to the terminal bronchioles, including respiratory bronchioles, alveolar ducts, alveolar sacs, and alveoli.

Respiratory bronchioles are lined with ciliated cuboidal epithelium and Clara cells (see Figure 1-5). Alveoli protrude intermittently from the respiratory bronchiole and participate in gas exchange.

Alveolar ducts arise from respiratory bronchioles. Alveoli protrude from the alveolar ducts. Arising from the alveolar duct are dilated pouches called alveolar sacs. Alveoli completely line the alveolar sac, giving an appearance of a grape cluster.

The most important structures in gas exchange are the alveoli. At birth approximately 24 million alveoli are present. By puberty the number of alveoli grows to 300 million, and it remains at this number throughout life. Normal alveoli range in diameter from 1 mm to 2 mm.

Alveoli comprise three types of cells: type I cells, type II cells, and alveolar macrophages (see Figure 1-5). Type I epithelial cells are composed of flattened nuclei and cytoplasm and are distinguishable because their cytoplasm does not respond to histologic stains. They form the monolayered alveolar epithelium. Pores of Kohn present in the epithelium allow collateral air exchange among neighboring alveoli.

The larger type II cells are present in the angles of the alveoli. Surfactant production is thought to be assumed by the type II cell. Pulmonary surfactant, a lipoprotein, is a surface-active material the function of which is to reduce alveolar surface tension and equalize intraalveolar pressure during inspiration and expiration. The effect of reduced surface tension is even distribution of ventilation in larger and smaller alveoli. The importance of surfactant often is not realized unless it is decreased or absent, as occurs in respiratory distress syndrome of the newborn. Recent research indicates a similar problem may be present in adult respiratory distress syndrome. It is unknown whether the adult form of the disease responds as positively to surfactant repletion.

The third type of alveolar cell is the macrophage. An alveolar macrophage is involved in phagocytosis, or ingestion of foreign material. The alveolar macrophage is important in preventing lung infection.

Gas exchange occurs in an area known as the alveolar capillary membrane. Air in the alveoli is separated from blood in the capillary by a membrane 1 μm thick. The alveolar capillary membrane has five layers, which are bathed in interstitial fluid. First there is a lining of squamous epithelium, which is less than 0.5 μm thick. This is followed by a fine basement membrane made up of elastic fibers and collagen, the basement membrane of the pulmonary capillary, a ground substance, and the endothelial lining of the capillaries. Oxygen must pass through all these layers for transfer into the blood at the same time that carbon dioxide leaves the blood to be exhaled.

PULMONARY CIRCULATION

The lungs receive blood from two distinct circulations, the pulmonary circulation and the bronchial circulation. The pulmonary circulation initiates in the right side of the heart. Blood from the systemic circulation flows into the right atrium, through the tricuspid valve, and into the right ventricle. Blood leaving the right ventricle passes through the pulmonary valve and into the right and left pulmonary arteries. Poorly oxygenated (mixed venous) blood is shuttled through a series of smaller arteries and arterioles until the blood reaches the pulmonary capillary, in which gas exchange takes place. Blood that is rich in oxygen leaves the lungs and returns to the heart through a system of progressively larger pulmonary veins. Blood enters the left atrium from the four main pulmonary veins, passes through the mitral valve into the left ventricle, and is pumped out the aortic valve into the aorta for distribution to the systemic circulation.

The bronchial circulation originates from the aorta or subclavian artery. At least three bronchial arteries (right bronchial artery and inferior and superior left bronchial arteries) supply blood to the perihilar region. The bronchial wall, the tracheobronchial lymph nodes, the midesophagus, and the mediastinal pleura are contained in the perihilar region. Blood returns from the bronchial circulation to the heart through the azygos vein into the left atrium.

THORACIC CAGE

The thorax, or thoracic cage, protects the lungs and heart from injury. The boundaries of the thorax are the 12 thoracic vertebrae posteriorly, the 12 ribs laterally, and the sternum anteriorly. The structure of the C-shaped ribs gives the thorax a vertical conical appearance. The first seven ribs, also called true ribs because they are attached directly to the sternum by costal cartilage, gradually increase in length and slant outward in the normal adult. The lower five ribs, also called false ribs because they are not attached directly to the sternum, gradually decrease in length and slant inward. Ribs 8 to 10 attach to the cartilage of the rib above, and ribs 11 and 12, also called floating ribs, are attached only posteriorly to the vertebrae.

The internal and external intercostal muscles help to form the anterior wall of the thorax, and the diaphragm forms the floor of the thoracic cavity. Together these muscle groups provide the forces necessary to overcome elastic recoil of the lung during inspiration.

The internal intercostal muscles extend from the sternum to the angle of the ribs. Internal intercostal muscles are directed downward and laterally. In contrast the external intercostal muscles angle downward and medially. Both the internal and external intercostal muscles connect adjacent ribs.

The diaphragm, which forms the floor of the conical thorax, separates the thorax from the abdomen. It is the primary muscle of breathing. The xiphoid process of the sternum, the lumbar vertebrae, and the lower six ribs are the anterior, posterior, and lateral origins of the diaphragm, respectively. Muscle fibers from the three origins converge with a sheet of connective tissue called the central tendon. Contraction of the dome-shaped diaphragm pulls the central tendon downward, increasing the volume of the thoracic cavity and initiating inspiration. At the same time, the external intercostal and scalene muscles contract. This increases the lateral and anteroposterior chest dimensions by elevating the anterior portion of the thoracic cage and ribs. This elevation is referred to commonly as the "bucket handle" motion.

Conversely, relaxation of the diaphragm decreases the volume of the thoracic cavity by releasing the central tendon and allowing passive exhalation. The elastic recoil of the lungs and chest wall allows the chest to come passively to its normal resting position. When exhalation is active, as in disease or during exercise, contraction of the internal intercostal muscles draws the ribs and sternum downward. Exhalation also can be enhanced by contraction of the rectus, external and internal oblique, and transverse abdominal muscles, which push the diaphragm higher in the thoracic cavity, squeezing air from the lungs. When muscles other than the diaphragm are used for inhalation or exhalation, the term *accessory muscle* is applied.

The diaphragm is innervated by the right and left phrenic nerves. The two phrenic nerves that feed each hemidiaphragm arise from the fourth cervical nerve, although the third and fifth cervical nerves also affect innervation. When a phrenic nerve is damaged by blunt, penetrating, or surgical trauma, the diaphragm is paralyzed, possibly permanently. Consequently, movement of the lung on the affected side is decreased.

The right and left pleural cavities each contain one lung (Fig. 1-7). The lung has a conical appearance, with a narrow apex and a wide base. Fissures divide the lungs into lobes. The right lung is divided into three lobes (upper, middle, and lower) by the horizontal and oblique fissures; the left lung is divided into two lobes (upper and lower) by the oblique fissure. Each lobe further subdivides into segments that correspond to bronchial airway segments. The medial portions of the right and left lungs are concave to accommodate the mediastinal structures, including the heart. The superior and inferior pulmonary veins, the pulmonary artery, and the main bronchi enter the lung at the hilum, or root.

The lungs are lined by two thin membranes, called pleura, a thin sheet of

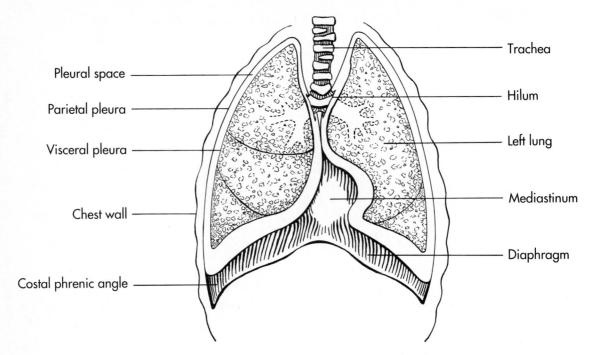

Fig. 1-7. Significant structural relationships of the thorax.

collagen, and elastic tissue. The visceral pleura encases each lung like a sac. The inside of the thoracic cavity is lined by the parietal pleura. Between the visceral and parietal pleura is a potential area called the pleural space. Approximately 25 ml of fluid occupies the pleural space. The purpose of this small amount of fluid is to decrease friction and allow the pleural surfaces to glide over each other during inhalation and exhalation. Because negative pressure exists in the intrapleural space, the lungs are unable to separate from the thorax. The function of pleural fluid can be simulated by wetting two pieces of glass. Placing one piece of glass on top of the other when they are wet allows the two pieces to slide but not to be pulled apart.

DEFENSE MECHANISMS

Both the upper and lower airways have defense mechanisms that help protect the lungs from harm. Upper airway defense mechanisms include the nose, pharynx, and larynx. Mucus secretion, ciliary activity, alveolar macrophages, lymphatics, cough, and airway reflexes are lower airway defense mechanisms.

The nose is the lungs' first defense against invading particles. The vibrissae, or stiff nasal hairs, filter particles larger than 10 μm. Particles approximately 10 μm also impact on the nasal septum, turbinates, tonsils, and adenoids. The carina and large airways also remove particles by impaction.

Once past the upper airway, smaller particles are deposited by sedimentation, brownian motion, and turbulent diffusion. Particles ranging from 0.2 μm to 5 μm are deposited by sedimentation in small airways. A slowing of air flow in the small airways allows sedimentation. Sedimentation occurs primarily in the tenth to twenty-third divisions of the bronchial tree. The mucociliary escalator removes particles trapped by impaction or sedimentation.

Brownian motion is the random movement of microscopic particles suspended in gases or liquids. It results from the bombardment of gas molecules and allows particles smaller than 0.1 μm to be deposited in the airways.

Turbulent diffusion is the final method of particle deposition in the lung. It occurs primarily in the larger airways.

Mucus production often is considered in tandem with ciliary function because the mucus is propelled continually out of the lung by the cilia. The lungs produce approximately 100 ml of watery, clear mucus daily in the healthy individual. In disease states, daily mucus production markedly increases, sometimes to 1000 ml. Sputum viscosity, which is determined by glycoproteins, also tends to increase in disease states.

Ciliary activity is a very important component of lung defense. Each ciliated cell contains approximately 200 cilia, which look like a shag rug moving in a waving motion. Cilia are covered by mucus, which consists of two layers. The lower layer, which consists of periciliary fluid, bathes cilia from the epithelial cell to the apex, and the upper layer, which is made up of gel, acts as a protective surface impermeable by water. The upper, gel layer also partially prevents penetration of toxic substances. The continuously moving blanket of mucus-coated hairs carries particles up to the trachea and through the epiglottis to the larynx. From there, secretions can be swallowed or expectorated. The ability of the mucociliary escalator to move secretions out of the lung is lessened by changes in mucus or in ciliary function. When mucus secretions are thickened or copious, the mucociliary escalator is less efficient. Similarly when ciliary function is paralyzed, damaged, or destroyed by air pollution, the most significant element of which is cigarette smoke, it is more difficult for the lung to dispose of secretions and particulate matter.

Alveolar macrophages are the "garbage disposal" of the lungs. The alveolar macrophage defends the lung by phagocytosis of particles that reach the acinus of the lungs. Alveolar macrophages are removed from the lung by the mucociliary escalator.

Lymph glands or nodes are found throughout the lungs. Although lymph glands are not located in the alveoli, the airway walls down to the level of the respiratory and terminal bronchioles are lined with lymphatics. Many intrapulmonary lymph nodes are located at bifurcations of the trachea and larger bronchi, including the subcarinal area. Peritracheal nodes are situated in front of the trachea and beside it. Hilar nodes are present where the main bronchi and vessels enter the lungs. The aortic arch and scalene area also contain lymphatics. In addition, lymph glands are located between plates of cartilage and are internal and external to the muscle layers.

Sneeze and cough are similar mechanisms of airway defense. Stimulation of a sneeze or cough can occur when irritation exists anywhere in the respiratory tract. A sneeze clears primarily the upper airway of trapped particulate matter, and a cough clears the lower airway of particulate matter and mucus. Loss or impairment of the cough reflex can result in aspiration. In the patient with a transplanted lung, the cough reflex is lost and must be replaced by other measures to clear the airway.

The final defense mechanism of the lungs is reflex bronchoconstriction. In response to mechanical or chemical irritants, the vagus nerve is stimulated.

This stimulation causes the smooth muscle lining of the airways to constrict and shorten, reducing airway diameter. Reflex bronchoconstriction can occur even when the concentration of the irritant is too low to stimulate a cough (Comroe, 1974).

CONCLUSION

This chapter provides an overview of anatomy and physiology of the pulmonary system, which are the foundation of pulmonary care. Assessment relies on knowledge of anatomy and physiology. A sound basis in anatomy and physiology is necessary to differentiate normal function from pathophysiology. It is also important for correct application of interventions, such as chest physical therapy. Because of the scope of this text, the nurse is encouraged to consult other, in-depth sources as needed.

BIBLIOGRAPHY

Baum GL, Wolinsky E: *Textbook of pulmonary diseases,* ed 3, Boston, 1983, Little, Brown & Co.

Borysenko M, Beringer T: *Functional histology,* ed 2, Boston, 1984, Little, Brown & Co.

Burki NK: *Pulmonary diseases: medical outline series,* Garden City, NY, 1982, Medical Examination Publishing.

Burton GC, Hodgkin JE: *Respiratory care: a guide to clinical practice,* ed 2, Philadelphia, 1984, JB Lippincott.

Cherniack NS, Widdicombe JG, eds: *Handbook of physiology, section 3: the respiratory system,* vol 3, Baltimore, 1986, Williams & Wilkins.

Clements JA, King RJ: *Composition of the surface active material.* In Crystal RG, ed: *The biochemical basis of pulmonary function,* New York, 1977, Marcel Dekker.

Comroe J: *Physiology of respiration: an introductory text,* ed 2, Chicago, 1974, Mosby–Year Book.

Gail D, Lenfant J: State of the art. Cells of the lung:biology and clinical implications, *Am Rev Respir Dis* 127(3):366-387, 1983.

Gray H, Clemente CD: *Anatomy of the human body,* American ed 30, Philadelphia, 1985, Lea & Febiger.

Guyton AC: *Textbook of medical physiology,* ed 6, Philadelphia, 1981, WB Saunders.

Hinshaw H, Murray J: *Diseases of the chest,* ed 4, Philadelphia, 1980, WB Saunders.

Janson-Bjerklie S: Defense mechanisms-protecting the healthy lung, *Heart Lung* 12(6):643-649, 1983.

Mackenzie CF et al: The shape of the human adult trachea, *Anesthesiology* 49(1):48-50, 1978.

Menkes HA, Traystman RJ: Collateral ventilation, *Am Rev Respir Dis* 116(2):287-309, 1977.

Mitchell RS, Petty TL, Schwarz MI: *Synopsis of clinical pulmonary disease,* ed 4, St. Louis, 1989, Mosby–Year Book.

Mountcastle VB, ed: *Medical physiology,* St Louis, 1980, Mosby–Year Book.

Murray JF: *The normal lung,* Philadelphia, 1986, W B Saunders.

Murray JF, Nadel JA, eds: *Textbook of respiratory medicine,* Philadelphia, 1988, WB Saunders.

Netter F: *The CIBA collection of medical illustrations,* vol 7: respiratory system, New York, 1979, CIBA Pharmaceutical Co.

Paré JAP, Fraser RG: *Synopsis of diseases of the chest,* Philadelphia, 1983, W B Saunders.

Proctor DF: The upper airways: 1. Nasal physiology and defense of the lungs 2. The larynx and trachea, *Am Rev Respir Dis* 115(1):97-129; 115(2): 315-342, 1977.

Shapiro B, Harrison R et al: *Clinical applications of respiratory care,* ed 3, St Louis, 1985, Mosby–Year Book.

Simmons DH, ed: *Current pulmonology,* vol 7, St Louis, 1986, Mosby–Year Book.

Slonim N, Hamilton L: *Respiratory physiology,* ed 5, St Louis, 1987, Mosby–Year Book.

Staub N: Lung structure and function-1982, *Basics Respir Dis* 10(3),1982.

Wade JF: *Comprehensive respiratory care: physiology and technique,* ed 3, St. Louis, 1982, Mosby–Year Book.

Wanner A, Sackner MA: *Pulmonary disease: mechanisms of altered structure and function,* Boston, 1983, Little, Brown & Co.

West J: *Respiratory physiology: the essentials,* ed 3, Baltimore, 1985, Williams & Wilkins.

West JB: *Pulmonary pathophysiology: the essentials,* ed 2, Baltimore, 1982, Williams & Wilkins.

2

Ventilation-Perfusion Relationships

Objectives:

- Differentiate among tidal volume, residual volume, inspiratory reserve volume, and expiratory reserve volume.
- Define inspiratory capacity, functional residual capacity, and total lung capacity.
- Discuss the significance of anatomical, alveolar, and physiological dead space.
- Discuss control of ventilation.
- Discuss the importance of position in determining distribution of ventilation and perfusion.
- Discuss the effects of compliance, elastic recoil, and resistance on ventilation.

Respiration, the exchange of oxygen and carbon dioxide across cell membranes, begins with ventilation, the exchange of air between the lungs and the atmosphere. An understanding of the different concepts related to ventilation is essential.

VENTILATION
Volumes and capacities

A complete pulmonary function test identifies four volumes and four capacities involved in ventilation (Fig. 2-1). Tidal volume (V_T) is the amount of air that is breathed in and out with a normal breath. V_T varies with the size of the person, but in the average young male adult it is about 500 ml. (Note: All volumes and capacities are approximately 25% less in women.)

When a person inspires as much air as possible after inhaling a normal V_T breath, the term *inspiratory reserve volume* (IRV) is used (see Fig. 2-1). In other words, IRV is the maximal volume of air that can be inspired from the end of a normal inspiration. IRV in the average young male adult is approximately 3000 ml.

The third volume, expiratory reserve volume (ERV), describes the amount of air that can be expired by forceful exhalation after exhaling a normal V_T (see Fig. 2-1). ERV is the opposite of IRV. The average young adult male has an ERV of approximately 1100 ml.

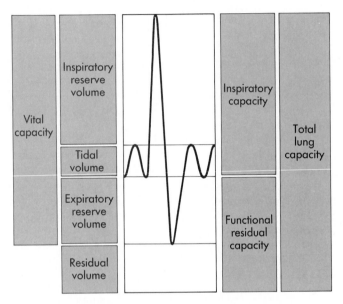

Fig. 2-1. Lung volume measurements. All values are approximately 25% lower in women. (From Pagana K, Pagana T: *Mosby's diagnostic and laboratory test reference,* ed 1, St. Louis, 1992, Mosby–Year Book).

Residual volume (RV) is the volume of air remaining in the lungs after the most forceful exhalation (see Fig. 2-1). The average young adult male has an RV of approximately 1200 ml. RV provides air to the capillary during exhalation and between breaths.

A pulmonary capacity is the sum of two or more volumes. Inspiratory capacity (IC) = V_T + IRV (see Fig. 2-1). IC is the maximum volume of air that can be inhaled after a normal exhalation. In the average young adult male IC is approximately 3500 ml.

Functional residual capacity (FRC), the sum of ERV and RV, is the amount of air remaining in the lungs at the end of a normal exhalation (see Fig. 2-1). The average young adult male has an FRC of approximately 2300 ml.

Forced vital capacity (FVC) is the amount of air a person can forcefully maximally exhale after a maximum inhalation (see Fig. 2-1). IRV, ERV, and V_T determine vital capacity. A vital capacity of 4600 ml is normal for the average young adult male. Vital capacity measurements in the same person differ depending on the position assumed during the measurement, that is, lying, sitting, or standing. Respiratory muscle strength and compliance also play a role.

Total lung capacity (TLC) is the maximum amount of air the lungs can hold (see Fig. 2-1). TLC is the sum of all four volumes: V_T, IRV, ERV, and RV. The average young adult male has a total lung capacity of approximately 5800 ml.

Dead space

As stated earlier, V_T is the amount of air inhaled during a normal breath. However, all of the V_T does not reach the alveoli for gas exchange. The amount of air that does not participate in gas exchange is termed ineffective, dead space, or wasted ventilation.

Three types of dead-space ventilation are present in the lungs: anatomical dead space (Vd anat), alveolar dead space (Vd alv), and physiological dead space (Vd p). Vd anat is the amount of V_T that remains in the conducting airways and does not participate in gas exchange. The conducting airways consist of the nose and mouth, pharynx, larynx, trachea, and bronchi to the level of the respiratory bronchioles. Vd anat is approximately 1 ml/lb (2.5 ml/kg) of ideal body weight. A value of 150 ml is common for Vd anat. Insertion of a tracheostomy tube that bypasses the upper airway can decrease Vd anat by approximately 50%.

Effective ventilation occurs when both ventilation and perfusion are adequate. Vd alv occurs when ventilation to the alveoli is ineffective. There are two causes of Vd alv. First, a portion of the V_T can reach alveoli with little or no perfusion. Ventilation is wasted because gas exchange does not occur or is inadequate. Second, when ventilation to the alveoli is excessive with regard to an adequate amount of perfusion to the capillary, Vd alv occurs.

Vd p is the sum of Vd anat and Vd alv. A measurement of Vd p assesses the total amount of wasted ventilation. In the normal individual, Vd p is considered equivalent to Vd anat because there is little or no Vd alv. In addition, because nearly all alveoli are functioning effectively, Vd anat usually accounts for all of the Vd p in the normal lung.

Vd p often is increased greatly in the diseased lung. Calculation of Vd p can be made at the bedside with measurement of exhaled carbon dioxide (using a Douglas bag), arterial carbon dioxide, and V_T. Following dead-space measurements can assist in developing treatment plans.

Frequency of breathing

Respiratory rate is the common term used for **frequency** of breathing. Although respiratory rate is measured routinely in patients, the information gained must be accompanied by other assessment data to assess patient status. Respiratory rate is an important factor in many calculations of respiratory function.

Minute ventilation

Minute ventilation ($\dot{V}_E$), or minute volume, is the amount of air that is inhaled into and exhaled from the lungs in 60 seconds. It usually is expressed as liters per minute (LPM). $\dot{V}_E$ is the product of V_T and respiratory rate.

$$V_T \times \text{frequency or rate of breathing (f)} = \dot{V}_E$$

The dot over the symbol for volume (V) indicates that the measurement occurs over time. An "E" is used to indicate that measurements of exhaled V_T were used in the measurement of $\dot{V}_E$.

Normal $\dot{V}_E$ in the young adult male is 6.0 LPM, assuming a V_T of 500 ml and a respiratory rate of 12.

$$500 \text{ ml} \times 12 = 6000 \text{ ml per minute}$$
$$(0.5 \text{ L}) \qquad (6.0 \text{ L})$$

$\dot{V}_E$ is calculated easily at the bedside with a hand spirometer and mouthpiece or 15 mm airway adapter. Many mechanical ventilators are designed to calculate $\dot{V}_E$ automatically.

Alveolar $\dot{V}_E$

Alveolar ventilation is one of the most important factors in determining oxygen and carbon dioxide concentrations in the alveoli and blood. Recall that the V_T that remains in conducting airways is Vd anat. The remaining V_T enters the alveoli and is available for gas exchange in the normal lung. (In the diseased lung additional V_T may be lost to Vd alv.) The amount of air that actually reaches the alveoli and participates in gas exchange is alveolar ventilation ($\dot{V}_A$). Measured in milliliters or liters per minute, $\dot{V}_A$ is dependent on V_T, frequency of breathing, and dead space. Using the previously stated normal values in a young adult male, $\dot{V}_A$ is 4.2 LPM as demonstrated below.

$$\dot{V}_A = (V_T - V_{DS}) \times f$$
$$4.2 \text{ LPM} = (500 \text{ ml} - 150 \text{ ml}) \times 12$$

An approximate value for alveolar $\dot{V}_E$ can be computed at the bedside using Vd anat, V_T, and respiratory rate. The need to measure dead space usually indicates that the patient also has a component of Vd alv. A better approximation of alveolar $\dot{V}_E$ can be made by calculating Vd p and then determining alveolar $\dot{V}_E$. A thorough nursing assessment can identify the presence of increasing Vd p by assessing changes in the patient's rate and depth of breathing in conjunction with the measurement of arterial blood gases. Either an increase in $\dot{V}_E$ to maintain the same arterial blood gases or a deterioration in blood gases with the same $\dot{V}_E$ is a sign of increased dead space.

Hypoventilation versus hyperventilation

The goal of ventilation is to produce a normal arterial carbon dioxide tension (Pa_{CO_2}) and aid in maintaining a normal arterial oxygen tension (Pa_{O_2}). Hypoventilation, or, more specifically, alveolar hypoventilation, occurs when ventilation of the alveoli is inadequate to meet the body's metabolic requirements. An elevated arterial carbon dioxide level, not the patient's breathing pattern, indicates that a patient has alveolar hypoventilation. Measurement of arterial blood gases is necessary to determine hypoventilation.

To demonstrate the concept of hypoventilation, a series of breathing patterns is given below. Note that assessing the rate or the V_T alone does not determine effective ventilation. It is the combined effect of respiratory rate and V_T that produce $\dot{V}_E$ and thus $\dot{V}_A$. An increase in V_T can offset a low respiratory rate. Similarly, a low V_T and an increased respiratory rate can produce normal $\dot{V}_E$. The main determinant of hypoventilation is the volume of air entering the alveoli.

	V_T	V_d	f	$\dot{V}_E$	$\dot{V}_A$	Pa_{CO_2}
A	500	150	12	6.0 LPM	4.2 LPM	40 mm Hg
B	300	150	12	3.6 LPM	1.8 LPM	65 mm Hg
C	500	150	20	10.0 LPM	7.0 LPM	27 mm Hg
D	300	150	20	6.0 LPM	3.0 LPM	45 mm Hg
E	500	150	8	4.0 LPM	2.8 LPM	60 mm Hg
F	300	150	8	2.4 LPM	1.2 LPM	100 mm Hg

Note: Vd = dead-space volume.

Cases A and D demonstrate normal $\dot{V}_A$ because Pa_{CO_2} is within the normal range of 35 to 45 mm Hg. Cases B, E, and F demonstrate hypoventilation because Pa_{CO_2} is above normal. Case C reflects hyperventilation because lower than normal Pa_{CO_2} is present.

Hypoxemia, below-normal arterial blood oxygen tension, and hypercapnia, above-normal arterial blood carbon dioxide tension, are the result of untreated hypoventilation. The treatment of hypoventilation is increasing $\dot{V}_A$ to eliminate carbon dioxide. Mechanical ventilation and respiratory stimulants may be used.

Hyperventilation is the opposite of hypoventilation. Hyperventilation occurs when alveolar $\dot{V}_E$ exceeds the body's requirement for eliminating carbon dioxide. A decreased level of carbon dioxide in the arterial blood demonstrates hyperventilation. Like hypoventilation, hyperventilation cannot be assessed by measuring respiratory rate and V_T. There are many physiological, metabolic, and psychological causes of hyperventilation. The treatment for hyperventilation is directed at treating the cause. Sedatives, diuretics, and insulin are just a few of the treatments.

Some nurses may confuse hypopnea with hypoventilation and hyperpnea with hyperventilation. Hypopnea and hyperpnea refer to the rate and depth of breathing. Case F above identifies a low rate and depth of breathing, or hypopnea. Case C may represent hyperpnea, a high rate and depth of breathing, if the patient is small.

Another term frequently confused with hypoventilation and hyperventilation is *tachypnea*. Tachypnea is defined as increased breathing rate. Depth of breathing is not defined in tachypnea. Both hypoventilation and hyperventilation are found in tachypneic patients. Consider the following cases.

Case	V_T	V_D	f	$\dot{V}_E$	$\dot{V}_A$	Pa_{CO_2}
G	500	150	30	15 LPM	10.5 LPM	25 mm Hg
H	300	150	30	9 LPM	4.5 LPM	42 mm Hg
I	200	150	30	6 LPM	1.5 LPM	70 mm Hg

All three cases are tachypneic; however, V_T is variable. $\dot{V}_A$ in Case G is excessive, reflecting hyperventilation. Case H demonstrates adequate ventilation, and Case I reflects hypoventilation even though $\dot{V}_E$ appears normal.

Control of ventilation

Metabolic needs vary throughout the day and night in healthy individuals and in ill individuals. Ventilation is increased or decreased as needed to maintain constant levels of arterial oxygen and carbon dioxide throughout awake and asleep periods. The control of ventilation is achieved by a complex network of receptors that sends impulses to the brain for processing. The brain in turn activates the muscles of breathing.

There are both involuntary and voluntary components of breathing. Involuntary control of breathing allows an individual to sleep or work without concentrating on the process of breathing. Voluntary breathing control permits breath-holding actions, such as singing, speaking, or swimming, and voluntary hyperventilation. Voluntary components of breathing override the involuntary components, except when carbon dioxide levels are excessive and stimulate spontaneous breaths. (Recall your efforts as a child to hold your breath until you turned blue in the face. Spontaneous involuntary ventilations overrode the attempt to not breathe.)

Central control. The control of breathing originates in the respiratory centers of the brainstem, that is, the medulla oblongata and pons. The medulla oblongata contains inspiratory and expiratory neurons, which are responsible for the inherent rhythmicity of breathing. The pons, located just above the medulla, contains the apneustic and pneumotaxic centers of ventilation. Ventilation initiated by the apneustic center consists of inspiratory gasps followed by expiratory efforts. The pneumotaxic center inhibits inhalation to regulate respiratory rate. Together the apneustic and pneumotaxic centers facilitate the transition from inhalation to exhalation.

Central chemoreceptors. Both chemical and neural stimuli enter the respiratory centers for processing. Chemosensitive areas near the ventral surface of the medulla are sensitive to ionized levels of carbon dioxide and hydrogen in the cerebrospinal fluid (CSF). Alterations in the concentrations of carbon dioxide, bicarbonate, and hydrogen ions increase or decrease respiratory rate. In general an acid environment stimulates respirations, and an alkaline environment inhibits respirations.

It is important to note that blood and CSF levels of carbon dioxide and hydrogen differ. A higher Pco_2 and lower pH (7.32), similar to venous blood, are present in CSF. Carbon dioxide easily diffuses across the blood-brain barrier. Low levels of carbon dioxide (respiratory alkalosis) or high levels (respiratory acidosis) alter pH and evoke an immediate decrease or increase in respiratory rate in acute situations, such as anxiety or fainting.

The blood-brain barrier is less permeable to both hydrogen and bicarbonate than to carbon dioxide. Buffering of hydrogen ions in the CSF depends primarily on bicarbonate because the protein content of CSF is less than that of blood. Metabolic, that is, non CO_2-related, increases (metabolic alkalosis) or decreases (metabolic acidosis) in blood pH are not immediately reflected in CSF pH like the respiratory changes seen above. Instead, active or passive transport of bicarbonate is necessary to alter the pH of the CSF. Hours to days are necessary to reestablish carbon dioxide/bicarbonate ratios.

A common situation seen in nursing practice that is affected by bicarbonate diffusion into and out of the CSF occurs in mechanically ventilated patients with chronic respiratory acidosis and resultant compensatory metabolic alkalosis. If the patient with chronic respiratory acidosis is overventilated so that the $Paco_2$ becomes "normal," the ratio of CO_2 and bicarbonate in the blood is altered. The kidney excretes bicarbonate to correct the alkalosis that occurs. The CSF must also excrete bicarbonate because the pH of the blood may now be lower than that in the CSF. Spontaneous ventilatory drive is depressed until pH, Pco_2, and bicarbonate levels in the blood and CSF are corrected to the patient's own "normals."

Peripheral chemoreceptors. Peripheral chemoreceptors are located in the carotid bodies at the bifurcation of the common carotid arteries and in the aortic bodies above and below the aortic arch. Decreases in Pa_{O_2} and increases in Pa_{CO_2} stimulate the aortic and carotid bodies. A decrease in pH also stimulates the carotid bodies. Stimulation of the peripheral chemoreceptors results in increased ventilation.

The peripheral chemoreceptors are responsible for all increases in ventilation that result from arterial hypoxemia. Increases in Pa_{O_2} decrease firing activity from the carotid and aortic bodies and ultimately decrease $\dot{V}_E$. Decreases in Pa_{O_2} increase firing activity from the peripheral chemoreceptors to stimulate increased ventilations. Maximum response from the carotid and aortic bodies occurs with a Pa_{O_2} between 30 and 50 mm Hg. Below 30 mm Hg and above 100 mm Hg, firing activity decreases.

A function of the carotid and aortic bodies that is less understood is stimulation of ventilation as a result of changes in arterial blood pressure. Increased blood pressure may result in reflex hypoventilation or apnea. Conversely, decreased blood pressure may stimulate ventilation.

Neural receptors. The lung contains three types of neural receptors: stretch, irritant, and juxtacapillary. There are also neural receptors in the nose and upper airway, joints, muscles, and arteries.

Pulmonary stretch receptors are reported to be present in the smooth muscle of the airways. The vagus nerve receives input from the stretch receptors in response to lung hyperinflation. Stimulation of the stretch receptor in the lung results in the Hering-Breuer inflation reflex, in which expiratory time is increased and inhalation is inhibited at large lung volumes. Stretch receptors are important in newborns, and they may also stimulate inhalation at very low lung volumes.

Irritant receptors are also located in the airways between epithelial cells. Noxious gases, cigarette smoke, inhaled dusts, and cold air are just a few of the irritants that may stimulate receptors.[1] Stimulated irritant receptors act through the vagus nerve to cause bronchoconstriction and hyperpnea. Irritant receptors may play a role in histamine-activated asthma attacks (Gold, 1973).

J receptors is the term commonly used for juxtacapillary receptors. J receptors are believed to be present in the alveolar walls near the capillary. Impulses occur as a result of increased interstitial fluid volume, as occurs in pneumonia or adult respiratory distress syndrome (ARDS). Apnea and rapid, shallow breathing are common responses to stimulation of the vagus nerve caused by J receptors, although hypotension and bradycardia can also occur (Widdicombe, 1977; Berger et al, 1977).

Other receptors outside the lung also affect ventilation. The nose, pharynx, larynx, and trachea contain receptors that respond to both mechanical and chemical stimulation, causing sneezing, coughing, bronchoconstriction, and laryngospasm. Muscle and joint receptors may increase ventilation during activity or exercise, even passive exercise, such as range of motion in the unconscious patient. Receptors in the intercostal muscles and diaphragm may contribute to the sensation of dyspnea.

Distribution of ventilation

Distribution of ventilation in the lung differs by region and position. In the normal upright lung, $\dot{V}_A$ increases from the apex to the base. That is, the bases of the lung receive a greater portion of the V_T than the apices. The bases are overventilated and compensate for the underventilated apices. In the supine lung the posterior segments receive more ventilation than the anterior segments. Similar ventilation changes occur when the patient is in the side-lying position, in that the dependent lung receives a greater portion of the V_T. Regardless of position, the most dependent areas of the lung receive the most ventilation.

The primary reason for unequal distribution of ventilation in the lung is gravity. It is known that intrapleural pressure is less negative at the bottom than at the top of an upright lung because of the weight of the lung. Alveoli closer to the base of the lungs are compressed by the weight of those above and therefore are smaller. At the apices of the lungs, there is less compression from above, and the alveoli are larger at a resting state. Assuming that all alveoli are capable of expanding to the same size, smaller alveoli located in the base of the lung need more air than the larger, apical alveoli to achieve identical size.

During inhalation the smaller alveoli at the base of the upright lung are much easier to distend than apical alveoli. At higher volumes, there is greater resistance to distention. An easy method to conceptualize this is the blowing up of a round balloon. Although it takes effort to overcome the initial elastic properties of a balloon, it takes little effort to add additional air once air begins to distend the balloon's elastic walls. As the balloon nears full capacity, it again takes great effort to add additional air.

MECHANICS OF BREATHING

Ventilation is affected by the mechanical properties of compliance, elastic recoil, and airway resistance of the lung and chest wall.

Elastic recoil

Elastic recoil is the tendency of the lung and chest wall to return to a resting state. It is measured when airflow is zero. The centripetal recoil of the lung is balanced by centrifugal recoil of the chest wall. The resting state for the lung is a collapsed state, but the resting state for the chest wall is a springing outward (Fig. 2-2). At FRC elastic recoil properties of the lungs and chest wall are equal but opposite. Above FRC, recoil pressure exceeds atmospheric pressure, and the chest pulls inward, forcing a decrease in lung volume. Below FRC, elastic recoil pressure (Pstl) is subatmospheric, and the chest recoils outward to pull air into the lungs.

For air to flow into the lung during inhalation, a transpulmonary pressure change occurs. Transpulmonary pressure (TPP), the pressure difference across the lung, is reflected by the difference between alveolar pressure (P_A) and pleural pressure (Ppl). At rest (no air flow), there is no pressure difference between the alveoli and the mouth. P_A equals mouth pressure (Pao) or atmospheric pressure. P_A is also equal to the sum of Ppl and Pstl. Therefore, as seen in the following equation, TPP is equal to Ppl because P_A is atmospheric or effectively zero. Pstl is also equal to TPP at rest.

$$TPP = P_A - Ppl$$
$$P_A = Ppl + Pstl$$
$$TPP = (Ppl + Pstl) - Ppl = Pstl$$

Compliance

Compliance (C) is a measure of the distensibility, or elastic properties, of the lungs and of the chest wall. Compliance is determined by the change in lung pressure (ΔP) produced by a change in volume (ΔV).

$$C = \Delta V / \Delta P$$

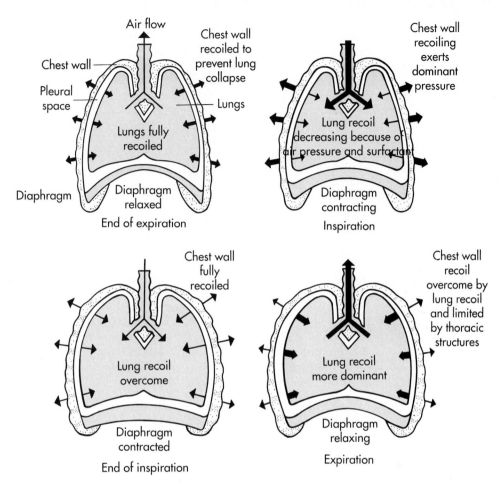

Fig. 2-2. Elastic recoil properties of the lungs.

Compliance of the lung is nonlinear. At higher lung volumes compliance is lower, meaning that less volume is achieved at the same pressure gradient. Therefore the lung is more difficult to inflate. As lung volumes near RV, compliance is increased; that is, greater volume per unit of pressure occurs, the lung or reduced compliance is easier to inflate.

The patient with ARDS or pulmonary fibrosis has a stiff lung or reduced compliance. Greater pressure is required to inflate the lungs with a V_T, and at exhalation the lung recoils quickly. Compliance and therefore ventilation are improved in the patient with ARDS by breathing shallowly and rapidly because elevated V_T increases work of breathing.

The typical patient with emphysema has increased lung compliance. Because elastic recoil is decreased, the lung readily accepts air. Inhalation produces greater increases in volume per unit of pressure. The lung is easily distensible; thus, compliance is increased. The net result is increased residual lung volume. Patients with increased RV, such as those with emphysema, breathe more efficiently at slower rates and deeper volumes.

There are two types of compliance: static (Cstat) and dynamic (Cdyn). Cstat is an indication of small-airway function, and Cdyn reflects large-airway function. Cstat is measured during periods of no air flow and therefore is not affected by airway resistance. Cdyn is determined from changes in lung volume and differences in Ppl at end-inhalation and end-exhalation. In the nonintubated patient an esophageal balloon records Ppl while a spirometer measures volume. In the intubated patient, peak and plateau pressures from the pressure manometer and the exhaled volume from the spirometer are used to calculate Cdyn and Cstat, respectively. If positive end-expiratory pressure (PEEP) is used in the mechanically ventilated patient, the level of PEEP is subtracted from the peak or plateau pressure before calculating compliance.

$$C = \Delta V/\Delta P$$
$$Cdyn = V_T/(Ppeak - PEEP)$$
$$Cstat = V_T/(Pplateau - PEEP)$$

In the normal individual, Cdyn and Cstat are nearly equal. In disease states a decrease in Cdyn reflects a change in the large airways, such as bronchospasm or excessive secretions. A decrease in Cstat is associated with an increase of fluid in the small airways, such as pneumonia or pulmonary edema.

Airway resistance

Any discussion of compliance must also include airway resistance. Airway resistance is the difference in pressures between the mouth and the alveoli divided by the flow rate ($\dot{V}$).

$$R = P/\dot{V}$$

Pressure at the mouth is measured with a manometer. At the alveoli, pressure is deduced from a body plethysmograph. The pressure differences depend on the rate and the pattern of flow. *Laminar flow* occurs at low flow rates (Fig. 2-3). Flow is streamlike and parallel to the sides of the tube. Unsteadiness, especially at the branches, develops as flow increases. Local eddies may form; this is termed *transitional flow*. As flow continues to increase, the stream lines of airflow become very disorganized; this is termed *turbulent flow* (see Fig. 2-3).

Airway resistance for laminar flow is described by Poiseuille's law, in which pressure is directly proportional to flow rate ($P = K \times \dot{V}$). In the following equation P is the change in pressure, r is the radius, n is the viscosity of the gas, and l is the length of the tube.

$$R = \frac{8nl}{\pi r^4}$$

As seen in the equation, radius is extremely important because decreasing the radius by one half increases resistance 16 times. Doubling the length of the tube only doubles the resistance. Density does not affect laminar flow.

Turbulent flow differs from laminar flow in that density is important in determining airway resistance. Increasing the density of a gas increases the pressure change between the mouth and the alveoli. A low-density gas, such as helium, is sometimes used clinically to overcome airway resistance induced by turbulent flow.

All three types of flow exist throughout the lung because airway diameter and length are constantly changing. Turbulent flow is more prominent in the

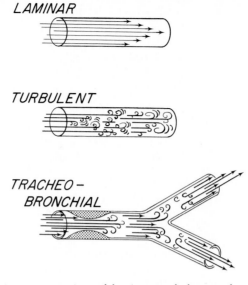

LAMINAR

TURBULENT

TRACHEO-
BRONCHIAL

Fig. 2-3. Schematic representation of laminar, turbulent, and transitional flow. In laminar flow, the center stream has the greatest velocity. In turbulent flow, flow is disorganized; there are eddies or whorls. Transitional flow has properties of both. (From Frownfelter D: *Chest physical therapy and pulmonary rehabilitation*, ed 2, St Louis, 1987, Mosby–Year Book).

trachea, and laminar flow occurs primarily in the very small airways. Most air flow in the lungs is transitional air flow. During exercise, when the flow rate increases, turbulent flow may increase. Airway resistance is lowest in the small airways and highest in the medium and large airways.

Lung volume is also important in determining airway resistance. At higher lung volumes, airway resistance is reduced. Airway diameter and length are both increased. The increase in airway diameter is primarily responsible for decreasing airway resistance. Applying this knowledge, the nurse identifies that a patient with increased airway resistance, such as bronchospasm, will breathe more effectively at higher lung volumes.

Airway resistance increases rapidly as lung volume decreases. Therefore with increased airway resistance the pressure gradient from the mouth to the alveoli must increase to maintain the same air flow. This is frequently demonstrated in patients receiving mechanical ventilation who develop bronchospasm or excessive secretions. Peak ventilating pressures elevate acutely, indicating increased airway resistance.

PERFUSION

As discussed earlier, pulmonary circulation begins in the pulmonary artery on the right side of the heart and ends in the pulmonary vein on the left side of the heart. Pressure in the pulmonary circulation is normally very low. Right atrial pressure is approximately 2 mm Hg, and left atrial pressure is about 5 mm Hg. Normal pulmonary artery pressure is $25/8$ mm Hg. Mean pulmonary artery pressure is therefore about 15 mm Hg. The pressure change from the pulmonary artery to the pulmonary vein is approximately 10 mm Hg (15 − 5 = 10). In contrast, the systemic circulation pressures are much higher—usually 120/80 is considered normal, although the range of normal is wide. Mean pressure in the systemic circulation, about 94 mm Hg, is about six times higher than that in the pulmonary circulation. The pressure drop in the systemic circulation is about 92 (94 − 2 = 92). The pressure change in the systemic circulation is 9 to 10 times greater than that in the pulmonary circulation.

Blood vessels in the pulmonary and systemic circulations have different characteristics. The walls of the pulmonary arteries are very thin. They contain little smooth muscle and are often mistaken for veins. Arteries in the systemic circulation are thick walled. Smaller arteries and arterioles are lined with smooth muscle and regulate flow to the various tissues of the body.

Pulmonary vascular resistance

Resistance in blood vessels is described as the difference in pressure divided by the volume of blood flow (Q) as seen in the following equation:

$$R = (\text{Input-output pressure})/Q$$

Using the pressures previously described and assuming a normal cardiac output of 5 LPM, a normal pulmonary vascular resistance is $^{10}\!/_5$, or approximately 2 mm Hg/liter/minute. When vascular resistance is expressed in the units dynes·sec·cm^{-5}, the mm Hg value is multiplied by 80. Systemic vascular resistance is much greater: 18.4 mm Hg/liter/minute or 1472 dynes·sec·cm^{-5}.

Although pulmonary vascular resistance is small, it may be decreased even further by the use of recruitment and distention of the pulmonary vessels (Fig. 2-4). In the normal lung some capillaries are open, with little or no blood flow, and some capillaries may be closed. As pulmonary capillary pressure rises, blood flow in the open capillaries increases, closed capillaries begin to open and accept blood flow, and pulmonary vascular resistance is lowered. This is termed *recruitment* and is the primary mechanism for decreased pulmonary vascular resistance.

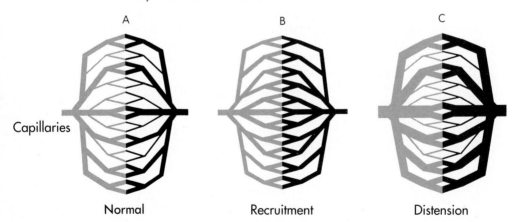

Fig. 2-4. Effects of increases in vascular pressures and pulmonary blood flow. **A,** Normal. Some pulmonary capillaries are closed, and no blood is conducting. **B,** Recruitment. As blood flow or pulmonary vascular pressure increases, more capillaries open. **C,** Distension. Capillaries widen and acquire a larger cross-sectional area when vascular pressures are high.

Distention of the pulmonary capillary occurs at higher vascular pressures. The diameter, or caliber, of pulmonary vessels increases. Pulmonary vascular resistance decreases as distention of the capillary increases. Distention is believed to be the primary mechanism for decreases in pulmonary vascular resistance at relatively high pulmonary pressures.

Pulmonary vascular resistance also is affected by lung volume. At high lung volumes vascular resistance is low because the caliber of extraalveolar vessels is increased as the lung expands. At low lung volumes smooth muscle and elastic tissue resist distention and increase vascular resistance. In atelectatic, or collapsed, lung areas, pulmonary blood pressure may increase several centimeters of water above downstream pressure before blood flow occurs. The latter is termed *critical opening pressure*.

Distribution of blood flow

Blood flow in the lung varies in a similar pattern to air flow. Blood flow is gravity dependent. In the upright lung blood flow increases almost linearly from the top to the bottom of the lung. At the apex of the upright lung, blood flow is minimal. The bases of the lung receive a greater portion of the cardiac output. In the supine lung, blood flow is almost equal in the apex and base and minimal in the anterior lung. Blood flow in the posterior, or dependent, regions of the lung exceeds that of the anterior lung. With exercise, blood flow increases to the apex and the base, and regional differences are less.

West (1985) describes three zones of pulmonary blood flow. The apical portion of the lung is termed *zone 1*. Here pulmonary artery pressure is less than PA. Capillaries are compressed, and blood flow is absent (Vd alv). Zone 1 is not present under normal conditions because pulmonary artery pressure is sufficient to deliver blood to the apex. When pulmonary artery pressure is reduced, such as in hypovolemic shock, or when PA pressure is increased, such as in positive pressure ventilation, zone 1 areas may exist.

Zone 2 encompasses the middle portion of the lung. Pulmonary artery pressure increases because of hydrostatic pressure changes. PA is less than pulmonary artery pressure. Because venous pressure is lower than PA, blood flow is determined by the difference between arterial pressure and PA, not by arterial-venous pressure differences. Arterial pressure increases down the zone, and PA remains unchanged. The pressure differences are responsible for increases in blood flow.

Zone 3 is described in the lower lung fields. Here venous pressure exceeds PA. Blood flow is determined by normal arterial-venous pressure differences. Although recruitment is the common mechanism to increase blood flow in zone 2, distention (along with some recruitment) is primarily responsible for the increase in blood flow in zone 3. Arterial-venous pressure differences increase down the zone, and PA remains constant. Blood flow increases down zone 3.

VENTILATION-PERFUSION MATCHING

If ventilation and perfusion were distributed evenly across the lung and diffusion were normal, arterial and alveolar carbon dioxide and oxygen levels would be identical. Regional differences in ventilation and perfusion do exist, as previously described. These differences are exaggerated in lung disease.

Ventilation-perfusion ($\dot{V}/\dot{Q}$) abnormalities occur when either ventilation or blood flow is altered. The rate of carbon dioxide and oxygen diffusion also is altered. Changes in arterial versus alveolar carbon dioxide and oxygen are observed.

In the normal lung the $\dot{V}/\dot{Q}$ ratio is approximately equal. Air entering the alveoli ($\dot{V}_E$) and blood flowing through the lung (cardiac output) determine the $\dot{V}/\dot{Q}$ ratio. In the normal lung, total $\dot{V}_A$ is usually slightly less than perfusion, making the normal $\dot{V}/\dot{Q}$ ratio 0.8.

Inspired air has a P_{O_2} of about 150 mm Hg and a P_{CO_2} of approximately 0 mm Hg. Blood entering the lung has a P_{O_2} of 40 mmHg and a P_{CO_2} of 45 mm Hg. After gas exchange, the alveolar and arterial P_{O_2} are approximately 100 mm Hg. The arterial and alveolar P_{CO_2} are 40 mm Hg. Calculation of alveolar oxygen tension at different levels of inspired oxygen is discussed in Chapter 6.

When ventilation is impaired, the $\dot{V}/\dot{Q}$ ratio is low and may approach zero if alveoli are completely obstructed (Fig. 2-5). The term *intrapulmonary shunt* is used when ventilation is absent but perfusion is present. In shunt areas of the lung, red blood cells in the capillary do not participate in gas exchange. Therefore the arterial and alveolar levels of oxygen are the same as those of mixed venous blood. The P_{O_2} of blood leaving the alveoli approaches 40 mm Hg, and the P_{CO_2} approaches 45 mm Hg. Because shunt is

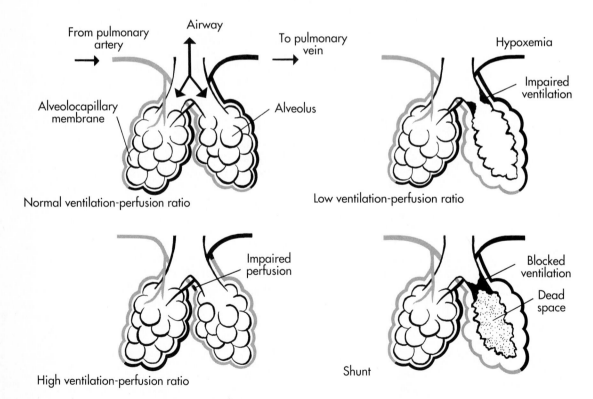

Fig. 2-5. Ventilation/perfusion abnormalities. Low $\dot{V}/\dot{Q}$ results from impaired ventilation, and high $\dot{V}/\dot{Q}$ results from impaired perfusion. Shunt is perfusion without ventilation.

rarely global, the arterial blood gas usually demonstrates various levels of hypoxemia with normal or slightly lowered P_{CO_2}. Ventilation increases to improve arterial oxygen tension (hypoxemic response). In clinical practice the nurse may see low $\dot{V}/\dot{Q}$ caused by a mucus plug, bronchospasm, ARDS, and other pulmonary disorders.

When perfusion is impaired, the $\dot{V}/\dot{Q}$ ratio is high (see Fig. 2-5), that is, ventilation exceeds perfusion. A high $\dot{V}/\dot{Q}$ ratio may be caused by either too much ventilation (wasted ventilation) or too little perfusion of alveoli. The term *dead space* is used when perfusion is absent but ventilation is present. Although the alveoli are being ventilated, the red blood cell in the capillary is not participating in gas exchange. Alveolar P_{O_2} and P_{CO_2} are normal: 150 mm Hg and 0 mm Hg, respectively. Arterial P_{CO_2} is usually lower, and arterial P_{O_2} is usually normal. A high $\dot{V}/\dot{Q}$ ratio may be caused by pulmonary emphysema, acute hemorrhage, anxiety, or pulmonary emboli.

CONCLUSION

This chapter reviews basic principles of ventilation and perfusion. The chapter begins by identifying various volumes and capacities used in caring for patients with pulmonary dysfunction. For instance, pulmonary function tests quantify the volumes and capacities and define the type of pulmonary dysfunction as restrictive, obstructive, or combined. The nurse uses this knowledge to teach pursed-lip breathing to the patient with obstructive problems as a means of improving ventilation. Lung volumes and principles of compliance and resistance are also important in weaning patients from mechanical ventilation. In addition, an understanding of ventilation/perfusion principles allows the nurse to apply nursing care scientifically, for example, patient positioning with the good lung down, to obtain maximum oxygenation.

BIBLIOGRAPHY

Baum GL, Wolinsky E: *Textbook of pulmonary diseases*, ed 3, Boston, 1983, Little & Brown.

Berger AJ, Mitchell RA, Severinghaus JW: Regulation of respiration, *N Engl J Med* 297, 1977.

Burki NK: *Pulmonary diseases: medical outline series*, Garden City, NY, 1982, Medical Examination Publishing.

Burton GC, Hodgkin JE: *Respiratory care: a guide to clinical practice*, ed 2, Philadelphia, 1984, JB Lippincott.

Cherniack NS, Widdicombe JG, eds: *Handbook of physiology, section 3: the respiratory system*, vol 3, Baltimore, 1986, Williams & Wilkins.

Comroe J: *Physiology of respiration: an introductory text*, ed 2, Chicago, 1974, Mosby–Year Book.

Fishman A: *Assessment of pulmonary function*, New York, 1980, McGraw-Hill Book Co.

Gold WM: *Cholinergic pharmacology in asthma*. In Austen KF, Lichtenstein LM, eds: *Asthma*, New York, 1973, Academic Press.

Gray H, Clemente CD: *Anatomy of the human body*, American ed 30, Philadelphia, 1985, Lea & Febiger.

Guyton AC: *Textbook of medical physiology*, ed 6, Philadelphia, 1981, WB Saunders.

Hedemark L, Kronenberg R: Chemical regulation of respiration: normal variations and abnormal responses, *Chest* 82(4):488-493, 1982.

Hinshaw H, Murray J: *Diseases of the chest*, ed 4, Philadelphia, 1980, WB Saunders.

Luce J, Culver B: Respiratory muscle function in health and disease, *Chest* 81(1):82-90, 1982.

Mitchell RS, Petty TL, Schwarz MI: *Synopsis of clinical pulmonary disease*, ed 4, St. Louis, 1989, Mosby–Year Book.

Mountcastle VB, ed: *Medical physiology*, St Louis, 1980, Mosby–Year Book.

Murray JF: *The normal lung*, Philadelphia, 1986, WB Saunders.

Murray JF, Nadel JA, eds: *Textbook of respiratory medicine*, Philadelphia, 1988, WB Saunders.

Netter F: *The CIBA collection of medical illustrations, vol 7, respiratory system,* New York, 1979, CIBA Pharmaceutical Co.

Pare' JAP, Fraser RG: *Synopsis of diseases of the chest,* Philadelphia, 1983, WB Saunders.

Pavlin E, Hornbein T: The control of breathing, *Basics Respir Dis* 7(2), 1978.

Shapiro B, Harrison R, et al: *Clinical applications of respiratory care,* ed 3, Chicago, 1985, Mosby–Year Book.

Simmons DH, ed: *Current pulmonology,* vol 7, Chicago, 1986, Mosby–Year Book.

Slonim N, Hamilton L: *Respiratory physiology,* ed 5, St. Louis, 1987, Mosby–Year Book.

Staub N: Lung structure and function—1982, *Basics Respir Dis* 10(3), 1982.

Wade JF: *Comprehensive respiratory care-physiology and technique,* ed 3, St. Louis, 1982, Mosby–Year Book.

Wanner A, Sackner MA: *Pulmonary diseases: mechanisms of altered structure and function,* Boston, 1983, Little & Brown.

West J: *Respiratory physiology: the essentials,* ed 3, Baltimore, 1985, Williams & Wilkins.

West JB: *Pulmonary pathophysiology: the essentials,* ed 2, Baltimore, 1982, Williams & Wilkins.

Widdicombe JG: Studies on afferent nerve innervation, *Rev Respir Dis* 115(6 pt 2):99-105.

Williams MH, ed: Disturbance of respiratory control: *Clin Chest Med* 1(1): 1-159.

C·H·A·P·T·E·R 3

Blood-Gas Transport and Acid-Base

Objectives:
_____

- Describe the importance of hemoglobin in oxygen transport.
- Discuss the actions of increased and decreased pH, Pa_{CO_2}, temperature, and 2,3-diphosphoglycerate (DPG) on oxygen delivery to the tissues.
- State the mechanisms for carbon dioxide transport in the blood.
- Differentiate acidemia, alkalemia, acidosis, and alkalosis.
- Describe respiratory control of pH, including P_{CO_2} and P_{O_2}.
- Describe renal control of pH with hypercapnia.

This chapter discusses the transport of oxygen and carbon dioxide in the blood. Because the transport of carbon dioxide is involved in controlling pH, acid-base concepts are presented. Both central nervous system and renal control of pH are presented.

The partial pressures of oxygen and carbon dioxide are determined by measurement of blood gases. Although both arterial and venous blood gases may be measured, arterial blood gases are used more frequently to evaluate a patient's status and are the primary focus of this section. The analysis of blood gases usually includes a determination of hydrogen ion concentration (pH), oxygen saturation of hemoglobin (S), and bicarbonate $H_{CO_3}^-$ levels. Although pH is measured directly, $H_{CO_3}^-$, and usually oxygen saturation (unless a cooximeter is used to measure S) are calculated values (see Chapter 6 for the assessment of arterial blood gases).

The pressure of oxygen in inspired air (P_{IO_2}) is 150 mm Hg at sea level. In the alveoli the pressure of oxygen (P_{AO_2}) is 100 mm Hg. Arterial oxygen tension (Pa_{O_2}) is usually 95 to 100 mm Hg, although normal Pa_{O_2} decreases with age. Arterial oxygen saturation is measured at 95% to 97% in the normal adult. The differences between the pressures of inspired air and alveolar air are primarily due to the effect of water vapor. The variance between alveolar and arterial oxygen tension is due to oxygen consumption and carbon dioxide elimination.

OXYGEN TRANSPORT

Oxygen is transported in the blood in two ways. A small amount of oxygen is dissolved in the plasma, but the chief means of oxygen transportation is chemical bonding to hemoglobin.

The amount of oxygen dissolved in the blood corresponds to Henry's law, which states that the amount dissolved is proportional to the partial pressure of oxygen in the blood (Po_2). About 0.003 ml of oxygen can be dissolved in 100 ml of blood. Identify the effect of Po_2 on the amount of dissolved oxygen in the following examples. Note that decreasing (or increasing) the Po_2 by 20 does not significantly alter the amount of dissolved oxygen.

$$100 \text{ mm Hg Po}_2 \times 0.003 \text{ ml} = 0.3 \text{ ml/100 ml}$$
$$80 \text{ mm Hg Po}_2 \times 0.003 \text{ ml} = 0.24 \text{ ml/100 ml}$$

(The term *vol%* may be used interchangeably with *ml/100 ml*.)

Based on the above examples, it is easy to see that dissolved oxygen is a very inefficient way to carry oxygen to the tissues. In contrast, the amount of oxygen that can be carried by hemoglobin is very large. Hemoglobin is the red-pigmented protein found in red blood cells (erythrocytes). Iron within the heme portion of hemoglobin combines with oxygen entering the erythrocyte. The result is oxygen-bound hemoglobin (oxyhemoglobin) described by the following chemical equation:

$$O_2 + Hg \circlearrowleft Hbo_2$$

Although oxyhemoglobin is the most common and most useful form of oxygen-bound hemoglobin, other forms do exist. Hemoglobin can also be oxidized to methemoglobin, carboxyhemoglobin, or sulfhemoglobin by various drugs and chemicals, including nitrites, sulfonamides, and acetanilide. Cigarette smoking and air pollution account for the majority of methemoglobin, carboxyhemoglobin, and sulfhemoglobin. Neither methemoglobin or sulfhemoglobin are useful for carrying oxygen to the tissues.

In the blood 1 g of hemoglobin can combine chemically with 1.34 ml O_2. This combination is termed the *oxygen capacity of blood*. Oxygen capacity reflects the maximum amount of oxyhemoglobin that 1 g of hemoglobin can carry, which is normally between 16 and 20 vol%. Oxygen capacity is dependent on the total amount of hemoglobin in the blood. The quality of the hemoglobin, such as sickle cell, is also important. In the following examples notice the effect of normal and reduced levels of hemoglobin on oxygen capacity.

$$15 \text{ gm Hb} \times 1.34 = 20.1 \text{ ml O}_2/100 \text{ ml blood}$$
$$10 \text{ gm Hb} \times 1.34 = 13.4 \text{ ml O}_2/100 \text{ ml blood}$$

Because hemoglobin is so important in oxygen transportation to the tissues, the nurse needs to differentiate between the oxygen capacity and the oxygen content. In calculating *oxygen content*, the actual saturation of oxygen carried as oxyhemoglobin, not methemoglobin, carboxyhemoglobin, or sulfhemoglobin, is multiplied by the oxygen capacity. Oxygen saturation reflects the ratio of oxygen content of blood to oxygen capacity, as demonstrated by the following equation:

$$S = 100 \times \frac{\text{Content} - \text{Dissolved O}_2}{\text{Capacity} - \text{Dissolved O}_2}$$

Normal arterial oxygen saturation is 97% with a Po_2 of 100 mm Hg, and normal venous oxygen saturation is 75% with a P_{O_2} of 40 mm Hg. In the following examples oxygen saturation has been decreased by the presence of excessive carboxyhemoglobin, methemoglobin, and sulfhemoglobin. Notice the effect of oxygen saturation in determining oxygen content.

$$15 \text{ g Hg} \times 1.34 \times 97\% = 19.5 \text{ ml O2/100 ml}$$
$$15 \text{ g Hg} \times 1.34 \times 87\% = 17.5 \text{ ml O2/100 ml}$$

It is important to understand the relationships among P_{O_2}, S, content, and capacity. Suppose a patient becomes anemic, with a hemoglobin concentration of 10 g/100 ml of blood. He has normal lungs, with a P_{O_2} of 100 mm Hg and a S of 97%. The nurse calculates the oxygen capacity to be $10 \times 1.34 = 13.4$ ml/100 ml, which is less than normal. Oxygen content from the P_{O_2} will be $100 \times 0.003 = 0.3$ ml/100 ml blood, and oxygen content from S will be $10 \times 1.34 \times 0.97 = 13.0$ ml/100 ml blood. Total oxygen content is $13.0 + 0.3 = 13.3$ ml/100 ml blood, slightly less than the oxygen capacity because lung function is normal.

Oxygen dissociation curve

Oxygen is released or dissociated to the tissues in a nonlinear fashion. The S-shaped curve commonly is referred to as the *oxygen dissociation curve*. It has several physiological advantages over a linear curve (Fig. 3-1). Notice

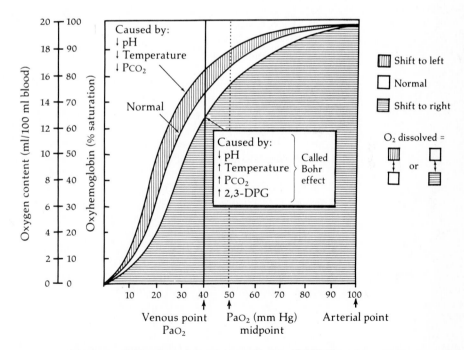

Fig. 3-1. Oxyhemoglobin dissociation curve at normal pH, Pa_{CO_2}, temperature, and 2,3-DPG. A shift to the right releases more oxygen to the tissues (lower oxygen content at any P_{O_2}). A shift to the left increases hemoglobin's affinity for oxygen, and less oxygen is released to the tissues (higher oxygen content at any P_{O_2}). (From Thompson J et al: *Mosby's manual of clinical nursing*, ed 2, St. Louis, 1989, Mosby–Year Book.)

Table 3-1. Oxyhemoglobin dissociation curve

Shift to the right (decreased oxygen affinity)	Shift to the left (increased oxygen affinity)
Increased H^+ (decreased pH)	Decreased H^+ (increased pH)
Increased $Paco_2$	Decreased $Paco_2$
Increased temperature	Decreased temperature
Increased 2,3-DPG	Decreased 2,3-DPG

that the top of the oxyhemoglobin dissociation curve is flat. Arterial Po_2 can decrease significantly with relatively little change in arterial oxygen saturation. For example, a patient develops pulmonary emboli with a sudden decrease in Pao_2 from 100 to 70 mm Hg. The arterial oxygen saturation decreases from 97% to 94%, a very small change. The hemoglobin remains saturated even when the Po_2 is reduced. The lower part of the curve becomes steep. Peripheral tissues can extract large amounts of oxygen from the hemoglobin with a small drop in Po_2.

Under the standard conditions of 7.4 pH, 40 mm Hg co_2, and 37° C, the curve demonstrates a few important points. A Po_2 of 60 mm Hg usually corresponds to an arterial saturation of 90%. When 50% of the hemoglobin is saturated with oxygen, the arterial Po_2 is approximately 27 mm Hg; this relationship is termed the P_{50}. It is used to express the affinity, or holding power, of hemoglobin for oxygen. A decrease in P_{50} shifts the oxyhemoglobin curve to the left. Oxygen affinity for hemoglobin is increased, and less oxygen is released to the tissues for metabolism. Therefore oxygen saturation is increased at any Po_2. Conversely, an increase in P_{50} shifts the curve to the right. Oxygen affinity for hemoglobin is decreased, and more oxygen is released to the tissues.

The position of the oxyhemoglobin dissociation curve, hence the affinity of hemoglobin for oxygen, is altered by four factors: pH, $Paco_2$, temperature, and 2,3-DPG. An increase in hydrogen ion concentration (decreased pH or acidemia), an increase in $Paco_2$, an increase in temperature, and an increase in 2,3-DPG cause the curve to shift to the right. Recall from basic physiology that 2,3-DPG is a product of erythrocyte metabolism and is increased in the presence of chronic hypoxemia, anemia, and alkalemia. Decreases in hydrogen ion concentration (increased pH or alkalemia), $Paco_2$, temperature, and 2,3-DPG cause a shift of the curve to the left (Table 3-1).

Oxygen dissociation also may be affected by the level of carbon monoxide in the patient's blood. Carbon monoxide has an affinity for hemoglobin that is 240 times greater than that of oxygen for hemoglobin. When carbon monoxide and hemoglobin bind together, the compound carboxyhemoglobin is formed. A healthy, nonsmoking adult has a carboxyhemoglobin level near 1%. In urban areas, where automotive pollution and industrial pollution are high, normal carboxyhemoglobin may increase to 3% to 5%. An active smoker frequently carries a carboxyhemoglobin level of 10% to 12%. The level of carboxyhemoglobin present in the blood is significant because small amounts of carbon monoxide can bind to very large amounts of hemoglobin. When this happens, Hb concentration and Po_2 are normal; however, oxyhemoglobin and therefore oxygen content are reduced. The oxyhemoglobin dissociation curve is shifted to the left, and less oxygen is released to the tissues.

CARBON DIOXIDE TRANSPORT

Carbon dioxide is produced by the mitochondria of metabolizing cells. Because the atmosphere contains minimal amounts of carbon dioxide (0.3%), all CO_2 in the body is the result of cell metabolism. Carbon dioxide production in normal adults is approximately 200 ml/min and is transported from the cells by diffusion for excretion by the lungs or kidneys. The gradient for diffusion is sometimes as small as 1 to 2 mm Hg, but diffusion can occur rapidly because CO_2 is 20 times more soluble than oxygen.

Carbon dioxide is carried in the blood as dissolved carbon dioxide (5% to 10%), as HCO_3^- (60% to 90%), and as a carbon dioxide-amino acid compound (5% to 30%), referred to as a *carbamino*. Dissolved carbon dioxide, like oxygen, corresponds to Henry's law of partial pressures. The partial pressure of CO_2 is 40 mmHg in arterial blood and 46 mmHg in venous blood.

Carbon dioxide is transported in the blood as dissolved CO_2 or HCO_3^- according to the following equation:

$$CO_2 + H_2O \xrightarrow{\text{CA}} H_2CO_3 \longleftrightarrow H^+ + HCO_3$$

As carbon dioxide diffuses into the blood, a small amount combines with water to form carbonic acid (H_2CO_3). Carbonic anhydrase (CA), a catalyst present in the erythrocyte but absent in the plasma, facilitates rapid combination of carbon dioxide and water in the erythrocyte. Carbon dioxide can diffuse from the cell to the erythrocyte in less than 1 second in the presence of CA. Without CA the reaction can take up to 200 seconds. The newly formed carbonic acid dissociates into hydrogen ions and HCO_3^-.

Carbon dioxide also is carried in the blood as a carbamino. Amino acids are composed of an amino group (NH_2), which is basic, and a carboxyl group (COOH), which is acidic. Amino acids are therefore amphoteric; that is, they can react with either acids or bases to neutralize or buffer an acid or base.

Proteins, composed of amino acids, are present in the plasma as well as in the hemoglobin in large amounts. The hemoglobin protein is composed of an alpha group containing 141 amino acids and a beta group containing 146 amino acids linked in a polypeptide chain. The most important protein is the globin of hemoglobin, which combines with carbon dioxide to form a carbamino compound called *carbamino-hemoglobin:*

$$HbNH_2 + CO_2 \circlearrowleft HbNH_2COOH$$

This rapid reaction allows the binding of more CO_2 to reduced (unloaded) hemoglobin than HbO_2. The unloading of oxygen and the loading of carbon dioxide onto the hemoglobin molecule occur simultaneously at the tissue level and in the lungs. The enhanced ability of deoxygenated blood to carry carbon dioxide is known as the *Haldane effect*. In other words, as the oxyhemoglobin saturation falls, the blood is able to carry more CO_2 for the same P_{CO_2}.

The dissociation of carbonic acid and carbamino compounds produces large amounts of H^+ and HCO_3^-, which must be excreted from the erythrocyte. Some of the liberated hydrogen ions are combined with hemoglobin to form $HHbo_2$. As $HHbo_2$ is reduced by the delivery of oxygen to the tissues, the compound HHb is formed. Buffering by hemoglobin is such that little pH change is observed, a process termed an *isohydric reaction*.

Bicarbonate ions are buffered similarly by potassium hemoglobin (KHb), forming potassium bicarbonate ($KHCO_3$) and reduced hemoglobin. As $KHCO_3$ ionizes, a HCO_3^- gradient between the erythrocyte and plasma occurs. HCO_3^- ions diffuse into the plasma until HCO_3^- equilibrium is achieved between the erythrocyte and the plasma. Chloride ions diffuse into the erythrocyte in exchange for HCO_3^- to maintain electrical neutrality in the plasma. Once in the cell, the chloride ion combines with potassium to form potassium chloride; in the plasma, HCO_3^- combines with sodium to form sodium bicarbonate. This phenomenon is known as the *chloride shift*.

The results of carbon dioxide transport are dissolved carbon dioxide, carbonic acid, and sodium bicarbonate. The sum of these three forms of carbon dioxide equals the carbon dioxide content of blood. In arterial blood a normal carbon dioxide content is 56.3 vol%. The carbon dioxide content includes carbon dioxide that is either transported in combined form or dissolved in plasma. Because the amount of carbon dioxide transported as sodium bicarbonate equals 53.5 vol%, the remaining 2.8 vol% of carbon dioxide represents the amount of carbonic acid and dissociated or dissolved carbon dioxide. The normal ratio of carbonic acid to sodium bicarbonate is 20:1.

The ability of the body to transport carbon dioxide in the blood is dependent on both the amount of carbon dioxide in the blood and integrity of the carbon dioxide transportation systems. Under normal conditions the lungs excrete approximately 13,000 mEq of carbonic acid daily, and the kidneys excrete 40 to 80 mEq of fixed acids daily. Increased carbon dioxide production yields increased amounts of carbonic acid and sodium bicarbonate that must be excreted efficiently by the body to maintain a normal carbonic acid/sodium bicarbonate ratio. Most of the excess carbon dioxide produced is excreted by the lungs through increased alveolar minute ventilation. Carbon dioxide transport provides the basis for acid-base balance.

ACID-BASE CONCEPTS

An acid is a substance that donates protons and increases hydrogen ion concentration. An acid may be weak or strong, depending on its ability to donate hydrogen ions in solution. Whereas hydrochloric acid is a strong acid and dissociates completely into free hydrogen ions, carbonic acid is a weak acid. Carbonic acid donates only half of its hydrogen ions in solution.

$$H_2CO_3 \circlearrowleft H_+ + HCO_3^-$$

Fixed or nonvolatile acids are present in plasma. The result of metabolism, fixed acids are buffered by HCO_3^- and plasma proteins. The most common fixed acids that affect acid-base status are lactate, inorganic phosphate, sulfate, and ketone bodies. Increases in these fixed acids result in metabolic acidosis, and decreases result in metabolic alkalosis.

A base is a substance that accepts protons and combines with the hydrogen ion. In solution a base dissociates into a hydroxyl ion (OH^-). Recall the structure of the carbamino compounds ($HbHN_2COOH$). A carbamino compound acts as a base in solution because the end unit is a hydroxyl that dissociates in solution.

A discussion of acid-base status includes the term *buffer*. A buffer is a weak acid or base solution that is able to prevent a significant change in pH. Buffering of a solution results in neutralization and equilibrium of the solution.

There are several acid-base buffering systems in the body. The most important buffer in the body is the carbonic acid-bicarbonate buffer. Other buffers in the body include intracellular and plasma proteins, hemoglobin, bone carbonate, phosphate, collagen, and other body solids.

The number of hydrogen and hydroxyl ions in a solution determines acid-base composition. Equal numbers of both hydrogen and hydroxyl ions in water at 24° C is termed *electrical neutrality*. Increased numbers of acids create acidity, and increased numbers of bases yield alkalinity. The acidity or alkalinity of a solution is determined by pH, *puissance hydrogène*, or the 'power of hydrogen.' Electrical neutrality is a pH of 7.0. An acid has increased numbers of hydrogen ions, decreasing the pH to under 7.0. A base has decreased numbers of hydrogen ions, and pH increases above 7.0.

Note: The terms *acidemia* and *acidosis* and the terms *alkalemia* and *alkalosis* are often confused. Acidemia refers to an increased concentration of acids (low pH) in the blood. Acidosis is the process that accompanies acidemia. Similarly, alkalemia refers to an increased concentration of base (high pH) in the blood. Alkalosis is the process that accompanies alkalemia.

The pH of a solution is determined by the Henderson-Hasselbalch equation. A simplified version of the equation reflects the ability of the kidney to excrete base and of the lung to excrete acid.

$$pH = pK + \log \frac{(base)}{(acid)} \text{ or } \frac{(kidney)}{(lung)}$$

pH is the negative logarithm of hydrogen ion concentration. The Henderson-Hasselbalch equation reflects the ratio of base to acid, or HCO_3^- to CO_2, which is 20:1. In the Henderson-Hasselbalch equation, pK, the dissociation constant of a buffer system, is 6.1. P_{CO_2} is converted to the same units (mM/L or mEq/L) as HCO_3^- by multiplying mm Hg by 0.03. The following example assumes a normal arterial bicarbonate of 24 mEq/L and a normal arterial carbon dioxide of 40 mm Hg.

$$pH = pK + \log \frac{(HCO_3^-)}{(CO_2)}$$
$$pH = 6.1 + \log \frac{24}{40 \times 0.03}$$
$$= 6.1 + \log \frac{24}{1.2}$$
$$= 6.1 + \log 20$$
$$= 6.1 + 1.30$$
$$= 7.40$$

As demonstrated by the above equation, the normal pH of arterial blood is 7.40. A change in arterial CO_2 or HCO_3 changes the pH. To maintain a normal pH, the lungs and kidneys increase or decrease excretion of carbon dioxide or bicarbonate.

RESPIRATORY CONTROL OF pH

Carbon dioxide is the most important factor in respiratory control of P_{CO_2} and H^+ concentration. When adequate, $\dot{V}_A$ maintains alveolar and arterial P_{CO_2} at 40 mm Hg. A decrease in alveolar $\dot{V}_E$ increases the carbon dioxide tension. As P_{CO_2} increases (hypercapnia), H^+ concentration increases, and the pH falls. When hydrogen ion concentration in the cerebrospinal fluid is increased, the respiratory chemoreceptors respond by increasing $\dot{V}_E$ to return the P_{CO_2} to normal. Respiratory rate or volume increases, which elevates $\dot{V}_A$ and restores the Pa_{CO_2} to a normal level. (Note: An acute high elevation in arterial carbon dioxide tension, especially above 80 mm Hg, has a narcotic effect on the central nervous system. The affected individual becomes drowsy or confused. If the elevation is prolonged, unconsciousness and coma can occur.)

An increase in $\dot{V}_A$ has the opposite effect: the P_{CO_2} decreases, and the pH increases. A decreased concentration of H^+ results in decreased $\dot{V}_E$ by slowing respirations. The P_{CO_2} is thus restored to a higher level. If an individual voluntarily hyperventilates, he or she will have no urge to breathe for a short time.

Most rapid decreases in pH result from inadequate $\dot{V}_E$ (increased Pa_{CO_2}), as occurs in drug overdose or excessive sedation. The brain responds, increasing $\dot{V}_E$. The addition of a large amount of fixed acids has the same effect on pH and ventilation as acutely increased P_{CO_2}. For instance, the patient with diabetic ketoacidosis has a large increase in the amount of fixed acids (metabolic acidosis). The compensatory respiratory response is to increase the rate and depth of respirations (Kussmaul's respirations). The increased $\dot{V}_E$ ventilation decreases the Pa_{CO_2}, which increases the pH.

The respiratory control of pH is also influenced by arterial P_{O_2} through the carotid and aortic bodies. Normal oxygen tension is associated with a regulated flow of low-frequency impulses to the respiratory centers in the medulla. The flow of impulses increases when arterial P_{O_2} falls below the normal range. When the respiratory centers are stimulated by hypoxemia, $\dot{V}_E$ increases to return the P_{O_2} to a normal level. As arterial P_{O_2} increases, the flow of impulses from the carotid and aortic bodies slows. $\dot{V}_E$ subsequently decreases. The increase in carbon dioxide and hydrogen ion concentrations, which results from less $\dot{V}_A$, stimulates respiration to return to normal. The respiratory control of pH by the hypoxemic drive becomes stronger than the carbon dioxide reflex when P_{O_2} falls below 60 mm Hg. The importance of the hypoxemic drive is especially important when hypercapnia and hypoxemia coexist.

RENAL CONTROL OF pH

The kidneys also play an important role in maintenance of pH by regulating the acidity or alkalinity of the urine. An increase in H^+ concentration in the blood from acidemia or hypercapnia results in increased renal tubular excretion of hydrogen ions, increasing the acidity of the urine. Conversely, when hydrogen ion concentration in blood is decreased, the excretion of HCO_3^- and reabsorption of hydrogen ions reestablishes acid-base balance. To understand this process, recall the equation of the dissociation of carbonic acid:

$$CO_2 + H_2O \circlearrowleft H_2CO_3 \circlearrowleft HCO_3^- - + H^+$$

In the kidney carbon dioxide and water diffuse from the capillary into the renal tubule cell, and sodium and HCO_3^- are absorbed selectively into the capillary. In the presence of carbonic anhydrase, carbonic acid is formed and dissociates into hydrogen and bicarbonate ions. The HCO_3^- is reabsorbed into the systemic circulation with sodium. At the same time the hydrogen ion is diffused into the proximal tubule. There the hydrogen ion recombines with HCO_3^- present in the filtrate to form carbonic acid, which again dissociates into carbon dioxide and water. The latter diffuse back into the renal tubule cell.

The hydrogen ion also may be buffered by phosphate (HPO_4^-) and ammonia (NH_3) present in the filtrate. Hydrogen ions may combine with sodium and phosphate to form NaH_2PO_4. In the tubular cell ammonia is formed from amino acids and glutamine. As it is excreted, the hydrogen ion combines with ammonia to form ammonium (NH_4).

Renal compensation to restore acid-base balance is much slower than respiratory control, which is caused almost instantly by peripheral chemoreceptors. The renal process takes several hours to days to completely restore acid-base balance by reabsorption or excretion of HCO_3^-. When persistent hypercapnia exists, the kidney excretes hydrogen ions and reabsorbs bicarbonate ions until arterial pH is normalized. If the carbon dioxide level is decreased suddenly, as sometimes occurs when a patient with chronic CO_2 retention is ventilated mechanically, the patient becomes acutely alkalemic. Similarly, the patient who is acutely acidemic from fixed acids often requires supplemental base, usually sodium bicarbonate, to restore acid-base balance because it may be days before the kidney can restore acid-base balance. It is important to note that excretion of the hydrogen ion is accompanied by retention of the cation potassium. The exchange of potassium and hydrogen ions is particularly evident in diabetic ketoacidosis, when the pH is often less than 7.25 and serum potassium is measured as high as 6 mEq/L to 7 mEq/L.

CONCLUSION

Understanding transport of oxygen and carbon dioxide in the blood is essential to care for patients with pulmonary dysfunction and other problems. Consider these compelling situations. A patient with chronic pulmonary dysfunction develops gastrointestinal bleeding. What effect will the decreased hemoglobin have on an already stressed system? Or a patient is admitted with hypothermia (postsurgical or caused by cold exposure). The nurse should interpret the patient's blood gases during warming with an understanding of the oxyhemoglobin dissociation curve. A patient develops sepsis. The nurse should predict the change in blood gases or pulse oximetry. Finally, what happens when a patient with pulmonary dysfunction causing chronic carbon dioxide retention receives an antibiotic that impairs renal function? These are real patients needing care. This chapter helps the nurse to understand the physiology necessary for applying the interventions.

BIBLIOGRAPHY

Baum GL, Wolinsky E: *Textbook of pulmonary diseases,* ed 3, Boston, 1983, Little & Brown.

Burki NK: *Pulmonary diseases: medical outline series,* Garden City, NY, 1982, Medical Examination Publishing.

Burton GC, Hodgkin JE: *Respiratory care: a guide to clinical practice,* ed 2, Philadelphia, 1984, J B Lippincott.

Cherniack NS, Widdicombe JG, eds: *Handbook of physiology, section 3: the respiratory system,* vol 3, Baltimore, 1986, Williams & Wilkins.

Comroe J: *Physiology of respiration: an introductory text,* ed 2, Chicago, 1974, Mosby–Year Book.

Davenport HW: *The ABC of acid-base chemistry,* ed 5, Chicago, 1971, The University of Chicago Press.

Guyton AC: *Textbook of medical physiology,* ed 6, Philadelphia, 1981, W B Saunders.

Harper R: *A guide to respiratory care-physiology and clinical applications,* Philadelphia, 1982, J B Lippincott.

Hinshaw H, Murray J: *Diseases of the chest,* ed 4, Philadelphia, 1980, W B Saunders.

Mitchell RS, Petty TL, Schwarz MI: *Synopsis of clinical pulmonary disease,* ed 4, St. Louis, 1989, Mosby–Year Book.

Mountcastle VB, ed: *Medical physiology,* St Louis, 1980, Mosby–Year Book.

Murray JF: *The normal lung,* Philadelphia, 1986, W B Saunders.

Murray JF, Nadel JA, eds: *Textbook of respiratory medicine,* Philadelphia, 1988, W B Saunders.

Netter F: *The CIBA collection of medical illustrations,* vol 7: respiratory system, New York, 1979, CIBA Pharmaceutical.

Paré JAP, Fraser RG: *Synopsis of diseases of the chest,* Philadelphia, 1983, W B Saunders.

Pavlin E, Hornbein T: The control of breathing, *Basics Respir Dis* 7(2), 1978.

Shapiro B, Harrison R et al: *Clinical applications of respiratory care,* ed 3, Chicago, 1985, Mosby–Year Book.

Simmons DH, ed: *Current pulmonology,* vol 7, Chicago, 1986, Mosby–Year Book.

Slonim N, Hamilton L: *Respiratory physiology,* ed 5, St. Louis, 1987, Mosby–Year Book.

Staub N: *Lung structure and function–1982, Basics Respir Dis* 10(3), 1982.

Wade JF: *Comprehensive respiratory care: physiology and technique,* ed 3, St. Louis, 1982, Mosby–Year Book.

Wanner A, Sackner MA: *Pulmonary diseases: mechanisms of altered structure and function,* Boston, 1983, Little & Brown.

West J: *Respiratory physiology: the essentials,* ed 3, Baltimore, 1985, Williams & Wilkins.

West JB: *Pulmonary pathophysiology: the essentials,* ed 2, Baltimore, 1982, Williams & Wilkins.

U·N·I·T T·W·O

Methods of Assessing Pulmonary Function

One of the most important components of caring for patients is the ability of the nurse to assess the patient thoroughly. Development of an accurate and complete health history is the foundation of an assessment. Although the nurse focuses primarily on the pulmonary system, she must not ignore other body systems. The concepts related to obtaining a health history are discussed in Chapter 4. Having completed a health history, the nurse performs a physical assessment of the patient. In Chapter 5 chest physical examination is discussed in detail. A brief discussion of related assessments, such as edema, is also included.

In Chapters 6 through 9 assessments of supplemental laboratory data are discussed. Arterial blood gas analysis is presented in Chapter 6. The nurse will learn not only simple identification of the disorder but also complex or advanced assessments of oxygenation. The analysis of a chest x-ray film is presented in Chapter 7. Major anatomical landmarks are identified, as is assessment of pathological conditions. Pulmonary function testing is another method to assess respiratory function, and it is discussed in Chapter 8. The final chapter in Unit II is focused on assessment of the critically ill patient. However, many concepts discussed in Chapter 9, such as oximetry, are also applicable to acutely ill patients.

C H · A · P · T · E · R *4*

Health History

*O*bjectives

- Identify environmental factors that enhance communication when taking a health history.
- Discuss the relationship of chief complaint to precipitating event.
- Discuss seven areas of questioning for each symptom.
- Discuss symptoms often seen in the patient with pulmonary dysfunction.
- Discuss the relevance of a complete health history in patients with pulmonary dysfunction.

A complete health history is essential to care of the patient with pulmonary dysfunction. From the history the nurse can identify the patient's problems and needs before physical assessment. Both subjective and objective data are necessary to identify problems, to generate nursing diagnoses, to set goals, and to plan and implement relevant interventions. (Note: For simplicity in reading, the terms *he, his, him* are used to refer to the patient, and *she, hers, her* are used to refer to the nurse. The author realizes that patients and nurses may be male or female.)

ENVIRONMENTAL FACTORS

Environment is an important consideration when obtaining a health history. The comfort of the patient and nurse is essential. The nurse should provide as relaxed and calm an environment as possible. An unhurried atmosphere helps to build confidence with the patient and allows him to know that he is most important at this time. Privacy should be provided within the constraints of the environment. A patient may be reluctant to reveal private, confidential information if he thinks people other than the nurse are able to hear his words. The patient should be reassured that information will be available only to individuals involved in his care. Rapport is often easier to attain when these environmental factors are controlled, and rapport promotes communication.

Effective communication is enhanced by the relative positions of the patient and the nurse. The nurse must demonstrate genuine interest in and concern for the patient. This demonstration can be achieved through use of face-to-face contact with the nurse and the patient at the same level, if such contact is not contraindicated by culture. The nurse should sit if a patient is lying in a bed or sitting in a chair. Standing over the patient can induce a superior-inferior nonverbal atmosphere.

The nurse also may facilitate communication with the patient by commenting on something in the near environment, such as a photograph or floral arrangement. All comments must be relevant and not superficial, for example, "What a nice photograph—who is this?" or "What beautiful flowers—who sent them?" The patient can then respond to the neutral comment as he desires. The nurse learns something about the patient's background as the patient explains who is in the photograph or who sent the flowers.

COMMUNICATION

When meeting a patient for the first time, the nurse introduces herself to the patient and family members. She states her role and the purpose of the interview. "Hello. My name is Mary Smith (Mrs. Smith or Mrs. Mary Smith, if preferred). I am a registered nurse at University Hospital and am here to obtain a history of your health." The nurse then asks the patient (and family members, as appropriate) how he wishes to be addressed. Some patients prefer formality (Mr., Mrs., Ms., Dr.), and others are more casual, asking to be addressed by their first names. If in doubt and until directed otherwise, always use a formal address; never assume that the patient prefers an informal address.

Because communication has both verbal and nonverbal components, the nurse must be aware of the body language of the patient and herself. Arms folded across the chest are a sign that communication may be ineffective. The listener is not receptive to words. If possible, the nurse should not write while the patient is talking because this may convey a sense of disinterest. When the patient finishes speaking, the nurse makes notations before asking a subsequent question.

Verbal communication is enhanced by talking to the patient at his own knowledge level. The nurse should replace complex medical terminology with ordinary terms or phrases that define words. The terms *hemoptysis* and *dyspnea* may have little meaning for the patient, although the patient clearly knows the meaning of the phrases *cough up blood* and *shortness of breath*.

Data collection is facilitated by helping the patient describe his health history. The nurse may choose open-ended or closed questions. An open-ended question encourages the patient to give basic information, as well as thoughts, feelings, opinions, and experiences. Although an open-ended question generates more information, the breathless patient often requires the use of more closed questions to conserve energy. Closed questions require a one-word or two-word answer, such as age, sex, occupation, marital status, number of children, or years as a smoker. The most common closed questions require a yes or no response.

Most interviews begin with general open-ended questions, such as "Why have you come here today?" or "How are you feeling today?" The use of phrases, such as "Tell me more," "I see," "I would like to hear about it," "This seems important to you," or "Tell me how you feel about this" encourage the patient to tell the story. Unfortunately, some patients tend to wander from the subject or problem being discussed when encouraging, open-ended phrases are used. The nurse must guide the patient back to pertinent facts with the use of more specific questions.

The nurse must avoid the use of biased questions in her interview with the patient. Use of biased questions implies a value judgment, suggests the desired answer, and impairs effective data collection. The patient may be reluctant to provide information that is not consistent with the expected response, especially when behavior is not consistent with social mores. For example, the question "You don't use street drugs or smoke marijuana, do you?" demonstrates expectation of a negative response. If the patient responds "yes," he may be concerned about alienating or prejudicing the nurse-interviewer against him.

The general appearance of the patient often provides clues that guide the nurse in her interview. Evidence of fatigue in the patient's appearance may indicate the need to limit questioning to pertinent facts or to end the interview soon. Tone of voice, fluctuations in voice, facial expression, body position, and body movements are important components of the patient's response to a question. The presence of abnormal positioning or expressions can precipitate questions related to the finding. For instance, perhaps the patient always leans to one side or has a facial droop that can be noticed only when he is smiling.

When the patient is unable to provide historical information, the nurse should seek responses from the patient's family or other individuals who are significant in the patient's life. Instances in which this may occur include patients on ventilators, patients who have inadequate memory, patients who cannot speak or cannot speak the same language as the nurse, and patients who have an altered level of consciousness.

THE INTERVIEW
Precipitating event and chief complaint

When obtaining a history, the first question the nurse usually asks pertains to the precipitating event or chief complaint for the admission to the hospital or home care agency or for the current illness. In effect the nurse wants to know why the patient needs or perceives a need for health care. The nurse later develops a plan of care that addresses the patient's chief complaint and other problems the nurse identifies in the interview. For instance, the nurse may observe the patient having problems performing activities of daily living or problems with medication administration secondary to forgetfulness, in addition to dyspnea, pain, and surgical wounds.

The nurse inquires what precipitating event brought the patient to the hospital or necessitated home health referral. The response may vary, from the patient's having been in an accident, to having an infection, to not being able to breathe, to having surgery. When inquiring about the precipitating event, the nurse may also learn of the chief complaint. If not, the nurse asks the patient about his chief complaint.

Chief complaint is the patient's perception of why he sought treatment. Occasionally the patient's chief complaint (arthritis pain) may not be congruent with his most pressing problem, such as an electrolyte disturbance, gastrointestinal bleeding, or dysrhythmias. The chief complaint is more likely to differ from what the nurse identifies as the chief problem when there is chronic illness overlying an acute event. Patients with chronic pain or chronic dyspnea often are focused on these problems to the exclusion of others. Consider the patient with chronic obstructive pulmonary disease, who has dyspnea, productive cough, and normal appetite. He then develops nausea and vomiting that do not respond to home remedies. Dyspnea worsens as the patient's electrolytes become more abnormal. The patient calls the hospital and says, "I can't breathe" (chief complaint). When asked what brought the patient to the hospital, he says, "I started vomiting yesterday. I thought I had the flu" (precipitating event). He may add that now he can't breathe. The precipitating event for the hospitalization was nausea and vomiting secondary to theophylline toxicity (which induced an electrolyte imbalance). After admission to a home health agency for follow-up, the precipitating event for this patient's home health referral is hospitalization. The chief complaint necessitating home health referral may differ from the discharge diagnosis of theophylline toxicity. Another example of this patient's chief complaint may be shortness of breath or inability to do activities of daily living, including proper medication administration.

Chronology

When obtaining a health history, it is important to identify how the illness developed. Identification of date of onset, duration, relationship to other occurrences, and treatment are important for each symptom or problem the patient identifies, especially in the patient with chronic lung disease. The patient with acute disease easily can relate the sequence of events surrounding the illness. The patient with chronic lung disease may have more difficulty remembering actual time sequences because he must remember years of time/event relationships. For instance, the patient who has suspected asbestosis or pneumoconiosis must recall employment history for more than 20 years. Similarly the patient with tuberculosis or bronchiectasis often has to relate events that occurred as a child. Recalling these time and event relationships is very hard to do.

A typical chronological history of a patient with chronic obstructive pulmonary disease may be similar to the following: "I began smoking at the age of 12 and have been smoking for 50 years. I did not have any problems with my breathing until 10 months ago, when I cut down my smoking. I got a real bad pneumonia then and was in the hospital for 3 weeks. I was even on a breathing machine. I never needed oxygen though until a year ago. I have been taking these pills since I was in the hospital, and they seem to make my breathing easier. My breathing is much worse now, and they tell me I have a spot on my lung." The nurse should clarify if the patient continued smoking while receiving supplemental oxygen.

Occupation and environmental history

Another important component of the health history is the occupation and environmental history. Many occupation-related pulmonary diseases are not apparent until 20 or more years after the exposure. This is particularly true of patients exposed to coal dusts (coal miners), silica particles (glass blowers and pottery crafters), asbestos particles (pipe workers, ship builders, brake liners, and elevator operators), and talc (mill workers). An occupation history is often difficult to obtain, especially when the patient worked out of a local union hall and went to a different job site frequently. At the minimum the nurse identifies the types of work that the patient has done in the past. Particular questions are asked related to pipe fitting, brake lining, glass working, mining, farming, and milling. Environmental history encompasses the following areas.

Geography. The first part of the environmental history is geography. Patients who live in or travel to certain areas of the country or the world are more prone to develop diseases indigenous to that area. Histoplasmosis is common in the farming states of the Midwestern river valley and among chicken farmers, and coccidioidomycosis is more common in the desert Southwestern states and northern Mexico. Parasitic infections commonly occur in Africa and South America. Schistosomiasis exposure occurs when traveling to Asia, Africa, the Caribbean, and South America. Although eradicated from the United States, smallpox is still prevalent in other areas of the world. Although it is always important to inquire about whether the patient has traveled out of the immediate area recently, it is especially important when a patient has an unusual pulmonary illness.

Tuberculosis is a disease people tend to think of as being uncommon and confined to Third World countries. This is untrue; tuberculosis is diagnosed frequently in many areas of the United States. In fact the American Lung Association is observing a rise in the number of reported cases of tuberculosis in the United States. A major outbreak of tuberculosis occurred in a Missouri school in 1990, with effects that will reach into the next century as screening and treatment are completed. The increase in patients with immune deficiency syndromes is reported to be a factor in the increase of tuberculosis.

Older patients may refer to tuberculosis as *consumption*. Some people believe falsely that the tuberculosis skin test is a vaccine. A positive tuberculosis skin test (10 mm induration with redness) indicates that the patient has been exposed to the tubercle bacillus and lymphocytes have been sensitized. The contact could have occurred recently or in the distant past, even during childhood. All persons having close contact with an individual with a positive tuberculosis skin test should be tested immediately. In selected exposed individuals with a negative skin test, the test is repeated in 3 to 6 months. Once an individual has tested positive, the skin test does not usually need to be repeated; serial chest x-rays and physical assessment are performed to assess for active disease. A patient with a positive skin test could have active or inactive tuberculosis. Patients with active tuberculosis usually complain of hemoptysis, fatigue, weight loss, and low-grade fevers, especially at night.

A negative skin test (less than 10 mm induration with or without redness) indicates that exposure to the tubercle bacillus has not occurred in a patient if, and only if, the patient's immune system is functioning properly. A falsely negative test can occur in an anergic or immune-suppressed patient who has active or inactive tuberculosis. (Anergy is determined at the time of the tuberculosis skin test by administering one or more skin-test controls, such as *Candida* or mumps. A positive skin-test control indicates properly functioning immune system and absence of anergy.) Note, there are few patients (less than 10%) with active tuberculosis who have a normal immune system but who have a negative skin test.

Smoking history. A smoking history is another facet of the environmental history. Exposure to smoke increases the susceptibility to respiratory infections from impaired mucociliary clearance. Individuals who smoke and their housemates may also demonstrate increased levels of carboxyhemoglobin and decreased levels of oxyhemoglobin from cigarette smoking. Theophylline metabolism also is affected by cigarette smoking; serum theophylline levels are decreased by smoking. Because the effects of second-hand, or sidestream, smoke are known to be as dangerous, if not more dangerous, than actually smoking the cigarette, the nurse must also inquire whether the patient is living with a smoker.

It is important to ascertain not only whether the patient is currently smoking but also whether he has ever smoked. A complete smoking history contains the number of cigarettes smoked in terms of pack years. To calculate pack years, the nurse identifies how many packs of cigarettes the patient smoked each day. The number of packs smoked each day is multiplied by the number of years as a smoker to obtain a smoking history in pack years. In some cases the patient has smoked varying numbers of cigarettes over his lifetime. The nurse attempts to identify each of these blocks of time at a given level of cigarette smoking. For instance, a patient tells the nurse he smoked 3 packs of cigarettes a day for 10 years, 2 packs of cigarettes a day for 10 years, and 1 pack of cigarettes a day for 15 years. He is currently smoking one half pack of cigarettes a day and has done so for 2 years. This patient has accumulated $30 + 20 + 15 + 1 = 66$ pack years of smoking history—a very significant number. The higher the number of pack years, the more damage may have occurred in the patient's lungs.

The nurse may also want to inquire about what kind of cigarettes the patient has smoked. Nonfiltered cigarettes allow more pollutants, including tar, carcinogens, and radioactive materials, to enter the patient's lungs. The amount of nicotine in a cigarette must also be ascertained. Nicotine is addictive; therefore a patient who smokes cigarettes with a higher nicotine content may have a more difficult time quitting smoking because of nicotine withdrawal.

In obtaining a smoking history, the nurse must include the use of marijuana, cigars, pipes, and chewing tobacco in her questioning. Marijuana smokers traditionally hold the smoke in their lungs to enhance the drug's effect. Content of marijuana cigarettes varies with the producer and packager of the marijuana because of the illegal nature of the drug and the subsequent lack of governmental control. Except for chronic bronchitis, risks to the marijuana-smoking patient are generally unknown. Inhaling smoke from all kinds of cigarettes into the lungs can produce chronic bronchitis, emphysema, and lung cancer. Holding the smoke in the upper airway can produce gum disease, tooth deterioration, mouth ulcers, and cancers of the tongue, neck, jaw, and throat. These diseases are not uncommon in the pipe-smoking, cigar-smoking, or tobacco-chewing individual.

A final component of the patient's smoking history is identification of attempts to quit smoking. The nurse asks the patient about types of cessation programs attempted and their effect. It is a fact that many patients quit and resume smoking several times before they actually quit completely. There are many types of programs that assist a patient to quit smoking, including abrupt cessation, behavior modification, hypnosis, group therapy, use of nicotine-containing substitutes, self-help books, and self-help tapes. Failure in one program does not preclude success in another program of the same or different type.

Alcohol history. Another component of the patient's environmental history is the use of alcohol. The nurse inquires about the type, amount, and frequency of alcohol consumption. Although alcohol ingestion does not cause lung disease directly, chronic alcohol use has the potential to affect the pulmonary system. The patient who uses alcohol chronically may have problems with adequate nutrition, general health maintenance, and finances. The chronic alcohol consumer often replaces balanced, nutritious meals with alcohol's empty calories. Personal hygiene may be sporadic. Routine health examinations are often omitted. Employment may be at risk because of tardiness, absenteeism, or poor work performance. Theophylline metabolism is altered by alcohol consumption. Less theophylline is cleared when alcohol is ingested, and a patient who binges occasionally is prone to swings from therapeutic to perhaps toxic levels of theophylline. A patient who drinks to a stuporous state may be unable to protect his lower airway from aspiration of oral or gastric contents.

Allergies. Allergies are often considered to be a part of the environmental history, especially in the patient with an asthmatic component to his lung disease. The nurse asks what allergies the patient experiences in his environment and if these allergies are seasonal. The areas of questioning include medications, foods, dyes, animals, dusts, pollens, and molds. Of particular importance is a food allergy to eggs because, like the flu vaccine, many vaccines involve the use of embryos or eggs. Because some patients confuse a true allergy with an adverse reaction, the nurse questions the patient to determine the response of the patient to the "allergen." Allergic reactions are characterized by hives, urticaria, bronchospasm, laryngospasm, or anaphylaxis. A rash may not be indicative of an allergic reaction, especially in children.

Significant past illnesses/injuries. The history should include significant past illnesses or injuries. Significant to the pulmonary history are medical events and surgical therapies, including tuberculosis, pneumonia (especially as a child), fractured ribs, spinal cord injuries, poliomyelitis, cancer, thoracoplasty, lobectomy, pneumonectomy, intubation, and tracheostomy. The nurse should also inquire about immunizations against diphtheria, pertussis, tetanus, measles, mumps, rubella, and *Haemophilus* influenza. Adult and sometimes pediatric patients also may have received a flu vaccine or a pneumococcal pneumonia vaccine.

Signs and symptoms

The patient with pulmonary dysfunction typically will present with one or more symptoms (subjective) or signs (objective and usually observed in physical examination). The most frequently occurring symptoms reported are cough, increased sputum production, dyspnea, wheezing, pain, edema, palpitations, and fatigue or weakness. Syncope and rhinitis are less common symptoms. These symptoms are going to be discussed even though there may be others. Each symptom (or sign) must be explored for the following: location, characteristics, chronology, setting, aggravating or alleviating factors, associated manifestations, exacerbations, and remissions. The box on p. 49 highlights each of these dimensions.

Cough. Cough is a key defense mechanism of the lower airway. A cough may be acute or chronic. A new cough usually accompanies an acute inflammatory or infectious process, such as bronchitis or pneumonia, but it also may be the first sign of chronic dysfunction of the air passages or lung tissue, such as chronic bronchitis or lung cancer.

Symptoms—seven areas of questioning

1. Location. Where is the symptom?
2. Characteristics. What is the quantity and/or quality of the symptom?
3. Chronology. What was the date of onset, and what course has the symptom followed?
4. Setting. What were the circumstances surrounding the occurrence of the symptom?
5. Aggravating and alleviating factors. What makes the symptom worse or better?
6. Associated manifestations. What other phenomena are associated with this symptom?
7. Exacerbations and remissions. What is the pattern for the symptom over time?

Cough is associated with many disorders of the upper and the lower airway, although nonpulmonary disorders also may initiate a cough (Table 4-1). A patient's cough may originate from deep in the chest or in the throat. A cough may be brief or prolonged. It may be paroxysmal or sporadic, hacking, coarse, barking, annoying, dry, or wet. Some coughs are associated with environmental or seasonal changes. Activities, such as running, and posture, such as lying down or sitting up, may also precipitate a cough. The coughs of some patients produce sputum, and other patients' coughs produce little or no sputum.

Sputum. Sputum is frequently difficult to evaluate because patients deny, overestimate, or underestimate the characteristics of the sputum. A thorough history of sputum characteristics includes exploration of color, consistency, quantity, odor, and taste. Normal mucus (or sputum) of healthy individuals is clear and thin and is similar in color and consistency to saliva. Most patients with chronic lung disease have a baseline sputum color and consistency that is slightly different from normal. The sputum is usually not clear; it may be gray, tan, or cream colored. The sputum also is usually not thin but is mucoid or thicker and souplike. These characteristics define "normal" or baseline color and consistency and are used as a reference for all subsequent comparisons.

Table 4-1. Origin of coughs

Upper airway	Postnasal drip
	Sinusitis
Lower airway	Abscess
	Aspiration
	Asthma
	Bronchitis
	Cystic fibrosis
	Fungal infection
	Pneumonia
	Smoking
	Toxic inhalation
	Tracheitis
Nonpulmonary	Aortic aneurysm
	Left ventricular failure

A white tissue routinely is used to assess color of sputum because it allows for easy visualization of color changes. Decorator tissues may conceal changes in the color of sputum. Infections frequently present themselves through a change in the color of sputum. Green, yellow, and rust-colored hues are signs that bacteria are present. When rust-colored or red sputum is present, the nurse is concerned about the presence of hemoptysis, another sign of infection, but hemoptysis is also present in cancer, heart failure, and pulmonary infarction. When evaluating sputum for hemoptysis, the nurse must remember that old blood appears dark brown or dark red, and fresh blood is bright red. Because patients tend to exaggerate when hemoptysis is present, all hemoptysis, whether blood streaked or frank blood, should be saved in a cup or basin for examination by the nurse, physician, or laboratory. Hemoptysis may be aggravated by vigorous coughing, chest trauma, chest physical therapy, anticoagulant therapy, and activity. True hemoptysis must be differentiated from hematemesis (vomiting blood) and epistaxis (bleeding from the nares). Hemoptysis comes from the lung, but hematemesis and epistaxis do not. Blood draining posteriorly from the nose may elicit coughing or vomiting of blood. Sometimes it is difficult to tell from the patient's description the origin of the bleeding.

Quantifying sputum is sometimes very difficult because many patients swallow rather than expectorate their sputum. Embarrassment may be a factor, especially in self-conscious patients. This is particularly true for women, who are taught not to cough sputum out and especially not to expose it to anyone else. Recall from physiology that normal sputum production is 100 ml per day. It usually goes unnoticed because it is swallowed. (This is one reason early morning gastric fluid reveals tuberculosis bacteria.) Sputum in excess of this amount occurs in many disease states either daily or periodically. Some patients cough out sputum primarily in the morning, and other patients expectorate sputum continuously. Sputum is quantified better in terms of teaspoons, tablespoons, or cups per day than in terms of small, moderate, or large amounts because perception of the latter measurements varies among individuals. In bronchiectasis, sputum production may exceed 1 to 2 cups a day.

Normal sputum is odorless. When infection is present, the sputum may be odorous and even rank. Different bacteria have characteristic odors. For example, bacteria in the *Pseudomonas* genus have one of the most characteristic odors.

The taste of the sputum to the patient can be an important diagnostic tool, especially in the patient with cystic fibrosis. Sputum of the patient with cystic fibrosis characteristically has a salty taste. Sputum that tastes "bad" may indicate the presence of infection.

Dyspnea. Dyspnea is one of the most common symptoms of pulmonary and cardiac disease. Often referred to as *shortness of breath* by the patient, dyspnea has both an objective and a subjective component. The nurse asks about the amount of difficulty the patient has in moving air in or out of the chest. Subjectively, the patient is asked to rate the degree of dyspnea using a numerical scale. Use of the terms *mild, moderate,* and *severe* is not recommended because of impreciseness and wide variability among measures used by different individuals. There are numerous rating scales in the literature, including numerical and vertical or horizontal visual analog. Perhaps the most used scale is a numerical scale from 0 (breathing normal) to 10 (unbearable). At a level of 5 the patient usually has reduced work performance.

The patient is asked about onset of the dyspnea. In chronic disease, such as chronic bronchitis or emphysema, the onset is usually insidious, but in acute disease, such as pulmonary edema, the onset is rapid. Sometimes the patient relates subtle breathing changes that have occurred over the years. In such cases it is difficult to pinpoint when dyspnea began.

The nurse also determines when dyspnea occurs. Some patients report intermittent dyspnea from hypoxemia or hypercapnia when performing activities of daily living, such as bathing, grooming, vacuuming, or climbing stairs. Other patients experience worsening dyspnea when anxious or when just sitting in a chair. Dyspnea also may be caused by severe anemia, fever, metabolic acidosis, weak respiratory muscles, pleural effusions, and chest wall abnormalities. The patient with a history of diseases that increase resistance to breathing, such as diffuse interstitial pulmonary fibrosis, left ventricular failure, and obstructive lung disease, frequently reports symptomatic dyspnea.

Dyspnea is used to identify worsening of the disease process. Exacerbations of diseases like chronic obstructive pulmonary disease and pulmonary edema are associated with worsening dyspnea, as is progression of the disease. The patient is able to perform fewer activities of daily living or is able to perform them less well. The distance a patient can walk without becoming dyspneic is often used as a gauge of an exacerbation or severity of the disease. For consistency the distance walked in 8 minutes is often measured and recorded at least annually.

Wheezing. The patient may identify a history of wheezing that frequently is accompanied by dyspnea. Wheezing is a high-pitched musical sound produced by air moving through narrowed airways. Patients often associate wheezing with tightness of the chest. Wheezing may occur episodically or continuously. It may develop gradually or abruptly, depending on the cause. In most patients a stethoscope is necessary to identify wheezing. However, in a few patients wheezing is audible without a stethoscope.

The primary cause of wheezing is bronchospasm, although aspiration, pulmonary embolism, tracheal stenosis, tumors, and anaphylaxis are also associated with wheezing (see the box below). Allergens, irritants, and body position often induce bronchospasm with wheezing, although anxiety and stress are other factors in its development.

Chest pain. Complaints of chest pain are common in patients with lung disease. The character of chest pain varies with its origin. The patient may

---

Causes of wheezing

Anaphylaxis
Anxiety
Aspiration
Bronchospasm (allergens, irritants, body position)
Mucus
Pulmonary embolism
Stress
Tracheal stenosis
Tumors

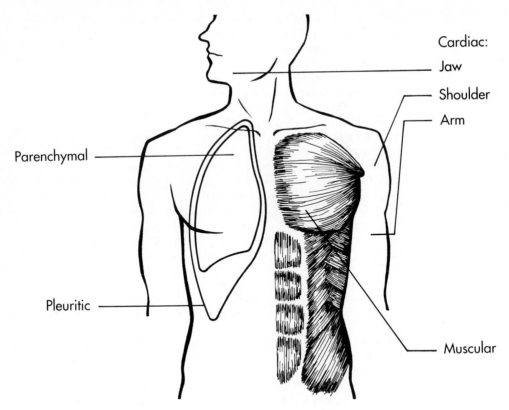

Fig. 4-1. Sites of chest pain.

experience chest pain of pulmonary, muscular, cardiac, or pleuritic origin (Fig. 4-1).

Pulmonary chest pain may originate in the airways or in the lung parenchyma itself. A patient with acute bronchitis frequently gives a history of raw or burning chest pain substernally or retrosternally. Usually associated with a dry, nonproductive cough, acute bronchitic pain is often present throughout respiration. When atelectasis is present, the patient reports a knifelike sensation (sudden intense pain followed by a sharp decrease in intensity), but the patient with pneumonia or a tumor may have a dull, aching pain in the chest.

Muscular chest pain often is caused by severe, paroxysmal, and uncontrolled episodes of coughing. Trauma (such as motor vehicle accidents) or overexertion also is associated with muscular chest pain. Usually worsened by deep inspiration, muscular chest pain may be continuous or intermittent. Muscular chest pain can be reproduced by direct pressure on the affected muscle groups.

Chest pain that originates in the heart frequently is referred to the shoulder, arm, or jaw; cardiac chest pain can be described as heartburn, heaviness, viselike pain, or stabbing pain. Most well known is severe pain or pressure just to the left of the sternum that is associated with a myocardial infarction. Cardiac chest pain may be intermittent, lasting only a few minutes, or continuous, lasting for several hours or days without treatment. Exertion-induced cardiac pain usually is relieved by rest.

Pleuritic pain is caused by inflammation or infection in the pleural space. Frequently confused with muscular pain, especially when associated with trauma, pleuritic chest pain is typically worse with inspiration. Yawning, coughing, and sneezing exacerbate pleuritic chest pain. A patient with pleuritic chest pain usually gives a history of severe, stabbing pain that is located over the affected area. Lasting several days to weeks, pleuritic chest pain is present until the inflammation or infection is resolved. Patients with pleural chest pain are prone to recurrence with subsequent infections, especially chest colds. Pleural infections frequently leave permanent pleural scars and sometimes chronic pain. The scars are seen on the chest x-ray film (sometimes) or at autopsy.

Pain, like dyspnea, is a symptom requiring grading by the patient. The use of a numerical scale, such as 0 to 10, is more useful than words, such as *mild, moderate,* or *severe* to gauge the severity of the chest pain. This is particularly true when cardiac chest pain is suspected. The nurse asks the patient to score numerically how various treatments tried by the patient have affected the pain.

Edema. Peripheral edema results from abnormal oncotic or hydrostatic pressure that allows fluid to exudate from the capillaries into the interstitial spaces. The most frequent cause of peripheral edema is right-sided congestive heart dysfunction (increased hydrostatic pressure), although low serum oncotic pressure (low albumin) is also a common cause. Right-sided heart dysfunction (failure) is fairly common in patients with chronic pulmonary dysfunction. Right-sided heart dysfunction develops when the right ventricle pumps against increased pulmonary vascular pressures (pulmonary vascular resistance). The heart works harder and harder until it is unable to compensate, resulting in a backup of fluid into the peripheral circulation. The most frequent cause of right-sided heart dysfunction is hypoxemia (which causes hypoxic pulmonary vasoconstriction), a common problem in patients with obstructive or interstitial pulmonary disease. Other factors that may precipitate right-sided heart dysfunction are massive pulmonary emboli, pulmonary fibrosis, primary pulmonary hypertension, and mitral stenosis. The nurse inquires about a previous history of any of these problems when edema is present.

Edema from right-sided heart dysfunction usually develops gradually over several days to months. The patient often notices that rings and shoes are more snug than usual, or the patient may mention overt edema of the legs and feet. When right-sided heart dysfunction is present, the patient also may complain of fatigue, angina pectoris (chest pain), anxiety, and weight gain. The nurse also may inquire about signs of liver engorgement (swollen abdomen), jugular venous distention (swollen neck), impaired cognition (thinking and concentrating), and renal insufficiency (color and frequency of urination or nocturia) to support the suspected problem of right-sided congestive heart dysfunction.

Pulmonary edema, fluid in the lungs, is caused by left ventricular dysfunction or left-sided congestive heart dysfunction. Left ventricular dysfunction develops when the heart pumps against increased systemic vascular resistance. The most frequent causes of left-sided heart dysfunction are hypertension and myocardial infarction. Dyspnea is the most common complaint of patients with left ventricular dysfunction. It is often difficult to distinguish between the dyspnea of lung dysfunction and dyspnea related to left heart dysfunction without laboratory tests of cardiac and pulmonary function (for example, chest x-ray, electrocardiogram, echocardiography). When left-sided heart dysfunction is present, the patient also may complain of fatigue, anxiety, angina pectoris, orthopnea, paroxysmal (suddenly occurring) nocturnal dyspnea, wheezing, cough, and hemoptysis.

Palpitations. Palpitations are described by the patient as "fluttering in the chest" or "heart jumping around." Excitement, exertion, and excessive caffeine or nicotine intake are common causes of palpitations, although palpitations are not unusual in the patient using bronchodilators, especially when toxic levels are present. The development of palpitations frequently is associated with minor dysrhythmias, such as premature systoles and paroxysmal tachycardias. Palpitations also may be the result of organic heart disease or thyrotoxicosis.

Palpitations typically have an abrupt onset and resolution. Although they are usually self-limiting and do not interfere with the patient's ability to perform usual activities, palpitations may be debilitating in the patient with little or no cardiac or pulmonary reserve. Palpitations also can impair ability to function when associated with extreme anxiety.

Fatigue and weakness. A history of fatigue or weakness is often one of the first signs of pulmonary dysfunction. The patient often complains of the inability to perform activities of daily living comfortably. This is especially true of activities that involve raising the arms above the head. The usual scenario when fatigue is present is a repetitive cycle of fatigue, rest, limited activity with muscle disuse, loss of muscle strength, and greater fatigue. Dyspnea often accompanies the fatigue and precipitates decreased exercise tolerance.

Fatigue or weakness also may signal the onset of an infection in many patients and may persist for days to weeks after the infection has resolved. Less obvious causes for complaints of fatigue include electrolyte disturbances (especially low levels of calcium, phosphate, potassium, and magnesium), inadequate nutrition, and neurological diseases affecting muscle use (myasthenia gravis, amyotrophic lateral sclerosis, muscular dystrophy, and poliomyelitis).

COMPLETE HEALTH HISTORY
Interrelationship between the pulmonary system and other systems

Symptoms of pulmonary dysfunction arise from and extend to origins other than those of the thorax. The interrelationship of the pulmonary system with other body systems necessitates obtaining additional historical information. The purpose of this section is not to provide the nurse with a comprehensive review of systems but to furnish the nurse with pertinent information to complement the pulmonary history. The systems are reviewed in this section in a head-to-toe manner.

Neurological history. Patients with airway dysfunction can exhibit changes in neurological function. Pertinent neurological history includes the dimensions of level of consciousness, orientation, mentation (ability to think), motor disturbances, sensory disturbances, and pupillary size. Each of these areas can suggest a problem with medications or arterial blood gases. Therefore a history of neurological symptoms is needed.

Level of consciousness is the patient's awareness of himself and his environment. Although the most common cause of impaired level of consciousness is central nervous system injury, drug or toxin overdose, endocrine disorders, cardiac disorders, hepatic disorders, renal disorders, and electrolyte disturbances also cause decreased level of consciousness. Hypoxemia, anemia, and respiratory failure can affect level of consciousness.

Orientation to time, place, and person suggests that cerebral oxygen saturation is adequate. The patient should be able to identify correctly the day of the week, month, date, year (time); address by number, street, city, state, and country (place); and their name and the names and relationships of individuals in the room (person). The names of elected officials, season of the year, temperature outside, healthcare institution, birthdays of relatives, and employment situation may be used to help clarify orientation.

Mentation often is assessed through the patient's response to questions. Incoherent words, inappropriate responses, and inability to concentrate indicate impaired mentation. Appropriate mentation also is assessed by asking the patient to count backward by multiples of numbers, such as seven. The patient's ability to receive, process, and respond to information is decreased when the patient is hypoxemic or hypercapnic.

Motor response, or appropriate movement of a muscle group on command, indicates intact and functioning nervous system to and from the muscle group and the brain. Impaired motor response may be exhibited by lack of motor control, tremors, or seizures. A central nervous system lesion that impairs phrenic nerve functioning limits or prohibits the diaphragm from contracting. The patient may complain of tremors, especially of the hands, while at rest. Static tremors often are associated with the use of theophylline. Action tremors, or inability to sustain a posture, are associated with carbon dioxide narcosis. Finally, seizures may be associated with severe theophylline toxicity.

Sensory disturbances are reflected by a history of paresthesias. When hyperventilation is present, the patient frequently complains of light-headedness, numbness, or tingling.

Pupillary changes may be observed in the presence of certain medications, especially narcotics and anticholinergics, which constrict the pupils, and amphetamines, which dilate the pupils. In the presence of hypercapnia or hypoxemia the pupils dilate. The presence of anisocoria, pupils of different sizes, is a common finding in 5% of the population and should be recorded in the patient's record.

Psychosocial history. Psychosocial problems are present in patients with chronic alterations in pulmonary function. The nurse determines the patient's psychosocial history as it pertains to the patient's ability to perform activities of daily living or to learn appropriate health behaviors. The most common psychosocial problems in the patient with pulmonary dysfunction are anxiety, depression, and denial. Anxiety often is accompanied by dyspnea. Similarly, dyspnea often is accompanied by anxiety. The cycle of dyspnea and anxiety can incapacitate the patient to the point of inactivity. Some patients with chronic pulmonary dysfunction become very anxious when leaving home, especially when supplemental oxygen is necessary. The patient may be afraid to run out of oxygen, or he may fear curious looks.

Depression is another common finding in the patient with chronic lung disease, especially in the terminal stages. Young patients often are concerned with inability to reach adolescent or adult milestones, including marriage and having children or grandchildren. Older patients often are depressed because the so-called "golden years" after retirement are not as they anticipated. Plans to travel often are hampered by the presence of a chronic disease.

Denial is a coping strategy used by many patients, especially when chronic disease is present. Acceptance of the diagnosis and lifestyle changes associated with cancer and chronic obstructive and restrictive lung diseases may take years, or acceptance may never occur.

Cardiovascular history. The cardiovascular history starts with identification of previous cardiac problems. Patients are familiar with the term *heart trouble*, which can range from hypertension to congestive heart failure, both of which are seen in patients with pulmonary dysfunction. The cardiac history of parents, siblings, and offspring often provides genetic clues to the patient's predisposition to heart disease. In this light the cause of death of closely related family members should be determined. The death of a 60-year-old father with heart disease is more significant than the death of a 90-year-old relative.

When a patient has a history of hypertension, the nurse also may obtain a history of headaches, blurred vision, and "seeing spots." The risk factors associated with hypertension are excessive stress, obesity, use of birth control pills, cigarette smoking, excessive use of alcohol, sedentary lifestyle, and genetics. Obesity also causes a restrictive ventilatory defect because the abdomen pushes up against the diaphragm and lungs, limiting expansion. Obesity may impair recovery from illness or surgery if the patient does not breathe deeply. Because patients with hypertension are often asymptomatic, compliance with the treatment plan is often a problem.

A history of congestive heart failure frequently is identified by sleep disturbances. Patients may complain of sudden awakenings with dyspnea, termed *paroxysmal nocturnal dyspnea,* or *PND.* Two or more pillow orthopnea with or without edema may be present. Remember that the patient may have right-sided, left-sided, or biventricular failure. The nurse does not usually diagnose heart failure, but she needs to know which symptoms to report to the physician for interpretation. The nurse may find it helpful to remember that *l*eft-sided heart failure backs fluid into the *l*ungs and *r*ight-sided heart failure backs up all 'round, including jugular veins, liver, and periphery (edema). In the patient with pulmonary dysfunction the right side of the heart often fails first because the right ventricle is pumping blood against increased pressure in the lung. Conversely, the patient with hypertension develops left ventricular failure from pumping blood against increased systemic pressure.

Gastrointestinal history. The gastrointestinal history concentrates on the areas of nutrition, weight, bowel habits, and the symptom of nausea. A precise nutritional history is often difficult to obtain. The underweight patient often overestimates intake, and the overweight patient tends to underestimate food intake. Perception of food quantities varies among individuals. A serving may be 2 to 6 tablespoons (as for vegetables or ice cream), 2 to 6 ounces (for protein), or 2 to 6 cups (for soup or coffee), depending on the patient's serving utensils and dishes. For patients receiving enteral alimentation (tube feeding) or parenteral nutrition, calculation of nutrient intake is performed more easily by the nurse or dietician. The nurse simply asks how many cans of supplement are consumed daily.

In the home environment the dyspneic patient may have limited ability to obtain and prepare foods. Convenience foods frequently contain excessive sodium and carbohydrates but little fiber. Gas-forming foods, such as cabbage and beans, limit diaphragmatic excursion by increasing abdominal size. A high-carbohydrate diet can increase carbon dioxide production as the sugar is metabolized to carbon dioxide and water. In some patients with carbon dioxide retention, a diet containing less carbohydrate and more fat is more appropriate.

One indicator of nutritional status is weight. In the hospital, daily weight measurements demonstrate fluid retention more than they demonstrate nutritional status. It is difficult to impossible to eat (or burn) enough calories to gain (or lose) several pounds overnight. In the home, weekly or monthly weight measurements demonstrate a trend of increasing or decreasing weight. The nurse must then decide if the weight change is due to fluid retention (caused by cardiac, neurological, or renal disease) or to nutritional status (affected by depression, malignancy, or advanced pulmonary dysfunction).

The nurse asks the patient about bowel habits. The color, consistency, and frequency of bowel movements indicate functioning of the gastrointestinal system. The presence of black stools is common in patients receiving iron supplements or bismuth (Pepto Bismol) but may also indicate occult gastrointestinal bleeding. Maroon or red stools are also representative of gastrointestinal bleeding, but they also can be caused by ingestion of red vegetables, such as beets, especially in children. Use guiac on the stool when the presence of blood is suspected. Occult or overt gastrointestinal bleeding decreases the amount of hemoglobin available for oxygen transport.

The consistency of stool varies among individuals. Diarrhea and constipation are two types of abnormal bowel habits. Diarrhea, or liquid stool, frequently occurs with viral or bacterial infections, although the use of certain antibiotics also may cause diarrhea. Some patients who have had bowel surgery may experience diarrhea from impaired water reabsorption. Tube-feeding administration generally decreases the consistency of stool to semisolid but not watery. Hard, dry stools associated with constipation are indicative of insufficient fluid or fiber intake and may result in bleeding from hemorrhoids. Diarrhea is associated with electrolyte disturbances, and constipation can limit diaphragmatic excursion. Straining to evacuate a constipated stool can increase the work of breathing significantly as a result of increased oxygen consumption and carbon dioxide production. The Valsalva maneuver is difficult to perform and especially to sustain in the presence of pulmonary and cardiac dysfunction. Increasing fluid intake or using bulk laxatives or stool softeners sometimes is done to avoid excessive cardiopulmonary strain during bowel movements. Stools of patients with cystic fibrosis tend to float because of the high fat content.

Finally, the nurse determines the frequency of bowel movements. The range of normal frequency is wide. The patient may evacuate stool once to several times daily or weekly. Some patients have stools on a regular schedule, but other patients are irregular.

Genitourinary history. The accurate reabsorption of fluid and electrolytes by the genitourinary system is important for proper pulmonary function. The patient's pulmonary status is affected by fluid volume by either increasing or decreasing the viscosity or the quantity of secretions or lung water (pulmonary edema). When fluid volume deficit, or dehydration, is present, the patient usually has thicker secretions. He may also experience orthostatic hypotension (feeling dizzy or light-headed after sitting or standing from a supine position), apathy, weakness, tachycardia, dry mucous membranes, and poor skin turgor. Fluid volume deficit should be suspected in patients with acute febrile illness, vomiting, diarrhea, or rapid weight loss.

Fluid volume excess accompanies renal and cardiac failure. An early sign of fluid volume excess is tightness of rings or shoes secondary to peripheral edema. Rapid weight gain, oliguria, jugular vein distention, increased dyspnea, copious frothy secretions (pulmonary edema), and hypertension are other signs of fluid volume excess.

The nurse also may identify a history of urinary frequency or nocturia from theophylline or nocturnal oxygen use. Theophylline has a weak diuretic effect. Failure of the right side of the heart from hypoxemia is treated with oxygen and also may induce diuresis of excess fluid volume.

When an electrolyte imbalance is present, the patient may experience respiratory muscle dysfunction that ranges from weakness to respiratory arrest. Symptoms of electrolyte imbalance are investigated when respiratory muscle dysfunction is present. The electrolytes most frequently involved in respiratory muscle dysfunction are potassium, calcium, magnesium, and phosphorus, the most important of which is phosphorus. Hypophosphatemia can cause respiratory failure and prevent weaning of a patient from mechanical ventilation. It also can induce cardiomyopathy. Table 4-2 identifies the most common causes of hypokalemia (low potassium), hyperkalemia (elevated potassium), hypocalcemia (low calcium), hypercalcemia (elevated calcium), hypophosphatemia (low phosphorus), hyperphosphatemia (elevated phosphorus), hypomagnesemia (low magnesium), and hypermagnesemia (elevated magnesium).

Musculoskeletal history. The musculoskeletal history has two specific areas for inquiry: muscle development and structural deformities. Muscle development may be normal, atrophied, or hypertrophied. The patient with chronic obstructive lung disease frequently has hypertrophied accessory muscles from increased work of breathing. Similarly, the patient with neuromuscular disease may have generalized atrophy, or atrophy may involve only specific extremities. Unilateral muscle atrophy is associated with stroke, and lower-extremity atrophy occurs in many patients with lower spinal cord injury.

Structural deformities, such as scoliosis, kyphosis, or rheumatoid arthritic joints, are sometimes obvious, although they may be obscure. Patients with scoliosis or kyphosis have a restrictive lung defect and impaired gas exchange, depending on the severity of the deformity. Some patients with rheumatoid arthritis develop a condition known as *rheumatoid lung*. Use of bone-wasting and muscle-wasting medications, particularly steroids, is associated with osteoporosis. Ribs and vertebrae fractured by coughing may be observed in patients with osteoporosis.

Clubbing is a structural deformity associated with interstitial or chronic suppurative lung diseases. Sometimes the patient observes the change in his fingertips and reports it to the nurse or physician. If possible, the nurse determines when the clubbing was first observed. Clubbing is assessed at the terminal phalanges of the fingers. Instead of the usual 160 degrees, the angle between the base of the nail and the skin is 180 degrees or more (Fig. 4-2). Table 4-3 lists the pulmonary and nonpulmonary causes of clubbing.

Medications. A health history is not complete without noting the patient's medications. Some pulmonary symptoms are the result of medications. Medications may be used to reduce one symptom with the potential to produce others. For instance, tremor is seen in patients taking theophylline for bronchospasm. The tremor increases in some patients as the theophylline level rises toward toxicity. At toxic theophylline levels, many patients develop nau-

Table 4-2. Electrolyte disturbances.

Disorder	Causes	Signs and symptoms
Hypokalemia	Increased pH or HCO_3, alcoholism, starvation, vomiting, diarrhea, diuretics	Ectopic beats, weakness
Hyperkalemia	Increased K^+ supplement, renal failure, metabolic acidosis, crush injury, hemolysis, absorbed hematoma	Cardiac dysfunction, weakness, paresthesia
Hypocalcemia	Decreased dietary calcium intake, hypoparathyroidism, hypomagnesemia, hyperphosphatemia, renal disease, liver disease, steroids, hypoalbuminemia,	Tetany, numbness/tingling of mouth or extremities, stiffness, muscle cramps, seizures, alopecia, psychoses, Chvostek's sign, Trousseau's sign
Hypercalcemia	Malignancy, hyperparathyroidism, granulomatous disease, thyrotoxicosis, thiazide diuretics, acute renal failure, Addison's disease, lithium, decreased excretion	Personality changes, lethargy, polyuria, polydipsia, short QT segment on ECG, constipation, nausea/vomiting, anorexia, hypertension, heart block, headache, soft-tissue calcification, pruritus, delirium, stupor/coma, bone pain
Hypophosphatemia	Alcoholism, refeeding after starvation, respiratory alkalosis, vitamin D deficiency, chronic diarrhea, diuretics, phosphate binding compounds, decreased intake, hypomagnesemia, decompensated diabetes, hypocalcemia	Hyperventilation, circumoral paresthesias, seizures, coma, muscle weakness, paralysis
Hyperphosphatemia	Renal failure, laxative abuse, phosphate enemas, rhabdomyolysis, antineoplastic chemotherapy, hypoparathyroidism, hyperthyroidism, acromegaly, severe volume contraction	No specific signs or symptoms although hypocalcemic signs are enhanced
Hypomagnesemia	Decreased intake, decreased absorption, increased excretion	Dysrhythmias, weakness, anorexia, nausea, mood alterations, tremor/seizures
Hypermagnesemia	Renal failure, magnesium antacids	Paresthesia, peripheral vasodilation, nausea/vomiting, progressive lethargy, progressive weakness, flaccid paralysis, hypotension, bradycardia, respiratory depression

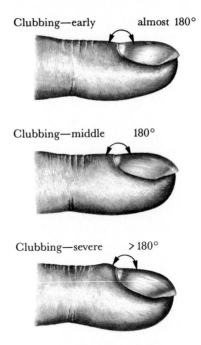

Clubbing—early   almost 180°

Clubbing—middle   180°

Clubbing—severe   > 180°

Fig. 4-2. Stages of clubbing in the fingers from infectious and noninfectious causes. (From Seidel H et al: *Mosby's guide to physical examination,* ed 2, St Louis, 1991, Mosby–Year Book.)

Table 4-3. Causes of clubbing

Pulmonary	Nonpulmonary
Infectious	
Tuberculosis	Infectious endocarditis
Empyema	
Lung abscess	
Bronchiectasis	
Noninfectious	
Lung cancer	Biliary cirrhosis
Interstitial lung disease	Hepatic cirrhosis
Cystic fibrosis	Hyperthyroidism
Lymphoma	Inflammatory bowel disease
Mesothelioma	Right-to-left cardiac shunts

sea and vomiting or seizures. Additionally, there are medications that produce undesirable side effects when taken together. Examples include decreased theophylline levels with cigarette smoking, elevated theophylline levels with some antibiotics, and swings in theophylline levels with alcohol ingestion.

A patient with pulmonary dysfunction frequently is prescribed a bronchodilator. Steroids, antibiotics, oxygen, decongestants, mucolytics, and antihistamines are other classes of medications that may be in use. Medications for other medical problems may include cardiotonics and diuretics. The nurse identifies the patient's knowledge of the name, dosage, action, and side effects of the medication. Inability to provide the requested information has implications for patient teaching (see Chapter 15 for a detailed discussion of medications).

CONCLUSION

The health history is an important component of patient care. A complete history prepares the nurse to perform a physical assessment. Based on the history and the physical assessment, the nurse identifies problems or potential problems on which to base nursing care. Environment is a very important facet of obtaining a history. Both the patient and the nurse must be in comfortable surroundings. The nurse uses various types of questions to elicit history from the patient, using verbal and nonverbal cues throughout the interview. The nurse is careful to question the patient about pulmonary specific symptoms, especially cough, sputum, dyspnea, wheezing, pain, edema, palpitations, and fatigue or weakness. It is important to remember that the lungs and other pulmonary structures do not exist in a void. The effects of pulmonary dysfunction are seen in other body systems, and disease in other body systems often affects the lungs. For this reason the nurse obtains a complete health history, including problems in other body systems.

BIBLIOGRAPHY

American Thoracic Society: Cigarette smoking and your health, *Am Rev Respir Dis*, 132(5):1133-1136, 1985.

Barbee R: The medical history in pulmonary disease, *Basics Respir Dis* 11(3), 1983.

Baum GL, Wolinsky E: *Textbook of pulmonary diseases*, ed 3, Boston, 1983, Little & Brown.

Billingsley J et al: Screening asymptomatic patients at risk, *Patient Care* 13(6):40-59, 1979.

Burton GC, Hodgkin JE: *Respiratory care: a guide to clinical practice*, ed 2, Philadelphia, 1984, J B Lippincott.

Dahms T, Bolin JF, Slavin RG: Passive smoking: effects on bronchial asthma, *Chest* 80(5):530-534, 1981.

Doyle NC: Marijuana and the lungs, American Lung Association bulletin, November 1979.

Hinshaw H, Murray J: *Diseases of the chest*, ed 4, Philadelphia, 1980, W B Saunders.

Loudon RG: Cough: a symptom and a sign, *Basics Respir Dis* 9(4), 1981.

Lyons H: Differential diagnosis of hemoptysis and its treatment, *Basics Respir Dis* 5(2), 1976.

Malasanos L et al: *Health assessment*, ed 2, St Louis, 1981, Mosby—Year Book.

Murray JF, Nadel JA, eds: *Textbook of respiratory medicine*, Philadelphia, 1988, W B Saunders.

Netter F: *The CIBA collection of medical illustrations, vol 7: respiratory system*, New York, 1979, CIBA Pharmaceutical Co.

Paré JAP, Fraser RG: *Synopsis of diseases of the chest*, Philadelphia, 1983, W B Saunders.

Shapiro B, Harrison R, et al: *Clinical applications of respiratory care*, ed 3, St Louis, 1985, Mosby—Year Book.

Simmons DH, ed: *Current pulmonology*, vol 7, St Louis, 1986, Mosby—Year Book.

Wade JF: *Comprehensive respiratory care: physiology and technique*, ed 3, St Louis, 1982, Mosby—Year Book.

Wanner A, Sackner MA: *Pulmonary diseases: mechanisms of altered structure and function*, Boston, 1983, Little & Brown.

5

Physical Assessment

*O*bjectives:

- Discuss the assessment of general appearance.
- Identify reference landmarks on the chest.
- Discuss the components of inspection of the chest.
- Discuss the technique of percussion.
- Identify the characteristics of pulmonary percussion notes: resonance, hyperresonance, flatness, dullness, and tympany.
- Discuss the technique of assessing diaphragmatic excursion.
- Differentiate vesicular breath sounds, bronchovesicular breath sounds, bronchial breath sounds, crackles, wheezes, and pleural friction rubs.
- Differentiate egophony, whispered pectoriloquy, and bronchophony.
- Identify normal and abnormal heart sounds.
- Discuss the assessment of fluid status.
- Identify pulmonary and nonpulmonary causes of clubbing.

The nurse is assessing the patient continually each time she interacts with him. In the hospital the nurse sees the patient for short intervals several times throughout the shift; in the home the nurse visits the patient for a longer time but less frequently. The nurse must assess the condition of many patients to become proficient in identifying what is normal, what is a normal variation, and what is an abnormal variation.

GENERAL OBSERVATIONS

Assessment begins with general observation. The nurse uses the senses of sight, hearing, touch, and smell to obtain information about the patient's condition. The nurse compares the current assessment with the patient's baseline to identify deviations. The assessments are categorized as the same as, better than, or worse than previous assessments. In some cases the baseline assessment and the current assessment are identical; many times there is a slight improvement or deterioration in the patient's condition. It is important to describe the patient's condition with each assessment rather than to write "no change" because some changes are subtle. Otherwise, the patient's record could read "no change" when there has been change that has gone unnoticed.

One of the first, obvious assessments the nurse makes is of the patient's general appearance. The nurse observes grooming, including condition of the hair and nails, body cleanliness and absence of odor, dental hygiene and tooth repair, facial hair growth, attire, posture, body movement, speech, and mental status. Dyspnea, lack of financial resources, lack of transportation, or depression can impair the ability of the patient to groom himself properly.

Assessing condition of the hair includes assessing not only the cleanliness of the hair but also whether the hair style is easy to maintain. Dyspneic patients need a hair style that is easy to comb and requires infrequent recombing, such as a short, straight cut or a permanent wave that requires just fluffing. The nurse assesses ability of the patient to comb and brush hair because raising the arms above the head is very energy-consuming.

The nurse assesses whether the patient's nails are manicured versus being chipped or broken. Nails also should be clean, with cuticles trimmed to prevent portals of infection. The nurse also may observe the patient for presence of nail biting. The patient suffering from malnutrition often has vertical ridges in the nails. Yellow stains on the nails suggest heavy cigarette smoking.

Body cleanliness may be difficult to achieve when soap and water are difficult to obtain. Perhaps the patient is too dyspneic to bathe or cannot get in and out of a tub or shower unassisted. (For such patients energy conservation techniques or a home health aide are needed.) The nurse assesses for body odor and for clean skin. In some cases a patient may try to hide body odor with the use of perfumes or colognes.

Dental hygiene is assessed by examining the teeth and gums for cleanliness and absence of disease. The patient with dental caries and gum infections may be prone to "seed" infections to the lungs. Clean teeth, whether natural or artificial, indicate good dental hygiene. Halitosis occurs with both infection and poor dental hygiene.

In the male patient, shaving and beard trimming are activities of daily living that reflect good grooming. The clean-shaven patient or the patient with a neatly trimmed or combed beard is groomed. Dyspnea may cause a man to omit facial-hair grooming from a daily routine.

Attire is another aspect of general appearance that the nurse assesses. Clothes should be clean and fit well. The patient may not be able to launder clothes if a convenient washing machine is not available because of stairs or lack of transportation. Clothes should be appropriate for the season, that is, lightweight for warm weather and multilayered or heavyweight for cool weather. Poorly fitting clothes may indicate weight loss or weight gain if too large or too small, respectively. The patient at home still may be in night wear during the day when he is ill.

Posture of the patient indirectly tells the nurse about how the patient is feeling or about past illnesses or injuries. A patient who is dyspneic often rests arms or elbows on the knees to help support the weight of the lungs. Inability to lie down may indicate congestive heart failure. A patient who is depressed, weak, or fatigued often slumps, whereas a patient who has had corrective spinal surgery may sit rigidly upright. Osteoporosis is evident in some patients with excessive spine curvatures, and peripheral vascular disease is evident in patients who continuously cross their legs.

Assessment of body movement is similar to assessment of posture. The nurse identifies how well the patient is able to move and to control different muscle groups. Moving slowly may be associated with stiff joints or pain.

The presence of a tremor may suggest adverse drug effects, such as theophylline toxicity, and neurological injury. Turning the head to one side selectively in a conversation is associated with hearing impairment. Stumbling and other gait abnormalities may accompany neurological diseases and alcohol use. Foot drop may be evident when the patient must lift and place each foot consciously; when walking, a slapping noise is heard.

Speech includes both verbal and nonverbal components. Careful listening to the character and manner of speech is revealing. A patient who can speak in uninterrupted, full sentences is not dyspneic, whereas the patient who speaks a few words at a time is extremely dyspneic. It is important to note how many words are spoken with each breath because this is a method of gauging improvement or deterioration of pulmonary function. Nasal quality of voice can indicate sinus abnormalities or presence of a cold. Improperly fitting dentures can impair both speech and eating. Anxiety is associated with a high-pitched voice, and fear may be accompanied by an excessively loud or excessively soft voice. A nurse whose primary language is not the same as that of the patient may have difficulty communicating and understanding.

The patient also may indicate nonverbally to affirm or negate spoken words. The nurse is encouraged to consult other sources for a complete explanation of nonverbal communication.

The mental status of the patient is another component of his general appearance. Confusion and disorientation are manifested by inappropriate responses to questions. Normal cognitive functioning allows the patient to comprehend questions and formulate answers. Mild degrees of dementia, limited intelligence, and mental retardation from congenital or acquired neurological insult can be assessed in the patient's response to questions. Depression sometimes is recognized by a dull affect, monotone speech, or lack of expression. In addition, irritability, common in chronic disease, also may be associated with inadequate gas exchange.

Other factors about the patient's appearance may be useful to assess. Black circles, or "bags," under the eyes occur in patients with vitamin deficiencies or inadequate sleep. Patients with sleep apnea also may have black circles under the eyes. Facial grimace usually is associated with pain, such as pleurisy, regardless of its origin. Steroid use, abnormal clotting factors, physical abuse, alcohol abuse resulting in liver failure, and falls may cause bruising of the skin (Fig. 5-1). The presence of corrective lenses or hearing aids has implications for patient teaching. Alcohol use may be suspected when alcohol is evident on the breath and present in the home.

PULMONARY EXAMINATION

After completing a general survey of the patient's appearance, the nurse performs a physical examination of the thorax. The room should be well lighted to enhance visibility, and the room should be at a temperature that is comfortable for the patient to prevent chilling or shivering. Extraneous noises should be prevented if possible. In some instances, such as when confidentiality and privacy are required, family members may be asked to leave the room. The nurse respects the privacy of the patient when performing a chest examination by shielding the patient from inadvertent exposure to the atmosphere or other individuals. This is accomplished through the patient's wearing a gown or robe and through use of doors or screens as available and necessary. Areas of the chest not being examined should be covered.

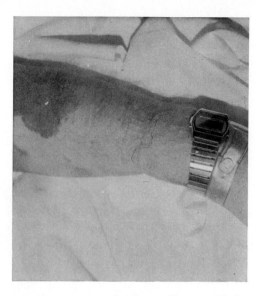

Fig. 5-1. Chronic steroid use causes fragile capillaries and skin bruising without known trauma.

A comprehensive chest examination has four components: inspection, palpation, percussion, and auscultation. Depending on the patient and on the circumstances, palpation or percussion may be limited to a specific area or may be omitted. The nurse should never omit inspection or auscultation.

The nurse performs the chest examination in a systematic manner from the apices to the bases. The left and right sides of the chest are compared with allowances for anatomical differences, including anterior, lateral, and posterior aspects. The nurse also uses standard reference points to describe the location of findings (Fig. 5-2). Named for landmarks, the reference points on the anterior chest include the midsternal line, the right and left midclavicular lines, and the right and left anterior axillary lines. Moving around to the lateral chest, there are the midaxillary and posterior axillary lines. Continuing to the posterior chest, the nurse locates the vertebral line and the right and left scapular lines.

Inspection

The first component of a comprehensive thoracic examination is inspection. The nurse assesses skin characteristics, muscle and body development, thoracic shape and movement, and respiratory pattern.

The nurse inspects the skin for the presence of scars from previous injuries or surgeries, moles, venous patterns, color, and irregular pigmentation. The presence of dryness, flakiness, red patches, or pustules is also noted.

Cyanosis. The color of the skin is specifically observed to determine cyanosis. Identification of cyanosis is dependent on tissue perfusion, cardiac output, rate of blood flow, skin thickness, skin color, and amount of hemoglobin, as well as the nurse's skill. When the nurse is assessing for cyanosis,

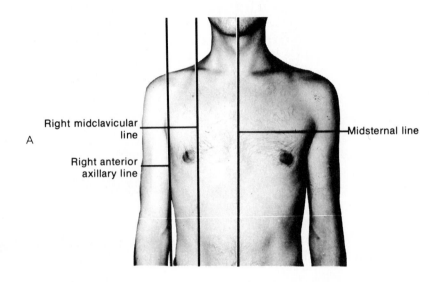

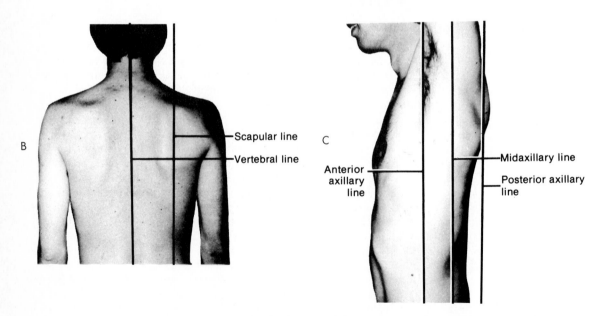

Fig. 5-2. Topographic landmarks of the (**A**) anterior thorax, (**B**) posterior thorax, and (**C**) lateral thorax. (From Bowers AC and Thompson JM: *Clinical manual of health assessment,* ed 3, St Louis, 1988, Mosby–Year Book.)

natural lighting should be used because artificial lighting may impart a bluish or greenish distortion to the skin. Cyanosis usually is assessed around the nares or lips, at the ear lobes, under the eyelids, and at the nail beds.

Cyanosis occurs when at least 5 g hemoglobin/100 ml blood is reduced, nonoxygenated. Cyanosis is an unreliable indicator of oxygen transport in both the anemic (hemoglobin less than 10 g/100 ml) and the polycythemic (hemoglobin greater than 17 g/100 ml) patient. The anemic patient may never become cyanotic in the face of severely decreased oxygen transport because approximately 50% (10 g − 5 g = 5 g) of the patient's blood would not be saturated before cyanosis occurred. Also, the polycythemic patient is often cyanotic in the presence of adequate oxygen transport because at least 5 g hemoglobin frequently is unsaturated.

Cyanosis is also an unreliable indicator of inadequate oxygen status in the patient with carbon monoxide poisoning. Patients with carbon monoxide poisoning typically have a cherry-red color to the mucous membranes even though oxygen saturation is frequently well below 80% and carboxyhemoglobin saturation is greater than 20%.

There are two classes of cyanosis: central cyanosis and peripheral cyanosis. The patient with central cyanosis has serious impairment of oxygen transfer in the lungs, and the patient's arterial oxygen saturation is abnormally low. The patient's skin has an overall bluish hue in the lips, the oral mucosa, the ear lobes, the sclera of the eye, and the extremities. The patient with peripheral cyanosis is exhibiting a local vasoconstrictor response to decreased blood flow. Peripheral cyanosis is common in cold temperatures and when vasoconstricting medications are used. Children commonly have peripheral cyanosis when swimming in a cool pool. The presence of peripheral cyanosis implies not impaired ability of the lungs to oxygenate blood but a localized impairment of blood flow. Arterial oxygen saturation is often normal when peripheral cyanosis is present.

Muscle and body development. Inspection of muscle and body development provides the nurse with information related to the patient's nutritional status and physical abilities. A thin patient with poor muscle tone may have limited physical abilities and inadequate calorie intake, in spite of indicating adequate nutrition in his patient history. Patients with chronic lung diseases, especially emphysema and bronchiectasis, are frequently thin and emaciated, with hypertrophy of respiratory accessory muscles. They often have limited ability to perform daily activities because of both peripheral and respiratory muscle fatigue. A patient with well-developed muscles usually has a strong cough (in the absence of pain) and can perform activities of daily living with minimal or no assistance. Obese individuals also may have weak muscles from disuse.

Anterior to posterior diameter. Determination of the anterior to posterior (A-P) diameter is the first component in assessing thoracic shape and movement. Normal A-P diameter is approximately 1:2. The distance from the anterior thorax to the posterior thorax is approximately half the distance from the left to the right lateral thorax, or the lateral diameter of the thorax is twice the A-P diameter (Fig. 5-3, *A*). A slightly increased A-P diameter occurs with normal aging. In conditions of chronic air trapping, such as emphysema, the A-P diameter is increased markedly, creating a round, or "barrel-chested," appearance. In some patients the A-P diameter is nearly 1:1 because of air trapping (Figure 5-3, *B*).

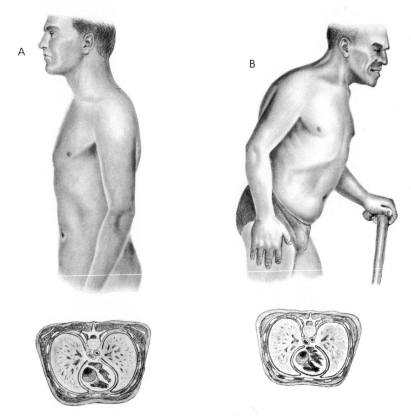

Fig. 5-3. (**A**) Thoracic diameter of normal healthy adult. The dotted lines represent abnormalities of (**B**) increased A-P diameter, or barrel chest, (**C**) pectus carinatum, or pigeon chest, and (**D**) pectus excavatum, or funnel chest. (From Seidel H et al: *Mosby's guide to physical examination,* ed 2, St Louis, 1991, Mosby—Year Book.)

Thoracic deformities. Pulmonary and cardiac functions can be impaired significantly by the presence of a chest or spine deformity. A protruding sternum is termed *pectus carinatum,* or "pigeon chest" (Figure 5-3, *C*). Conversely, a "sunken," or inwardly angled, sternum is termed *pectus excavatum,* or "funnel chest" (Figure 5-3, *D*). *Kyphosis* is the term given to an exaggerated outward curve of the posterior spine that is referred to commonly as "hunchback," and the term *scoliosis* is used to describe an abnormal lateral curve of the spine. Kyphosis is seen commonly in patients with osteoporosis resulting in vertebral decalcification. The combination of kyphosis and scoliosis yields the thoracic deformity kyphoscoliosis. Finally, an abnormally straight spine is termed "poker spine."

The normal thorax moves symmetrically. The thorax expands and contracts equally. Asymmetrical movement of the thorax reflects underlying pneumothorax, severe atelectasis, pleural disease, skeletal abnormalities, or surgical removal of lung tissue. Flail chest, a skeletal abnormality caused by trauma, causes asymmetrical paradoxical thoracic movements. A flail chest

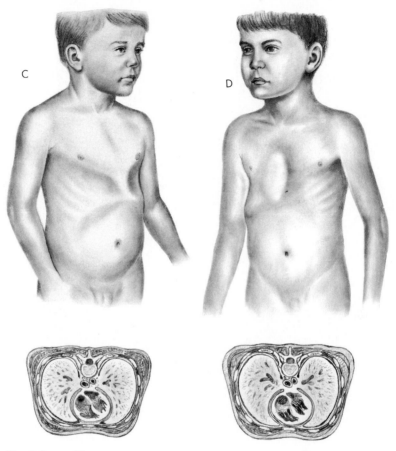

Fig. 5-3, cont'd.

occurs when two or more ribs are fractured in two or more places. The disconnected rib segments move opposite to normal inhalation and exhalation. A flail chest segment moves in during inhalation and out during exhalation (Fig. 5-4).

The most common technique to assess symmetry is visual examination. The nurse also may place a sheet of paper across the patient's chest and observe for its symmetrical movement. The assessment of symmetry is more difficult when the nurse is positioned at the patient's side. The nurse should stand directly in front of or behind the patient to assess symmetry. In the reclining patient, the nurse often can assess symmetry more effectively by standing at the foot of the bed.

Examination of the thorax for movement includes an assessment of muscles used for inhalation and exhalation, as well as time spent in each phase. The diaphragm is the primary muscle of inhalation. When the diaphragm contracts during inhalation, it can be seen moving down and out. After relaxation the diaphragm rises. During strenuous exercise the diaphragm may facilitate exhalation. Lower levels of exercise, even walking, in the patient with lung disease may require the use of the diaphragm as an expiratory muscle. Patients with air trapping should have a prolonged expiratory phase.

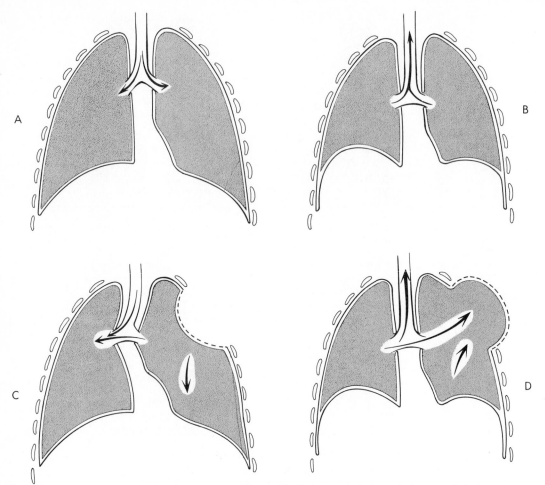

Fig. 5-4. Normal ventilation: (**A**) inhalation and (**B**) exhalation. Flail chest: (**C**) inhalation, the area of lung underlying the flail chest sucks in, and (**D**) exhalation, the same area balloons out. Note movement of the mediastinum toward opposite lung on inhalation. (From Phipps W et al: *Medical-surgical nursing,* ed 4, St Louis, 1991, Mosby–Year Book.)

The nurse may observe abnormal diaphragmatic movement. Instead of moving out during inhalation, the diaphragm moves up or in. This is called a *paradoxical diaphragm.* The nurse also may observe that the patient alternates between breathing with the diaphragm and breathing with the upper chest. This pattern of breathing is termed *respiratory alternans.*

Accessory muscles. The nurse observes for the presence of accessory muscle use in the neck, shoulder, back, and intercostal areas. Retractions, an excessive pulling of the muscles usually during inhalation, may be located in the substernal, suprasternal, or intercostal spaces. Retractions are a sign of increased work of breathing. The nurse also may assess bulging in the intercostal (IC) spaces. Bulging is usually due to prolonged exhalation in patients with obstructive lung diseases. It also may result from tumor bulk, aneurysm, or cardiomegaly.

Other accessory muscles are distant from the thorax. Nasal flaring, grunting, mouth breathing, and movement of the abdominal muscles are examples of nonrespiratory accessory muscle use. Use of these muscles indicates increased work of breathing or respiratory distress.

Respiratory pattern. The assessment of respiratory pattern involves analysis of the rate, depth, and rhythm of breathing. When observing respiratory pattern, it is also important for the nurse to note if the patient is using pursed-lip breathing or has noticeable prolonged exhalation. The normal respiratory rate of 12 to 20 breaths per minute at rest is determined by the patient's metabolic demands. (Note: Normal respiratory rate varies with the source. Some sources allow a minimum respiratory rate of 8 breaths per minute and a maximum of 24.) *Tachypnea*, a respiratory rate above 20 breaths per minute, is associated with many disorders (Fig. 5-5). Interstitial pulmonary fibrosis, anxiety, fever, and infectious processes account for most tachypnea. The patient who is tachypneic frequently breathes shallowly. *Bradypnea*, a respiratory rate less than 12 breaths per minute, also is associated with a multitude of disorders. The most common causes of bradypnea are neurological and cardiovascular diseases. *Apnea*, absence of respiratory rate, can be intermittent or complete. Intermittent apnea occurs in patients with neurological, pulmonary, and cardiac diseases. Sleep apnea is a condition of intermittent apnea, and cardiopulmonary arrest is a condition of complete apnea.

The terms *hyperventilation* and *hypoventilation* often are confused with the terms *tachypnea* and *bradypnea*. Hyperventilation and hypoventilation are assessed through arterial blood gases (ABGs), although clinical observation often can suggest their presence. Low carbon dioxide tension in arterial blood reflects a condition of hyperventilation, and elevated carbon dioxide tension indicates hypoventilation.

Similarly, depth of breathing is determined by metabolism. The normal depth of breathing also is determined by the size of the patient. Larger patients generally have a greater tidal volume (V_T). Eupnea is normal breathing. When a patient is breathing shallowly, the term *hypopnea* is used. *Hyperpnea* describes deep, and usually rapid, respirations.

The rhythm of breathing in conjunction with rate and depth of breathing provides a complete assessment of respiratory pattern. Several types of rhythmic and dysrhythmic patterns of breathing may be observed. *Kussmaul breathing*, seen in metabolic acidosis, such as diabetic ketoacidosis, is characterized by regular, deep, and rapid breaths. *Cheyne-Stokes* respirations are irregular. The patient demonstrates a repeating cycle of increasing rate and depth of breathing followed by decreasing rate and depth of breathing and periods of apnea. Patients with congestive heart failure, acute cerebral vascular accident, uremia, and terminal conditions frequently exhibit Cheyne-Stokes respirations. *Biot's breathing* is another type of irregular breathing pattern. The patient with Biot's breathing demonstrates unpredictable irregularities in the rhythm, rate, and depth of breathing, and apnea may occur. Impaired medullary control of breathing most commonly is found in patients with Biot's breathing, although other central nervous system disorders also may precipitate this pattern.

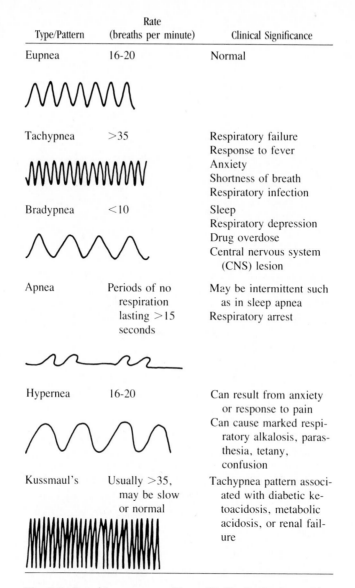

Type/Pattern	Rate (breaths per minute)	Clinical Significance
Eupnea	16-20	Normal
Tachypnea	>35	Respiratory failure Response to fever Anxiety Shortness of breath Respiratory infection
Bradypnea	<10	Sleep Respiratory depression Drug overdose Central nervous system (CNS) lesion
Apnea	Periods of no respiration lasting >15 seconds	May be intermittent such as in sleep apnea Respiratory arrest
Hypernea	16-20	Can result from anxiety or response to pain Can cause marked respiratory alkalosis, parasthesia, tetany, confusion
Kussmaul's	Usually >35, may be slow or normal	Tachypnea pattern associated with diabetic ketoacidosis, metabolic acidosis, or renal failure

Fig. 5-5. Breathing patterns. (From Weilitz P: *Pocket guide to respiratory care,* ed 1, St Louis, 1991, Mosby–Year Book.)

Type/Pattern	Rate (breaths per minute)	Clinical Significance
Biot's	Variable	Periods of apnea and shallow breathing caused by CNS disorder; found in some healthy clients
Apneustic	Increased	Increased inspiratory time with short grunting expiratory time; seen in CNS lesions of the respiratory center

Fig. 5-5, cont'd.

Palpation

Palpation, the first "hands-on" component of physical assessment, is used to assess abnormalities of skin texture and composition, thoracic structure, and tracheal deviation, as well as thoracic excursion and fremitus. The technique of palpation varies with the purpose and site of assessment and with the nurse's preference. Some nurses use the ball of the hand, and other nurses prefer to use the side of the hand. Sometimes the nurse uses her fingers. The nurse places her hands firmly on the patient's chest wall throughout the respiratory pattern. The nurse moves her palpating hands from side to side, progressing from top to bottom. The two sides of the thorax are compared simultaneously. An alternate method for palpation is to use one hand and compare right side with left side.

Skin. When assessing skin for abnormalities, the nurse first identifies temperature. Skin that is feverish or excessively warm also may be flushed or diaphoretic. Causes of excessively warm skin include improper room temperature (too warm), fever, hypoxemia, anxiety, embarrassment, and infection. Feeling warm may also be a sign of carbon dioxide retention. Decreased skin temperature, or cool skin, most frequently is associated with a cool environment, circulatory impairment, or chilling with fever.

Skin turgor is assessed to identify a patient's fluid status. The nurse can assess for fluid volume deficit and for fluid volume excess. Skin turgor is assessed by pinching or tenting skin over bony prominences. The nurse determines the time required for the skin to return to its original position. Tented skin in a patient without fluid volume deficit returns to normal promptly, but tented skin in a patient with fluid volume deficit remains tented for several seconds. Because elderly patients often have thinner, drier, and less elastic skin than younger patients, the use of the patient's hand or forearm to assess skin turgor is less accurate than use of the forehead or sternum.

Because skin turgor in a patient with fluid volume excess usually is compressed instead of tented, the nurse often is unable to tent the skin. The nurse exerts gentle but direct pressure with the thumb over a bony prominence for 2 seconds. In a patient with fluid volume excess, the impression remains for several seconds to a minute or more. Edema is graded by the depth of the impression in millimeters. An impression of 1 mm is 1+ edema, 2 mm is 2+ edema, 3 mm is 3+ edema, and up to 4+ edema. Edema may be caused by low oncotic pressure and by fluid volume excess. Because edema accumulates in dependent areas, the most common site to assess edema is the lower leg, just above the ankle, although other sites may be used. In the patient who remains supine, the edema must be assessed over the lower spine. When edema involves the trunk and the limbs, the term *anasarca,* or total body edema, is used.

Trachea. A normal trachea is positioned in the midline and is freely moveable to the left and right about 1 cm. When a patient has atelectasis, pleural effusion, tumor, or enlarged thyroid gland, the trachea shifts to the side (Table 5-1). With severe tracheal deviation, as occurs with tension pneumothorax, the mediastinum may be displaced, and the great vessels may be compressed.

Table 5-1. Tracheal displacement

Toward the affected side	Toward the opposite side
Atelectasis	Tension pneumothorax, pleural effusion, unilateral tumor, enlarged thyroid gland, thyroid lymph nodes

To assess tracheal deviation, the nurse positions the thumbs or the second and third fingers in the suprasternal notch (Fig. 5-6). Care is taken to not obstruct blood flow through the jugular vein or carotid arteries. The fingers are gently moved to the left and to the right as the patient swallows. This movement determines position and mobility of the trachea. Deviation usually is noticed during this maneuver. Alternately, the nurse may gently apply downward tension on the skin over the trachea to identify midline or abnormal position. An enlarged trachea or the presence of tracheal nodes is assessed when the patient swallows.

Chest wall. The chest wall is palpated to assess for rib fractures, abscesses, tumors, and strained muscles. The nurse identifies areas of tenderness or swelling. Less commonly, bulges or masses also may be observed when palpating the chest wall. When rib fractures puncture the pleura, the nurse frequently palpates *crepitus* or subcutaneous emphysema. Caused by air escaping from the lung into the subcutaneous area, crepitus is described as sounding like cellophane crackling or bubbles popping under the skin. Crepitus also may be observed after a tracheostomy when skin sutures are too tight. Crepitus itself is harmless to the patient but may frighten the patient and visitors. Because the underlying process, such as pneumothorax or tension pneumothorax, can compromise the patient's gas exchange, crepitus must be evaluated thoroughly.

The nurse assesses anterior and posterior *chest excursion* by palpation (Fig. 5-7). The nurse can identify unilateral and bilateral lung problems that impede full chest excursion. In the normal adult the chest expands equally on the left and right sides. Asymmetrical movement, one side moving less than the other, is associated with a unilateral problem. A bilateral decrease from normal in the amount of excursion is usually a sign of bilateral disease (see box on p. 76). Bilateral pleural effusions and obesity are common causes of decreased bilateral chest excursion.

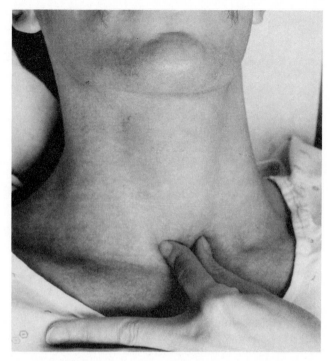

Fig. 5-6. Tracheal position is assessed in the suprasternal notch with thumbs or second and third fingers. (From Potter P and Perry A: *Fundamentals of nursing*, ed 2, St Louis, 1989, Mosby–Year Book.)

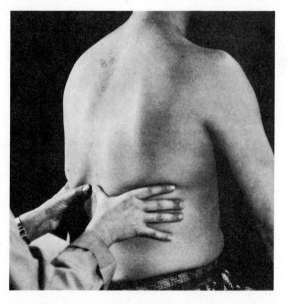

Fig. 5-7. Thumbs are placed at the level of the tenth rib for palpating thoracic expansion. (From Malasanos L et al: *Health assessment*, ed 4, St Louis, 1990, Mosby–Year Book.)

Table 5-2. Causes of fremitus

Increased	Decreased
Consolidation, pneumonia	Bony structures, empyema, pleural thickening, pleural effusion, pneumothorax, thick chest wall, tumor

To assess anterior chest excursion, the nurse lightly places the thumbs at the costal angle, spreading and firmly pressing the fingers over the lateral chest wall. Asking the patient to inhale deeply, the nurse observes the movement of her thumbs. In the normal patient the nurse's thumbs should move apart equally. Posterior chest excursion is assessed similarly, except the thumbs are centered over the patient's spine. The nurse assesses separation of the thumbs as the patient inhales. As the patient inhales and exhales, the nurse's thumbs move in unison with thoracic excursion.

Fremitus assessment is the final technique of palpation. Fremitus is palpable when sound vibrates through fluid rather than through air. Caused by sound (the patient's voice) vibrating through fluid, fremitus assists the nurse to identify secretions in the airways because water is a much better conductor of sound than air. Fremitus assessment can be inaccurate when air movement is impaired by tumor growth or mucus plugs. The amount of fremitus transmitted is dependent on the proximity of the airways to the surface of the lung, the thickness of the chest wall, and the location of the bones. Abnormal increases in vibrations occur when sound transmission is enhanced (Table 5-2). Abnormal decreases in vibrations occur when sound transmission is impaired, such as when air is increased.

The nurse can assess tactile or vocal fremitus, or both. To palpate fremitus, the nurse places the ulnar or palmar aspect of one or both hands gently but firmly on the patient's chest. In some instances the nurse actually may feel secretions moving within the patient's chest; this is tactile fremitus. At other times the nurse may need to use additional techniques to identify fremitus.

Vocal fremitus is assessed by asking the patient to repeat in a monotone voice phrases such as "99, 99, 99," "How now, brown cow," or "blue moon, blue moon, blue moon" each time the nurse repositions her hands.

Causes of decreased chest excursion

Atelectasis	Pneumonectomy
Lobectomy	Pneumonia
Pleural effusion	Pneumothorax
Pleural plaques	Rib fractures
Pleuritis	Splinting from pain

The nurse moves from the apices to the bases on the anterior, lateral, and posterior aspects of the lungs. The nurse feels increased vibrations (vocal fremitus) over affected areas. Fremitus findings are assessed further with auscultation.

Percussion

Percussion is useful for determining the boundaries of organs surrounding the chest and for identifying densities of air and fluid in the chest. Percussion is most useful for determining air trapping, pleural effusion extent, and diaphragmatic excursion. The sounds of percussion notes are altered by a thick chest wall, the presence of excessive muscle or adipose tissue, poorly developed muscles in the extremely thin individual, and large bones or dense organs.

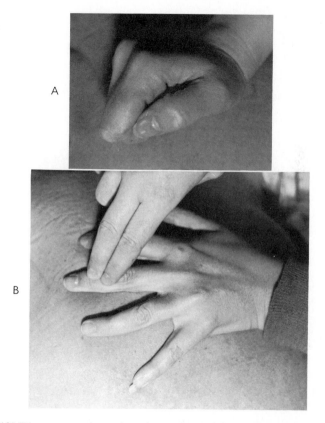

Fig. 5-8. (A) Direct percussion using ulnar aspect of fist or **(B)** indirect percussion using fingers.

The technique of percussion is easy to learn but more difficult to perfect than other techniques of physical assessment. The chest is percussed directly or indirectly (Fig. 5-8). Direct percussion is performed by striking the chest with the ulnar surface of a fisted hand. The nurse performs indirect percussion by placing the distal portion of the third finger of the nondominant hand firmly in an intercostal space. The nurse uses the tip of the middle finger of the dominant hand to strike firmly or tap over the nail bed (not the nail) of the finger on the chest, using a quick motion of wrist flexion and extension. The nurse must be careful to place only one finger on the chest because sound

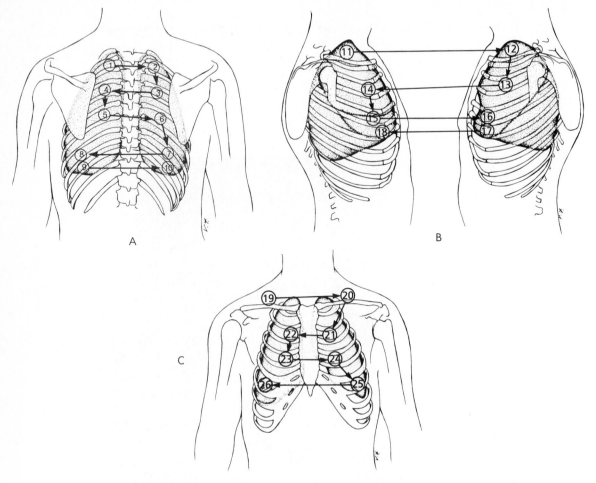

Fig. 5-9. A systematic sequence is used to assess percussion and auscultation of the thorax: (**A**) posterior chest, (**B**) right and left lateral chest, and (**C**) anterior chest. (From Perry A and Potter P: *Clinical nursing skills and techniques,* ed 2, St Louis, 1990, Mosby–Year Book.)

transmission is dampened by the addition of more fingers or the hand. The nurse performs percussion in each interspace on one side and then the other in succession from the apices to the bases (Fig. 5-9).

Short nails facilitate percussion and decrease nurse discomfort. The nurse who experiences discomfort because of longer nails may prefer to use a percussion hammer to deliver the strike. Use of a percussion hammer is also helpful in patients with thick chest walls.

The nurse can elicit five percussion notes on the thorax: resonance, hyperresonance, flatness, dullness, and tympany (Table 5-3). Tympany is rarely heard in the thorax unless the bowel herniates through the diaphragm. The percussion notes are described according to intensity, pitch, timbre, and duration. Intensity is the loudness or amplitude of the percussion note, and pitch refers to the frequency or number of vibrations produced per second. A

Table 5-3. Percussion notes

Sound	Intensity	Pitch	Timbre	Duration	Cause
Resonance	Moderate/loud	Low	Hollow	Long	Normal
Hyperresonance	Very loud	Low	Booming	Very long	Emphysema, pneumothorax, acute asthma, cystic fibrosis
Flatness	Soft	High	Very dull	Short	Pleural effusion, pleural thickening
Dullness	Soft/medium	Medium/high	Thudlike	Moderate	Atelectasis, consolidation, pneumonia, pulmonary edema (massive)
Tympany	Loud	High	Drumlike	Moderate	Large pneumothorax, herniated bowel

Table 5-4. Diaphragmatic excursion

Unilateral decrease	Bilateral decrease
Ascites, enlarged liver, paralyzed diaphragm (unilateral), pneumothorax (large), large unilateral pleural effusion	Acute asthma attack with air trapping, ascites, cystic fibrosis, large bilateral pleural effusions, bilateral massive pleural thickening, pregnancy, obstructive lung disease with hyperinflation, bilateral paralyzed diaphragms

low-pitched sound occurs when vibrations are few, and a high-pitched sound occurs when vibrations are increased. Timbre describes the degree of hollowness or dullness created by the sound. Finally, duration is the length of time that the note is audible.

Percussion notes other than resonance and hyperresonance often are learned best over body parts peripheral to the lung. The percussion notes dullness, flatness, and tympany can be remembered when compared with more common sites. For instance, dullness is the sound heard when percussing over the liver or heart, and flatness occurs when percussing large muscle groups, such as the thigh, or bones, such as the scapula. The sound of tympany is heard when percussing the gastric air bubble in the stomach.

Percussion is used to determine diaphragmatic excursion or the distance the diaphragm moves from inhalation to exhalation, or vice versa. (Table 5-4 lists causes of decreased diaphragmatic excursion.) Assessment of diaphragmatic excursion usually is performed on the posterior thorax because major organs do not interfere with percussion. Diaphragmatic excursion is assessed on both the right and the left chest. Because the resting diaphragm is usually at the level of the eighth rib, percussion for diaphragmatic excursion starts at that level. Contraction of the diaphragm (inhalation) positions the diaphragm at the level of the tenth to twelfth ribs; hence normal diaphragmatic excursion is 3 to 6 cm (Fig. 5-10). Excursion on the right side of the chest is frequently slightly less (approximately 1 cm) than that of the left, possibly because of the location of the liver.

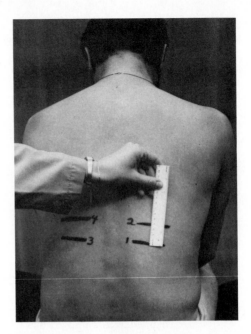

Fig. 5-10. Diaphragmatic excursion, usually measured on the posterior chest with the patient sitting upright, is normally 3 to 6 cm. (From Malasanos L et al: *Health assessment*, ed 4, St Louis, 1990, Mosby–Year Book.)

To assess diaphragmatic excursion, the nurse asks the patient to breathe normally as she percusses down the midscapular line. The patient should be sitting upright. At the point that resonance changes to dullness, the nurse is over the diaphragm or abdominal contents. The nurse mentally notes or draws a line on the patient's chest with a pen, marker, or fingernail at the point of change in percussion note. The nurse instructs the patient to breathe deeply and hold the inhalation as she continues percussing downward until she hears dullness. The distance between the two points of dullness is diaphragmatic excursion.

Auscultation

Auscultation of the thorax, the final component of chest assessment, requires the use of a high-quality stethoscope. The ideal stethoscope has binaural (double) tubing, is less than 20 inches long, and has an internal diameter at least ³/₁₆ inches to enhance acoustics and minimize interference. The earpieces should be comfortable and snug to reduce external noise (Prior and Silberstein, 1977). The diaphragm of the stethoscope is used to assess higher-pitched lung sounds, and the bell of the stethoscope is used to identify lower-pitched lung sounds.

Auscultation, like inspection, palpation, and percussion, is performed from apex to base and side to side, covering anterior, lateral, and posterior areas of the lung (see Fig. 5-9). The nurse can perform auscultation with the patient in a sitting or reclining position, although a sitting position is preferred. When the patient is reclining, the nurse must roll the patient from side to side to

Table 5-5. Auscultation of breath sounds

Sound	Bronchial	Bronchovesicular	Vesicular
Where heard	Trachea, sternum	Major bronchi, sternal border, 1-2 ICS anteriorly at the apices and between scapula posteriorly	Periphery
Quality	Tubular, hollow, loud intensity, high pitch	Inspiratory are like vesicular; expiratory are like bronchial. Moderate to loud intensity, medium to high pitch	Quiet, breezy, moderate intensity, low pitch
I:E	E > I (3:2), pause between I:E	E = I (1:1)	E > I (2:5)
Sounds like	Blowing through a hollow tube		Wind rustling through leaves

perform auscultation. It is important to remember that ventilation and perfusion are altered in the recumbent patient. In addition, pleural fluid moves to the most dependent area of the lung, which is the base in the upright lung and the lateral area in the side-lying lung. Sound transmission is enhanced and noise transmission is reduced by placing the stethoscope directly on the patient's skin and not over clothing. Chest hair and clothing sometimes can simulate crackles with movement of the stethoscope. Auscultating the lungs of a patient on mechanical ventilation is difficult because water and air moving in the tubing often interfere with breath-sound transmission.

Normal breath sounds. The chest is auscultated for both normal and abnormal lung sounds. Normal breath sounds are characterized as bronchial, bronchovesicular, and vesicular (Table 5-5). Auscultation of the lungs over the main airways produces bronchial breath sounds. Moving further away from the main airways, the nurse hears bronchovesicular sounds. Vesicular lung sounds are heard in the periphery.

Adventitious breath sounds. Abnormal breath sounds are termed *adventitious*. Terminology used to describe adventitious breath sounds varies among practitioners. The American Thoracic Society, the medical branch of the American Lung Association, recommends the use of standardized nomenclature. Nurses are encouraged to adopt the terms *crackles* and *wheezes* in place of *rales* and *rhonchi*, respectively. An alternative suggestion is to describe the sound if a label cannot be applied.

Crackles. Crackles are short, discontinuous sounds produced either by secretions popping or exploding during inhalation, exhalation, or cough or by alveoli snapping open during inhalation. Thus crackles usually are heard in the peripheral airways and alveoli. Crackles usually are caused by atelectasis, consolidation, pulmonary edema, bronchitis, or pulmonary fibrosis.

Assessment of crackles can be defined further as coarse, medium, or fine. A coarse crackle is low-pitched and resembles the sound produced by blowing through a straw into a glass of thick syrup. Coarse crackles usually are caused by resolving pneumonia, pulmonary edema, and bronchitis. A medium crackle is medium-pitched and is similar to the fizzing sound produced by the opening of a carbonated beverage. Finally, fine crackles are high-pitched and parallel the sound of rubbing hair between the thumb and forefinger. Atelectasis usually produces fine crackles.

Other terms used to describe crackles are *wet* or *dry*. The term *wet crackles* is used to describe secretions (mucus, pulmonary edema fluid, or fluids produced by atelectasis), and *dry*, or *Velcro*, crackles refers to interstitial fibrosis.

Wheeze. The term *wheeze* is used to identify a high-pitched or a low-pitched sound that is produced by air moving turbulently through a narrowed airway. (The former term for *wheeze* varied among *sibilant, musical,* or *sonorous* rhonchi and gurgles.) High-pitched wheezes have a whistling or squeaking character; low-pitched wheezes resemble a moaning or snoring sound. The most common cause of wheezes is bronchospasm, although inflammation, obstruction of the airway by tumor or foreign body, bronchial stenosis, and secretions are also factors. Low-pitched wheezes frequently are associated with secretions and usually resolve with coughing or suctioning.

Pleural friction rub. Another adventitious sound assessed by auscultation is pleural friction rub. Caused by inflamed parietal and visceral pleura rubbing together, pleural friction rub is a coarse, grating, or scratching sound. A pleural friction rub can resemble a pericardial friction rub or medium crackles. The difference between a pericardial friction rub and a pleural friction rub is that a pericardial friction rub is continuous in spite of breath-holding, and a pleural friction rub is heard during inhalation and exhalation. The most common causes of pleural friction rub are pneumonia, tuberculosis, cancer, pulmonary infarction, and chest-tube insertion.

Voice sounds. Voice sounds are similar to fremitus except voice sounds are assessed with a stethoscope. Three voice sounds may be assessed, although usually only one or perhaps two are used at a time. The voice sounds are bronchophony (words), whispered pectoriloquy (whispers), and egophony (letters). In the normal lung, voice is transmitted poorly through air; words heard through the stethoscope are unclear and muffled. When fluid accumulates, sound-wave transmission is enhanced, and words are heard more clearly. This is the principle of voice sounds.

Bronchophony is assessed by asking the patient to repeat a monotone phrase each time the stethoscope is repositioned. The most frequently used phrases include "How now, brown cow" and "99, 99, 99." Over areas of consolidation the nurse can distinguish the words clearly because they are not muffled.

Whispered pectoriloquy is assessed by asking the patient to whisper a monotone phrase. The nurse hears the whispered phrase clearly and loudly over areas of consolidation.

Egophony is assessed by asking the patient to say *ee, ee, ee* each time the stethoscope is moved to a new position. Over normal lung areas the nurse auscultates a muffled *ee*. The *ee* sound is heard as *aa, aa, aa* over areas of consolidation. Most nurses find that egophony is the easiest of the three voice sounds to assess.

Cardiac assessment

Because the cardiac and pulmonary systems are intertwined by the continual exchange of blood, the nurse also must be able to perform a cardiac assessment. Measurement of pulse, blood pressure, heart sounds, and fluid status contributes to a cardiopulmonary data base. Abnormalities in these measurements may be the result of muscle deconditioning or cardiac dysfunction, such as congestive heart failure, cardiomyopathy, myocardial ischemia or infarction, or hypertension, as well as pulmonary diseases, such as ventilation-perfusion mismatching (hypoxemia), pulmonary emboli, and obstructed airways or interstitial lung dysfunction.

Pulse. The nurse most often assesses pulse by placing the second and third fingers medial to the radial prominence and distal to the thumb. When the nurse does not palpate a radial pulse, she may use the brachial pulse in the antecubital fossa, the carotid pulse in the angle of the jaw, the temporal pulse just distal to the outer eye above the ear, the femoral pulse in the groin, or the popliteal pulse behind the knee. Ideally, all pulses should be assessed. Presence of a femoral pulse in the absence of a measurable blood pressure indicates a systemic blood pressure of approximately 60 mm Hg.

When assessing the pulse, the nurse observes rate, regularity, and strength. A normal pulse ranges from 60 to 100 beats per minute, which varies from baseline during periods of exertion or exercise. The nurse may assess *tachycardia*, that is, rate greater than 100 beats per minute, or *bradycardia*, that is, rate less than 60 beats per minute.

The normal pulse has a regular rhythm. An alteration in electrical pathway produces premature or late beats and an irregular pulse. An electrocardiogram reveals the origin of the extrasystole. The patient may have ectopic atrial beats, ectopic ventricular beats, atrial fibrillation, atrial flutter, or sinus arrhythmia.

A normal pulse is strong but not bounding. Patients may have a bounding pulse, weak pulse, or pulse that alternates in strength. A bounding pulse *(pulsus magnus)* may indicate patent ductus arteriosus, hypertension, thyroid storm, aortic insufficiency, or arteriovenous fistula. *Pulsus parvus*, a small, weak pulse, is found with mitral and aortic valve stenosis and with cardiac tamponade and pericarditis. When the pulse alternates between weak and strong beats *(pulsus alternans)*, left ventricular failure or severe hypertension is a possible cause.

Blood pressure. Blood pressure is assessed most frequently in the upper arm. When arm pressures are unobtainable or when lower extremity arterial insufficiency is suspected, the upper-leg blood pressure is assessed. A blood pressure measurement is only as accurate as the equipment and the examiner allow. The ideal blood pressure cuff completely encircles the extremity 1.5 to 2 times without compressing blood flow or slipping off. Properly placed, the ideal blood pressure cuff covers two thirds of the upper arm or thigh, with the lower edge 1 inch above the point of auscultation or palpation and the zero value of the mercury or aneroid manometer at the level of the aorta. A cuff that is too small or narrow measures the blood pressure as falsely high, and a cuff that is too large or wide measures the blood pressure as falsely low. The use of a quality stethoscope in conjunction with a properly fitted blood pressure cuff enhances the auscultation of blood pressure.

The proper technique to assess blood pressure once the cuff is properly applied is first to palpate the pulse while inflating the cuff. When the pulse is obliterated, the nurse notes the manometer reading and releases all air from the cuff. After waiting 15 seconds, the nurse again inflates the cuff 20 to 30 mm Hg higher than the palpated value. Releasing the air from the cuff at a rate of 2 to 3 mm Hg per second, the nurse listens or palpates for the first pulse beat, termed *Korotkoff sounds*. The point where Korotkoff sounds are observed first is the systolic blood pressure. Korotkoff sounds traditionally become muffled at the point of the first diastolic blood pressure. The second diastolic pressure is measured when Korotkoff sounds disappear. The nurse may hear Korotkoff sounds to zero (second diastolic pressure) in a few people. An example of a complete blood pressure is 100/70/60 instead of 100/60.

Pulsus paradoxus. At the same time that she measures blood pressure, the nurse also may assess for pulsus paradoxus. An abnormal fall in blood pressure during inhalation, pulsus paradoxus is assessed by inflating the blood pressure cuff 5 to 10 mm Hg above the patient's systolic blood pressure. While very slowly releasing air from the cuff, the nurse listens for the first Korotkoff sound only during exhalation and then throughout inhalation and exhalation. The difference between the two points is pulsus paradoxus and is usually less than 10 mm Hg. An increase in the measured pulsus paradoxus is seen in cardiac tamponade and chronic pulmonary diseases.

A systolic blood pressure of 90 to 140 mm Hg and a diastolic blood pressure of 60 to 90 mm Hg are considered normal in the adolescent and adult, but normal blood pressure in the neonate ranges from 20 to 60 mm Hg. Controlled by the renin-angiotensin system, blood pressure is affected by many factors: cardiac output, peripheral vascular resistance, O_2 tension, arterial elasticity, blood volume, exercise, emotions, weight, position, and age. The presence of acute, mild arterial hypoxemia causes hypertension. Hypotension occurs when hypoxemia is prolonged or severe. Hypovolemia also is associated with hypotension. Congestive heart failure may increase or decrease the blood pressure, depending on severity. Anxiety usually increases the blood pressure. Obese or overweight patients often develop hypertension. Sepsis or sepsis syndrome is accompanied by low systemic vascular resistance and low blood pressure. Conversely, blood pressure increases several hours after awakening (in the late afternoon for day workers or in the morning for night workers) and decreases during sleep. Going from a supine position to a sitting position or from a supine or sitting position to a standing position causes a small decrease in systolic and diastolic blood pressure. A decrease of 10% to 12% is considered normal, but a decline of 15% or more is termed *orthostatic hypotension.* Aortic stenosis and partial or complete peripheral arterial occlusion cause blood pressure differences between the right and left extremities. Blood pressure that is higher in the arms than in the legs is seen in coarctation of the aorta.

Heart sounds. Heart sounds are another component of the physical assessment that the nurse must repeat frequently to become proficient at evaluating. Different heart sounds are produced when the tricuspid, pulmonic, mitral, and aortic valves open and close in conjunction with muscular contraction. Table 5-6 lists the causes of each heart sound and identifies the best position of the stethoscope to auscultate valvular heart sounds.

Fluid status. Fluid status assessment is another component of the cardiac evaluation. The nurse assesses fluid status through the estimation of jugular venous pressure and peripheral edema and the presence of adventitious lung sounds, especially crackles, and abnormal heart sounds.

Table 5-6. Heart sounds

Heart sound	Cause	Stethoscope	Area
S_1, **normal**	Closure of mitral, tricuspid valves	Diaphragm	4 ICS left of sternum 5 ICS left midclavicular
S_2, **normal**	Closure of aortic, pulmonic valves at end of ventricular systole*	Diaphragm	2 ICS right and left sternal borders
S_3, **normal (children)**	Ventricular contraction	Bell	4 ICS and 5 ICS midclavicular
S_3, **abnormal (adult)**	Increased volume, decreased compliance†	Bell	3 ICS and 4 ICS left sternal border, lateral decubitus
S_4, **abnormal**	Atrial contraction, ventricular overload, increased diastolic pressure‡	Bell	Apex of heart

*S_2 may be split physiologically when pulmonic valve closure is delayed during inhalation because of increased venous return and slowed right ventricular contraction. Persistent splitting during inhalation and exhalation is abnormal and may be due to atrial septal defect, pulmonary stenosis, pulmonary hypertension, severe mitral insufficiency, aortic stenosis, and bundle branch block.

†S_3, a ventricular gallop, accompanies congestive heart failure, tricuspid insufficiency, and left-to-right shunts. It sounds like *Ken-tuc-ky*.

‡S_4 is associated with myocardial infarction, pulmonary hypertension, aortic stenosis, pulmonary stenosis, heart failure, and hyperthyroidism. S_4 sounds like *Ten-nes-see*.

Jugular venous pressure can be estimated fairly accurately in most patients. The types of patients in whom the assessment of jugular venous pressure is less accurate include those with short, fat necks and superior vena cava syndrome. The jugular vein usually is visible in the supine patient, but it disappears or is barely visible when the head is elevated. A flat jugular neck vein is present in patients with normal fluid volume or fluid volume deficit. When the jugular vein is distended, that is, more than 3 cm above the angle of Louis, fluid volume excess or right heart failure should be suspected. Application of pressure over the liver that results in filling of the jugular veins in right-sided heart failure is termed the *hepatojugular reflex.*

Jugular venous pressure can be estimated in the following manner. The nurse positions the patient supine in the bed and elevates the head of the bed 30 to 45 degrees (the reverse Trendelenburg position may be used in patients requiring spinal cord precautions). Sometimes it is necessary for the nurse to ask the patient to turn his head away from her for easier visualization of the internal jugular vein. Alternately, the nurse assesses jugular venous pressure using the external jugular vein. The nurse measures the distance in centimeters between the angle of Louis (sternal angle) and the top of the jugular vein to obtain jugular venous pressure.

CONCLUSION

Accurate thoracic assessment is critical to developing an appropriate plan of care. This chapter presents thoracic assessment of a patient, beginning with the most basic of concepts, general appearance. Thoracic assessment focuses on the lung and then the heart. Each component of lung assessment (inspection, palpation, percussion, and auscultation) is discussed in detail with references to possible causes of abnormalities. Because cardiac function greatly affects the lung, assessment of cardiac status, including pulse, blood pressure, and heart sounds, is reviewed.

BIBLIOGRAPHY

American College of Chest Physicians— American Thoracic Society: Pulmonary terms and symbols, *Chest* 67(5):583-593, 1975.

Bates B: *A guide to physical examination and history taking,* ed 4, Philadelphia, 1987, JB Lippincott.

Baughman R, Loudon R: Lung sound analysis for continuous evaluation of airflow obstruction in asthma, *Chest* 88(3):364-368, 1985.

Baum GL, Wolinsky E: *Textbook of pulmonary diseases,* ed 3, Boston, 1983, Little & Brown.

Broughton J: Chest physical diagnosis for nurses and respiratory therapists, *Heart Lung* 1(2):200-206, 1972.

Burton GC, Hodgkin JE: *Respiratory care: a guide to clinical practice,* ed 2, Philadelphia, 1984, JB Lippincott.

Cohen CA, Zagelbaum G et al: Clinical manifestations of inspiratory muscle fatigue, *Am J Med* 73(3):308-316, 1982.

Cugell D: Lung sounds: classifications and controversies, *Semin Respir Med* 6(3):180-182, 1985.

Forgacs P: Applied cardiopulmonary physiology: the functional basis of pulmonary sounds. *Chest* 73(3):399-405, 1978.

Fraser R, Paré J: *Diagnosis of diseases of the chest,* vol 3, ed 2, Philadelphia, 1979, WB Saunders.

Hinshaw H, Murray J: *Diseases of the chest,* ed 4, Philadelphia, 1980, WB Saunders.

Krumpe P: Practical application of lung sounds research, *Semin Respir Med* 6(3):229-237, 1985.

Loudon R, Murphy R: State of the art: lung sounds, *Am Rev Respir Dis* 130(4):663-673, 1984.

Malasanos L et al: *Health assessment,* ed 4, St Louis, 1990, Mosby–Year Book.

Murphy R, Holford S: *Basics Respir Dis* 8(4), 1980.

Murray JF, Nadel JA, eds: *Textbook of respiratory medicine,* Philadelphia, 1988, WB Saunders.

Netter F: *The CIBA collection of medical illustrations,* vol 7: respiratory system, New York, 1979, CIBA Pharmaceutical.

Paré JAP, Fraser RG: *Synopsis of diseases of the chest,* Philadelphia, 1983, WB Saunders.

Petty T: Clinical evaluation of patients with chronic respiratory insufficiency, *Semin Respir Med* 1(1):1-8, 1979.

Ploysongsang Y, Paré JA, Macklem PT Lung sounds in patients with emphysema, *Am Rev Respir Dis* 124(1):45-49, 1981.

Ploysongsang Y, Schonfeld SA: Mechanism of production of crackles after atelectasis during low-volume breathing, *Am Rev Respir Dis* 126(3):413-415, 1982.

Prior J, Silberstein J, Stang J: *Physical diagnosis: the history and examination of the patient,* ed 6, St Louis, 1981, Mosby–Year Book.

Shapiro B, Harrison R et al: *Clinical applications of respiratory care,* ed 3, Chicago, 1985, Mosby–Year Book.

Simmons DH, ed: *Current pulmonology,* vol 7, Chicago, 1986, Mosby–Year Book.

Stright PA, Soukup SM: How to hear it right: evaluating and choosing a stethoscope, *Am J Nurs* 77(9):1477, 1977.

Thompson D: *Cardiovascular assessment: guide for nurses and other health professionals,* St Louis, 1981, Mosby–Year Book.

Wade JF: *Comprehensive respiratory care: physiology and technique,* ed 3, St Louis, 1982, Mosby–Year Book.

Waring W, Beckerman R, Hopkins R: Continuous adventitious lung sounds: site and method of production and significance, *Semin Respir Med* 6(3):201-209, 1985.

CHAPTER 6

Arterial Blood Gas Analysis

Objectives:

- Describe the technique of arterial blood gas (ABG) sampling by direct puncture and from an indwelling arterial catheter.
- State the values of a normal arterial and mixed venous blood gas.
- Differentiate assessment and causes of respiratory alkalosis, respiratory acidosis, metabolic alkalosis, and metabolic acidosis.
- Calculate the alveolar/arterial oxygen gradient, Pao_2/Fio_2 oxygen ratio, and arterial/alveolar oxygen ratio.
- Calculate shunt using the classic shunt equation, clinical shunt equation, and alternate clinical shunt equation.

A patient's oxygenation and ventilation status can be assessed accurately only through ABG analysis. Maintenance of ABGs at the optimal level for an individual depends on ventilation, perfusion, and diffusion. Measurement of ABGs provides the nurse with information about each of these processes. When ventilation is adequate, the inspired air comes into contact with the alveolar capillary membrane, effectively removing carbon dioxide from the blood as oxygen enters the blood. Inadequate ventilation, decreased perfusion, or impaired diffusion (cardiac output) are recognized by increased carbon dioxide tension or by decreased oxygen tension.

DRAWING ARTERIAL BLOOD GASES

In many hospitals the nurse obtains the blood gas sample. The proper technique to obtain an ABG sample is presented first because ABG analysis results depend on the quality of the blood obtained. Analysis of an ABG follows. The importance of being able to interpret blood gas values accurately cannot be overstressed. On the patient floor or in the critical care unit, the nurse is often the first person to see the results of a blood gas analysis. The nurse must be able to recognize deviations from normal and to interpret these deviations. At the minimum the blood gas is classified. There are other, more sophisticated methods of assessing oxygenation based on ABG analysis. These concepts also are presented in this chapter.

The technique of ABG sampling is similar to venipuncture with a few differences. The systemic circulation is under high pressure rather than low pressure; therefore extra care is needed to prevent complications, especially hematoma formation or arterial occlusion. A hematoma is prevented most effectively by direct puncture of the artery followed by pressure over the puncture site for at least 5 minutes after the needle has been removed. Arterial occlusion can be prevented by use of the proper puncture technique, prevention of a hematoma, and rotation of the puncture site with subsequent samples between the left to right extremities.

Once the sample has been obtained, several precautions must be taken in handling the ABG sample to ensure an accurate patient profile. For accurate blood gas analysis the sample must not clot; therefore, an anticoagulant, such as liquid sodium heparin or dry lithium heparin, should be added to the syringe to prevent clotting. Some syringes are preheparinized, but other syringes require the nurse to coat the inside of the syringe with a liquid heparin solution. A common source of error in manually heparinized syringes is that too much heparin is left in the syringe. Because the pH of heparin is 7.0, this may lower blood pH falsely. Care must be taken to avoid excess heparin in the syringe.

Another consideration is that the sample is placed on ice immediately to slow cellular metabolism. Failure to ice the sample allows cellular metabolism to continue, which alters blood gas values. Oxygen consumption and carbon dioxide production, especially by the white blood cells, continue in the blood sample after removal from the body. Reducing the temperature of the blood by submersing the syringe in ice reduces the metabolic rate of the blood, but the ice must come into direct contact with the syringe. A delay in placing the sample on ice can lower oxygen levels and increase carbon dioxide values in the blood sample. Once obtained and placed on ice, a sample should be analyzed within 1 hour.

For accurate ABG analysis, the nurse should assess the patient's body temperature very near the time of the arterial blood sample and report the temperature to the blood gas laboratory. In some institutions the temperature is written on the slip that accompanies the sample; in other institutions it is entered into a computer. Arterial blood samples are analyzed at 37° C. If the patient's temperature is above 37° C, arterial P_{O_2} and P_{CO_2} are higher than reported, if the blood gas laboratory automatically uses a reference temperature of 37° C (the nurse should review the concepts of oxyhemoglobin dissociation). The P_{O_2} and P_{CO_2} are lower than reported, assuming a reference temperature of 37° C, in hypothermic patients. The change in P_{O_2} is approximately 6% for each degree change (celsius).

Finally, the sample is obtained anaerobically, and air must be evacuated rapidly from the syringe to prevent an alteration in the ABG values. When an air bubble reacts with the blood gas sample, the P_{O_2} is increased and the P_{CO_2} is lowered because room air P_{O_2} is approximately 150 mm Hg, and P_{CO_2} is 0 mm Hg.

An ABG sample may be obtained either from an indwelling arterial catheter or from percutaneous puncture of an artery. The easier technique is to obtain the sample from an indwelling arterial line. When frequent arterial blood samples are needed, the physician usually inserts an arterial line. The boxes on p. 90 and p. 89 describe the techniques of arterial line and percutaneous puncture sampling of ABGs.

The radial artery is the most common site of arterial puncture because of accessibility and excellent collateral circulation from the ulnar artery. The brachial (second choice) and femoral arteries (not used unless there is no

Obtaining an ABG sample by direct puncture

- Explain the procedure to the patient with emphasis on normal, quiet breathing.
- Identify site of puncture and collateral circulation.
- For radial artery, hyperextend the wrist by positioning over a rolled towel (Fig. 6-1). For brachial artery, fully extend the arm, and support the elbow with a firm towel or pillow. Obtain a heparinized syringe (3 ml) with a 1 inch, 25-gauge needle. (A 1.5 to 2 inch 22-gauge needle may be used for the femoral artery. Blood gas analysis is not affected by the size of the needle, although the smaller the hole made in the artery, the less the chance for bleeding complications.)
- Apply gloves.
- Cleanse the puncture site and glove tips with alcohol or povidone-iodine according to protocol.
- A local anesthetic may be used to decrease pain and subsequent hyperventilation, to stabilize the artery when injected bilaterally, and to reduce arterial spasm. Because most punctures are successful on the first attempt and use of a local anesthetic requires two sticks, an intradermal or subcutaneous anesthetic usually is omitted unless an indwelling arterial catheter is being inserted.
- Palpate and stabilize the artery with the second and third fingers.
- Slowly insert the needle, bevel up, at a 30 to 45 degree angle to the artery until blood flashes into the hub. The artery should be entered at an oblique angle so that circular smooth muscle fibers seal the hole when the needle is removed.
- Withdraw 1 to 3 ml arterial blood.
- Quickly remove the needle from the artery and apply direct pressure for at least 5 minutes (depending on the patient's hematological status).
- Expel air from the syringe immediately after withdrawing from the artery. Some ABG kits include a plastic cube in which to stick the needle. Air is expelled from the back of the syringe by pressing on the plunger. The help of a second nurse may be necessary.
- Rotate the syringe between your palms or your palm and a hard surface to mix the heparin with the blood.
- Cap the sample and place on crushed ice.
- At the end of 5 minutes, apply a nonobstructing pressure dressing or Band-Aid, according to protocol, over the site.
- The puncture site is assessed every 5 minutes for up to 30 minutes for bleeding, hematoma and pulse.

other arterial access) are used less frequently. The foot does not have collateral circulation by a second artery like the hand has; occlusion of the femoral artery usually results in amputation. The femoral artery lies adjacent to a large nerve and vein, and errors of venous sampling can occur. In emergencies the femoral artery may be used because of its large size and the subsequent ease of palpating the pulse when blood pressure is low.

Before an arterial puncture is performed, the nurse must assess for collateral circulation in case the artery becomes occluded. The Allen test is a technique used to assess patency and collateral circulation of the ulnar artery before the radial artery is used for sampling arterial blood. Modification of the

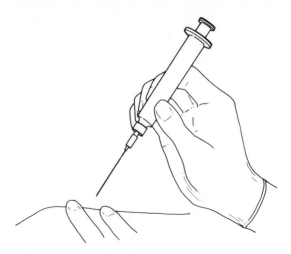

Fig. 6-1. Technique for puncture of the radial artery. (From Wade JF: *Comprehensive respiratory care*, ed 3, St Louis, 1982, Mosby–Year Book.)

Obtaining an ABG sample from an indwelling arterial catheter

- Obtain a 3 ml heparinized syringe and a 6 to 12 ml nonheparinized syringe.
- Apply nonsterile gloves.
- Remove protective dead-end cap from stopcock and place in clean, safe place. Take care not to contaminate cap.
- Place nonheparinized syringe in stopcock.*
- Turn stopcock off to pressure manometer and on to artery.
- Withdraw 3 to 5 ml blood from arterial line with nonheparinized syringe.
- Turn stopcock partially off to artery.
- Remove syringe from stopcock and discard into appropriate receptacle.
- Place heparinized syringe in stopcock.
- Turn stopcock on to artery.
- Withdraw 1 to 3 ml blood.
- Turn stopcock off to artery.
- Remove syringe and flush air from syringe.
- Immediately cap and place on crushed ice.
- Flush arterial line with heparinized or nonheparinized saline flush according to protocol.
- Flush stopcock with saline to clear blood and replace protective dead-end cap.

---

*To conserve the patient's blood, use the stopcock closest to the transducer to withdraw waste, and use the stopcock proximal to the artery to obtain the arterial sample. Pull fluid into the waste syringe until blood flows past the stopcock closest to the artery (about 6 ml). After removing the sample, slowly inject the fluid and blood back into the patient.

When this technique is used, the line is easily flushed and the patient loses less blood. However, some institutions do not allow this procedure. If the fluid is injected too rapidly, capillary pressure increases, and blood vessels in the hand can rupture spontaneously.

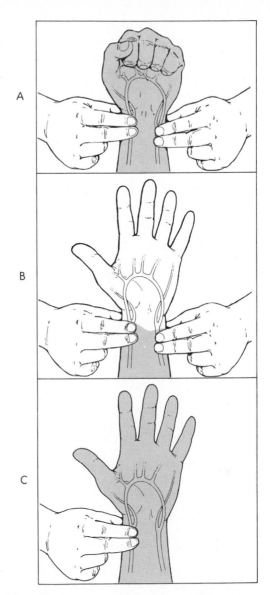

Fig. 6-2. Allen test assesses collateral circulation in ulnar artery. (**A**) The nurse occludes both arteries with firm pressure until (**B**) the hand blanches and then (**C**) releases pressure from ulnar artery to assess for return of normal hand color. (From Weilitz P: *Pocket guide to respiratory care*, ed 1, St Louis, 1991, Mosby–Year Book.)

technique by applying direct pressure over the femoral artery can be used to identify collateral arterial blood flow in the leg.

The Allen test is performed by one of two methods. The first method is to compress the radial artery for 3 minutes. If the palmar surface of the hand remains pink, the ulnar artery is patent. In the interest of time an alternate method may be used (Fig. 6-2). While the nurse compresses both the radial and the ulnar arteries with her thumbs, the patient rapidly opens and closes

Table 6-1. ABG analysis

Normal factors	Arterial	Mixed venous
pH	7.35-7.45	7.30-7.40
P_{CO_2}	35-45 mm Hg	40-46 mm Hg
P_{O_2}	80-100 mm Hg	35-42 mm Hg
S_{O_2}	95%-100%	70%-76%
HCO_3^-	22-26 mEq/L	22-26 mEq/L
Base excess	−2 to +2 mEq/L	

his fist, usually with the hand elevated, for about 30 to 60 seconds until the hand becomes white. The nurse releases pressure only from the ulnar artery, and the hand flushes within 10-15 seconds, indicating adequate collateral circulation. If the hand does not become pink, collateral circulation is inadequate, and another site should be chosen.

Interpretation of ABGs is based on memorization of the normal values for each of the components. Table 6-1 lists normal values for the most important elements obtained from an arterial and a mixed venous blood gas analysis. Having memorized normal values or with the values nearby, the nurse begins interpretation.

VENTILATION

Ventilatory or acid-base status is the first component of the blood gas to be evaluated. This is accomplished by assessing first the CO_2 and then the pH. Unfortunately, many nurses and physicians tend to look first (or only) at the P_{O_2} and often miss signs of acidosis or alkalosis. As evidenced by an elevated Pa_{CO_2}, hypoventilation can cause hypoxemia or a low Pa_{O_2}.*

Guideline 1: Whenever the Pa_{CO_2} is less than 35 mm Hg, the patient is in a state of respiratory alkalosis from alveolar hyperventilation. Conversely, any time the Pa_{CO_2} is greater than 45 mm Hg, the patient is in a state of respiratory acidosis from alveolar hypoventilation, that is ventilatory failure. Respiratory acidosis and respiratory alkalosis may be primary, or they may occur in response to a metabolic derangement.

Respiratory alkalosis

Alveolar hyperventilation is the cause of respiratory alkalosis. When CO_2 is blown off, as occurs in respiratory alkalosis, less H^+ and HCO_3^- are produced, causing an increase in pH. When respiratory alkalosis is acute, the kidneys have not had time to compensate. Although the CO_2 is decreased, the HCO_3^- remains normal. With prolonged respiratory alkalosis the kidneys excrete HCO_3^- and retain chloride to normalize the pH. With chronic respiratory alkalosis, pH is normal, and CO_2 and HCO_3^- are decreased.

The treatment for respiratory alkalosis depends on the cause. Sedation, decreased minute-ventilation ($\dot{V}_E$) on the mechanical ventilator, antipyretics, antibiotics, and oxygen are among the therapies that may be used.

---

*Note: A lowercase "a" is used to denote arterial (such as in Pa_{O_2}), an uppercase "A" is used to denote alveolar (such as in PA_{O_2}), and a lowercase "v" is used to denote venous (such as in Pv_{O_2}). A line over the lowercase "v" (such as in $P\bar{v}_{O_2}$) indicates mixed venous, usually from the pulmonary artery.

Respiratory acidosis

Alveolar hypoventilation is the primary cause of respiratory acidosis, which may be acute or chronic. Respiratory acidosis can be combined with metabolic acidosis or with metabolic alkalosis. When respiratory acidosis is acute, the pH is low. This occurs because an elevated CO_2 (as carbonic acid) causes an increase in H^+, thus a decreased pH. In acute respiratory acidosis the kidneys do not have time to compensate, and the HCO_3^- remains in the normal range. Respiratory acidosis that persists for more than a few days is termed *chronic*. The patient is unable to blow off the CO_2. The renal response to respiratory acidosis is to retain $NaHCO_3^-$ to buffer the increased acid. H^+ is excreted in the urine as HCl and NH_4Cl. Renal compensation of respiratory acidosis results in an increase in serum HCO_3^- and normal or near-normal pH, depending on the degree of compensation.

The primary treatment for respiratory acidosis is increased alveolar ventilation ($\dot{V}_A$). Sometimes this can be achieved with respiratory stimulants, although in severe cases mechanical ventilation may be necessary.

Having identified whether Pa_{CO_2} is in the normal range, the nurse identifies the effect of the carbon dioxide on the pH. A pH less than 7.35 indicates the presence of acidemia, and a pH greater than 7.45 signifies alkalemia. With acute changes in Pa_{CO_2}, the pH is abnormal in the opposite direction of the Pa_{CO_2}. Chronic changes in Pa_{CO_2} usually are accompanied by a normal or near-normal pH.

Guideline 2: A pH less than 7.35 is acidemia. A pH greater than 7.45 is alkalemia. Acidemia or alkalemia may be due either to respiratory or metabolic conditions or to combined metabolic and respiratory conditions. When pH and either P_{CO_2} or HCO_3^- are abnormal, the factor (other than pH) that is abnormal defines the origin. For instance, an abnormal pH and P_{CO_2} define a respiratory condition, and an abnormal pH and HCO_3^- define a metabolic condition.

A normal pH can be achieved when respiratory alkalosis and metabolic acidosis are present or when respiratory acidosis and metabolic alkalosis are present. The pH is abnormal in acute disorders and normal or near normal in chronic disorders. A normal pH in the presence of abnormal P_{CO_2} or HCO_3^- indicates compensation.

Interpretation of HCO_3^- can help differentiate an acute respiratory process from a chronic one. Because the HCO_3^- level is calculated from a blood gas, serum CO_2 level from a chemistry panel is more accurate. The calculated (blood gas) and measured (serum) values are often close, within 2 mEq/L. Base excess or deficit, a measurement of the amount of acid or base necessary to reestablish a pH of 7.40, can be used instead of HCO_3^-. A normal HCO_3^- value is seen in an acute respiratory process. When Pa_{CO_2} elevation is prolonged, the kidney retains HCO_3^- as reflected by an increase in serum HCO_3^-. Chronic hyperventilation results in elimination of HCO_3^- to reestablish acid-base balance.

Guideline 3: If the HCO_3^- is less than 22 mEq/L, metabolic acidosis is present. If the HCO_3^- is greater than 26 mEq/L, metabolic alkalosis is present.

Metabolic acidosis

Whereas respiratory acidosis is caused by an increase in volatile carbonic acid, metabolic acidosis is caused by an increase in fixed body acids. The most common causes of increased fixed acids are sepsis, circulatory failure (increases lactic acid), diabetes or starvation (increases ketone acid), and renal disease (increases inorganic phosphate or sulfate acids). Chronic metabolic acidosis is accompanied by a decrease in HCO_3^- in an attempt to buffer the increase in fixed acids, which cannot be blown off. Depending on the amount of fixed acids, HCO_3^- may or may not be able to buffer the fixed acid adequately. Hyperventilation occurs almost immediately as a response of pH-sensitive receptors in the carotid and aortic bodies to an increase in circulating H^+. Because the lungs compensate so rapidly for an increase in the amount of fixed body acids, it is rare to see an acute metabolic acidosis with a normal CO_2 level.

The treatment for metabolic acidosis is twofold: immediately restore the pH and treat the underlying cause. The acid must be neutralized, and acid-base values must be normalized. Sodium bicarbonate ($NaHCO_3^-$) is the drug used most frequently to nullify immediately the effects of increased H^+. It is important to remember that if the cause is not identified and treated, metabolic acidosis is likely to recur. In the case of increased lactic acid, medications and other therapies to improve cardiac output are indicated. With ketoacidosis, insulin is used for diabetes, and nutrition is used for starvation. Patients with renal disease often require the addition of phosphate-binding medications to their treatment regimen.

Metabolic alkalosis

The most common cause of metabolic alkalosis is potassium depletion. Prolonged diuretic therapy, gastrointestinal disorders, and excessive gastric drainage are usually the origin of excessive K^+ loss. Increased potassium excretion causes a decrease in circulating chloride. In metabolic alkalosis low levels of K^+ (hypokalemia) usually are accompanied by low levels of chloride (hypochloremia). Cl^- also may be excreted excessively as HCl. As HCl is excreted, less H^+ and Cl^- are available to bind with Na^+ and HCO_3^-. The amount of $NaHCO_3^-$ increases in the blood, and metabolic alkalosis results. The same outcome occurs when excessive $NaHCO_3^-$ is administered, such as in a cardiac arrest. When metabolic alkalosis is present, the pH-sensitive carotid and aortic bodies reduce respiratory drive and $\dot{V}_E$. CO_2 levels frequently are elevated, although the CO_2 usually does not increase above 45 mm Hg.

The treatment for metabolic alkalosis is correction of the cause. Potassium repletion is frequently necessary. Also, nasogastric drainage can be decreased through intermittent clamping, the amount or frequency of diuretics can be decreased, or the kind of diuretic can be changed (usually to acetazolamide [Diamox], an angiotensin-converting enzyme inhibitor).

To help differentiate how much of the change in the pH from baseline is due to respiratory conditions and how much is related to metabolic conditions, the nurse uses one of the following formulas.

Guideline 4: For every 10 mm Hg change in $Paco_2$ from 40 mm Hg, there is a corresponding change in pH of 0.08 from 7.40 in the opposite direction. An increase in $Paco_2$ results in a decrease in pH.

Guideline 5: For every 0.1 change in pH from 7.40, there is a corresponding change in HCO_3^- from 24 mEq/L of 1.2 in the same direction. An increase in HCO_3^- results in an increase in pH.

To help explain Guidelines 4 and 5 consider the following blood gas values: pH 7.28, $Paco_2$ 50, HCO_3^- 24. The nurse determines that the patient has a respiratory acidosis and acidemia. The pH seems lower than it should be for a $Paco_2$ of 50 mm Hg. The nurse wants to determine whether there is also a metabolic cause in addition to the respiratory cause. Using Guideline 4, the nurse calculates that there is a 10 mm Hg increase in $Paco_2$, for which the nurse anticipates a 0.08 decrease in pH. The actual pH is 0.12 lower than normal. The remaining 0.04 change in pH is due to metabolic causes. This patient is in a state of mixed respiratory and metabolic acidosis.

The blood gas change is not always exactly 10 mm Hg as in the above example. To determine the amount of pH change for less or more CO_2, a mathematic equation can be used:

$$\frac{\text{Actual } Paco_2 \text{ change}}{10} = \frac{\text{X (anticipated pH change)}}{0.08}$$

For instance, if the $Paco_2$ change is 14 less than 40 (26 mm Hg), then the following mathematic equation would apply:

$$\frac{14}{10} = \frac{X}{0.08} \text{ then } 1.4 = \frac{X}{0.08} \text{ and X} = 1.4 \times 0.08$$

$$\text{or } 0.112 \text{ (e.g., } 7.40 + 0.112 = 7.512)$$

It is essential for the nurse to have grasped the concept of assessing ventilatory and acid-base status before progressing to interpreting other components of the ABG. Table 6-2 identifies the mechanisms for acid-base abnormalities and possible causes for each of them. Table 6-3 lists the characteristics of $Paco_2$, pH, and HCO_3^- for naming acid-base abnormalities. The following examples are provided for the self-assessment.

pH	$Paco_2$	HCO_3^-	Disorder
7.27	56	24	Acute respiratory acidosis
7.49	30	21	Chronic respiratory alkalosis
7.29	47	24	Respiratory/metabolic acidosis
7.33	28	20	Chronic metabolic acidosis
7.40	40	24	Normal
7.52	44	28	Acute metabolic alkalosis
7.41	55	30	Chronic respiratory acidosis
7.58	18	24	Acute respiratory alkalosis
7.44	45	27	Chronic metabolic alkalosis
7.25	36	20	Acute metabolic acidosis

ASSESSING OXYGENATION

Once the nurse has evaluated ventilatory and acid-base status, the next step is to assess the patient's oxygenation status. To assess oxygenation status the nurse evaluates Pao_2 and Sao_2. As stated in previous chapters, oxygen saturation is the most important component of oxygenation because Pao_2 is altered by age, altitude, and ventilation-perfusion abnormalities.

Guideline 6: Any time the Pao_2 is less than 80 mm Hg in patients younger than 60 years, hypoxemia is present. In patients older than 60 years a predicted Pao_2 at sea level should be calculated using the following formula: $109 - (0.43 \times \text{age}) +/- 4$. *A Pao_2 that is greater than 100 mm Hg is clinically not necessary and may harm the patient if high levels of supplemental oxygen are in use.*

Guideline 7: Whenever the arterial saturation falls below 90%, the patient is on the steep curve of the oxyhemoglobin dissociation curve, and small decreases in Pao_2 can result in large decreases in arterial saturation.

Table 6-2. Acid-base disturbances

Disturbance	Mechanism	Cause
Respiratory acidosis	*Acute*—Increase in CO_2, thus $H_2CO_3^-$ and H^+ cause decreased pH *Chronic*—Renal response to increased CO_2 is excrete more H^+: $NaHCO_3$ reabsorbed to restore pH; increased HCO_3^-	Alveolar hypoventilation caused by pulmonary disease, drugs, metabolic alkalosis response (tempered), sleep, obesity
Respiratory alkalosis	*Acute*—Less CO_2 (blown off), excess base, increased pH *Chronic*—Renal response to decreased CO_2 is excrete HCO_3^-, retain Cl^- to restore pH; thus less CO_2 and less HCO_3^- are present	Alveolar hyperventilation caused by excess mechanical ventilation, metabolic acidosis response, hepatic failure, bacteremia, fever, thyrotoxicosis, hysteria, anxiety, hypoxemia response
Metabolic acidosis	Increased acids in blood, causes loss of base and decreases pH; respiratory response is to blow off CO_2 and increase pH	Increases in fixed acids: lactic acid caused by circulatory failure, ketoacid caused by diabetes or starvation, phosphate or sulfate caused by renal disease, acid ingestion, caused by salicylates, respiratory alkalosis response
Metabolic alkalosis	Retention of base or loss of acid results in increased pH and HCO_3^-; minimal CO_2 response results in slightly elevated CO_2	Retained base or acid loss caused by excess gastric drainage, vomiting, burns, K^+ depletion (from diuretics), excessive $NaHCO_3$ use

Table 6-3. Acid-base analysis

Classification	Pa_{CO_2}	pH	HCO_3^- or base excess*
Simple disorders			
Acute respiratory acidosis	I	D	N
Acute respiratory alkalosis	D	I	N
Acute metabolic acidosis	N	D	D
Acute metabolic alkalosis	N	I	I
Mixed disorders			
Chronic respiratory acidosis	I	N	I
Chronic respiratory alkalosis	D	N	D
Chronic metabolic acidosis	D	N/D	D
Chronic metabolic alkalosis	I	N/I	I

I = Increased, D = Decreased, N = Normal.
*Either HCO_3^- or base excess can be used.

Both the Pa_{O_2} and the Sa_{O_2} must be interpreted in relationship to the amount of oxygen the patient is receiving. The age-based formula given in Guideline 6 applies only to gases drawn on room-air oxygen. Many ill patients receive supplemental oxygen, which complicates assessment of oxygenation.

Alveolar air equation

There are several methods of correlating the amount of oxygen inhaled with that in arterial blood oxygen. One technique is to calculate the difference between the amount of air inhaled and the amount of air in arterial blood, termed the *alveolar-arterial oxygen difference* or *gradient (A-aD$_{O_2}$)*. The alveolar-air equation is used to calculate the A-aD$_{O_2}$ and other equations that follow.

The first step of the alveolar air equation is to calculate the amount of oxygen in inspired air (Pi_{O_2}). For dry gas the Pi_{O_2} is equal to the fraction of oxygen in the air multiplied by the barometric pressure (P_B).

$$Pi_{O_2} = P_B \times Fi_{O_2}$$

The Fi_{O_2} is expressed as a decimal; that is, 21% Fi_{O_2} is 0.21. At sea level the room-air Pi_{O_2} is $760 \times 0.21 = 159$ mm Hg. (Note: The actual concentration of oxygen in room air is 20.94%, but it has been rounded to 21%.) However, air in the lung is humidified, and the amount of pressure exerted by water vapor PH_2O must be subtracted. The pressure exerted by water vapor at body temperature is 47 mm Hg. Therefore, the Pi_{O_2} of humidified room-air oxygen is $(760 - 47) \times 0.21 = 149$ mm Hg. Table 6-4 contains the Pi_{O_2} for different levels of Fi_{O_2}.

$$Pi_{O_2} = (P_B - PH_2O) \times Fi_{O_2}$$

Table 6-4. Pi_{O_2} for different levels of Fi_{O_2}

Fi_{O_2}	Pi_{O_2} mm Hg (humidified and at sea level)
0.21	149
0.25	178
0.30	214
0.35	250
0.40	285
0.45	321
0.50	356
0.55	392
0.60	428
0.65	463
0.70	499
0.75	535
0.80	570
0.85	606
0.90	641
0.95	677
1.0	713

The alveoli also contain CO_2, which exerts a pressure. The amount of pressure exerted by CO_2 is equal to the $Paco_2$ divided by the respiratory-exchange ratio (R). The respiratory-exchange ratio represents the ratio of CO_2 production to O_2 consumption. In normal, healthy individuals the respiratory-exchange ratio is considered to be 0.8 (CO_2 production of 200 ml/min and O_2 consumption of 250 ml/min), although diet plays a role. When a high-carbohydrate diet is consumed, the respiratory-exchange ratio is closer to 1.0. A high-fat diet can lower the respiratory-exchange ratio to 0.7. For most patients the nurse uses a respiratory-exchange ratio of 0.8 or 1.0 for simplicity, although the nurse realizes that assumption of any value in the absence of mass spectrometry and exhaled-gas analysis may not accurately reflect the patient's changing status and alters the alveolar gas equation.

Following is the complete alveolar gas equation, taking into consideration water-vapor pressure and CO_2 pressure:

$$PAo_2 = [(P_B - PH_2O) \times Fio_2] - Paco_2/R$$

Assuming a R of 0.8, the equation can be simplified to $Pao_2 = Pio_2 - (Paco_2 \times 1.25)$. If a patient's $Paco_2$ is a normal 40 mm Hg on room air, $PAo_2 = 149 - (40 \times 1.25) = 149 - 50 = 99$ mm Hg.

Oxygen gradient. Once the alveolar gas equation has been determined, the nurse can calculate the $A-aDo_2$. A normal $A-aDo_2$ is 10 to 15 mm Hg. As age increases, the Pao_2 decreases, and the normal $A-aDo_2$ widens. The following formula can be used to calculate the normal $A-aDo_2$ in older adults: $2.5 + (0.43 \times age)$. For example, to calculate the normal $A-aDo_2$ of an 80-year-old patient, the equation is $2.5 + (0.43 \times 80) = 2.5 + 34.4 = 37$. In an 80-year-old person, a normal $A-aDo_2$ is less than 37 mm Hg.

The $A-aDo_2$ also widens with lung disease or respiratory failure. Ventilation-perfusion imbalances, alveolar hypoventilation, physiological shunts, and diffusion defects result in widening of the $A-aDo_2$. It is important for the nurse to calculate the patient's $A-aDo_2$ to observe for trends. When the $A-aDo_2$ for a particular patient widens, the nurse assesses for deteriorating pulmonary function. Conversely, narrowing of the $A-aDo_2$ indicates that the patient's pulmonary status is improving.

One of the problems in calculating the $A-aDo_2$ is that the relationship between increasing Fio_2 and alveolar oxygen tension is nonlinear. In addition, the difference between alveolar and arterial blood oxygen is wider at higher levels of supplemental oxygen because the PAo_2 is higher. As Fio_2 is decreased, it is difficult to discern whether the patient is actually improving, as indicated by a decreasing $A-aDo_2$, or whether the change in $A-aDo_2$ is just a function of decreasing Fio_2. For instance, a patient has a Pao_2 of 150 on 60% Fio_2. He is decreased to 50% Fio_2 with a resultant Pao_2 of 125 mm Hg. The $Paco_2$ is 40 mm Hg. The $A-aDo_2$ on 60% Fio_2 is $428 - 40 (1.25) - 150 = 228$ mm Hg; on 50% Fio_2 the $A-aDo_2$ is $356 - 40 (1.25) - 125 = 181$ mm Hg.

Ratio of Pao_2 to Fio_2. Some nurses assess gas exchange by using the ratio of Pao_2 to Fio_2 (P/F), which is simpler to calculate at the bedside than the $A-aDo_2$. This ratio has problems similar to those of the $A-aDo_2$, although they are much less pronounced. The P/F ratio is fairly consistent at the lower range of Fio_2. Using the above values on 60% Fio_2, the P/F is $150/0.6 = 250$, and on 50% Fio_2 the P/F is 125/0.5 = 250. A normal P/F is 475.

Oxygen ratio. Perhaps the most useful method to compare Pao_2 at varying levels of Fio_2 is the arterial/alveolar ratio, abbreviated a/Ao_2. Although the $A\text{-}aDo_2$ widens at increasing levels of Fio_2, the a/Ao_2 remains relatively stable. Using the same examples cited above, the a/Ao_2 at 60% Fio_2 is 150/378 = 0.399, and at 50% Fio_2 it is 125/306 = 0.406. Observe that the $A\text{-}ao_2$ suggested improvement in gas exchange, the P/F and a/Ao_2 demonstrate no change in gas exchange. A normal a/Ao_2 is 0.8. The box below demonstrates the comparison of $A\text{-}aDo_2$, P/F, and a/Ao_2 for the same patient at two levels of O_2.

Comparison of $A\text{-}aDo_2$, P/F, and a/Ao_2

Mr. Doe is in the intensive care unit. He became acutely short of breath, and the following ABGs were obtained on room air: pH 7.53, $Paco_2$ 25, Pao_2 66, Sao_2 91. Several hours later on 60% Fio_2 ABGs were repeated and demonstrated the subsequent values: pH 7.49, $Paco_2$ 29, Pao_2 188, Sao_2 98 (P_B 760 mm Hg). The nurse calculated $A\text{-}ao_2$, P/F, and a/Ao_2 for the two sets of ABGs. Although the $A\text{-}ao_2$ suggests that the patient's gas exchange has worsened, the P/F suggests the opposite, that is, that the patient's gas exchange has improved. According to the a/Ao_2 the patient's gas exchange is actually unchanged.

	$A\text{-}ao_2$	P/F	a/Ao_2
Room air	119 − 66 = 53	66/0.21 = 314	66/119 = 0.56
60% Fio_2	392 − 220 = 172	220/0.6 = 367	220/392 = 0.56

One of the advantages of calculating the a/Ao_2 is that a patient's Pao_2 at a given Fio_2 can be predicted. This is especially important when weaning a patient from supplemental oxygen and mechanical ventilation or when increasing the amount of Fio_2 quickly and safely is necessary. The use of the a/Ao_2 in predicting Pao_2 assumes that the patient's cardiac output, ventilation-perfusion matching, shunt, O_2 consumption, and $Paco_2$ remain constant. Continuing with the above patient, assume that the physician wants to decrease the patient's Fio_2 to obtain a Pao_2 of 80 mm Hg. Using the following formula, the nurse calculates the amount of Fio_2 to be used:

$$PAo_2 \text{ required} = \frac{Pao_2 \text{ desired}}{a/Ao_2}$$

$$PAo_2 = 80/0.406 = 197 \text{ mm Hg}$$

Assuming that the patient has a respiratory-exchange ratio of 0.8, then

$$PAo_2 = [(P_B - PH_2O) \times Fio_2] - [Paco_2 \times 1.25]$$
$$197 = (713 \times Fio_2) - (40 \times 1.25)$$
$$197 = 713 \times Fio_2 - 50$$
$$247 = 713 \times Fio_2$$
$$247/713 = Fio_2$$
$$0.346 = Fio_2 \text{ (approximately 35% } Fio_2)$$

A similar benefit is being able to calculate the patient's A-aDo$_2$ for different altitudes. As the altitude increases from sea level, the P$_B$ becomes progressively less. The P$_B$ at 5000 feet is approximately 600 mm Hg. When patients who use supplemental O$_2$ travel to high altitudes or fly, their O$_2$ needs change because less inspired O$_2$ is available. Some patients who do not require O$_2$ at sea level may require the use of supplemental O$_2$ when flying or traveling to high altitudes. Flying is equivalent to traveling to high altitudes because most planes are pressurized between 5000 and 8000 feet above sea level. Airplanes are pressurized at different altitudes, depending on the airline, the pilot, the weather, and other factors.

To help explain how the A-aDo$_2$ can be used to predict O$_2$ needs when flying, consider the following patient.

Mr. Jones has chronic obstructive pulmonary disease (COPD). He uses 2 LPM (about 28% Fio$_2$) supplemental O$_2$ and is flying to Miami to board a cruise ship. His ABG readings demonstrate a Pao$_2$ of 65 mm Hg and a Paco$_2$ of 45 mm Hg with a normal pH and Sao$_2$. Using the alveolar air equation, the nurse calculates the PAo$_2$ to be 713 (0.28) − 45 (1.25) = 200 − 56 = 144 (sea level). The A-aDo$_2$ is 144 − 65 = 79 (sea level). If the P$_B$ is 600 mm Hg, then the patient's PAo$_2$, assuming no further CO$_2$ retention, would be (600 − 47) 0.28 − 45 (1.25) = 155 − 56 = 99. Subtracting the patient's known A-aDo$_2$ from the available PAo$_2$ gives the patient a Pao$_2$ of 99 − 79 = 20 mm Hg, which is not compatible with life. The a/Ao$_2$ can be used to estimate the amount of O$_2$ that the patient requires. In this instance the patient needs about 36% Fio$_2$ (5 to 6 LPM) to maintain the same 65 mm Hg Pao$_2$. (PAo$_2$ = 65/0.451 = 144 mm Hg and 144 = 553 × Fio$_2$ − 56. Therefore, 144 + 56 = 553 × Fio$_2$ and 200 = 553 × Fio$_2$. Fio$_2$ = 200/553 = 36.1%.)

Shunt equation

An understanding of ventilation-perfusion abnormalities and O$_2$ content is essential. The nurse is encouraged to review necessary content in previous chapters before proceeding.

The physiological shunt is calculated frequently in critically ill patients. The nurse should recall that a physiological shunt refers to the amount of blood that never comes in contact with alveoli. Venous blood bypasses ventilated lung and mixes with arterial blood. Therefore, blood shunted past alveoli and not oxygenated has characteristics similar to those of mixed venous blood. The overall arterial oxygen content is lowered. The greater the area of shunt, the lower the overall arterial O$_2$ content. A 1% to 2% physiological shunt is normal and results from the bronchial circulation and the Thesbian veins from the myocardium. In critically ill patients physiological shunt often is increased. The most frequent causes of increased physiological shunt are atelectasis and alveolar congestion, which are associated with myriad pulmonary conditions.

For the nurse to calculate shunt, the patient breathes a high concentration of O$_2$, typically 100%. Care must be exercised when administering 100% O$_2$. The nurse should recall that N$_2$ is necessary for alveolar stability. Unstable alveoli may collapse because N$_2$ is washed out with the administration of "pure" O$_2$. This is referred to as *absorption atelectasis* and can cause increased intrapulmonary shunting.

After the patient has breathed the increased O$_2$ concentration for 15 to 30 minutes, samples of arterial blood and mixed venous blood are drawn, and the patient is returned to his previous Fio$_2$. Any artery may be used for sampling arterial blood. The mixed venous sample should represent the sum of all metabolic demands. Thus a pulmonary artery catheter should be used, and the sample should be obtained from the most distal port. A mixed venous blood sample from a central venous catheter is not recommended because venous O_2 tensions from the superior and inferior vena cava may differ, depending on upper and lower body metabolisms.

Several different equations are available to calculate shunt. The most accurate method to calculate the amount of intrapulmonary shunting is to use the classic shunt equation (see the box below). The *classic* shunt equation identifies the relationship between total cardiac output and shunted cardiac output (Shapiro and Harrison, 1985). A simpler shunt equation (the *clinical* shunt equation) assumes that hemoglobin is saturated completely with O_2 in capillary and arterial blood. The clinical shunt equation assumes the only difference between capillary and arterial blood is the amount of dissolved O_2; the latter varies with O_2 tension (see box on p. 102). When the PaO_2 is greater than 150 mm Hg, hemoglobin is considered to be fully saturated with O_2. The clinical shunt equation is less accurate because the difference in arterial-venous content in critically ill patients is usually not in the normal range of 4.5 to 6 vol% but is closer to 2.5 to 4.5 vol% (Shapiro and Harrison, 1985). A greater margin of error is introduced into the calculation because the user must assign a value to the difference in arterial-venous content. The clinical shunt equation is useful when a pulmonary artery catheter is not available.

A third shunt equation useful in the clinical area is depicted in the box on p. 102. The alternate shunt equation is more accurate than the clinical shunt equation previously described. It is useful when $S\overline{v}O_2$ is monitored continuously. The $P\overline{v}O_2$ can be calculated from a nomogram when a blood sample is not available. Either clinical shunt equation may be used as long as the limitations are recognized.

Classic shunt (QS/QT) equation

$$\frac{QS}{QT} = Cco_2 - \frac{Cco_2 - Cao_2}{Cco_2 - C\overline{v}o_2}$$

$Cco_2 \qquad\qquad = (Hb \times 1.34) + (PAo_2 \times 0.003)$

$\qquad\qquad\qquad$ where $PAo_2 = (P_B - PH_2O) \times Fio_2$

$Cao_2 \qquad\qquad = \dfrac{Hb \times 1.34 \times Sao_2}{100} + (Pao_2 \times 0.003)$

$C\overline{v}o_2 \qquad\qquad = \dfrac{Hb \times 1.34 \times S\overline{v}o_2}{100} + (P\overline{v}o_2 \times 0.003)$

Cco_2 = Calculated content of alveolar O_2 (ideal).

Cao_2 = Calculated content of arterial O_2 (actual).

$C\overline{v}o_2$ = Calculated content of mixed venous O_2 (actual).

Clinical shunt equation

$$\frac{QS}{QT} = \frac{(PAo_2 - Pao_2) \times 0.003}{(Cao_2 - C\bar{v}o_2) + (PAo_2 - Pao_2) \times 0.003}$$

$PAo_2 = (P_B - PH_2O) \times Fio_2$

Pao_2 measured on ABGs

$Cao_2 - C\bar{v}o_2$ assumed to be below normal (such as 3.5 vol%) in the critically ill patient

---

Alternate clinical shunt equation

$$\frac{(Hb \times 1.34)(1 - Sao_2) + (0.003)(PAo_2 - Pao_2)}{(Hb \times 1.34)(1 - S\bar{v}o_2) + (0.003)(PAo_2 - P\bar{v}o_2)}$$

The following examples demonstrate use of the classic and clinical shunt equations. Note that in both examples shunt is underestimated grossly, using the clinical shunt equation. The variance between the classic and alternate clinical shunt equations is less than 1% at the same time.

Example 1: Mr. Jones is in the intensive care unit after a coronary artery bypass graft surgery. He is on a ventilator with the following ABG values on 50% Fio_2: pH 7.40, $Paco_2$ 40, Pao_2 98, Sao_2 97%. Mixed venous blood gases revealed $P\bar{v}o_2$ 35, $S\bar{v}o_2$ 75%. His hemoglobin is 12.1 g, and the P_B is 747 mm Hg. Measurements have been rounded to two decimal places.

$$PAo_2 = (747 - 47) \times 0.50 = 350$$

$$Cco_2 = (12.1 \times 1.34) + (350 \times 0.003) = 16.21 + 1.05 = 17.26$$

$$Cao_2 = \frac{12.1 \times 1.34 \times 97}{100} + (98 \times 0.003) = 15.75 + 0.29 = 16.04$$

$$C\bar{v}o_2 = \frac{12.1 \times 1.34 \times 75}{100} + (35 \times 0.003) = 12.16 + 0.10 = 12.26$$

$$\text{Classic shunt } \frac{QS}{QT} = \frac{17.26 - 16.04}{17.26 - 12.26} = \frac{1.22}{5.00} = 24.5\%$$

$$\text{Clinical shunt } \frac{QS}{QT} = \frac{(350 - 98)(0.003)}{3.5 + (350 - 98)(0.003)} = \frac{0.76}{4.26} = 17.8\%$$

$$\text{Alternate clinical shunt } \frac{QS}{QT} = \frac{(16.21)(1 - 0.97) + (0.003)(350 - 98)}{(16.21)(1 - 0.75) + (0.003)(350 - 35)}$$

$$= \frac{0.49 + 0.76}{4.05 + 0.94} = \frac{1.25}{4.99} = 25.0\%$$

Example 2: Mrs. Smith is admitted to the intensive care unit after a motor vehicle accident, in which she sustained blunt chest trauma. She has the following ABG values: pH 7.35, $Paco_2$ 46, Pao_2 72, Sao_2 93%, and MVGs $P\bar{v}o_2$ 30, $S\bar{v}o_2$ 62 on 40% Fio_2. Her hemoglobin is 10 g. The P_B is 700 mm Hg.

$$PA_{O_2} = (700 - 47) \times 0.40 = 261$$

$$Cc_{O_2} = (10 \times 1.34) + (261 \times 0.003) = 13.4 + .78 = 14.18$$

$$Ca_{O_2} = \frac{(10 \times 1.34 \times 93)}{100} + (72 \times 0.003) = 12.46 + 0.22 = 12.68$$

$$C\bar{v}_{O_2} = \frac{(10 \times 1.34 \times 62)}{100} + (30 \times 0.003) = 8.31 + 0.09 = 8.4$$

$$\text{Classic shunt } \frac{QS}{QT} = \frac{14.18 - 12.68}{14.18 - 8.4} = \frac{1.5}{5.78} = 25.9\%$$

$$\text{Clinical shunt } \frac{QS}{QT} = \frac{(261 - 72)(0.003)}{3.5 + (261 - 72)(0.003)} = \frac{0.57}{4.07} = 14\%$$

$$\text{Alternate clinical shunt } \frac{QS}{QT} = \frac{(13.4)(1 - 0.93) + (261 - 72)(0.003)}{(13.4)(1 - 0.62) + (261 - 30)(0.003)}$$

$$= \frac{0.94 + 0.57}{5.09 + 0.69} = \frac{1.51}{5.78} = 26.1\%$$

CONCLUSION

Assessment of ABGs is essential to understanding the patient's ventilatory, oxygenation, and metabolic states. At the most basic level the blood gas is classified into one of four categories: respiratory or metabolic, acidosis or alkalosis. ABGs also are assessed at a higher level, as appropriate. The amount of O_2 inhaled is compared to the amount present in arterial blood. There are multiple ways to determine the relationship of arterial and alveolar O_2. The best way in critically ill patients is to calculate the a/A_{O_2}. Consistently calculating the relationship of inhaled (alveolar) O_2 to arterial O_2 demonstrates clinical stability, deterioration, or improvement in the patient's condition.

BIBLIOGRAPHY

Bageant R: Variation in arterial blood gas measurements due to sampling techniques, *Respir Care* 20(6):565-570, 1975.

Baum GL, Wolinsky E: *Textbook of pulmonary diseases*, ed 3, Boston, 1983, Little & Brown.

Burton GC, Hodgkin JE: *Respiratory care: a guide to clinical practice*, ed 2, Philadelphia, 1984, JB Lippincott.

Cohen A, Taeusch HW, Stanton C: Usefulness of the arterial/alveolar tension ratio in the care of infants with respiratory distress syndrome, *Respir Care* 28(2):169-173, 1983.

Davenport HW: *The ABC of acid-base chemistry*, ed 5, Chicago, 1971, University of Chicago Press.

Demers R, Irwin R: Management of hypercapnic respiratory failure: a systematic approach, *Respir Care* 24(4):328-335, 1979.

Fromm G: Using basic laboratory data to evaluate patients with acute respiratory failure, *Crit C Q* 1(4):43-51, 1979.

Guyton AC: *Textbook of medical physiology*, Philadelphia, 1981, WB Saunders.

Hess D et al: The validity of assessing arterial blood gases 10 minutes after an F_{IO_2} change in mechanically ventilated patients without chronic pulmonary disease, *Respir Care* 30(12), 1037-1041, 1985.

Hinshaw H, Murray J: *Diseases of the chest*, ed 4, Philadelphia, 1980, WB Saunders.

Keyes JL: Blood gas analysis and assessment of acid-base status, *Heart Lung* 5(2):247-255, 1976.

Morrison M: *Respiratory intensive care nursing*, ed 2, Boston, 1979, Little, Brown & Co.

Murray JF, Nadel JA, eds: *Textbook of respiratory medicine*, Philadelphia, 1988, WB Saunders.

Narins R, Emmett M: Simple and mixed acid-base disorders: a practical approach, *Medicine* 59(3):161-187, 1980.

Netter F: *The CIBA collection of medical illustrations*, vol 7: respiratory system, New York, 1979, CIBA Pharmaceutical.

Norkool DM: Current concepts in hyperbaric oxygenation and its application in critical care, *Heart Lung* 8(4):728-735, 1979.

Paré JAP, Fraser RG: *Synopsis of diseases of the chest,* Philadelphia, 1983, WB Saunders.

Shapiro B, Harrison R et al: *Clinical applications of respiratory care,* ed 3, St Louis, 1985, Mosby–Year Book.

Shoemaker WC, Thompson WL, Holbrook PR: *The Society of Critical Care Medicine textbook of critical care,* Philadelphia, 1984, WB Saunders.

Simmons DH, ed: *Current pulmonology,* vol 7, St Louis, 1986, Mosby–Year Book.

Simmons D: Evaluation of acid-base status, *Basics Respir Dis* 2(3), 1974.

Slonim N, Hamilton L: *Respiratory physiology,* ed 4, St Louis, 1981, Mosby–Year Book.

Sue D: Measurement of shunt in respiratory failure, *Chest* 78(6):898-9, 1980.

Swearingen PL, Sommers MS, Miller K: *Manual of critical care: applying nursing diagnoses to adult critical illness,* St Louis, 1988, Mosby–Year Book.

Wade JF: *Comprehensive respiratory care: physiology and technique,* ed 3, St Louis, 1982, Mosby–Year Book.

West J: *Respiratory physiology: the essentials,* ed 3, Baltimore, 1985, Williams & Wilkins.

White K: Completing the hemodynamic picture: $S\bar{v}o_2$, *Heart Lung* 14(3):272-280, 1985.

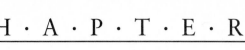

C·H·A·P·T·E·R   7

Interpretation of a Chest X-ray Film

Objectives

- Compare and contrast portable, anterior-posterior, and decubitus chest x-ray films.
- Identify the following structures on a chest x-ray film: carina, heart, aorta, diaphragm, costophrenic angle, and ribs.
- Discuss the density differences of metal, fat, water, and air on a chest x-ray film.
- Identify proper position in a patient by examining the chest x-ray film of an endotracheal tube, pulmonary artery catheter, intraaortic balloon pump, central venous catheter, or chest tube.
- Differentiate a pleural effusion from a pneumothorax on a chest x-ray film.

Until recently it was not necessary for the nurse to be able to assess a chest x-ray film. With the increase in technology and acuity of patients' conditions, it is helpful if not essential for the nurse, especially the critical care nurse, to understand the basic principles of interpretation of a chest x-ray film. The purpose of this chapter is to familiarize the nurse with characteristics of the normal chest x-ray film. After reading this chapter, the nurse will be able to identify landmarks that aid in assessing for abnormalities. The most common abnormalities found in chest x-ray films are discussed.

TYPES OF X-RAY EXAMINATIONS

A chest x-ray examination is usually done with the patient standing, although a sitting position may also be used. The patient places his anterior chest firmly against a plate or cassette that holds the film. The x-ray machine is positioned 6 feet behind the patient, who is instructed to take a deep breath and hold it for a few seconds as the x-ray beam is delivered. This is a posterior-anterior (PA) chest x-ray examination and provides the physician with the most accurate view of the patient's chest. The images produced on the film are generally less magnified but sharper in a PA chest x-ray film.

In some instances the patient is unable to be transported to the radiology

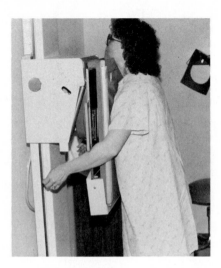

Fig. 7-1. Position of the patient for a posterior-anterior chest x-ray film.

department. In such cases an anterior-posterior (AP) chest x-ray examination may be done. The patient is usually supine or is sitting upright in a bed for convenience. Placed approximately 3 feet in front of the patient, the x-ray beam passes through the patient from the anterior to the posterior (Fig. 7-1). The patient is asked to take a deep breath, or the nurse delivers a manual breath through the ventilator as the x-ray beam is delivered. An AP film is less sharp than a PA film. Images are more magnified but less sharp in an AP film.

When a portable chest x-ray examination or other x-ray examination is done, the nurse is careful to prevent self-exposure. Whenever possible, the nurse should leave the room. At least 8 feet should separate the nurse from the patient and x-ray beam. When the patient's condition does not permit the nurse to leave the room, the nurse (and radiology technician if present) should wear a lead apron. Ideally the apron should cover the chest and abdomen, as well as the neck. This prevents excessive radiation of the nurse. Some patients, especially women who are pregnant or of child-bearing potential, should have their abdomens shielded during a chest x-ray examination.

The physician frequently orders a lateral chest x-ray film to be taken at the same time as a PA film. Unless specified, the patient is positioned with his left side against the plate. The x-ray beam passes through the patient from right to left. A lateral x-ray examination is helpful in identifying abnormalities behind the heart, along the spine, or at the base of the lung. If the physician suspects an abnormality in the right chest, he may order a right lateral chest x-ray examination, in which the patient's right chest is placed against the plate. When the right side of the chest is against the plate, images in the right lung are less magnified but sharper.

An oblique chest x-ray examination, or visualization of the chest at an angle, may be used to localize lesions without interference from bony or overlying structures. This technique is used when the physician needs to visualize the trachea or when an anterior lesion is differentiated from a posterior lesion when bilateral lung disease is present. A right oblique film is taken with the

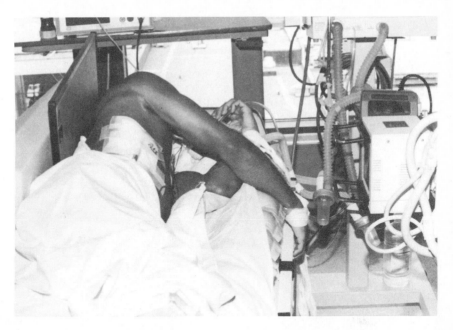

Fig. 7-2. Position of the patient for a decubitus chest x-ray examination.

right-front area of the patient's chest against the plate. The patient is positioned with his left-front chest against the plate for a left oblique film. The physician determines whether a left or right oblique film is necessary, depending on the position of the suspected lesion.

The lateral decubitus, or side-lying, position is used to assess for air fluid levels or free-flowing pleural fluid (Fig. 7-2). When the patient is upright, gravity pulls the fluid to the bases of the lungs, where pleural fluid frequently obscures the diaphragm. In a supine patient, free-flowing pleural fluid settles posteriorly along the dependent regions of the lungs, where visualization is frequently impossible, especially when bilateral pleural effusions are present. Pleural fluid gravitates laterally toward the dependent lung when the patient is positioned on his side. To do a lateral decubitus chest x-ray examination, the patient is positioned on his side. The x-ray beam is positioned horizontal to the patient and parallel to the floor. A decubitus x-ray examination done with the patient supine is called a *cross-table lateral x-ray examination.*

When the physician needs to better visualize the apices of the chest, a lordotic chest x-ray examination is ordered. The clavicles are projected above the apices in a lordotic view. The left lingula and right middle lung fields are also better identified on a lordotic chest x-ray film. For a lordotic chest x-ray examination the patient is positioned as for a PA or AP chest x-ray examination. The x-ray machine is elevated or lowered and angled downward or upward 45 degrees.

NORMAL STRUCTURES

Knowledge of anatomy is used to identify normal and abnormal structures on a chest x-ray film. Fig. 7-3 shows the normal position of anatomical structures observed on an anterior or posterior chest x-ray film. The corresponding normal PA film also is shown in Figure 7-3.

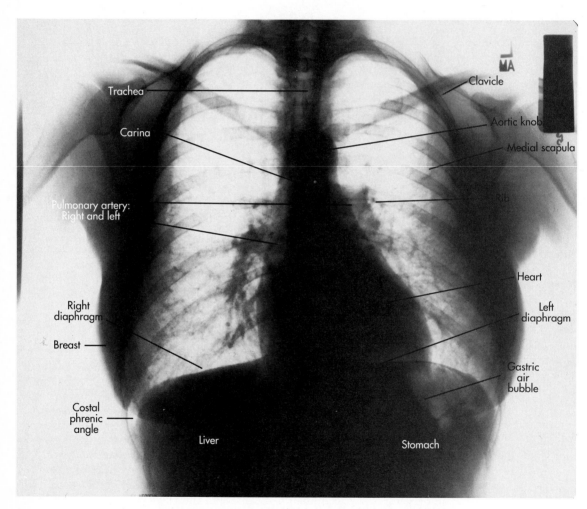

Fig. 7-3. Normal position of anatomical structures on a posterior or anterior chest x-ray film.

The nurse should recall that the visceral pleura covers each lobe of the lung. An interlobar fissure separates one lobe of the lung from another on a chest x-ray film. The major fissure separates the upper and lower lobes (see Fig. 7-3). The major fissure runs obliquely from posterior to anterior, beginning approximately at the level of the fifth thoracic vertebra. The major fissure extends down to the diaphragm. It is usually not visible on a PA projection because it is not parallel to the x-ray beam.

The minor fissure separates the right upper lobe from the right middle lobe and is visible in both the PA and the lateral x-ray film (see Fig. 7-3). The minor fissure is not visible on the chest x-ray films of 44% of adults (Felson, 1965). On a lateral chest x-ray film the minor fissure extends from the anterior chest wall and intersects the major fissure. The minor fissure usually is seen at approximately the level of the fourth rib, although it may appear as high as the second or as low as the sixth rib. The lower the minor fissure, the smaller the right middle lobe.

Position of the major and minor fissures is important to note on every chest x-ray film. Displacement of the fissure from normal position on a chest x-ray film often indicates the presence of lobar collapse. When atelectasis or collapse is present, the fissure is pulled toward the collapsed area. The identification of the affected lobe or segment on a chest x-ray film aids in proper positioning for chest percussion and postural drainage.

Anatomical structures are identified on a chest x-ray film by their densities. As the radiographical beam passes through the patient, the denser tissues absorb more of the beam, and the less-dense tissues absorb less of the beam. Tissues that are denser (such as subcutaneous tissue or the heart) and absorb more of the x-ray beam appear opaque, or white, on the x-ray film. Less-dense tissues (such as the lungs) are radiolucent and appear dark on x-ray films.

Densities

Four densities are identified on a chest x-ray film: metal, fat, water, and air (Fig. 7-4). Bones are rich in calcium and are often designated as metal density. More dense metals, such as bullets, shotgun pellets, coins, teeth, and ECG electrodes, may be identified in some patients. Metal density appears bright white on an x-ray film. Fat appears less white than metal. Fat density is readily apparent in breast tissue and fat surrounding the rib cage. Water density appears white on a chest x-ray film, but it is less white than metal density. Blood in the heart and blood vessels is characteristic of water density. Lung tissue is filled with air in the normal lung. It is radiolucent and should appear black on a normal chest x-ray film.

When analyzing a chest x-ray film, the nurse should develop a systematic approach. The nurse first analyzes the quality of the film and then assesses lung structures. If possible, the nurse uses a previous film for comparison. When films are compared to each other, differences in technique and penetration often make interpretation difficult. Differences in technique and penetration are more common with portable or AP films than with PA films.

Thorax

In general an x-ray film should be viewed from the lateral to medial. The soft tissues surrounding the lungs are briefly assessed for normalcy. Breast shadows are outlined. Unilateral absence of a breast can make one lung appear

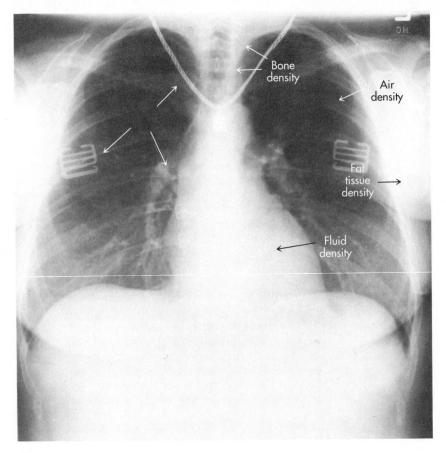

Fig. 7-4. Densities on a chest x-ray film.

radiolucent and one radiopaque. Subcutaneous emphysema is identified in the fatty tissues surrounding the lung and can signal the x-ray film reader to look closely for a pneumothorax.

The bony thorax is inspected for intactness of the ribs, clavicles, scapulae, spine, and manubrium. The nurse counts the ribs, following the curve of each rib from the anterior around posteriorly to the spine. Eight or more ribs overlie the lung in an inspiration chest x-ray film. The position of the clavicular heads and medial ends of the clavicles is assessed. The clavicular heads should be centered over the midline (spine). When the clavicular heads are not centered, the patient is rotated or turned slightly when the chest x-ray examination is done. Rotation of the patient can drastically alter the assessment of fluid status and infiltrates. A common error of the novice viewer is to mistake the scapulae for pneumothorax. This is one reason the PA chest x-ray examination is more desirable. The shoulders are rotated forward, pulling the scapulae apart. In a well-penetrated chest x-ray film, the viewer is able to count the thoracic vertebrae and the ribs.

The diaphragm is assessed for contour. A normal diaphragm is rounded with sharp, pointed costophrenic angles. The right diaphragm is approximately 1 to 2 cm higher than the left diaphragm. The dome of the diaphragm is frequently identified at the level of the sixth rib.

The appearance of the mediastinum is assessed. The normal mediastinum is in the midline position. Cardiomegaly may be present. The heart is enlarged when it occupies space equivalent to more than one third of a hemithorax in a PA film or one half of a hemithorax in an AP film. The nurse also inspects the chest x-ray film for abnormalities in position or size of the large vessels, for mediastinal widening, and for the presence of air or calcium in the mediastinum.

The hili are inspected for size and position. An enlarged hilum is not uncommon in lung cancer. The right hilum is usually about 2 cm lower than the left hilum. The nurse traces the pulmonary vessels from the hili to the periphery. Vessel size normally diminishes in the periphery although prominent vessels are common in congestive heart failure.

Finally, the nurse assesses the lung fields. The right and left sides are compared from top to bottom as in chest assessment. The lungs should be radiolucent. Diffuse or localized areas of increased radiopacity or increased translucency indicate an abnormality.

When diffuse increased radiopacity is present, the nurse may identify an *alveolar pattern,* an *interstitial pattern,* or a *vascular pattern.* The alveolar pattern is characterized by fluffy, soft, poorly demarcated opacifications, which are usually less than 1 cm in diameter. The normal vascular pattern is blurred as the alveoli fill with water-density material. An air bronchogram may be present when the alveolar pattern is identified. An air bronchogram is the outline of a bronchus on chest x-ray film that is caused by fluid surrounding the airway. The most common cause of an alveolar pattern on chest x-ray film is cardiogenic or noncardiogenic pulmonary edema, although it is also associated with some viral pneumonias, pneumocystis, alveolar cell carcinoma, and other causes.

An interstitial pattern results from consolidation of interstitial tissue, that is, alveolar walls, intralobular vessels, interlobar septa, and connective tissue, that surrounds the pulmonary vessels and bronchial tree. Pulmonary fibrosis and interstitial pneumonitis are the most common causes of an interstitial pattern on a chest x-ray film. An interstitial pattern is characterized by a branching line with multiple thin strands that radiate toward the periphery of the lung. Often referred to as Kerley lines, these linear streaks may intersect to form a reticular network. The most common feature of interstitial lung disease on x-ray film is the appearance of honeycombing. Multiple round, translucent areas up to 1 cm in diameter are surrounded by dense, interstitial consolidations.

Recognizing the pattern of the pulmonary vessels on a chest x-ray film can assist in identifying left ventricular failure, pulmonary hypertension, and emphysema. Pulmonary vessels typically decrease in size from the hilum to the periphery. Enlarged pulmonary vessels near the periphery are associated with left ventricular failure. In some cases, increased prominence of the apical vessels, termed *cephalization,* may be present. Pulmonary hypertension is identified by an increase in the size of the hilar vessels. A generalized decrease in the size of pulmonary vessels is observed in pulmonary stenosis and emphysema, and an isolated decrease in pulmonary vessels is seen in large pulmonary embolism.

ABNORMALITIES
Atelectasis and infiltrates

Atelectasis is collapse of the alveoli, causing loss of volume in a segment or lobe and opacification on a chest x-ray film. Three causes of atelectasis are obstruction, compression, and contraction. Obstruction may be central, as occurs after aspiration of a foreign body or when the bronchus is obstructed by a tumor, or peripheral, as occurs with postoperative atelectasis and pneumonia. Compression atelectasis develops when alveoli are squeezed by an external source, such as a pneumothorax or pleural effusion. The last form of collapse, contraction atelectasis, results from scarring that causes a decrease in lung volume. Contraction atelectasis is common in patients with tuberculosis, silicosis, or pulmonary fibrosis.

When atelectasis is present, the nurse uses several techniques to localize the area. The most reliable technique is to first identify proper placement of the fissures, hili, and mediastinum. Displacement of a fissure, a hilum, or mediastinal structures indicates that collapse is present. When a lobe collapses, the fissure, hilum, and mediastinal structures are often pulled *toward* the area of atelectasis. An area of atelectasis also appears more radiopaque, or dense. Unilateral atelectasis elevates the diaphragm on the side of the collapse. (The nurse should recall that the right diaphragm is normally slightly higher than the left.) Narrowing of the rib cage and air bronchograms may also be present when atelectasis is identified.

Bronchi are not seen on a normal chest x-ray film because they have thin walls, contain air, and are surrounded by air in the alveoli. When the physician wants to study the structure of the bronchi, such as in bronchiectasis, he orders a bronchogram, or chest x-ray examination that follows bronchoscopic instillation of an opaque contrast material. When bronchi can be seen on a chest x-ray film without use of opaque contrast material, the term *air bronchogram* is used to describe the occurrence. An air bronchogram is air showing through a greater density, such as water.

Presence of an air bronchogram in older children and adults is abnormal and indicates that the bronchi are surrounded by a water density. In infants and young children the proximal portions of the lobar bronchi may lie within the soft tissues of the mediastinum. An air bronchogram is frequently seen in pneumonia and pulmonary edema, although it may also be observed in pulmonary infarcts and in some chronic lung diseases, such as bronchiectasis. An air bronchogram is one technique used to identify collapse, or atelectasis, of a segment or lobe. When air bronchograms are crowded together, the nurse should suspect collapse of a segment or lobe. As long as the bronchi contain air and the surrounding lung tissue does not, an air bronchogram is present. When bronchi are filled with secretions, an air bronchogram is not present. Air bronchograms are also not present with extrapulmonary abnormalities, such as pleural, mediastinal, or chest wall disease, because these structures do not contain air-filled bronchi.

Infiltrates are fluid-filled airways (Fig. 7-5). When one water density, such as the heart, is in anatomical contact with another water density, such as an infiltrate, the interface between the two areas is obliterated. Water in the airway in anatomical contact with the heart or diaphragm obliterates the border along the area of contact. Radiologists refer to the loss of a normal cardiac or diaphragmatical border or outline as a *silhouette sign*. Use of the silhouette sign enables the nurse to better identify specific areas of infiltrate and then to direct chest therapy more efficiently.

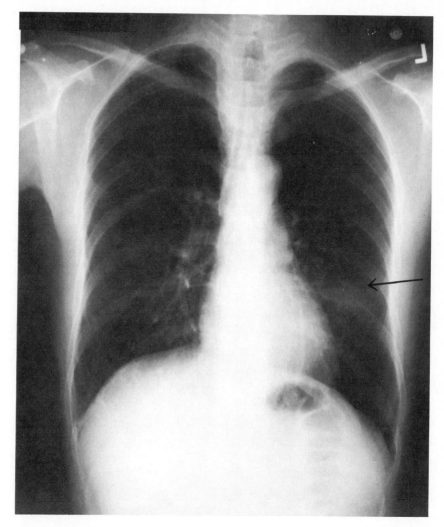

Fig. 7-5. Infiltrate (arrow).

The diaphragm is an anterior structure, as are the heart (both right and left borders) and the ascending aorta. The right middle lobe of the lung is also anterior and is in contact with all but the uppermost portion of the right heart border. If the right heart border is obliterated, the silhouette sign indicates that the infiltrate is in the right middle lobe. The upper portion of the right heart border and the ascending aorta are in anatomical contact with the anterior segment of the right upper lobe. A silhouette sign involving the upper portion of the right heart border or the ascending aorta indicates an infiltrate in the anterior segment of the right upper lobe. The lingula is in anatomical contact with most of the left heart border. An infiltrate that obliterates the left heart border is in the lingula. Similarly, an infiltrate that obscures the upper portion of the left heart border is in the anterior segment of the left upper lobe.

The aortic knob (see Fig. 7-3) and the descending aorta are posterior structures. (The aortic knob is the point at which the ascending, transverse, and descending aortas converge in the chest. The name is appropriate because the knob sticks out of the area around the thoracic vertebrae like a doorknob.) The right and left lobes of the lungs are also posterior and are not in contact with the heart borders. The apical posterior segment of the left upper lobe is in anatomical contact with the aortic knob. When the silhouette sign involves the aortic knob, disease is present in the apical posterior segment of the left upper lobe. Infiltrates in the lower lobes do not obliterate the heart borders, although the diaphragm is often obscured. When the lower lobes of the lungs are diseased, the heart border can be seen through the infiltrates. Presence of an infiltrate in the superior segment of the right or left lower lobe overlaps the middle portion of the heart border. The heart border is not obliterated because the superior segments are posterior structures. Disease in the superior segment of the left lower lobe may also obliterate the descending aorta just below the aortic knob.

Pneumonia. Atelectasis can develop into pneumonia, an inflammatory consolidation of the lung. Pneumonia can be isolated to a segment or generalized to one or more lobes. When aspiration is responsible for pneumonia, the most common site of infiltration is the right lower lobe. The right lower lobe is more susceptible to aspiration than the left lower lobe because of the less sharp angle of the bronchus. An alveolar or interstitial pattern is present on the chest x-ray film. Air bronchograms are present in many types of pneumonia. Some pneumonias, especially those caused by staphylococcus, aerobic gram-negative bacilli, and anaerobes, may cause necrosis of lung tissue. Cavities, or holes in the lung, can develop and are identified on chest x-ray film by the appearance of air-filled hyperlucent areas sometimes surrounded by a "white ring." If fluid is present in the cavity, it settles to the bottom of the cavity, and an air fluid level is seen on the chest x-ray film.

Lung abscess. A lung abscess is a localized area of lung destruction caused by necrosing bacteria. On a chest x-ray film a lung abscess that is full of suppurative material may appear to be a solid mass. As the lung abscess drains, air enters the cavity. The characteristic appearance of a lung abscess on a chest x-ray film is a thick-walled round shadow with an air fluid level.

Pleural effusions

Pleural effusions are fluid accumulations in the pleural space. When the fluid is blood, the term *hemothorax* is used. An *empyema* is fluid that is composed of pus, and a *chylothorax* contains chyle or lymphatic fluid. Because fluid is heavier than air, free pleural fluid falls by gravity to the most dependent area of the lungs. In the supine patient, free pleural fluid gravitates posteriorly. The presence of a unilateral pleural effusion in a supine patient makes the affected lung appear less radiolucent. The chest x-ray film of the affected side appears to have a homogeneous opacification, which some clinicians refer to as ground glass. In the upright patient free pleural fluid gravitates to the bases of the lungs, where it obscures the costophrenic angle. (Note: The costophrenic angle has four sections: anterior, posterior, medial, and lateral. The posterior angle is not visible on a PA film because the dome of the diaphragm extends above it. The lateral costophrenic angle is referenced most frequently when chest x-rays examinations are discussed).

Pleural fluid that accumulates below the lung and above the diaphragm is termed a *pleural effusion*. Approximately 300 ml of pleural fluid must accumulate before the lateral costophrenic angle is obliterated on a chest x-ray

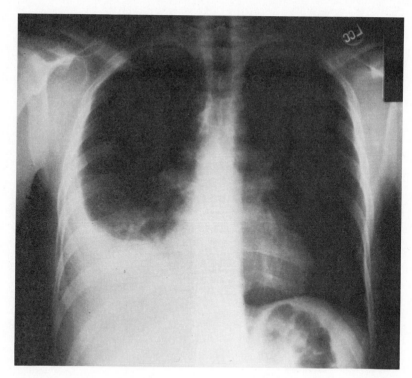

Fig. 7-6. Large pleural effusion in the right lung. (From Mitchell R et al: *Synopsis of clinical pulmonary disease,* ed 4, St Louis, 1989, Mosby–Year Book.)

film. A pleural effusion is identified on a chest x-ray film by appearance of a high diaphragm, by apparent separation of the gastric air bubble from the diaphragm, or by presence of shallow costophrenic angles. A meniscus is frequently seen at the lateral costophrenic angle. In some patients the fluid can be seen "tracking" up the lateral rib cage. The most common causes of pleural effusions are congestive heart failure and infection. Figure 7-6 demonstrates presence of a pleural effusion.

The physician usually orders a lateral decubitus chest x-ray examination to assess for the presence of a pleural effusion and to determine if the fluid is free flowing or loculated. When a patient is positioned on his side, free-flowing pleural fluid gravitates to the dependent area and forms a layer that is visible on the chest x-ray film. In the critically ill patient who is unable to go to the radiology department for a lateral decubitus examination, the physician frequently orders bilateral lateral decubitus chest x-ray examinations. A high-quality lateral decubitus film is technically more difficult to obtain when the patient is positioned on a soft mattress rather than on a hard x-ray table. The nondependent costophrenic angles are assessed for clearing, and the dependent lung is assessed for fluid layering.

A loculated pleural effusion is one that is encapsulated by pleural adhesions, that is, not free flowing, and is localized to a particular area. Other radiographical signs used to identify a loculated pleural effusion are absence

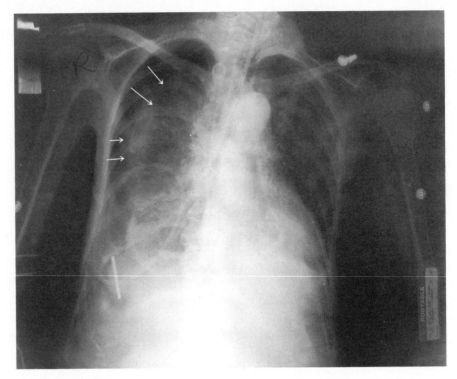

Fig. 7-7. Pneumothorax. Arrows indicate lung borders.

of an air bronchogram and presence of pleural thickening elsewhere in the same border. In congestive heart failure, loculated pleural effusions usually are found in the fissures. Infectious causes of loculated pleural effusions may be found anywhere on the pleural surface.

Pneumothorax

Pneumothorax is air in the thorax, specifically the pleural space. Air may enter the pleural space through the chest wall, mediastinum, visceral pleura, or diaphragm. A pneumothorax is usually caused by blunt or penetrating trauma, although it may be spontaneous. The most common causes of iatrogenic or nosocomial pneumothorax are insertion of central venous catheters via the subclavian vein, diagnostic procedures of the lung in which needles are used, and barotrauma from positive-pressure mechanical ventilation.

The identification of a pneumothorax on a chest x-ray film depends on the size of the pneumothorax and the subsequent loss of lung volume (Fig. 7-7). The typical pneumothorax is identified by a hairline shadow (the visceral pleura) that follows the chest wall. The hairline shadow is separate from the chest wall. Beyond the hairline shadow no vascular markings are visualized. A pneumothorax usually is identified near the apex of the lung, especially when the chest x-ray examination is done with the patient in the upright position. Sometimes a pneumothorax is identified by a thin line of air surrounding the mediastinum, termed the *pneumomediastinum*. The presence of air in the subcutaneous tissues, termed *subcutaneous emphysema*, is another sign

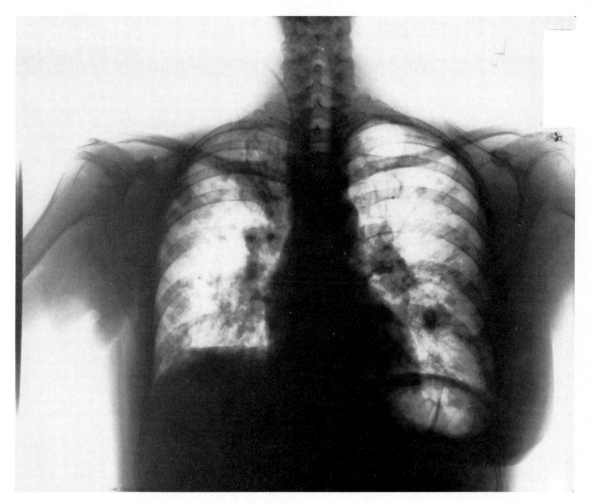

Fig. 7-8. Lung mass or tumor.

that pneumothorax may be present. Because the lung is more inflated on inspiration, a pneumothorax may be difficult to identify on an inspiration x-ray film. The physician orders an expiration chest x-ray examination when in doubt because the smaller, less inflated lung makes the pneumothorax apparent.

Tumors

Tumors appear on chest x-ray film as a dense opacification (Fig. 7-8). A tumor may be located in any area of the lung. The lateral chest x-ray examination is usually necessary to localize the tumor to a particular segment of the lung. A tumor is usually not visible on chest x-ray film until it is approximately 1 cm in size. Endobronchial tumors are often not evident on the chest x-ray film. A tumor in the hilum may be difficult to localize although the hilum usually appears enlarged and the trachea may be displaced.

Pulmonary edema

The most common cause of an alveolar pattern on chest x-ray film is pulmonary edema, of which there are two primary types: cardiogenic and noncardiogenic. (A third type of pulmonary edema, which rarely is seen, is reexpansion pulmonary edema, which occurs secondary to overly rapid inflation of the lungs after aspiration of a pneumothorax or pleural effusion.)

Cardiogenic pulmonary edema results from left ventricular failure or pulmonary venous hypertension. In early cardiogenic pulmonary edema, an opaque "butterfly" pattern can be observed in the hilum. A patient with cardiogenic pulmonary edema has a diffuse interstitial pattern followed by an alveolar pattern that ascends from the bases and does not usually involve the apices. The patient's state of fluid overload determines the height of the interstitial and alveolar patterns. Kerley lines are often present when the intralobular septa are thickened. The pulmonary vessels near the apices are increased in size and are more visible (cephalization). With the presence of the other radiographic signs, the enlarged heart usually seen on the chest x-ray film is diagnostic of a patient in cardiogenic pulmonary edema (see Fig. 12-1 for an x-ray film of cardiogenic pulmonary edema).

Conversely, in noncardiogenic pulmonary edema or adult respiratory distress syndrome (ARDS), the infiltrates are diffuse, bilateral, and nondependent. The infiltrate affects the apices and the bases equally, unlike cardiogenic infiltrates. The heart and hilar structures are also normal size in noncardiogenic pulmonary edema and differentiate cardiogenic from noncardiogenic pulmonary edema (see Fig. 12-2 for an x-ray film of noncardiogenic pulmonary edema).

Chronic obstructive pulmonary disease

The characteristic radiographic change of chronic obstructive pulmonary disease (COPD) is hyperinflation, or increased lung volume, secondary to air trapping. Obstructive lung disease may also be recognized on chest x-ray films by flattened, depressed diaphragms and generalized increased translucency of the lung fields. In some patients, increased lung markings, commonly referred to as "dirty lungs," are perceptible. Loss of interstitial tissue and pulmonary vessels is apparent. In many patients, excessive interstitial-tissue loss results in the observation of bullae. (Refer to Chapter 10.)

A bulla is a thin-walled area of emphysema. Because a patient usually has more than one bulla, the term *bullae* is used. Bullae vary in size and may involve an entire lobe of the lung. A bulla appears on x-ray film as a hyperlucent area with a partially or completely visible hairline shadow surrounding the area.

Invasive lines

In the critical care patient the nurse is concerned with the proper placement of invasive lines and tubings. Although a physician must interpret the chest x-ray film for proper placement of invasive lines and tubings, the nurse should be familiar with proper placement to alert the physician and prevent serious complications. The most common invasive lines and tubings are central venous catheter, pulmonary artery catheter, intraaortic balloon pump, endotracheal tube, and chest tube.

Following insertion of a central venous catheter, particularly with the subclavian vein approach, the chest x-ray film is assessed for pneumothorax.

When a central venous catheter is inserted into the internal jugular vein, a radiopaque line is observed extending from near the jaw into the superior vena cava. A central venous catheter that originates in the subclavian vein lies under the clavicle and extends into the superior vena cava. In some rare cases the tip of the catheter is seen extending up into the head. In such cases the nurse should alert the physician for prompt removal and reinsertion. A femorally placed central venous catheter is in proper position when the tip of the catheter is in the inferior vena cava. The tip of any central venous catheter should not extend into the right atrium.

A pulmonary artery catheter is usually inserted through the internal jugular or subclavian vein, which necessitates examination of the chest x-ray film for a pneumothorax. The catheter enters the right atrium and continues through the tricuspid valve into the right ventricle and out the pulmonic valve into the pulmonary artery. Some catheters coil in the right atrium or ventricle, increasing the risk of ectopic foci. The tip of the catheter may enter either the right (usual) or left pulmonary artery. When the left pulmonary artery is catheterized, the catheter may appear to double back on itself and is sometimes better visualized on a lateral chest x-ray film. A pulmonary artery catheter should not extend past the inner (medial) one third of the lung diameter (Figure 7-9, A). A catheter that extends further out into the periphery of the lung places the patient at high risk for pulmonary infarction.

Insertion of an intraaortic balloon pump through the femoral artery and into the aorta does not place the patient at risk for a pneumothorax. A balloon pump is in proper position when the tip of the catheter is just distal to the origin of the left subclavian artery. Positioning distal to this point may cause inadequate augmentation. The tip of the intraaortic balloon pump also can migrate into the aortic arch and occlude the left subclavian artery. More proximal positioning increases the risk of cerebral embolization and arterial laceration. When the left radial artery pulse is absent, the nurse should suspect migration past the left subclavian artery.

An endotracheal tube has a radiopaque line that extends the entire length, including the tip. Inserted nasally or orally, an endotracheal tube is in proper position when the tip of the tube is 2 to 3 cm above the carina and 3 cm below the vocal cords in an adult (Figure 7-9, B). The carina may be difficult to visualize on some chest x-ray films. If the carina cannot be seen, the position of the tube can be estimated to be in proper position when the tip of the tube is at or just slightly below the clavicles (at the second or third rib) in an upright or supine nonrotated, nonlordotic chest x-ray film. The nurse should recall that the tip of the endotracheal tube is approximately 1 cm below the lower edge of the cuff. Depending on the size of the endotracheal tube, the cuff is approximately 2 to 3 cm long. If the tip of the tube is above the clavicles, the likelihood of the cuff's being in the vocal cords is enhanced because the distance between the vocal cords and clavicles is about 4 cm. Position of the patient's head during the chest x-ray examination is noted because a change in position of the head alters the tracheal position of the endotracheal tube. Flexion of the head forces the endotracheal tube closer to the carina, and extension of the head pulls the endotracheal tube closer to the vocal cords.

Chest tube position is variable because a chest tube may be placed anterior or posterior to the lung. The chest tube may be inserted through an incision in the anterior chest or through an incision in the lateral chest wall. A chest

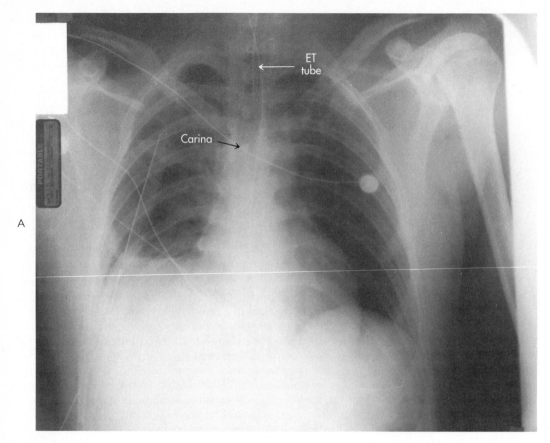

ET
tube

Carina

A

Fig. 7-9. A, Correct position of an endotracheal tube.

tube has several holes to facilitate drainage of air and fluid. Each chest tube
has a radiopaque line that extends the entire length of the chest tube, with the
exception of breaks in the radiopaque line, in which there are holes. When a
chest tube is in proper position, the most distal or last hole of the chest tube,
that is, the break in the line, is positioned within the rib cage (Figure 7-9, C).
When a break in the line extends outside the rib cage in the subcutaneous

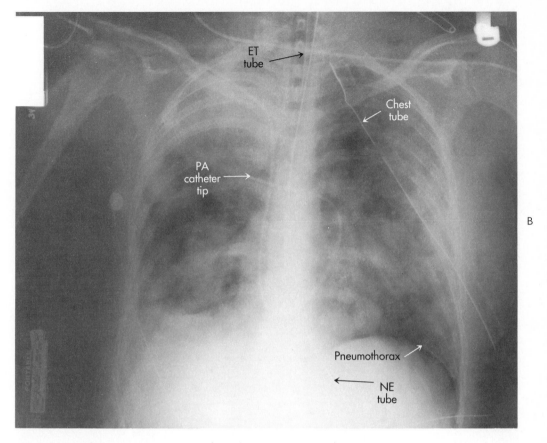

ET
tube

Chest
tube

PA
catheter
tip

Pneumothorax

NE
tube

B

Fig. 7-9, cont'd. B, Correct position of a pulmonary artery catheter.

tissue or when it cannot be seen, the physician is notified to reposition the chest tube because air can enter the chest through the distal hole if it is not in the chest. A pneumothorax may occur, and vigorous bubbling throughout inhalation and exhalation is seen in the chest drainage bottle. The nurse also assesses the chest tube position for kinks that impede drainage. A chest tube should appear as a relatively straight line.

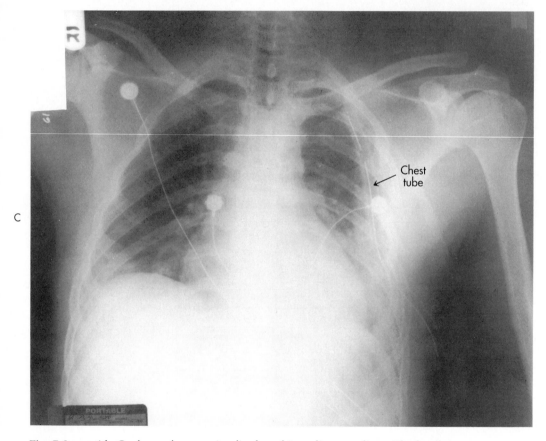

C

Fig. 7-9, cont'd. C, chest tubes are visualized as thin radiopaque lines. The break in the line indicates a hole is positioned inside the rib cage in the pleural space.

CONCLUSION

The role of the nurse in assessing chest x-ray films is changing. Although the nurse is not responsible for diagnostic interpretation of a chest x-ray film, patient care is improved when the nurse understands major normal and abnormal findings on a chest x-ray film. Increased awareness of radiographic findings helps the nurse to understand physical assessment better. For instance, the nurse may assess a change in breath sounds that suggests misplacement of an endotracheal tube. She then can intervene quickly to prevent complications from accidental intubation of a mainstem bronchus. The nurse also may apply chest therapy more effectively by identifying position of an infiltrate on a chest x-ray film. The nurse should remember that this chapter is only an introduction to assessing chest x-ray films. Being able to accurately interpret a chest x-ray film requires systematic review of many x-ray films with a qualified individual, such as another nurse or a physician or radiologist.

BIBLIOGRAPHY

Baum GL, Wolinsky E: *Textbook of pulmonary diseases,* ed 3, Boston, 1983, Little, Brown.

Burton GC, Hodgkin JE: *Respiratory care: a guide to clinical practice,* ed 2, Philadelphia, 1984, J B Lippincott.

Canobbio M: Chest x-ray film interpretation, *Focus Crit Care* 11(2):18-24, 1984.

Felson B, Weinstein AS, Spitz HB: *Principles of chest roentgenology: a programmed text,* Philadelphia, 1965, W B Saunders.

Felson B: The chest roentgenologic workup: what and why? Conventional methods, *Basics Respir Dis* 8(5):1-5, 1980.

Felson B: *Chest roentgenology,* Philadelphia, 1973, W B Saunders.

Fraser R, Pare J: *Diagnosis of diseases of the chest,* vol 1-3, ed 2, Philadelphia, 1977-1979, W B Saunders.

Guenter C, Welch M: *Pulmonary medicine,* ed 2, Philadelphia, 1982, J B Lippincott.

Hinshaw H, Murray J: *Diseases of the chest,* ed 4, Philadelphia, 1980, W B Saunders.

MacMahon H, Montner SM, Doi K, et al: The nature and subtlety of abnormal findings in chest radiographs, *Med Phys* 18(2):206-210, 1991.

Murray JF, Nadel JA, eds: *Textbook of respiratory medicine,* Philadelphia, 1988, W B Saunders.

Netter F: *The CIBA collection of medical illustrations,* vol 7, respiratory system, New York, 1979, CIBA Pharmaceutical.

Pare JAP, Fraser RG: *Synopsis of diseases of the chest,* Philadelphia, 1983, W B Saunders.

Prior J, Silberstein J, Stang J: *Physical diagnosis: the history and examination of the patient,* ed 6, St Louis, 1981, Mosby–Year Book.

Thompson D: *Cardiovascular assessment: guide for nurses and other health professionals,* St Louis, 1981, Mosby–Year Book.

Tinker J: Understanding chest x-rays, *Am J Nurs* 76(1):54-58, 1976.

Wade JF: *Comprehensive respiratory care: physiology and technique,* ed 3, St Louis, 1982, Mosby–Year Book.

Wanner A, Sackner MA: *Pulmonary diseases: mechanisms of altered structure and function,* Boston, 1983, Little, Brown.

H·A·P·T·E·R   8

Pulmonary Function Testing

Objectives:

- Identify environmental factors that enhance or detract from pulmonary function testing.
- Discuss the rationale for withholding systemic and inhaled bronchodilator medications.
- Discuss the preparation of the patient for pulmonary function testing.
- Identify four lung volumes and four lung capacities.
- Differentiate between inspiratory vital capacity and forced vital capacity.
- Differentiate between obstructive and restrictive lung disease by pulmonary function testing.
- Discuss the measurement of residual volume.
- Differentiate spirometry, nitrogen washout, helium dilution, and plethysmography.
- Discuss the significance of closing volume and diffusing capacity.

Pulmonary function tests (PFTs) are an important component of patient assessment in health and disease. Used in conjunction with clinical symptoms and physical assessment, PFTs are useful diagnostic and prognostic tools for patient care. The presence and extent of lung diseases, such as asthma or asbestosis, frequently are identified by PFT screening after complaints of chest tightness or shortness of breath. PFTs can distinguish between obstructive and restrictive lung diseases and are valuable in directing therapy. Intermittent serial PFTs are used to follow progression of chronic diseases, such as COPD or sarcoidosis, and are useful in determining extent of disability. PFTs are also useful in screening patients at risk for postoperative pulmonary complications.

PFTs require full cooperation from the patient to be a valid assessment parameter. The nurse, especially in the long-term clinic or with the newly hospitalized patient, is usually the most knowledgeable about the patient's ability to follow instructions and the patient's strength to perform the tests. Therefore the nurse is important not only in scheduling the patient for PFTs but also in preparing the patient for PFTs.

This chapter discusses PFTs that are performed in a pulmonary function laboratory or at the bedside. Nursing care of the patient having PFTs is examined.

LABORATORY PFT

Complete PFTs provide the best information when the patient is in a steady state. The patient should be free of acute infection and breathing in a normal pattern. Distractions may alter the patient's breathing pattern and subsequently affect the outcome of the PFT. Therefore a conducive laboratory environment is essential for obtaining an accurate test. Although there are individual differences in pulmonary function laboratories, all laboratories must comply with standards to be accredited.

Several factors about the laboratory testing site may or may not be alterable. Because the patient must hear and respond to commands, the testing site should be situated away from high-traffic areas. A closed door and a "Test in Progress" sign on the door help to deter visitors during the test. Extraneous noises, such as ringing telephones or background conversations, may be distracting and should be prevented. The PFT area should be pleasant and should exude a calm, relaxed, and unhurried atmosphere.

Individuals performing complete PFTs are respiratory therapists in some institutions and trained technicians in others. (Bedside PFTs are also performed in some cases by a nurse, especially in a clinic.) Because many PFTs are effort-dependent, staff of the laboratory develop rapport with the patient and give clear, concise directions to perform accurately each independent test. Coaching and enthusiasm by the staff for proper patient performance of the test are critical in obtaining an accurate reflection of the patient's pulmonary function. In some institutions PFT staff also take a history and perform a limited physical assessment before testing. By conveying pertinent history and physical information to the staff, the nurse aids in streamlining patient care.

A pulmonary function laboratory has a medical director who is usually a pulmonary physician or clinical physiologist. The director is responsible for accurate standardized testing of the patient and for staff training in some laboratories. The medical director knows the proper function and maintenance of the equipment and often interprets the PFTs. When the medical director is unavailable to interpret the PFTs, another pulmonary physician frequently performs the task. Because the average physician or nurse is unfamiliar with interpretation of PFTs, a full report that explains abnormalities in familiar terms is written and is placed on the patient's chart (Fig. 8-1). The written report usually gives an impression, similar to a diagnosis, classifying the abnormalities as obstructive or restrictive or a combined obstructive-restrictive pattern and indicating severity, such as mild, moderate, or severe.

Preparing the patient for PFT

Scheduling concerns. Scheduling the patient for PFT often is performed by the unit secretary or nurse. In many institutions PFTs may be scheduled as early as 7 or 8 AM and through the lunch period. The patient should receive a light or clear-liquid meal 1 hour before the test. A full stomach limits lung expansion, which alters PFT results. After the test the patient may resume a normal diet.

The use of systemic and inhaled bronchodilator medications improves pulmonary function and affects the outcome of the test. Accurate baseline PFTs usually require withholding long-acting systemic bronchodilators, such as theophylline, for at least 24 hours and short-acting systemic bronchodilators, such as somophyllin or elixophyllin, for at least 12 hours before the test. Inhaled bronchodilators should not be administered for a minimum of 6 hours

SEX: M   PRED COLLINS1
AGE: 68   RM#: 918-2
HT: 71.0 in
WT: 225.0 lb

SMK HX: Quit   OY; (CIGS 50y 90d) OCC: RET TRUCK DR 40 Y HAZARD: FUMES

Spirometry		Pre-Drug* Pre	%Pre	Predicted	Post-Drug* ALBUTEROL Post	%Post	%Chg
FVC	(L)	1.84	40	4.57	2.00	43	9
FEV1	(L)	0.76	24	3.09	0.93	29	22
FEV3	(L)	1.43	32	4.44	1.51	34	5
FEF25-75%	(L/S)	0.37	13	2.79	0.36	12	–3
FEFmax	(L/S)	3.03	34	8.81	3.03	34	0
FEF25%	(L/S)	0.63	8	7.79	0.99	12	56
FEF50%	(L/S)	0.38	7	4.96	0.36	7	–5
FEF75%	(L/S)	0.25	14	1.71	0.19	11	–25
FEV1/FVC	(%)	41.26	61	67.62	46.21	68	11
FEF50/FIF50	(%)	8.57			9.24		7

Spirometry		Pre-Drug* Pre	%Pre	Predicted	Post-Drug* ALBUTEROL Post	%Post	%Chg
MVV	(L/MIN)	35.76	29	121.62	35.55	29	0

Lung Volumes		Pre-drug* Avg Pre	%Pre	Predicted
TLC	(L)			
FRC	(L)	6.39	89	7.15
RV	(L)	5.00	122	4.07
VC	(L)	4.35	168	2.58
IC	(L)	2.03	44	4.57
ERV	(L)	1.39	45	3.08
RV/TLC	(%)	0.64	43	1.50
He Equil	(MIN)	68.15	189	36.05
		5.00		

Plethysmography	Pre-Drug* Avg Pre	%Pre	Predicted
TLC (L)	6.86	95	7.15
FRC (L)	5.17	126	4.07
RV (L)	4.93	191	2.58
VC (L)	1.93	42	4.57
IC (L)	1.70	55	3.08
ERV (L)	0.23	15	1.50
RV/TLC (%)	71.00	196	36.05
VTG (L)	5.13		
Raw (Cm H20/L/SEC)	3.55		(0.20-2.50)
SGaw (L/SEC/Cm H20)	0.06		(0.11-0.40)

Diffusion		Pre-Drug* Avg Pre	%Pre	Predicted
Dsb	ml/min/mmHg	15.69	61	25.64
VA(sb)	(L)	4.30		
D/VA		3.65		

DLCO CORRECTED FOR HEMOGLOBIN OF 13.7

Lung volumes: Decreased vital capacity with normal TLC. The FRC and residual volume are increased. Flow rates: All flows are reduced. Specific conductants: Reduced. Diffusing capacity: Reduced.
Interpretation: Severe obstructive ventilatory defect with airtrapping and impaired gas transfer. There is a significant improvement in flow rates following inhaled bronchodilators.

Fig. 8-1. A full PFT and interpretation.

before PFTs. If the PFTs demonstrate obstruction, the patient usually is given an inhaled bronchodilator, such as metaproterenol sulfate or albuterol. PFTs are then repeated to determine the amount of reversible airway obstruction. The physician is consulted regarding holding bronchodilator medications before the test.

Because fatigue may impair PFT, activities that tire the patient are postponed. Physical therapy, such as flexibility, strengthening, or endurance exercises, should be rescheduled well before PFT to allow sufficient rest or delayed until after the test. Chest physical therapy, including postural drainage and percussion, is performed at least 1 hour before PFT to promote airway clearance. In this instance, bronchodilators are not given before chest physical therapy. In the postoperative patient pain medications should be administered 1 hour before the test so that lung expansion is not limited by pain. Because PFTs are altered by overmedication, care should be taken to avoid administering excessive analgesics or oversedating the patient.

Patients with communicable respiratory infections, such as pseudomonas, tuberculosis, staphylococcus, or pneumocystis, should not be scheduled for PFT until the infection is resolved. Because alveolar clearing is slow, PFTs are usually scheduled 6 weeks after an acute infection or exacerbation of disease. When PFTs are performed on an infected patient, the inside of the spirometer becomes contaminated with contagious organisms that can be transmitted to other patients. The inside of the spirometer is clean, not sterile, and is difficult and expensive to disinfect once contaminated.

Psychological concerns. When scheduling concerns have been addressed, the patient is psychologically prepared for PFT. The nurse teaches the patient that PFTs are not painful although the nose clip may be uncomfortable. The nurse informs the patient that he will be asked to breathe in as deeply as possible and to exhale as fully as possible through a machine. The nurse also informs the patient that he will be asked to hold his breath or to pant on command. Most PFTs require the patient to perform maneuvers as rapidly as possible to identify decreased airway flows that are important in the diagnosis of disease of the small airways. Because performing these maneuvers rapidly is exhausting for many patients, recovery time is allowed between each test, especially for dyspneic patients. It is not unusual for the test to take an hour or more. Perhaps the most frightening part of complete PFT is getting in the body plethysmography box. Although the sides are clear, patients often feel confined and sometimes claustrophobic.

Special considerations. Some patients require special preparation or testing procedures. Children, patients with language problems, patients with continuous supplemental oxygen, patients with intravenous catheters, and patients with tracheostomies are examples.

Children. Children present a special challenge in obtaining accurate PFTs reflective of lung function. Children of the same chronological age have differing ability to perform various tests. The ability of the child to follow directions and cooperate is more important than age. A parent or adult caregiver usually accompanies the very young child and acts as interpreter for instructions although this is usually left to the discretion of the PFT technician. An experienced PFT technician puts the child at ease and makes the testing a game. Noncomputerized equipment makes games easier. For example, the technician can ask the child to see how high he can make the pin go on the spinning paper. Nose clips may be too large or too frightening for some children and therefore may be omitted. Fortunately, children requiring frequent PFT, such as children with cystic fibrosis, lung transplantation, or asthma, usually become acclimated to the testing procedure quickly.

Language. Language problems of patients vary, from not being able to speak English or other native languages to being deaf. Depending on the area, patients or nurses who do not speak a common language may present a problem. The testing of patients who speak different languages is facilitated by the aid of an interpreter who speaks the patient's native language. The interpreter should be present during pretesting preparation and during the testing. When deaf patients are studied, one of several communication techniques may be used, depending on the patient. Some patients are experienced in sign language, and other patients are adept at lip reading. The patient who can read lips usually presents no special problem to the PFT technician, depending on placement of equipment and location of the technician. The PFT technician is advised to look at the patient when speaking and to speak slowly and clearly. A signing interpreter, often a family member, is used when the patient is experienced in sign language. When the patient neither reads lips nor signs, flash cards are used to explain the patient's participation.

Supplemental O$_2$. The patient who requires continuous O$_2$ is at risk for hypoxemia during PFT administration because supplemental O$_2$ is not usable during testing. Depending on the amount of O$_2$ used and on the patient's overall cardiopulmonary status, the patient may be able to perform one or more maneuvers without oxygen. The patient uses oxygen and rests between testing efforts. Some patients require several minutes between tests to reoxygenate.

Intravenous catheters. Patients with intravenous catheters require additional planning by the nurse before sending the patient for PFT. If possible, fluids are discontinued, and a heparin lock is inserted. When intravenous fluids must be administered, the nurse provides sufficient volume in the bag or bottle for several hours although the patient is usually gone for about an hour. Intravenous piggyback medications may need to be rescheduled either before or after PFT.

Tracheostomy tubes. Patients with tracheostomy tubes can be tested in many but not all pulmonary function laboratories. Special adapters are necessary for PFT equipment when a test is performed with the tracheostomy tube in place. At the discretion of the physician, in some patients a metal tracheostomy tube is replaced by a cuffed plastic tube for the PFT. The cuff is inflated during PFT to prevent or at least minimize air leakage. Because some patients develop bronchospasm after inflation of the cuff, the cuff should be inflated before the patient arrives for the test to allow the spasm to resolve. Because air leakage occurs around the tracheostomy tube, even in a cuffed tube, measurements are not totally accurate.

For other patients the physician requests PFT without the tracheostomy tube. The tracheostomy tube is removed before the test, and the stoma is sealed with an occlusive dressing. Some physicians use petrolatum-impregnated gauze to seal the stoma. In patients at risk of developing permanent stoma closure or respiratory distress, a Kistner or Olympic button may be used to keep the stoma patent. The button is occluded with tape or a plastic plug that can be removed rapidly if the patient develops respiratory distress.

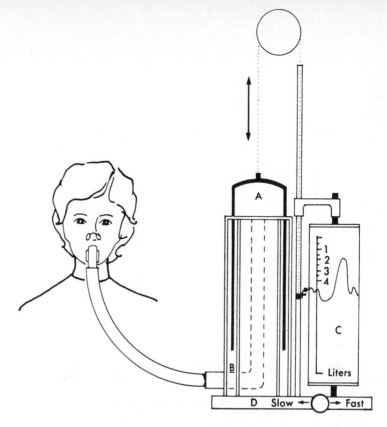

Fig. 8-2. A patient performs spirometric pulmonary function tests. The bellows (**A**) move in a water-filled area (**B**) that rotates a drum (**C**) at variable speed (**D**) to make a spirogram.

Types of pulmonary function tests

PFTs are grouped into three categories: spirometry, gas dilution, and body plethysmography. Of the three, spirometry is most frequently ordered because the machine is portable and the tests are simple to perform. Spirometry may be performed at the bedside or in the clinic. Gas dilution and body plethysmography are generally available only in the pulmonary function laboratory.

Spirometry testing. A spirometer is used to determine lung capacities, lung volumes, and flow rates (Fig. 8-2). There are many types of spirometers, including water seal, dry rolling seal, and bellows. Modern spirometers are connected to a computer that calculates volumes and flows automatically. Not all tests are available with each spirometer. Ruppel (1990) discusses differences in spirometers. The spirometer is usually attached to a writing device or printer, such as a two-channel or four-channel recorder, x-y plotter, or kymograph, that provides graphic representation of inhalation/exhalation volumes. The graphic tracing of lung volumes is called a *spirogram*.

Upon arrival at the pulmonary function laboratory for spirometry, the patient usually is seated in a chair although some portable spirometers require a standing position. Tight clothing can impede movement of the thorax and alter PFT results. Therefore belts and constrictive undergarments are loosened.

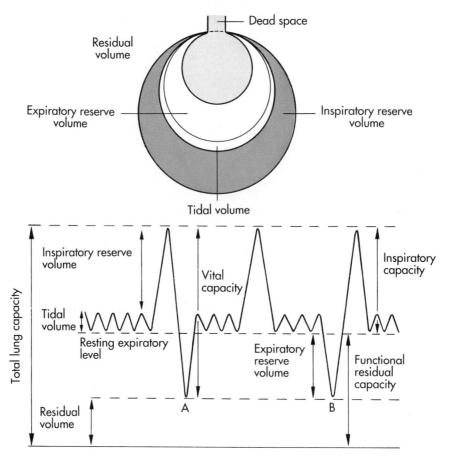

Fig. 8-3. Spirogram of lung volumes and capacities and corresponding alveolar size. An upward deflection reflects exhalation, and a downward deflection indicates inhalation. Vital capacity is determined by (**A**) maximal exhalation from total lung capacity or (**B**) maximal inhalation from residual volume.

After the patient is briefly interviewed, a mouthpiece is inserted, and nose clips are applied. For accurate testing, there must be no air leaks from the patient or from the system. A perforated eardrum may allow leakage of air and is noted on the patient's chart and test record. The patient breathes normally for a time to determine **tidal volume** (V_T), that is, the amount of air that the patient inhales and exhales with each breath. Then the patient either breathes out completely followed by a maximal inhalation or breathes in as deeply as possible and then exhales completely to determine **vital capacity** (**VC**) (Fig. 8-3). The patient takes as long as necessary to perform the exhaled vital capacity maneuver. For this reason it is sometimes termed *slow vital capacity*. In patients with air trapping, the former technique, which measures inspiratory vital capacity, is preferred over the latter slow vital capacity technique, which measures expiratory vital capacity and may enhance air trapping. Figure 8-4 shows a normal spirogram of V_T and forced vital capacity

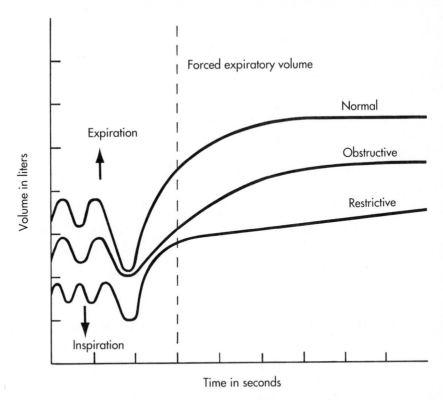

Fig. 8-4. Top, Typical spirogram from a patient with normal, obstructive, and restrictive lung function: The dashed line represents the FEV_1. FVC is measured at the end of maximal exhalation (far right). Note the $FEV_{1\%}$ is normal in restrictive lung disease and decreased in obstructive lung disease.

(FVC) and spirograms of patients with obstructive and restrictive lung diseases.

The knowledge that is gained from the vital capacity maneuver includes determination of inspiratory and expiratory reserve volumes and inspiratory capacity and is dependent on the effort of the patient performing the maneuver (Table 8-1, see Fig. 8-3 for illustration). A good effort produces more accurate values. **Inspiratory reserve volume (IRV)** is the amount of air breathed in from end inhalation of a resting V_T to maximal inhalation. **Expiratory reserve volume (ERV)** is the difference between the amount of air exhaled after a normal V_T and maximal exhalation. The nurse should recall that a capacity is the sum of two or more volumes. **Inspiratory capacity (IC)** is the sum of the inhaled V_T and IRV. **Vital capacity (VC)** is the sum of IRV, ERV, and V_T. Another way to define VC is the sum of IC and ERV. In normal individuals IC is equal to two thirds of VC, leaving one third of VC resulting from ERV.

Some air remains in the patient's lungs to support body metabolism even after a maximal exhalation. Termed **residual volume (RV)**, the air remaining in the patient's lungs after a maximal exhalation is not measured by spirom-

Table 8-1. Pulmonary function test volumes

Volume	Abbreviation	Definition
Tidal volume	V_T	Amount of air normally inhaled and exhaled with each breath
Inspiratory reserve volume	IRV	Maximum amount of air inhaled in addition to normal V_T
Expiratory reserve volume	ERV	Maximum amount of air exhaled in addition to normal V_T
Inspiratory capacity	$IC = V_T + IRV$	Maximum amount of air inhaled from resting expiratory level
Vital capacity	$VC = V_T + IRV + ERV$ $VC = IC + ERV$	Maximum amount of air inhaled (exhaled) after a maximal exhalation (inhalation)
Residual volume	RV	Amount of air remaining in the lungs at the end of a *maximal* exhalation
Functional residual capacity	$FRC = RV + ERV$	Amount of air remaining in the lungs at the end of a *normal* exhalation
Total lung capacity	$TLC = RV + VC$ $TLC = IC + FRC$	Volume of air contained in the entire thorax

etry. RV is measured by gas dilution. The sum of RV and VC is **total lung capacity (TLC)**. RV and ERV make up **functional residual capacity (FRC)**, that is, the amount of air remaining in the patient's lungs at the end of a normal V_T breath.

Gas dilution. Helium dilution and nitrogen washout are techniques that measure only ventilated lung areas to determine FRC and RV. In patients with air trapping from tumor or emphysema, FRC is underestimated with gas-dilution techniques.

Helium dilution. In helium dilution a known concentration of helium, a gas relatively insoluble in blood, is mixed with a known volume of air and breathed by the patient for about 10 minutes through a closed circuit. Air is exchanged exclusively between the patient and the spirometer without contact with outside air. Equilibration of the helium mixture takes longer for patients with larger lung volumes or diseased lungs than for those with smaller lung volumes or healthy lungs. When the helium mixture is equilibrated between the patient and the spirometer, FRC can be calculated from the concentration of helium and the volume of gas absorbed by the patient.

Nitrogen washout. Conversely, nitrogen washout is an open-circuit technique of estimating FRC. The nitrogen washout technique assumes that the lungs, like the environment, contain 80% nitrogen. The patient breathes 100% oxygen for 7 minutes to wash nitrogen from his lungs. Exhaled gases are gathered in a collecting bag for analysis of nitrogen content and computation of FRC. Normal lungs excrete all but approximately 2.5% nitrogen in 7 minutes (Ruppel, 1990). Diseased lungs with uneven ventilation require longer than 7 minutes to excrete the same percentage of nitrogen.

Because small amounts of nitrogen also are washed out from the blood and tissues, allowances must be made in the interpretation of results. The major disadvantage to calculating FRC from nitrogen washout is that the exhaled concentration of nitrogen is very low. Therefore small errors in measurement lead to large errors in calculated lung volume (West, 1985).

Body plethysmography. Body plethysmography uses an air-tight wooden, metal, or plastic box, commonly called the *body box*, which is shaped to accommodate the seated individual. The body plethysmography box looks like an individual sauna bath with a transparent top. Although both the helium and nitrogen washout techniques measure air from ventilated airways only, body plethysmography measures total lung volume, including air trapped by closed airways. Body plethysmography estimates fairly accurately and rapidly the entire thoracic volume by measuring pressure changes during panting (or a suck-blow technique) against an occluded airway at the end of a normal exhalation. As the patient tries to inhale, gas in the lungs expands, lung volume increases, and box pressure rises as its volume decreases. Boyle's law, which states that the volume of gas varies inversely with pressure at constant temperature, is used to calculate FRC. Although FRC is nearly the same in most patients when helium dilution, nitrogen washout, or body plethysmography are used, it is significantly higher when body plethysmography is used for patients who have lung areas trapped by closed airways (emphysematous bullae or occlusion of an airway by tumor).

Mechanical properties

Spirometry measures not only lung volumes but also flow rates and other tests of mechanical function to evaluate the performance of the patient's muscles, thorax, and lungs in moving air. Mechanics deal with energy and force and require the patient to move air as rapidly as possible. Tests of mechanical function aid in the diagnosis of diseases of the small airways.

The FVC maneuver is the primary test of mechanical function performed during spirometry. This maneuver quantifies the maximum amount of air available for ventilation. Additional calculations are made from the effort-dependent FVC maneuver, which differs from a normal VC maneuver primarily in speed of exhalation. The patient takes in a maximal breath and forcefully exhales it as rapidly as possible until all air is exhaled. The amount of FVC exhaled over a specified period, that is, FEV, is calculated from the paper spirogram or by the computer. Commonly reported intervals are one half, one, two, and three-second periods, also termed $FEV_{0.5}$ (forced expiratory volume in one half second), FEV_1, FEV_2, and FEV_3, respectively (see Fig. 8-4). An individual with normal lungs exhales 75% to 80% of the VC in 1 second and 90% to 100% in 3 seconds with maximal effort (Burton and Hodgkin, 1984). Patients with airway obstruction may take as long as 20 to 30 seconds to exhale completely.

In addition to FEV, measurement of the FVC also provides **forced expiratory flow (FEF)** rates. Formerly termed the **maximal midexpiratory flow rate (MMEF)**, FEF commonly is measured between 25% and 75% of the FVC

($FEF_{25\%-75\%}$) because the middle portion of the FVC is believed to be the least effort-dependent portion of the maneuver (Burton and Hodgkin, 1984; Sobol, 1978). Because the $FEF_{25\%-75\%}$ is relatively effort-independent, a change in the caliber of the small airways indicating airways obstruction is observed as a decreased $FEF_{25\%-75\%}$. In asthma and other diseases with small-airways obstruction, the $FEF_{25\%-75\%}$ is used as a screening or diagnostic tool.

Another test of pulmonary function is **maximal voluntary ventilation (MVV)**, which measures function of the respiratory muscles, lung compliance, and airways resistance. The patient is asked to inhale and exhale as rapidly and deeply as possible for 15 seconds. Healthy young men can breathe approximately 170 LPM (Ruppel, 1990). Because the MVV maneuver can increase air trapping and exertion of respiratory muscles, it may not be performed in patients with severe obstructive airways disease. The MVV can be estimated by multiplying the $FEV_1 \times 30$ (Hodgkin, 1984).

Small airways disease also may be assessed by the measurement of **closing volume (CV)**, that is, the lung volume at which small airways begin to close. **Closing capacity** = CV + RV. Airway closure is related to the effects of gravity and to pressure-volume changes during exhalation. A single-breath nitrogen washout test is one method of determining CV. The first exhaled gas is from dead space areas and contains no nitrogen. As alveoli empty, nitrogen concentration increases and then plateaus. Toward the end of exhalation the concentration of nitrogen sharply increases as basal alveoli close and more poorly ventilated apical alveoli contribute nitrogen-rich gas to the airways. In young, healthy individuals, CV is approximately 10% of VC and increases with age, smoking, and disease (West, 1985; Ruppel, 1990).

Flow-volume properties

Complete assessment of PFT includes the determination of flow-volume properties. Flow-volume loops are produced during FVC maneuvers by recording flow rates against lung volumes. The patient exhales maximally then inhales maximally. The inspiratory and expiratory components of the flow-volume loop have characteristic shapes, which aid in the diagnosis of restrictive disorders from obstructive disorders and intrathoracic disorders from extrathoracic disorders (Fig. 8-5).

In patients with obstructive airway disease, airways close at higher lung volumes, and expiratory flows are reduced. The flow-volume loop of a patient with obstructive airway disease typically has a flattened or "scooped out" expiratory limb compared with that of normal individuals. In patients with restrictive lung disease, lung volumes are decreased overall although flows are normal or somewhat higher than normal. The flow-volume loop of a patient with restrictive lung disease is higher and narrower than a normal flow-volume loop. Variable intrathoracic large airway obstruction, such as a tracheal tumor, produces a plateau on the expiratory limb of the flow-volume loop, and the inspiratory limb of the flow-volume loop remains somewhat normal. Variable extrathoracic large airway obstruction, such as a laryngeal tumor, produces a characteristic plateau on the inspiratory limb of the flow-volume loop because the trachea tends to collapse on inhalation, reducing inspiratory flow. When a fixed large airway obstruction, such as tracheal stricture, is present, both the inspiratory and expiratory limbs of the flow-volume loop demonstrate a plateau (Burton and Hodgkin, 1984).

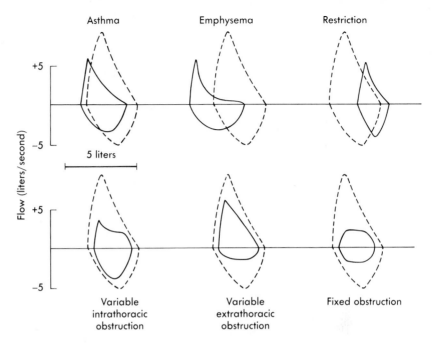

Fig. 8-5. Flow-volume loops. Normal loops are shown by dashed lines overlying the abnormality. Inhalation is below the zero line, and exhalation is above the line. Note that with obstructive lung diseases, the expiratory limb of the loop is "scooped out." With restrictive lung diseases the shape of the curve is normal although volumes are reduced. Variable intrathoracic obstruction is identified by near-normal inhalation and reduced flows on exhalation, and variable extrathoracic obstruction causes an opposite pattern. When there is fixed large airway obstruction, inspiratory and expiratory flows are reduced equally. (From Ruppel G: *Manual of pulmonary function testing*, ed 5, St Louis, 1991, Mosby–Year Book.)

Measurement of **diffusing capacity of the lung (D_L)** is standard in many pulmonary function laboratories both for screening and for following therapy. A test of D_L assesses the ability of gases to cross the alveolar-capillary membrane in the presence of normal hemoglobin and ventilation. A highly soluble gas, such as carbon monoxide (CO), is used to assess D_L. Oxygen also can be used, but because CO has 210 times the affinity of oxygen for hemoglobin, it is preferred. Because CO can be lethal, a very small quantity is used in testing diffusing capacity of the lung for carbon monoxide ($D_L CO$).

Several techniques exist to assess D_L (Ruppel, 1990). The most common technique is the single-breath method of measuring $D_L CO$ because of its simplicity and noninvasive nature. The patient inhales a known volume of CO and holds his breath for 10 seconds to allow the gas to diffuse across the alveolar-capillary membrane. CO is measured in the patient's exhaled breath and compared to the initial volume. A normal D_{LCO} by the single-breath method is 25 ml/min/mm Hg. D_{LCO} is reduced by decreased hemoglobin (anemia) and in diseases causing thickening of the alveolar-capillary membrane or alveolar fibrosis, such as sarcoidosis or edema. Tumors, subsequent lung resection, and emphysema also reduce D_{LCO}. Conversely, D_{LCO} is increased by elevated alveolar CO_2 tension, polycythemia, and supine position (Table 8-2).

Table 8-2. Changes in $D_L CO$

Increased	Decreased
Exercise, hypervolemia, increased PA_{CO_2}, polycythemia, supine position	Alveolar-capillary membrane thickening or fibrosis (e.g., pulmonary edema, interstitial fibrosis, and sarcoidosis), cigarette smoking, decreased hemoglobin (e.g., anemia), loss of effective gas-exchanging surfaces (e.g., emphysema, lobectomy, pulmonary emboli, and tumors)

Interpretation of results

PFTs are altered by many elements. VC is a dynamic volume that changes daily, depending on the time of day, level of fatigue, and other factors. A change in position from upright to supine decreases VC because the diaphragm shifts upward and ventilation decreases at the bases. Similarly, obesity and pregnancy both push the diaphragm upward and decrease ERV and VC. Age is another factor that determines VC. As age increases, VC decreases. VC also is decreased as elastic properties of the lung decrease and the thoracic cage becomes more rigid.

The value of PFTs lies not only in the production of raw numbers but also in the comparison of the raw numbers to preestablished normals, also referred to as *predicted values*. Each volume or capacity measured by PFT has a normal range determined by age, height, sex, race, and weight of the patient. When compared with pulmonary function in other individuals with the same characteristics, alterations in pulmonary function are often more meaningful. For instance, FVC of 3.21 L may be normal for a 21-year-old woman who is 5 feet tall but low for a 21-year-old man who is 5 feet, 10 inches tall. Table 8-3 contains the normal predicted percentages for common PFTs although the derivation of individual predicted values is beyond the scope of this text. Table 8-3 also contains classification of pulmonary dysfunction as mild, mod-

Table 8-3. Pulmonary function tests

Test	Classification of predicted percentages			
	Normal	Mild	Moderate	Severe
FVC	≥80			
FEV_1	≥80	79-65	64-50	<50
FEV_1/FVC*	≥75	74-60	59-40	<40
$FEF_{25\%-75\%}$	≥80	79-60	59-40	<40
TLC	80-120			

*Not recorded as percentage of predicted but as actual percentage.

erate, or severe according to PFTs. (Note: There are many guidelines for interpretation of pulmonary function tests as mild, moderate, or severe. In addition, the values for disability vary from those commonly used for interpretation.)

The terms *obstructive* and/or *restrictive ventilatory defect* are used to describe a pattern of PFT results. When these results are combined with clinical and other laboratory evidence, the physician classifies the patient as having obstructive, restrictive, or combined obstructive-restrictive lung disease. Obstructive lung diseases narrow air passages, creating turbulence, increasing resistance to air flow, and producing an obstructive ventilatory defect. Patients experience difficulty exhaling through narrowed airways, and air trapping may result.

Obstructive lung patterns. One of the earliest signs of small airways obstruction on PFTs is a decrease in the $FEF_{25\%-75\%}$. This is accompanied or followed by a decrease in FEV. Because the patient cannot empty the lungs completely at the end of a breath, both FRC and RV increase. Evidence of air trapping is suggested by a difference in inspiratory VC (IVC) and FVC. It is thought that when FVC is smaller than IVC, obstruction with air trapping occurs during the forced-exhalation maneuver.

VC may be normal or decreased as a result of increased RV in patients with obstructive lung disease. Also, **the ratio of FEV_1 to FVC ($FEV_{1\%}$) is reduced.** When air trapping is persistent, TLC increases, and the patient develops a barrel-chested appearance. Patients with bronchospastic obstructive lung diseases, like asthma or bronchitis, respond to the administration of bronchodilators by demonstrating a 15% or greater improvement in FVC or FEV_1. Because emphysema is not always associated with bronchospasm, patients may not demonstrate significant improvement with inhaled bronchodilators. In patients with suspected asthma and normal PFT results, a methacholine challenge may be performed to exacerbate the asthma.

Restrictive lung patterns. In restrictive lung diseases lung expansion may be prevented by either internal or external forces (also termed *intrinsic* and *extrinsic*, respectively). Pneumonia, pulmonary edema, and interstitial fibrosis are examples of internal conditions that prevent lung expansion. External forces that prevent or limit lung expansion include obesity, pleural effusions, scoliosis, and myasthenia gravis. Regardless of the cause, patients with restrictive lung diseases have reduced inspiratory volumes and capacities, including VC, FEV_1, and TLC. RV and $FEF_{25\%-75\%}$ are normal unless obstruction is concurrent. Because flows are normal in pure restrictive lung disease, **the ratio of FEV_1 to FVC is usually normal or increased.**

Bedside pulmonary function tests

Bedside PFTs are useful in patients who are too ill or debilitated to be transported to the pulmonary function laboratory. Bedside PFTs are also useful in semiemergent situations, such as for the asthmatic patient in the emergency room or the patient undergoing major surgery with a full PFT laboratory schedule. Serial PFTs in the emergency room direct therapy by indicating increasing or decreasing obstruction or restriction in susceptible patients. Intubation is performed in a more controlled environment when the PFTs suggest increasing obstruction (as in asthma) or increasing restriction (as in progressive muscle weakness with Guillain-Barré syndrome). Intubation is prevented when PFTs demonstrate improvement in pulmonary function (see Table 8-4 for an analysis of PFT patterns).

Table 8-4. Analysis of PFT patterns

Test	Obstructive	Restrictive	Obstructive-restrictive combined
FEV_1/FVC	Decreased	Normal or increased	Normal or decreased
FVC	Decreased	Decreased	Decreased
FEV_1	Decreased	Decreased	Decreased
$FEF_{25\%-75\%}$	Decreased	Normal	Decreased
Bronchodilator response	Increased*	None	Increased

*No response in pure emphysema.

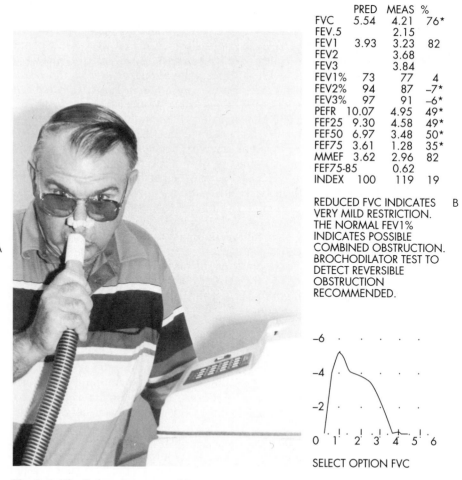

DATE 08/13/91   22°C
AGE HGT SEX RACE
54   75"   M   CAUC

	PRED	MEAS	%
FVC	5.54	4.21	76*
FEV.5		2.15	
FEV1	3.93	3.23	82
FEV2		3.68	
FEV3		3.84	
FEV1%	73	77	4
FEV2%	94	87	–7*
FEV3%	97	91	–6*
PEFR	10.07	4.95	49*
FEF25	9.30	4.58	49*
FEF50	6.97	3.48	50*
FEF75	3.61	1.28	35*
MMEF	3.62	2.96	82
FEF75-85		0.62	
INDEX	100	119	19

REDUCED FVC INDICATES
VERY MILD RESTRICTION.
THE NORMAL FEV1%
INDICATES POSSIBLE
COMBINED OBSTRUCTION.
BROCHODILATOR TEST TO
DETECT REVERSIBLE
OBSTRUCTION
RECOMMENDED.

A

B

SELECT OPTION FVC

Fig. 8-6. The Robert-Jones portable spirometer assesses spirometric pulmonary function (**A**) and is capable of determining many volumes and flows (**B**).

Baseline spirometry before surgery aids in predicting potential for postoperative complications and inability to wean from mechanical ventilation in patients with actual or suspected preexisting lung disease. Bedside PFTs also assist in the postoperative care of patients by identifying restrictive and obstructive defects in ventilation.

Bedside PFTs assist the physician to identify appropriate inhaled bronchodilator therapy in patients with obstructive airway disease. The physician determines effectiveness of beta-adrenergic and anticholinergic medications in a patient by testing pulmonary function after each medication is given independently several hours or a day apart (to allow the effect of the first medication to subside). If a bronchodilator response is noted with only one medication or both medications, the physician writes appropriate orders. If no response is observed with one of the medications, it may be discontinued.

The tests available at the bedside depend on the machine. Older bedside PFT machines may be capable only of printing an expiratory curve on graph paper. FVC, FEV_1, and $FEF_{25\%-75\%}$ are calculated manually. Some models also may have a digital display. Newer bedside or portable PFT machines perform a complete set of spirometry tests and print the patient's values compared with predicted and postbronchodilator values (Fig. 8-6). Flow-volume loops and MVV are measured with many newer models. In addition, modern computerized models provide an immediate interpretation comparable to current electrocardiographic machines.

CONCLUSION

PFTs are useful in assessing health and disease in conjunction with history and physical assessment. This chapter describes the types of PFTs available in a pulmonary function laboratory or at the bedside. Although nurses are not responsible for interpretation of PFTs, it is important for them to understand how the tests are performed and what the reported values mean. With this knowledge the nurse is better able to prepare the patient for the test, to help the patient understand implications of an abnormal test, and to direct nursing care, including patient teaching. For instance, if the test indicates an obstructive pattern of dysfunction, the nurse instructs the patient in techniques, such as pursed-lip breathing or proper inhaler administration, that minimize obstruction.

BIBLIOGRAPHY

American College of Chest Physicians: Statement on spirometry: a report of the section on respiratory pathophysiology, *Chest* 83(3):547-550, 1983.

American Thoracic Society: Guidelines for bronchial challenges with pharmacologic and antigenic agents (position paper), *ATS News* 6(2):11-19, spring 1980.

American Thoracic Society: ATS statement: snowbird workshop on standardization of spirometry, *Am Rev Respir Dis* 119(5):831-838, 1979.

American Thoracic Society: Standardization of spirometry: 1987 update, *Am Rev Respir Dis* 136:1285-1298, 1987.

Baum GL, Wolinsky E: *Textbook of pulmonary diseases,* ed 3, Boston, 1983, Little, Brown.

Bhagat RG, Grunstein MM: Comparison of responsiveness to methacholine, histamine, and exercise in subgroups of asthmatic children, *Am Rev Respir Dis* 129(2):221-224, 1984.

Burki NK: *Pulmonary diseases: medical outline series,* Garden City, NY, 1982, Medical Examination Publishing.

Burton GC, Hodgkin JE: *Respiratory care: a guide to clinical practice,* ed 2, Philadelphia, 1984, J B Lippincott.

Cary J, Huseby J, Culver B: Variability in interpretation of PFTs, *Chest* 76(4):389-90, 1979.

Cherniack NS, Widdicombe JG, eds: *Handbook of physiology, section 3: the respiratory system,* vol 3, Baltimore, 1986, Williams & Wilkins.

Cherniack R: Pitfalls in pulmonary function testing, *Respir Care* 28(4):434-441, 1983.

Comroe J: *Physiology of respiration: an introductory text,* ed 2, St Louis, 1974, Mosby—Year Book.

Fishman A: *Assessment of pulmonary function,* New York, 1980, McGraw-Hill.

Forster RE: *The lung: clinical physiology and pulmonary function tests,* ed 3, St Louis, 1986, Mosby—Year Book.

Fraser R, Paré J: *Diagnosis of diseases of the chest,* vol 1-3, ed 2, Philadelphia, 1977-1979, W B Saunders.

Gelb A, Williams A, Zamel N: Clinical significance of pulmonary function test: spirometry FEV_1 vs FEF_{25-75} percent, *Chest* 84(4):473-474, 1983.

Girard WM, Light RW: Should the FVC be considered in evaluating response to bronchodilator? *Chest* 84(1):87-89, 1983.

Harper R: *A guide to respiratory care: physiology and clinical applications,* Philadelphia, 1982, J B Lippincott.

Hinshaw H, Murray J: *Diseases of the chest,* ed 4, Philadelphia, 1980, W B Saunders.

Hyatt RE, Black LF: The flow-volume curve, *Am Rev Respir Dis* 107:191-199, 1973.

Kanner R, Renzetti A: Predictors of spirometric changes and mortality in obstructive airway disorders, *Chest* 85(6):15S-19S, 1984.

Morgan WKC: Pulmonary disability and impairment: can't work? won't work? *Basics RD,* American Thoracic Society 10(5), 1982.

Murray JF, Nadel JA, eds: *Textbook of respiratory medicine,* Philadelphia, 1988, W B Saunders.

Netter F: *The CIBA collection of medical illustrations, vol 7, respiratory system,* New York, 1979, CIBA Pharmaceutical.

Paré JAP, Fraser RG: *Synopsis of diseases of the chest,* Philadelphia, 1983, W B Saunders.

Ruppel G: *Manual of pulmonary function testing,* St Louis, 1990, Mosby–Year Book.

Shapiro B, Harrison R et al: *Clinical applications of respiratory care,* ed 3, St Louis, 1985, Mosby–Year Book.

Shoemaker WC, Thompson WL, Holbrook PR: *The Society of Critical Care Medicine textbook of critical care,* Philadelphia, 1984, W B Saunders.

Simmons DH, ed: *Current pulmonology,* vol 7, St Louis, 1986, Mosby–Year Book.

Slonim N, Hamilton L: *Respiratory physiology,* ed 5, St Louis, 1987, Mosby–Year Book.

Solomon DD: Are small airways tests helpful in the detection of early airflow obstruction? *Chest* 74(5):567-569, 1978.

Taussig LM: Standardization of lung function testing in children: Proceedings and recommendations of the GAP Conference Committe, Cystic Fibrosis Foundation. *J Pediatr* 97(4):668-676, 1980.

Tisi GM: Preoperative evaluation of pulmonary function: validity, indications and benefits, *Am Rev Respir Dis* 119(2):293-310, 1979.

Wade JF: *Comprehensive respiratory care: physiology and technique,* ed 3, St Louis, 1982, Mosby–Year Book.

Wanner A, Sackner MA: *Pulmonary diseases: mechanisms of altered structure and function,* Boston, 1983, Little & Brown.

West JB: *Pulmonary pathophysiology: the essentials,* ed 3, Baltimore, 1987, Williams & Wilkins.

West J: *Respiratory physiology: the essentials,* ed 3, Baltimore, 1985, Williams & Wilkins.

C H · A · P · T · E · R 9

Bedside Monitoring of Acutely Ill Patients

O*bjectives*

- Critique the components of breathing frequency.
- Assess the components of weaning parameters and discuss their significance.
- Identify various clinical applications for capnography.
- Examine the assessment of dead space and dead space to tidal volume ratio.
- Determine the measurement of dynamic and static compliance.
- Summarize the measurement of resistance.
- Analyze a normal capnogram and differences observed with ventilator circuit leak, cardiopulmonary arrest, and airway obstruction.

Invasive and noninvasive techniques are used to assess the ability of the patient to exchange air with the environment and to exchange gases between the lungs and blood. Although most equipment used to monitor the patient's respiratory status was formerly reserved for the intensive care unit, technology has advanced to allow application on general floors also. This chapter is devoted to bedside monitoring of ventilation and oxygenation in acutely ill patients, beginning with basic monitoring and progressing to more advanced methods of respiratory assessment. Ventilation is discussed first because air must get into the lungs before it can be oxygenated (oxygenation is dependent on ventilation). Some concepts examined in assessing ventilation (and possibly oxygenation) are unfamiliar to many nurses and are difficult to grasp without repeated application. In addition, some parts of the chapter are very technical and are intended for the nurse desiring advanced knowledge to assess ventilation and oxygenation.

The basic or simple methods discussed in this chapter to assess ventilation include breathing frequency and other measurements commonly referred to as weaning parameters, although they also have many other applications. Advanced or more complex methods to assess problems with ventilation include alveolar minute ventilation ($\dot{V}_A$), dead space, dead space (V_D) to tidal volume (V_T) ratio, compliance, pressure-volume curves, resistance, and capnography.

Unfortunately the simple bedside methods to assess oxygenation are fewer than those of ventilation. This chapter explains the role of vital signs and hemodynamics in assessing oxygenation. Oxygen transport, oxygen delivery, and oxygen consumption are examined as more complex methods of assessing problems with oxygenation. Finally, this chapter presents the role of pulse oximetry in assessing oxygenation in critically and noncritically ill patients.

VENTILATION
Characteristics of breaths

Frequency. Ventilatory assessment begins with evaluation of respiratory rate, also termed *frequency of breathing*. Although it often is overlooked, breathing frequency provides clues to the patient's ventilatory status. When assessing breathing frequency, the nurse also notes the sound, pattern, and depth of the breaths because rate alone, unless it is zero, tells little about the patient's ventilatory status. The nurse should recall that a normal respiratory rate varies from 12 to 20 breaths per minute. Because lung compliance is enhanced at lower frequencies in patients with obstructive lung disease, these patients are often observed breathing at lower rates (and increased depths). Conversely, patients with restrictive lung disease breathe more rapidly (and shallowly) to improve compliance. In patients receiving mechanical ventilation, both the spontaneous and ventilator breaths are counted to determine breathing rate. A significant increase in breathing frequency, especially in nonmechanically ventilated patients, warns of respiratory compromise from various conditions, including atelectasis, bronchospasm, air trapping, or pulmonary edema.

Sounds of breaths. Normal breathing is quiet. Adventitious sounds (reviewed in Chapter 5) are associated with many lung diseases. Secretions cause both wheezing and crackles and bronchospasm causes wheezing and decreased breath sounds. Noisy breaths or snoring is common in obstructive sleep apnea.

Pattern of breaths. The pattern or rhythm of breathing changes in many illnesses (see Chapter 5). For instance, in sleep apnea many different patterns of breathing are observed. Snoring is commonly accompanied by periods of shallow respirations, which are followed by apneas. The apneic intervals are subsequently replaced by deep breathing to restore oxygen and carbon dioxide to baseline levels. In mechanically ventilated patients asynchronous spontaneous breaths and ventilator breaths may occur. Frequently the patient tries to exhale as the ventilator is forcing air into his lungs. Some patients attempt to initiate a breath before the ventilator is ready to deliver one. Pressure alarms are usually activated, and the patient is reported to be "fighting the ventilator."

Another abnormal respiratory pattern is paradoxic diaphragm, sometimes termed *Hoover's sign*. Instead of the diaphragm descending on inspiration, it ascends. During expiration, when the diaphragm normally ascends, it is seen descending.

The nurse may also observe use of alternating muscles of respiration. The patient uses the upper chest muscles to inhale for a time. As these muscles fatigue, the patient begins to use the lower chest or abdominal muscles to inhale. In effect the patient is alternating between upper chest muscles and lower chest muscles to breathe. The pattern, sometimes termed *respiratory alternans,* is usually somewhat cyclic and is associated with respiratory muscle fatigue.

Depth of breaths. Depth of breathing, or tidal volume (V_T), varies among individuals and states of health and wakefulness. Depth of breathing is difficult to assess consistently by simple observation (objective measurement of V_T is discussed below). Reliability and consistency of measurement are a concern when nurses hold a hand in front of the patient's mouth to feel the volume of air moved. The use of palpation (see physical assessment section of Chapter 5) to measure uniformity and degree of respiratory excursion is a useful adjunct.

Breathing is usually more shallow during periods of rest or sleep. Acidosis is often countered by deep ventilations (Kussmaul respirations) to blow off the excess acid. Pain, especially from chest trauma, angina, or thoracic or abdominal surgery, is often accompanied by decreased depth of breathing. A significant change in the depth of breathing, such as excessively deep or shallow breathing, requires further investigation.

Weaning parameters

The term *weaning parameters* refers to a group of tests that are commonly used to assess the patient's readiness to be removed, or weaned, from mechanical ventilation. Depending on the institution, weaning parameters may include a few tests or a long list of tests. Traditional weaning parameters include measurement of vital capacity (VC), negative inspiratory force, $\dot{V}_E$, V_T, and frequency. (Techniques of weaning and the implementation of weaning parameters are discussed in Chapter 14.)

Tidal volume. Accurate, objective measurement of V_T is required in many instances. Either inhaled or exhaled V_T is measured in most circumstances. In mechanically ventilated patients, exhaled V_T is compared to inhaled V_T to determine cuff integrity and inflation.

To measure inhaled V_T, a device, such as an incentive spirometer, is used. Accuracy varies, depending on the incentive spirometer device. (Incentive spirometers are discussed in Chapter 13.)

Exhaled V_T is accurately measured with the use of a Wright respirometer or similar device. Resembling a hand-held stopwatch or clock, a Wright respirometer consists of a vane connected to a series of gears. Air rotates the vane, and volume is calculated. The Wright respirometer is accurate when air flows through it between 3 and 300 LPM (Ruppel, 1990). To measure volume, the Wright respirometer is connected to the mouth with a mouthpiece or to the endotracheal tube with an adapter (Fig. 9-1). The Wright respirometer may also be positioned in the exhalation tubing of the ventilator circuit. Used to assess one breath or a series of breaths, the Wright respirometer contains two scales: a scale calibrated in $\frac{1}{10}$ L (10 ml) increments up to 1 L and another scale calibrated in 1 L increments up to 100 L.

In severe restrictive lung disease, V_T is reduced markedly. The patient compensates by increasing rate of breathing. When V_T is decreased unexpectedly, the nurse assesses for the cause. Common reasons for decreased V_T are accumulation of secretions or fluid in the airways or alveoli, increased airway resistance from bronchospasm or pain, and leaks in the ventilator circuit.

Minute ventilation. $\dot{V}_E$ is the sum of all of the air inhaled or exhaled in 1 minute. Assessment of $\dot{V}_E$ is more useful than either frequency (f) or V_T. $\dot{V}_E$ is the product of frequency and V_T. Changes in either f or V_T alter $\dot{V}_E$. Reciprocal changes in both f and V_T are necessary to maintain a normal $\dot{V}_E$. For instance, $\dot{V}_E$ may remain constant if f increases even though V_T is

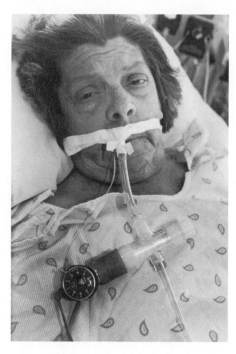

Fig. 9-1. The Wright respirometer connects to the endotracheal tube with an adapter containing one-way valves to measure weaning parameters.

decreased significantly.

$$\text{Normal } V_T \ 500 \times f \ 12 = \dot{V}_E \ 6 \text{ LPM}$$
$$\text{Example } V_T \ 250 \times f \ 24 = \dot{V}_E \ 6 \text{ LPM}$$

$\dot{V}_E$ is measured using a Wright respirometer or an air bag (such as Douglas or Hudson). The Wright respirometer is commonly used to measure $\dot{V}_E$ in spontaneously and mechanically ventilated patients. Instead of assessing a single V_T breath, the Wright respirometer accumulates V_T breaths for 1 minute before being turned off or disconnected. When the Douglas air bag is used, exhaled gases are collected over a period, usually 1 to 5 minutes. The volume of air in the bag is measured. $\dot{V}_E$ is obtained by dividing the volume of air measured in the bag by the collection time. Use of the Douglas air bag technique to measure $\dot{V}_E$ usually is reserved for simultaneous measurement of exhaled-gas components to quantify dead space or measure oxygen consumption. Usually used in the home, a Hudson bag is used to assess $\dot{V}_E$, particularly of a patient on a mechanical ventilator. A Hudson bag contains markings to indicate volume and is inexpensive, but it is also less precise than a Wright respirometer.

Vital capacity. VC is the maximum amount of air that can be forcefully exhaled after a maximum inhalation. The VC of a particular patient is based on height, weight, gender, position, and age of the patient. Nomograms are usually used to determine predicted VC for a given patient although calculations can be performed that are based on regression analysis. Although it is useful to compare the patient's measured VC to predicted values, it is often more useful to relate consecutive measurements of VC in the same patient.

The trend of VC measurements is particularly useful in assessing progression of neuromuscular disease. As the muscles of inspiration weaken, ability to perform a VC maneuver decreases. Similarly, stabilization of or improvement in neuromuscular function is observed by the patient's improved ability to perform a VC maneuver. VC measurement is also useful in the postoperative thoracotomy or laparotomy patient. Development of atelectasis or pneumonia is associated with a decrease in VC. Inability of the patient to inhale to VC may be associated with impaired ability to cough and clear secretions. The value of VC in weaning patients from mechanical ventilation is controversial but usually is assessed.

VC is measured with a Wright respirometer or similar bedside device (such as a portable or incentive spirometer). The patient is positioned in semi-Fowler's position or an upright sitting position to enhance diaphragmatic function. At least three VC measurements are made at each testing, depending on the patient's compliance, effort, and condition. The patient's best effort is recorded on the chart although it is useful and accepted to record all efforts. In patients with bronchospasm or weakened muscles, the first effort is frequently the best. VC measurements decrease as bronchospasm or respiratory muscle fatigue increases.

Inspiratory and expiratory force. Another measure of the patient's muscular ability to move a volume of air and to maintain adequate alveolar ventilation is inspiratory force. Negative inspiratory force (NIF), or the ability to breathe in, measures diaphragmatic strength. Unlike VC, NIF does not require patient cooperation for accurate measurement. Therefore NIF is more useful in uncooperative and obtunded patients, in whom VC cannot be measured.

A procedure to measure NIF is performed by occluding the patient's airway with an adapter for approximately 20 seconds while an inspiratory force or pressure manometer measures NIF (Fig. 9-2). Unless the patient is apneic, he will make respiratory efforts and generate subatmospheric pressure (hence the term *negative*).

NIF is reduced in cases of decreased respiratory muscle function. Diminished respiratory muscle function has many causes. The most frequent cause of diminished respiratory function and decreased NIF in mechanically ventilated patients is muscle disuse, which leads to atrophy and reduced lung compliance.

Similar to VC, following consecutive measurements or trends of NIF guides patient care. When used to assess ability of the patient to be weaned from mechanical ventilation, NIF of at least −20 cm water pressure is desired. Values below −20 cm water pressure are associated with inability to sustain adequate spontaneous ventilation over time. Healthy individuals are able to generate at least −80 cm water pressure.

Caution must be exercised when measuring NIF in patients receiving mechanical ventilation with high levels of supplemental oxygen or positive end-expiratory pressure (PEEP). Removal of the oxygen and PEEP for even 20 seconds may compromise the patient's cardiopulmonary status. Similarly, NIF should be measured cautiously in patients with unstable cardiovascular status, including congestive heart failure.

Positive expiratory pressure. Positive expiratory pressure (PEP), the opposite of NIF, sometimes is termed *positive expiratory force (PEF)*. It is not to be confused with PEEP, which is used in mechanical ventilation. As in NIF

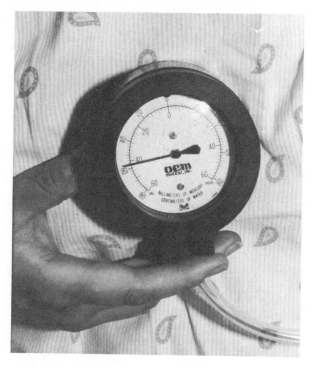

Fig. 9-2. Measuring negative inspiratory force with pressure manometer while the airway is occluded.

PEP measures muscular strength. PEP commonly is assessed in patients with neuromuscular diseases to assess the progression or remission of the disease. The technique of assessing PEP is similar to the technique of assessing NIF. A pressure manometer is inserted in the airway, but the patient exhales instead of inhaling. As the patient exhales, the manometer records PEP.

Maximum voluntary ventilation. Maximum voluntary ventilation (MVV) is the maximal volume that can be breathed per minute by voluntary effort. It is another technique that assesses status of the respiratory muscles and is affected by changes in compliance and resistance, which are discussed later in this chapter. The patient breathes in and out as rapidly and deeply as possible for a specified interval, up to one minute; most clinicians use 15-second intervals. Actual values are extrapolated to 1 minute when lesser times are used. For example, a 15-second measurement is multiplied by 4. Normal values vary greatly, up to 30% (Ruppel, 1990). Therefore only profound reductions in MVV are clinically significant. The MVV maneuver exaggerates air trapping and respiratory muscle fatigue and should be used cautiously in susceptible patients. In patients being weaned from mechanical ventilation, the ability to double measured $\dot{V}_E$ with the MVV maneuver indicates adequate ventilatory reserve.

Peak flow. Peak flow is the maximum flow rate generated during a forced-exhalation maneuver. Most hand-held devices, such as the Wright or Assess peak flow meters (Fig. 9-3), record flow in liters per minute although some devices record flow in liters per second. Although most peak-flow devices

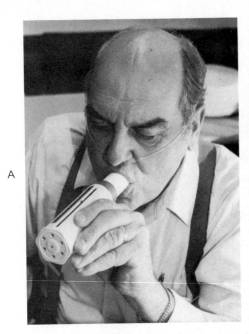 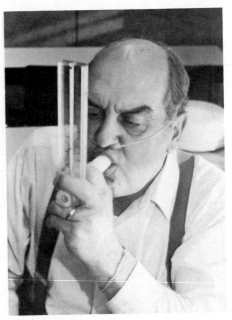

A   B

Fig. 9-3. Patients measure peak flow with the use of a portable peak flow meter. (**A**) mini-Wright and (**B**) Assess.

measure peak flow up to 500 LPM, newer models assess peak flows up to 800 LPM. Sophisticated devices to measure peak flow are also available and include pneumotachometers and computer-assisted pulmonary function machines.

Peak flow is an effort-dependent test that demonstrates in numerical form the ability of the patient to "get the air out." Physicians commonly use peak flow meters in patients with bronchospastic obstructive airways disease to monitor the effectiveness of bronchodilator therapy. Peak flow measurements are made and recorded in a diary immediately before and 30 to 60 minutes after inhaled bronchodilator treatments. An improvement in peak flow is associated with a positive response to therapy. However, because patients with obstructive lung disease may develop initially high peak flows before airway closure occurs, peak flows should be correlated with other assessments.

Alveolar minute ventilation

Alveolar minute ventilation, $\dot{V}_A$, is the portion of inhaled air that participates in gas exchange ($\dot{V}$ is the abbreviation for volume and A is the abbreviation for alveolar). Alveolar ventilation depends on a variety of factors, the most important being V_T, frequency, dead space (Vd), and metabolic factors, such as oxygen consumption and carbon dioxide production.

The easiest method to calculate alveolar minute ventilation assumes that alveolar dead space (Vd alv) is zero; in other words, physiological dead space (Vd p) is equal to anatomical dead space (Vd anat).

$$\dot{V}_A = f \, (V_T - V_d)$$

where f = respiratory rate. This equation is not useful in patients with ventilation-perfusion mismatching because Vd alv is not zero.

Alveolar minute ventilation is assessed more accurately by measuring volume and concentration of CO_2 in exhaled gases because all carbon dioxide in exhaled gases comes from alveoli:

$$\dot{V}_A = \frac{\dot{V}_{CO_2}}{F_{A}CO_2}$$

CO_2 production ($\dot{V}_{CO_2}$) is the volume (milliliters per minute) of CO_2 exhaled in one minute, and $F_A CO_2$ is the fraction of CO_2 in alveolar gas. When an end-tidal CO_2 monitor (capnography) is used, the concentration of CO_2 is read from the monitor, and the equation is simplified:

$$\dot{V}_A = \frac{\dot{V}_{CO_2}}{F_{E}CO_2}$$

where $F_E CO_2$ is the fractional expired concentration of CO_2 in percent stated as a decimal. Because $F_E CO_2$ is indirectly proportional to alveolar CO_2 (Pa_{CO_2}) and to arterial CO_2 (Pa_{CO_2}) and directly proportional to the volume of CO_2 exhaled, alveolar minute ventilation is calculated in the following manner:

$$\dot{V}_A = \frac{\dot{V}_{CO_2}}{Pa_{CO_2}} \times 0.863$$

Dead space. In measuring $\dot{V}_E$, the amount of air that ventilates both functioning and nonfunctioning alveoli are measured. The most important component of $\dot{V}_E$ is the portion that participates in gas exchange. The rest, Vd, is approximately 1 ml per pound of ideal body weight in the normal individual (see the physiology section of Chapter 2 as needed for understanding Vd). Because Vd anat is constant while Vd alv (thus Vd phy) varies, a change in the measurement of Vd implies a change in Vd alv.

Measuring the amount of Vd is important in many lung conditions and can be expressed as a ratio of Vd phy to V_T (Vd/V_T). The Vd/V_T ratio tells exactly how much of the ventilation is being wasted. Normal Vd/V_T is 0.2 to 0.35. Vd/V_T is calculated using the following equation:

$$Vd/V_T = \frac{Pa_{CO_2} - P_{E}CO_2}{Pa_{CO_2}}$$

where $P_E CO_2$ is the amount of CO_2 measured from exhaled gases. The nurse should recall that because there is essentially no CO_2 in inspired air, all CO_2 from expired air comes from the alveoli as a result of gas exchange. The $P_E CO_2$ contains CO_2 from only Vd alv.

Exhaled CO_2 may be reported as either a percentage of exhaled CO_2 ($F_E CO_2$) or in mm Hg. When reported as a percentage, the alveolar air equation is used to convert CO_2 to mm Hg. For instance, the nurse should assume that in the following example the patient's exhaled CO_2 has been reported as 4% and the Pa_{CO_2} from ABGs is 40 mm Hg.

$$
\begin{aligned}
P_{E}CO_2 &= (P_B - PH_2O) \times F_E CO_2 \\
&= (760 - 47) \times 4\% \\
&= 28 \text{ mm Hg}
\end{aligned}
$$

Using the equation above, then

$$\frac{Vd}{V_T} = \frac{40 - 28}{40} = 0.3$$

If the amount of CO_2 in the patient's exhaled gases were decreased by half to 2% without a reciprocal change in the Pa_{CO_2}, then Vd/V_T would be as follows:

$$P_{E_{CO_2}} = (P_B - P_{H20}) \times F_{E_{CO_2}}$$
$$= (760 - 47) \times 2\%$$
$$= 14 \text{ mm Hg}$$

Using the equation above, Vd/V_T doubles.

$$\frac{Vd}{V_T} = \frac{40 - 14}{40} = 0.65$$

If the patient in the above examples is breathing 12 times per minute at a volume of 500 ml, the $\dot{V}_E$ is 6 LPM. In the first example, 70% of 500 ml (350 ml) participates in gas exchange, and 30% (150 ml) is Vd. In the subsequent example, 35% of 500 ml (175 ml) is ventilating functioning alveoli and participating in gas exchange, and 65% of 500 ml (325 ml) is wasted ventilation.

Normal Vd/V_T is usually about 30% because, in the normal individual, Vd is equal to about 30% of V_T and is composed primarily of Vd anat. An increase in measured Vd is then attributable to Vd alv. For instance, if a patient has V_T of 500 ml and Vd of 150 ml as shown above, Vd is calculated as follows:

$$\frac{Vd\ 150\ ml}{V_T\ 500\ ml} = 0.3$$

Assume that the patient has pain and breathes more shallowly. V_T drops to 300 ml. Vd anat is constant. Vd/V_T increases, demonstrating an increase in Vd alv or alveoli that are not being ventilated.

$$\frac{Vd\ 150\ ml}{V_T\ 300\ ml} = 0.5$$

Assume instead that the patient develops a ventilation-perfusion abnormality that increases wasted ventilation with respect to blood flow or reduces blood flow with respect to ventilation. V_T is constant at 500 ml. Vd ventilation increases to 250 ml.

$$\frac{Vd\ 250\ ml}{V_T\ 500\ ml} = 0.5$$

Whether V_T decreases or Vd ventilation increases, the end result is increased Vd/V_T.

Compliance. Compliance, a measure of work of breathing, was described in Chapter 2. In the laboratory, compliance is measured by controlling lung volume and observing pressure changes that are measured with an esophageal balloon. Airway resistance is not a factor because the measurements are made under static conditions at points of zero air flow. In the nonintubated, nonmechanically ventilated patient, compliance can be estimated by following changes in the VC. As compliance decreases, work of breathing increases to inspire the same volume of air. Inability to overcome deteriorating compliance results in lowered VC.

Two types of compliance are measured easily at the bedside of a patient on mechanical ventilation: dynamic (Cdyn) and static (Cstat). The terms *effective dynamic compliance* and *effective static compliance* are used frequently to differentiate estimated bedside measurements from actual measurements made in the laboratory with an esophageal balloon. The terms *dynamic* and *static* compliance used here imply effective dynamic or static compliance.

Cdyn is measured by dividing the patient's exhaled V_T in milliliters by the peak airway pressure (P_P) in cm H_2O − the baseline pressure (P_b).

$$Cdyn = \frac{V_T}{P_P - P_b}$$

Baseline pressure is the level of PEEP. Exhaled V_T is measured with the spirometer attached to the ventilator or with a Wright respirometer positioned in the expiratory limb of the ventilator circuit. In many instances the inhaled or delivered V_T is used. Using the delivered V_T is inaccurate when a cuff leak is present or when the patient has an air leak from chest tubes.

Peak airway pressure is directly observed on the peak airway pressure manometer of the ventilator, or it can be obtained by connecting a pressure manometer to the ventilator circuit. After the breath is delivered by the ventilator, the nurse observes the highest point (at the end of inspiration) reached by the pressure gauge pointer, that is, peak airway pressure. This number is used in calculating Cdyn. Cdyn is normally greater than 50 ml/cm H_2O although the trend of measured compliance is more important than the actual number. When PEEP and V_T remain constant, simply observing the variance in peak pressures indicates stability of Cdyn and work of breathing. A patient with decreasing Cdyn (or increasing peak pressures when PEEP and V_T are constant) over the course of several hours to days should be assessed for respiratory compromise. He may have a mucus plug or bronchospasm. Compliance measurements should be made with the patient in the same position, usually supine or semiFowler's position, and at the same peak flow rate.

Cstat is also easily assessed at the bedside. The patient's exhalation tubing is temporarily occluded at the end of inspiration, or an inspiratory pause or hold is set on the ventilator. Following the peak pressure measurement, the pointer falls to a new level, where it momentarily pauses or plateaus before falling to baseline. The point of pause after peak pressure measurement is termed the *plateau pressure* (P_{pl}) and is used for Cstat measurements. As in Cdyn the actual value of Cstat is often not as important as the trend. A trend of decreasing compliance (or increasing P_{pl} in the presence of stable PEEP and V_T) is cause for warning. Further assessment to determine the cause is warranted. Pneumonia, pulmonary edema, and noncardiogenic pulmonary edema are frequent causes.

Although compliance is easy to measure, it does not encompass all factors that can increase work of breathing. Airway resistance is another factor.

Example 1:

A 70 kg patient receives mechanical ventilation for pulmonary edema at a V_T of 700 ml (0.7 L), ventilatory rate of 10, and PEEP 5 cm H_2O. Peak flow on the ventilator is set to deliver the V_T in 1 second (0.7 L/sec). The nurse measures peak pressure 50 cm H_2O and P_{pl} 40 cm H_2O. The nurse calculates the patient's Cdyn and Cstat.

$$Cdyn = \frac{V_T}{P_P - P_b} = \frac{700}{50 - 5} = \frac{700}{45} = 15.5 \text{ ml/cm } H_2O$$

$$Cstat = \frac{V_T}{P_{pl} - P_b} = \frac{700}{40 - 5} = \frac{700}{35} = 20 \text{ ml/cm } H_2O$$

The patient's lungs are said to be stiff or noncompliant because great pressure is required to deliver the volume.

Pressure-volume curves. Determining Cdyn and Cstat at various V_Ts is the basis for developing a pressure-volume curve. In PEEP or V_T-sensitive patients, compliance is significantly different with volume changes as low as 200 ml and PEEP changes as low as 2 cm H_2O. Under the direction of the physician, the nurse alters in sequence either the V_T or the PEEP and measures Cdyn and Cstat. If the pressure suddenly increases 10 to 15 cm H_2O, the patient's compliance has decreased significantly. The nurse returns the patient to the previous area of best compliance and notifies the physician.

Resistance. The nurse may need to assess resistance to air flow. Secretions and bronchospasm are frequent causes of airways resistance. In addition to compliance resistance may be calculated to determine the optimal level of pressure-support ventilation. Resistance is the pressure required to deliver a volume of air in a specified period. The following equation is used to calculate airways resistance:

$$R = \frac{P_{P-Pl}}{F}, \text{ where F (flow)} = \frac{V_T}{Ti} \text{ and Ti = inspiratory time}$$

Using the data above in example 1, the nurse calculates resistance.

$$R = \frac{P_{P-Pl}}{F} = \frac{50 - 40}{0.7/1} = \frac{10}{0.7} = 14.3 \text{ cm } H_2O/l/sec$$

As with compliance, the trend of airway resistance is often more important than a single measurement. A resistance trend is identified by assessing the peak and plateau pressures over time. Assuming that the patient's V_T and peak flow do not change, resistance increases when the peak pressure increases without a change in plateau pressure. Compliance is altered when the plateau pressure also changes.

Capnography. Capnography is a relatively new method of assessing ventilation by measuring the amount of CO_2 in exhaled gases with an infrared analyzer in either intubated or nonintubated patients. By assessing each individual breath and observing the trend of breathing over time, the nurse learns useful information about cardiopulmonary function. Capnography is clinically useful in recognizing critical incidents, preventing intubation and anesthetic mishaps, and identifying failure to ventilate. The effects of nursing interventions, such as suctioning or positioning, on ventilation can be assessed by capnography. When assisting with intubation or resecuring an endotracheal tube, the nurse is assured of correct placement of the artificial airway by the presence or maintenance of end tidal CO_2 levels. Nurses rely on capnography during periods of weaning to identify hypoventilation and ineffective breathing patterns that impede weaning from mechanical ventilation. Patients can frequently be spared drawing of numerous ABG samples during weaning from mechanical ventilation or cardiopulmonary arrest with the use of capnography.

Capnography is an analysis of the patient's respiratory pattern obtained by continuously monitoring exhaled carbon dioxide. With capnography both the waveform, analogous to an electrocardiogram or pulmonary artery catheter tracing, and a digital value of exhaled CO_2 are assessed. Capnography is not to be confused with capnometry, which is only a digital expression of exhaled carbon dioxide and not accompanied by a waveform. A capnogram is the graphic display of continuous exhaled CO_2 assessment.

To understand capnography, pertinent physiology is reviewed briefly. Oxygen supplied by inspiration is necessary for the production of adenosine triphosphate (ATP). When ATP is consumed in cellular function, CO_2 is produced ($\dot{V}CO_2$). The amount of carbon dioxide produced is a measure of body metabolism. The carbon dioxide waste gas is picked up by the circulating red blood cells and transported to the lungs for elimination. Whereas respiration is the exchange of gases at the cellular level, ventilation is the exchange of air with the environment. The nurse should recall that increased ventilation decreases the amount of CO_2 in the blood, and decreased ventilation increases the amount of CO_2 in the blood. Assessing the amount of exhaled CO_2 provides information about metabolism, circulation, and ventilation.

A normal capnogram has a characteristic waveform (Fig. 9-4). At the start of exhalation CO_2 is essentially zero because air is coming from Vd anat, including the mouth, trachea, and bronchi. As carbon dioxide leaves the alveoli, a sharp upstroke followed by a slowly rising plateau, termed the *alveolar plateau,* is noted on the capnogram. With the onset of inspiration the capnogram quickly returns to baseline, where it remains until the next breath. End tidal CO_2 ($EtCO_2$) is measured at the point just before inspiration. In the normal capnogram $EtCO_2$ is maximal just before inspiration.

The normal capnogram is assessed for five characteristics: height, frequency, rhythm, baseline, and shape. End-tidal CO_2 ($EtCO_2$) determines the height. Respiratory rate determines the frequency. Medullary and ventilator functions characterize rhythm. Baseline should be zero. Finally, metabolism, circulation, and ventilation define shape.

Capnography can usually be observed in two forms. The monitor may be set to view each capnogram on the screen in real time, similar to an ECG. The number of capnograms observed on the screen depends on the patient's respiratory rate. Alternately, the monitor may be set to view in the split-screen mode, where all end tidal points over the last minute, termed *compressed respiration cycles,* and the most recent (last breath) capnogram are observed on the screen. In most situations the split-screen mode, which identifies trends in the patient's $EtCO_2$, is preferred for identifying time-related problems.

Carbon dioxide gradient. Alveolar CO_2 is estimated by the $EtCO_2$ measured by capnography. Normal $EtCO_2$ is equivalent to $PaCO_2$ in healthy individuals. A gradient of 1 to 5 mm Hg from $EtCO_2$ to $PaCO_2$ is considered normal variation (the $PaCO_2$ is higher). Increased ventilation-perfusion mismatching or shunt is responsible for greater increases in the $EtCO_2$ to $PaCO_2$ gradient. CO_2 that does not participate in gas exchange builds up in the blood. The size of the gradient provides useful information about the extent of shunt. Increases in the gradient are associated with increased shunting, and decreases in the gradient are associated with decreased shunting. Increased gradients are observed in pulmonary embolism and other cardiopulmonary diseases (Hatle and Rokseth, 1974).

Analysis of waveform. Several guidelines assist in analyzing the capnogram (Table 9-1). Both individual and trending capnogram waveforms are

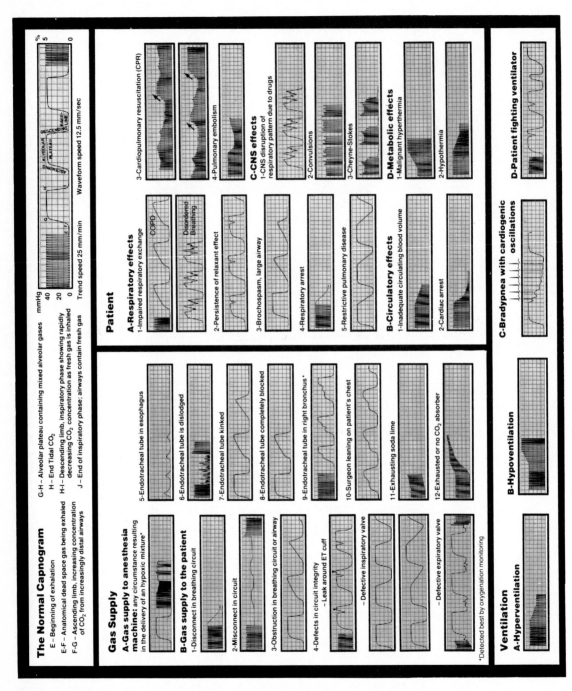

Fig. 9-4. Examples of normal and abnormal capnograms. (Courtesy Hewlett–Packard, Andover, Md.)

Table 9-1. Capnogram

Alveolar plateau level falls	Alveolar plateau level rises

Increased ventilation
  Central, peripheral
	Decreased ventilation
	Depressed respiration
	  Central, peripheral

Decreased CO_2 production
  Hypothermia
	Increased CO_2 production
	  Rewarming, hyperthermia, increased
	  motor tone, convulsions

Impaired CO_2 transportation
  Elimination defects,
  technical defects
	Increased CO_2 transportation
	  Improved circulation after shock,
	  increased blood pressure after hypotension
	Increased CO_2 absorption
	  Laparoscopy

Impaired circulation
  Shock, pulmonary embolism,
  cardiac arrest
	Infused intravenous bicarbonate
	  solutions
	Rebreathed CO_2
	Condensed water in analyzer

evaluated for slope of the alveolar plateau, height, and baseline. The slope of the alveolar plateau depicts condition of the airways and lung tissue. The nurse should recall that the alveolar plateau is almost horizontal in the normal capnogram. When expiration is impaired, the slope of the alveolar plateau is altered. When a leak is present in the ventilator circuit, including ruptured endotracheal tube cuff, the alveolar plateau does not develop. If a mechanically ventilated patient tries to inhale during exhalation, a cleft is seen in the alveolar plateau.

A high $Etco_2$ may be seen in patients with normal respiratory rate, and alveolar plateau may be seen in patients receiving insufficient $\dot{V}_E$ from the mechanical ventilator. It is also seen in patients with increased body temperature. Patients unable to compensate for respiratory depression (increased intracranial pressure, narcotic respiratory depression, and pharmacological paralysis) will also have an elevated $Etco_2$ and a normal capnogram.

A low $Etco_2$ may be seen in patients receiving excessive $\dot{V}_E$ from the mechanical ventilator. Patients with low body temperature, metabolic acidosis, central neurogenic hypoventilation or hypoxemia and patients in shock or pain may also have a low $Etco_2$.

A sudden drop in the height of the $Etco_2$ to a low level or to zero indicates a technical disturbance or defect, such as patient disconnection from the capnography system or from the mechanical ventilator, defective $Etco_2$ analyzer, or defective mechanical ventilator. A sudden decrease in the $Etco_2$ value (but not to zero) indicates a leak in the mechanical ventilator system (usually accompanied by a low-pressure alarm) or airway obstruction (usually accompanied by a high-pressure alarm). Gradual lowering of the $Etco_2$ is associated with decreased CO_2, as occurs in gradual hyperventilation, decreasing body temperature, and decreasing body or lung perfusion. However, an exponential decrease in $Etco_2$ within 1 to 2 minutes indicates a sudden disturbance in circulation or ventilation, including circulatory arrest, embolism, shock, and sudden severe hyperventilation.

Sudden increases in the height of the alveolar plateau occur when CO_2 rapidly enters the bloodstream. Three causes of sudden increase in the alveolar plateau are injection of $NaHCO_3^-$, quick release of a tourniquet, and abrupt increase in blood pressure, as occurs after use of intravenous epinephrine. Gradual increase in the alveolar plateau in either the spontaneously breathing or mechanically ventilated patient is a sign of increased CO_2 or hypoventilation. This pattern is also seen in patients with rapidly increasing body temperature (fever from sepsis or postoperative warming) and postlaparoscopy (CO_2 absorbed from peritoneal cavity).

Disturbances in respiratory rhythm are responsible for alternating increases and decreases in alveolar plateau height. The capnogram observed in Cheyne-Stokes respirations, seen in conditions such as cerebral arteriosclerosis, brain damage, congestive heart failure, and drug intoxication, is shown in Figure 9-4. The alveolar plateau appears as a half-moon or quarter-moon shape followed by rapidly decreasing alveolar plateau. During apnea the capnogram returns to zero. As respiration resumes, the moon-shaped alveolar plateau returns.

When the baseline suddenly increases, with or without changes in the alveolar plateau level, there is usually calibration error, CO_2 absorber saturation, water buildup in the analyzer, or condensation in the airway adapter. Gradual increases in both the baseline and alveolar plateau are also associated with increasing Vd.

OXYGENATION

Techniques to assess ventilation have been covered in some detail. The second half of this chapter discusses assessment of oxygenation. (Please review concepts of oxygenation presented in Chapters 3 and 6.) Inadequate oxygenation is often difficult to recognize because the body efficiently distributes available O_2 to vital areas (Bryan-Brown, 1982). In the presence of hypoxemia, sympathetic output is increased. Subsequently, skin, skeletal muscle, and splanchnic blood flow is decreased, and coronary and brain flow is increased. Compensatory mechanisms, such as increased $\dot{V}_E$ and increased cardiac output, are activated.

One of the major determinants of oxygenation is the ability of the heart to eject a volume of blood through the body, that is, cardiac output. Four factors affect cardiac output: preload, afterload, contractility, and heart rate.

Preload is the degree of myocardial fiber stretch at the end of diastole. In the absence of tricuspid valve disease, preload is clinically estimated in the right heart by central venous pressure (CVP) or right atrial pressure (RAP). Left heart preload is assessed by the measurement of pulmonary artery wedge pressure (PAWP) or left atrial pressure (LAP). Because preload is affected by circulating blood volume, atrial contraction, and ventricular contraction, alteration in one or more of the factors can ultimately change cardiac output.

Afterload, tension in the myocardium during systole, is affected by blood viscosity, distensibility of the vascular system, and valvular function. Afterload is assessed by the determination of systemic vascular resistance (SVR) and pulmonary vascular resistance (PVR) for the left and right heart, respectively. Increased afterload may result in cardiac ischemia or injury.

Contractility functions independently of preload and afterload. Contractility is the ability of the heart to contract effectively. Contractility is assessed indirectly by the presence of low cardiac output with normal preload, afterload, and heart rate. Preload, afterload, and contractility determine stroke volume, that is, the amount of blood that is ejected with each contraction.

Heart rate or pulse can adversely affect cardiac output. When the rate is sufficiently elevated to impair diastolic filling of the chambers, cardiac output is decreased.

Vital signs

Cardiac output is determined by stroke volume and heart rate. One of the earliest signs of impaired oxygenation is an increased heart rate because stroke volume remains stable for a time. When the heart is no longer able to compensate by increasing heart rate, the stroke volume falls. The best bedside estimate of stroke volume is blood pressure. An increase in heart rate is usually followed by a decrease in blood pressure when hypoxemia is severe.

In some instances, mean arterial blood pressure is assessed. Mean arterial blood pressure represents the average of systolic and diastolic blood pressure. Because systole accounts for almost one third of the cardiac cycle and diastole for two thirds, mean arterial pressure (MAP) is calculated according to one of the following formulas:

$$MAP = \frac{\text{Systolic pressure} - \text{Diastolic pressure}}{3} + \text{Diastolic pressure}$$

$$MAP = \frac{\text{Systolic pressure} + (2 \times \text{Diastolic pressure})}{3}$$

Hemodynamics

A common method of assessing cardiopulmonary function is via insertion of arterial and central venous catheters for monitoring heart pressures, commonly referred to as *hemodynamic monitoring*. The use of intraarterial and pulmonary artery catheters also allows easier blood sampling and calculation of many other hemodynamic parameters (Table 9-2).

Intraarterial catheters continuously assess arterial blood pressure, which is especially important in the patient with low cardiac output and peripheral vasoconstriction. Intraarterial pressure assessment is essential in critically ill patients receiving intravenous vasodilator or vasopressor medications.

In most instances the physician inserts an intraarterial catheter in the radial artery or, rarely, the femoral artery; care of the catheter and assessment of the blood pressure are the nurse's responsibility. Reliable blood pressure measurements are obtained when the arterial waveform has a sharp, rapid upstroke, clear dicrotic notch, and definite end diastole (Fig. 9-5). Impaired left ventricular outflow, as occurs in aortic stenosis, slows the upstroke. Accurate readings are obtained with the transducer at the level of the aortic valve (Fig. 9-6). Dampened waveforms and falsely low blood pressure readings occur as a result of clot formation at the catheter tip, bubbles in the pressure tubing or dome, or location of the catheter tip against the arterial wall (Daily and Schroeder, 1989).

Central venous pressure. Intermittent measurement of CVP was the norm until the invention of the pulmonary artery catheter. With its introduction medical and nursing professions realized the inadequacies of merely monitoring CVP, which often inaccurately predicted fluid volume status, especially in patients with lung disease or heart failure. CVP measures only right-sided heart pressure, which contributed to its inadequacy. Although the original pulmonary artery catheter was able to assess only pulmonary artery pressure,

Table 9-2. Calculation of hemodynamic parameters

Name	Formula	Normal range
MAP	$\dfrac{S + 2D}{3}$ or $\dfrac{S - D}{3} + D$	60-100 mm Hg
Mean pulmonary artery pressure (MPAP)	Same as for MAP using pulmonary artery pressures	10-15 mm Hg
SVR	$\dfrac{MAP - RA}{CO} \times 80$	900-1600 dynes/sec/cm^{-5}
Cardiac output (Fick equation)	$\dfrac{\dot{V}O_2}{a - vDO_2 \times 10}$	4-8 L/min
Cardiac index (CI)	$\dfrac{CO}{\text{Body surface area (BSA)}}$	2.5-4 L/min/m^2
Stroke volume	$\dfrac{CO}{HR}$	55-100 ml/beat
PVR	$\dfrac{MPAP - PAWP}{CO} \times 80$	20-120 dynes/sec/cm^{-5}
O$_2$ consumption ($\dot{V}o_2$)	$\dfrac{Cao_2 - C\bar{v}o_2}{Cao_2}$	200-300 ml/min
Arteriovenous O$_2$ difference (a-vDo$_2$)	$Cao_2 - C\bar{v}o_2$	3.0-5.5 vol %
Arterial O$_2$ content (Cao$_2$)	$(Pao_2 \times 0.003) + (Hgb \times 1.34 \times Sao_2)$	20 vol %
Venous O$_2$ content (C$\bar{v}$o$_2$)	$(P\bar{v}O_2 \times 0.003) + (Hgb \times 1.34 \times S\bar{v}o_2)$	15 vol %
O$_2$ delivery	$Cao_2 \times CO$	1000 ml/min

recent technology makes possible continuous assessment of mixed venous O$_2$ saturation (S$\bar{v}o_2$), right ventricular ejection fraction, and continuous cardiac output (Segal, 1989). Pulmonary artery pressure monitoring has become the standard for assessing cardiopulmonary fluid status.

Pulmonary artery catheter. The flow-directed, balloon-tipped pulmonary artery catheter is inserted by the physician with the assistance of the nurse. The most common sites for insertion of the pulmonary artery catheter are the internal jugular and the subclavian arteries. Rarely are the femoral or brachial arteries used. With the femoral approach the catheter has to come up through the inferior vena cava and then descend into the right ventricle. This is often difficult to accomplish. It is also difficult to stabilize the leg, and movement of the leg can cause the catheter position to change. In addition, the groin is considered a "dirty" area and thus is more prone to catheter contamination. However, the groin may not be less clean than the neck or chest, which are prone to contamination by oral and gastric secretions. When using the smaller brachial artery, there is concern for venous insufficiency. It is also technically more difficult for the catheter to make the sharp angle at the shoulder and to prevent catheter migration as the patient moves his arm.

When a pulmonary artery catheter is inserted, it is attached to a transducer that displays a wave form on the monitor. Characteristic wave forms are assessed to identify position of the catheter (Fig. 9-7). The catheter enters the

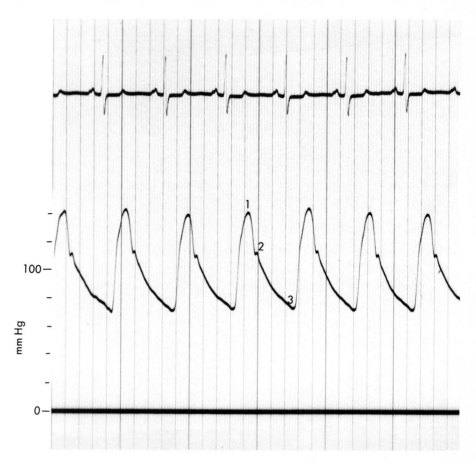

Fig. 9-5. Normal arterial pressure tracing. Systole *(1)*, dicrotic notch *(2)*, diastole *(3)*. (From Daily E and Schroeder J: *Hemodynamic waveforms: exercise in identification and analysis,* ed 2, St Louis, 1983, Mosby–Year Book.)

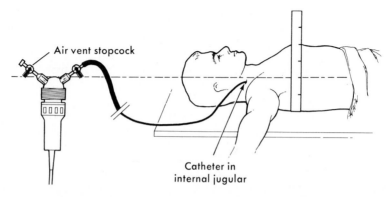

Fig. 9-6. The transducer for arterial pressure monitoring is leveled at the aortic knob. When pulmonary artery pressures are also measured, the reference point is the right atrium. (From Daily E and Schroeder J: *Techniques in bedside hemodynamic monitoring,* ed 4, St Louis, 1989, Mosby–Year Book.)

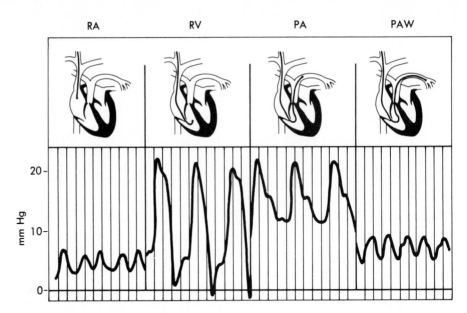

Fig. 9-7. Position of flow-directed pulmonary artery catheter and corresponding pressure tracings. Right atrium *(RA)*, right ventricle *(RV)*, main pulmonary artery *(PA)*, and pulmonary artery wedge *(PAW)*. (From Wade J: *Comprehensive respiratory care,* ed 3, St Louis, 1982, Mosby–Year Book.)

right atrium and travels through the tricuspid valve into the right ventricle. From the right ventricle the catheter flows through the pulmonic valve into the pulmonary artery. The catheter is floated into the pulmonary artery with the balloon inflated until it wedges. The balloon is then deflated, and the catheter is secured. Proper positioning of the catheter in a West zone 3 is essential for accurate recording of pulmonary pressure (Darovic, 1987). The nurse records the pressure when the catheter is in the right atrium, the right ventricle, the pulmonary artery, and the pulmonary artery wedge position. Some physicians may also request blood samples at each measurement to identify O_2 step-up abnormalities.

The pulmonary artery catheter is associated with several risks and complications. During insertion of the pulmonary artery catheter the patient may develop atrial or ventricular dysrhythmias from mechanical irritation. Although most dysrhythmias are usually transient and limited to the period of insertion, some dysrhythmias are persistent and may require pharmacological treatment or catheter removal. Sudden development of ventricular dysrhythmias after catheter insertion usually signals migration of the catheter into the ventricle. The right ventricular wave form is usually present. The physician repositions the catheter into the pulmonary artery.

The catheter may also migrate further into the pulmonary artery, causing pulmonary infarction or pulmonary hemorrhage. Either of these complications is very serious. The nurse observes a "wedged" tracing on the monitor. The patient may develop hemoptysis or occasionally complain of pain when either of these conditions occurs. Pulmonary hemorrhage or pulmonary infarction may also occur when the balloon is overinflated or left inflated for a prolonged period. The catheter must be pulled back into proper position to prevent further damage.

Pulmonary air embolism may occur if the balloon ruptures and air is injected into the catheter. When the balloon ruptures, normal resistance is not felt when air is inserted into the balloon. Blood may be withdrawn into the syringe when the balloon port is aspirated. The port is closed securely and tied in a knot to prevent more air from entering the chest until the catheter is removed. The catheter should be replaced without delay by the physician.

As is true for all invasive devices, a pulmonary artery catheter predisposes the patient to infection. Bacteria may enter the insertion site, migrate down the catheter, and enter the blood. Bacteria may also enter stopcocks used for administering medications, drawing blood, or obtaining cardiac outputs. When bacteria are present in the blood, endocarditis is a concern. Vigilance and strict asepsis when dressing the site and using stopcocks prevent infection.

Wave form measurement and assessment. Like the intraarterial catheter, the pulmonary artery catheter has a distinct wave form for each pressure tracing: right atrial, pulmonary artery, and PAWP tracings. Right atrial (RA) pressure is the CVP of the past. The RA pressure wave form has three positive waves that correspond to events in the ECG. (Fig. 9-8, *A*). An *a* wave corresponds to the P-R interval on the ECG, which is atrial systole. Following the *a* wave is a decline in pressure that reflects atrial relaxation and is termed the *x descent*. The *c* wave corresponds to the S-T segment, which is produced by closure of the tricuspid valves. It sometimes appears as a notch on the *a* wave, or it sometimes is absent. The *v* wave corresponds to the interval between the *T* and *P* waves. The *v* wave represents ventricular systole. The *y* descent immediately follows the *v* wave and is caused by opening of the tricuspid valve. Normal RA pressure is 2 to 8 mm Hg. Table 9-3 lists causes of increases in RA pressure.

The pulmonary artery pressure wave form is similar to the arterial wave form. Systolic and diastolic phases correspond to blood flow through the pulmonic valve. Systolic pressure is the peak pressure generated by the right ventricle. Diastolic pressure is the lowest pressure in the pulmonary artery. In

Table 9-3. Causes of increases in RA and PA pressures

RA pressure increases (normally 2 to 8 mm Hg)	PA pressure increases (normal pulmonary artery systole/pulmonary artery diastole (PAS/PAD) 20-30/5-15 mm Hg; normal PAWP 4-12 mm Hg)
RV failure	Left-to-right shunt
Tricuspid stenosis	Ventricular or atrial septal defect
Tricuspid regurgitation	Chronic obstructive pulmonary diseases
Constrictive pericarditis	LV failure
Pulmonary hypertension	Pulmonary hypertension
Chronic LV failure	Mitral stenosis
Chronic mitral stenosis	Mitral insufficiency
Cardiac tamponade	Volume overload
Volume overload	PEEP
	Pulmonary embolism

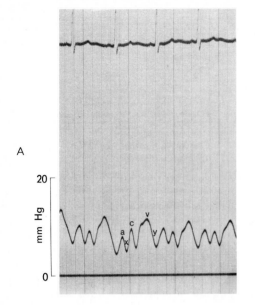

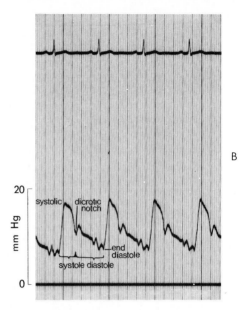

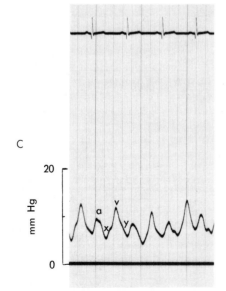

Fig. 9-8. A, RA pressure waveform showing *a, c,* and *v* waves with *x* and *y* descents. The recorded waveforms follow the corresponding electrical event because of the delay in recording pressures through a long catheter. **B,** Normal PA waveform showing systole, dicrotic notch, and end diastole. In normal patients PA end diastole closely correlates with left ventricular end-diastolic pressure. **C,** Normal PAW pressure waveform with *a* and *v* waves and *x* and *y*. (From Daily E and Schroeder J: *Techniques in bedside monitoring,* ed 4, St Louis, 1989, Mosby–Year Book.)

preatrial systole the mitral valve is open, allowing the ventricle to fill with blood. Pressures are equalized between the left heart and the pulmonary circulation in the absence of mitral valve disease. Therefore pulmonary artery end-diastolic pressure is used to assess left ventricular end diastolic pressure. After opening of the pulmonic valve, blood is ejected, causing a sharp rise in pulmonary artery pressure. When the pulmonary valve closes, a dicrotic notch is seen (Fig. 9-8, **B**). After the dicrotic notch, pressure continues to fall until the next systole occurs. The point just before the next systole is end-diastolic pressure.

Pulmonary artery diastolic pressure is measured at end diastole. At this point pulmonary diastolic pressure is an indirect measurement of left ventricular end diastolic pressure. Estimation of left ventricular end diastolic pressure assesses left ventricular performance according to the Frank-Starling ventricular function curve. Normal end diastolic filling pressure is low. In the diseased or poorly functioning left ventricle, a higher pressure is required to maintain stroke volume.

The PAWP is a reflection of left atrial pressure. The pulmonary catheter is wedged tightly in a small branch of the pulmonary artery by inflating the balloon. Left atrial pressure, hence left ventricular end diastolic pressure, is reflected across the pulmonary bed. The wave form of the pulmonary artery is similar in form to the right atrial pressure. There are *a, c,* and *v* waves (Fig. 9-8, C). The *a* wave is produced by atrial systole and coincides with the *P* wave on the ECG. Closure of the mitral valve at the beginning of systole is associated with the *c* wave. In most instances, the pressure change is so small that the *c* wave is not observed. The *v* wave occurs during ventricular systole as the mitral valve bulges back into the atrium. On the ECG, the *v* wave occurs at the same time as the *T* wave. Timing of both the *a* and *v* wave is slightly delayed because of the interval for the pressure to be recorded by the transducer. When assessing PAWP, the nurse occludes the catheter for a time as short as possible. Occluding the pulmonary artery for longer than 3 to 4 breaths or 10 to 15 seconds places the patient at risk for pulmonary artery infarction.

In patients with normal cardiac and pulmonary function, the gradient between the pulmonary artery diastolic pressure (PADP) and the PAWP is 1 to 3 mm Hg. The PADP is slightly higher than the PAWP. This pressure gradient is necessary for forward flow through the pulmonary circulation. When the PADP/PAWP gradient is greater than 4 to 5 mm Hg, PVR is increased. When the PADP/PAWP gradient is constant, only the PADP is assessed; the wedge reading is not performed. Reducing the number of balloon wedgings limits the risks of pulmonary infarction and balloon rupture.

When measuring pulmonary artery pressures, the nurse assesses respirations. Because changes occur in intrathoracic pressure during breathing, pulmonary artery pressure is consistently measured at end-expiration. Normal breathing is initiated by negative intrathoracic pressure. Measuring pulmonary artery pressure at end-expiration is relatively easy in the nonmechanically ventilated patient. Negative pressure breaths are easy to identify. In the mechanically ventilated patient, negative pressure breaths are interspersed with positive pressure breaths. Analysis of end-expiration is often difficult. In addition, increases in West zones 1 and 2 are possible. If this occurs, measurement of the PAWP is influenced by alveolar pressure.

When tachypnea is present, when work of breathing is increased, or when assistive modes of mechanical ventilation are used, digital pulmonary catheter readings may be inaccurate. The nurse assess end-expiration pressure more accurately by recording the pressure tracing on a strip recorder for analysis. It is good practice to assess the pressure at end-expiration for several cycles.

Fig. 9-9, *A* demonstrates the interpretation of PAP in the patient receiving controlled or assist-control modes of ventilation. Because all breaths are delivered by the ventilator, the point of end-expiration occurs between two breaths. Measurement of pulmonary artery pressure is often direct.

Fig. 9-9, *B* demonstrates the difficult interpretation of pulmonary artery pressure in the patient receiving intermittent mandatory ventilation (IMV). Some of the breaths are initiated by the patient (negative pressure); other breaths are initiated by the mechanical ventilator (positive pressure). When assessing pulmonary artery pressure, the nurse evaluates pressure at end-expiration for both spontaneous and mechanical ventilator breaths. The nurse notes in the patient's record whether spontaneous or mechanical ventilator pressure is recorded.

In some institutions the patient is removed from the mechanical ventilator for measurement of pulmonary artery pressure. Unfortunately, this practice places the patient at risk for hemodynamic compromise, especially when positive end-expiratory pressure (PEEP) is applied. Removing the patient from the ventilator to measure pulmonary artery pressure has several effects. Venous return is suddenly increased, and capillary compression is relieved, causing increased blood emptying into the left ventricle. In addition, alveolar stability is lost, causing airway collapse. Because the patient spends only a few minutes a day without the mechanical ventilator or PEEP, pulmonary artery pressure measured in this way do not reflect steady state.

Some institutions estimate actual pulmonary artery pressures in the patient receiving mechanical ventilation with high levels of PEEP. The accuracy of the technique is unproved, and the technique is not recommended. To estimate PAWP, the nurse should subtract one third to one half of the PEEP from the measured PAWP. She should remember to convert centimeters of water to mm Hg by multiplying the level of PEEP by 1.36.

Oxygen transport and delivery

The terms O_2 *transport* and O_2 *delivery*, often used interchangeably, encompass all processes involved in getting O_2 from the environment to the tissues for utilization. The processes involved in O_2 delivery include pulmonary gas exchange, O_2 binding to hemoglobin, cardiac output, distribution of cardiac output, and distribution of microvascular flow. The O_2 delivery system is adaptable to supply sufficient O_2 in periods of increased demand and to overcome inadequacies in a particular component. Approximately 1000 ml/min of O_2 is transported in the blood.

The amount of O_2 transported to the tissues is more important than partial pressure of O_2 (Pao_2) alone although the Pao_2 is the most commonly assessed parameter of oxygenation. The amount of O_2 available for transport to the tissues is characterized by Cao_2. An arterial blood gas (ABG) sample is necessary to calculate Cao_2. The nurse should recall that O_2 content is dependent on Pao_2 and Sao_2.

$$Cao_2 = (Pao_2 \times 0.003) + (\text{Hemoglobin [Hgb]} \times 1.34 \times Sao_2)$$

O_2 delivery to the tissues depends on O_2 content and the ability of the heart to transport oxygenated blood to the tissues (cardiac output). An ABG sample alone is insufficient to calculate O_2 delivery to the tissues; cardiac output is required. Either measured (pulmonary artery catheter) or calculated (Fick equation) cardiac output may be used. Following is the formula for calculating O_2 delivery:

$$O_2 \text{ delivery} = Cao_2 \times \text{Cardiac output}$$

When cardiac output is decreased, O_2 delivery is impaired. A disruption in O_2 transport can have a variety of causes, from anemia to low cardiac output.

Oxygen consumption

The amount of O_2 actually consumed by tissues is calculated with the following equation:

$$\dot{V}o_2 = \frac{Cao_2 - C\bar{v}o_2}{Cao_2}$$

($\dot{V}o_2$ is O_2 consumption, and $C\bar{v}o_2$ is venous O_2 content). Normal $\dot{V}o_2$ is approximately 250 ml/min (3 to 4 ml O_2/kg/min). When O_2 delivery is inadequate, such as in low cardiac output, $\dot{V}o_2$ is significantly higher than normal. More O_2 is extracted to meet metabolic needs. An abnormally low $\dot{V}o_2$ is seen in excessively high cardiac output states (sepsis) and shunting.

If necessary, the nurse should review calculation of arterial and venous content (for consistency use the patient examples from Chapter 6). O_2 consumption is calculated below for both patients. The nurse should notice that in Example 1, O_2 consumption is normal, and in Example 2, O_2 consumption is increased.

Example 1. Mr. Jones is in the intensive care unit after surgery to install a coronary artery bypass graft. He is on a ventilator with the following ABG values on 50% fraction of inspired O_2 (Fio_2): pH 7.40, $Paco_2$ 40, Pao_2 98, Sao_2 97%. Mixed venous blood gases revealed $P\bar{v}o_2$ 35, $S\bar{v}o_2$ 75%. His Hgb is 12.1 g, and the barometric pressure is 747 mm Hg. Cao_2 = 16.04. $C\bar{v}o_2$ = 12.26.

$$\dot{V}o_2 = \frac{16.04 - 12.26}{16.04} = 235 \text{ ml/min}$$

Example 2. Mrs. Smith is admitted to the intensive care unit after a motor vehicle accident, in which she sustained blunt chest trauma. She has the following ABGs: pH 7.35, $Paco_2$ 46, Pao_2 72, Sao_2 93% and the following mixed venous blood gases (MVGs): $P\bar{v}o_2$ 30, $S\bar{v}o_2$ 62 on 40% Fio_2. Her Hgb is 10 g. The P_B is 700 mm Hg, Cao_2 = 12.68, and $C\bar{v}o_2$ = 8.4.

$$\dot{V}o_2 = \frac{12.68 - 8.4}{12.68} = 337 \text{ ml/min}$$

Oximetry

The use of oximeters as an assessment parameter has expanded in the past few years. First used noninvasively in patients in 1940, oximeters measure either arterial or mixed venous blood saturation continuously. In brief an oximeter uses spectrophotometric techniques to measure Hgb O_2 saturation. Pulse oximeters use red and infrared wavelengths of light to measure the intensity of light. Differences in oxygenated and reduced Hgb determine arterial saturation. Pulse oximetry calculates arterial saturation based on the difference between the light transmitted and the light absorbed by red blood cells. The resultant saturation is displayed digitally.

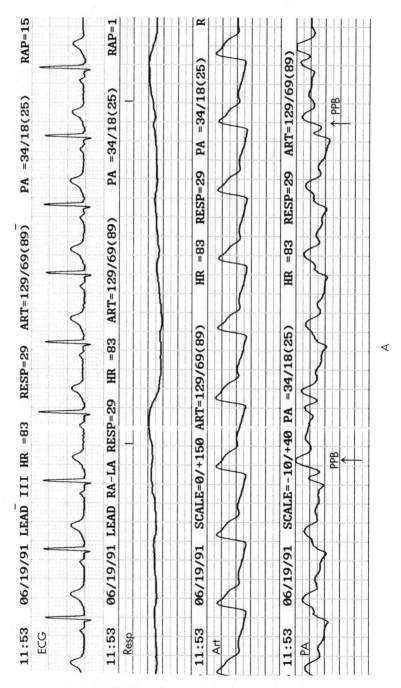

Fig. 9-9. A, Controlled breathing with mechanical ventilator. **B,** Intermittent positive-pressure breathing (PPB). SB is spontaneous breathing.

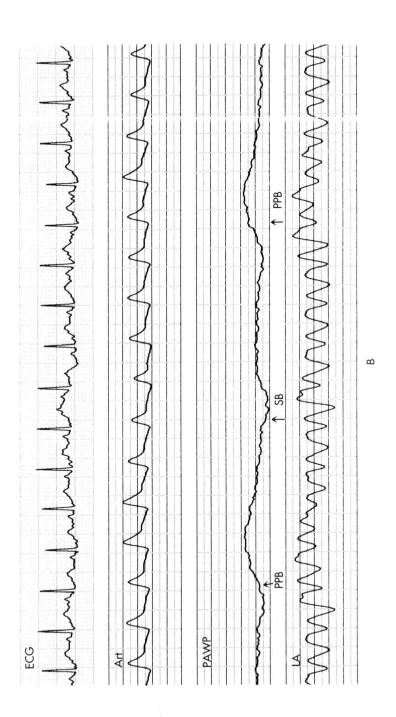

B

The accuracy of arterial saturation measured by pulse oximetry, sometimes referred as SpO_2, is within approximately 2% when SaO_2 is above 50% (Taylor and Whitham, 1986). Factors that alter the oxyhemoglobin dissociation curve and O_2 delivery affect accurate measurement (Tremper et al, 1985; Brunel and Cohen, 1988). These factors include temperature, pH, $PaCO_2$, hemodynamic status, and anemia.

Accuracy of pulse oximetry readings is also affected by the types of Hgb. Differences between measured O_2 saturation using ABG and pulse oximetry O_2 saturation are often due to other forms of Hgb, primarily carboxyhemoglobin and methemoglobin. The nurse should recall that carboxyhemoglobin is a byproduct of smoking and smoke. Methemoglobin is formed with the use of drugs such as lidocaine and nitroglycerine. When O_2 is not bound to true Hgb, the oximeter reading is higher than SaO_2 measured by arterial puncture. In other words arterial saturation is actually lower than that shown on the pulse oximeter.

Pulse oximetry provides a safe, noninvasive, and easy alternative to frequent ABG samples in the critically and noncritically ill patient. The uses of pulse oximetry are varied. Pulse oximetry is used in the hospital or home for determining nocturnal O_2 desaturation in the patient with sleep-disordered breathing. The pulse oximeter probe is applied before the patient goes to sleep. Usually a paper recorder or pulse oximeter with memory is used to assess nocturnal O_2 desaturation.

Pulse oximetry is invaluable in the weaning of patients from O_2 and PEEP when pH and $PaCO_2$ are stable. As the FiO_2 or PEEP is decreased, significant decreases in SaO_2 are reflected by the pulse oximeter, indicating the need to not further wean the patient from O_2 or PEEP. Pulse oximetry also aids in increasing supplemental O_2 or PEEP when needed. It is also useful in routine performance of suctioning and positioning, both of which may cause hypoxemia. In some cases hypoxemia indicates the need for suctioning. In other cases nurses use oximetry to assess presence and extent of hypoxemia during suctioning. The nurse times suction passes to maintain adequate O_2 saturation. She may need to hyperinflate or perhaps hyperoxygenate the patient before or after suctioning.

In patients with lung dysfunction the nurse assesses the effect of the position changes on oxygenation. Positions that seriously decrease oxygenation may not be used or may be limited in time.

Physicians frequently use pulse oximetry when performing bronchoscopy and during and after other diagnostic procedures. Continuous arterial saturation is frequently assessed during pulmonary exercise testing. Pulse oximetry is also used effectively in assessing patient response to pulmonary rehabilitation exercises and in the recertification of need for home O_2. Some physicians use pulse oximetry to assess successful replantation of traumatically amputated extremities (see box on p. 169).

For pulse oximetry to assess arterial saturation accurately, several nursing and technical considerations are necessary. Depending on the pulse oximeter and the condition of the patient, a sensor is applied to the finger, ear, toe, or nasal bridge. With some oximeters, especially older models, skin pigment, nail polish, and bilirubin alter saturation readings. This is not true with the improved technology found in newer models. Use of vasoconstricting medications, such as dopamine, may impair arterial pulsations in the extremity and prevent accurate reading of arterial saturation. Cooling blankets similarly af-

---

Uses of pulse oximetry

Bronchoscopy
Nocturnal O_2 desaturation
Positioning
Pulmonary rehabilitation exercises
Pulmonary exercise testing
Replantation of amputated extremities
Suctioning
Titrating supplemental O_2
Titrating PEEP

---

fect pulse oximetry because of peripheral vasoconstriction. The use of warming mittens may improve accuracy. Incorrect application of the pulse oximetry sensor prevents accurate assessment of saturation. Loose application allows extraneous light to enter the sensor. Conversely, positioning the sensor too snugly may result in venous pulsations being read in addition to arterial pulsations.

When pulse oximetry is initiated, an ABG sample is usually drawn. Arterial saturation by pulse oximetry is compared to the Sao_2 obtained on the ABG. The nurse also assesses body temperature, pH, and $Paco_2$. A common error made in the use of pulse oximeters for assessment of oxygenation is forgetting that pulse oximetry only measures functional Sao_2. It does not imply delivery of adequate O_2 to the tissues. In addition, other measurements obtained by ABG analysis are unknown. Shifts in CO_2 tension or arterial pH that dramatically affect saturation may unknowingly affect O_2 delivery to the tissues.

A safe Sao_2 is considered to be 90% or higher. Recalling the shape of the oxyhemoglobin dissociation curve, the nurse realizes that at or above 90% Sao_2, small increases in Sao_2 occur, for an increase in Pao_2. Below 90% Sao_2 the Sao_2 falls rapidly with relatively small decreases in Pao_2. When the oximeter saturation falls below 90%, the nurse assesses the patient for impaired oxygenation. In some cases the sensor is improperly positioned. When a technical cause, such as displaced sensor, is not the problem and other methods of assessing oxygenation indicate deterioration, the physician is notified immediately. (The nurse should remember to assess the effect of position changes.) ABG samples are frequently drawn to confirm the abnormality before or while immediate treatment is initiated.

Mixed venous O_2 saturation

Continuous assessment of $S\bar{v}o_2$ is available with specialized pulmonary artery catheters. The same principles of light transmission and absorption discussed above apply. $S\bar{v}o_2$ is an indicator of O_2 exchange at the alveolar capillary membrane in the lung; $S\bar{v}o_2$ is also an indicator of cardiac output and peripheral O_2 utilization. When $S\bar{v}o_2$ decreases, one of several problems of O_2 transport, O_2 delivery, or O_2 utilization is present. The lungs may not be exchanging O_2 efficiently at the alveolar level. In some cases anemia may be the cause of inefficient gas exchange; in other cases airway obstruction, pulmonary edema, or fibrosis may be the cause. O_2 transport may be impaired from decreased cardiac output, shock, hypovolemia, dysrhythmias, or other causes. Metabolic demands, such as shivering, suctioning, positioning, or fever, have also resulted in increased tissue utilization.

Increased $S\overline{v}o_2$ is associated with improved gas exchange in the lungs and improved cardiac output. A negative cause of increased $S\overline{v}o_2$ is impaired peripheral utilization of O_2. Hypothermia, cyanide poisoning secondary to nitroprusside, and sepsis are common causes of impaired peripheral O_2 utilization. The relationship of $S\overline{v}o_2$ to cardiopulmonary function is demonstrated by rearranging the Fick equation as follows:

$$C\overline{v}o_2 = Cao_2 - \frac{\dot{V}o_2}{CO}$$

Continuous assessment of mixed venous O_2 is frequently used in the critically ill patient to titrate multiple vasoactive medications. $S\overline{v}o_2$ is also instrumental in choosing the position that promotes optimal ventilation and perfusion in the lung. As a general rule, when the $S\overline{v}o_2$ acutely changes 10% from baseline or falls below 60%, the nurse performs a complete hemodynamic assessment of the patient. Below 40% $S\overline{v}o_2$, circulatory failure is present. Conversely, when the $S\overline{v}o_2$ increases above 85%, the nurse suspects distal migration of the catheter, which may ultimately cause pulmonary infarction. Wedging of the catheter results in a transient increase in $S\overline{v}o_2$ from reflection of left atrial saturation. The nurse should remember that wedging of a pulmonary artery catheter reflects left atrial pressures. The left atrium contains oxygenated blood, which is the reason a wedged catheter reflects a high saturation. The nurse notifies the physician of changes in the patient's condition.

CONCLUSION

This chapter examines basic and advanced concepts of assessing problems with ventilation and oxygenation. Concepts discussed in this chapter are designed to improve assessment skills already practiced. For instance, nurses unconsciously assess ventilation and oxygenation with each measurement of vital signs. What do the changes mean? If a patient is breathing faster, is he also breathing more shallowly? These signs together may indicate a decrease in $\dot{V}_A$ or an increase in Vd ventilation. Similarly, the nurse assesses a change in blood pressure. With the use of current technology, such as pulse oximetry, the nurse is often able to identify when the patient has a problem with oxygenation. If the patient has a pulmonary artery catheter, the nurse can identify if the problem is due to fluid overload, low cardiac output, increased O_2 utilization, or another problem. The nurse integrates physical assessment findings with technology and laboratory analysis of the patient's exhaled gases and blood (arterial and venous) samples to improve patient care.

BIBLIOGRAPHY

Ahrens TS: Concepts in the assessment of oxygenation, *Focus Crit Care* 14(1):36-44, 1987.

Ahrens T, Rutherford K: The new pulmonary math: applying the a/A ratio, *Am J Nurs* 87(3):337-40, 1987.

Ahrens T: Blood gas assessment of intrapulmonary shunting and deadspace, *Crit Care Nurs Clin North Am* 1(4):641-648, 1989.

Ahrens T: $S\bar{v}o_2$ monitoring: is it being used appropriately? *Crit Care Nurse* 10(7):70-72, 1990.

Baum GL, Wolinsky E: *Textbook of pulmonary diseases*, ed 3, Boston, 1983, Little, Brown.

Bellamy P, Mercurio P: An alternative method for coordinating pulmonary capillary wedge pressure measurements with the respiratory cycle, *Crit Care Med* 14(8):733-734, 1984.

Bodai B: Use of the pulmonary arterial catheter in the critically ill patient, *Heart Lung* 11(5):406-416, 1982.

Boyd K, Thomas S, Gold J, Boyd A: A prospective study of complications of pulmonary artery catheterizations in 500 consecutive patients, *Chest* 84(3):245-249, 1983.

Brunnel W, Cohen NH: Evaluation of the accuracy of pulse oximetry in critically ill patients, *Crit Care Med* 16(4):432, 1988.

Bryan-Brown CW: *Oxygen transport and the oxyhemoglobin dissociation curve.* In *Handbook of Critical Care Medicine*, Boston, 1982, Little, Brown.

Bryan-Brown CW et al: The axillary artery catheter, *Heart Lung* 12(5):492-497, 1983.

Burki NK: *Pulmonary diseases: medical outline series*, Garden City, NY, 1982, Medical Examination Publishing.

Burton GC, Hodgkin JE: *Respiratory care: a guide to clinical practice*, ed 2, Philadelphia, 1984, JB Lippincott.

Carlon GC, Ray C, Miodownik SM, Kopec I, Groeger LS: Capnography in mechanically ventilated patients, *Crit Care Med* 16(5):550-556, 1988.

Cengiz M, Crapo R, Gardner R: The effect of ventilation on the accuracy of pulmonary artery and wedge pressure measurements, *Crit Care Med* 11(7):502-507, 1983.

Cohen A, Taeusch HW, Stanton C: Usefulness of the arterial/alveolar tension ratio in the care of infants with respiratory distress syndrome, *Respir Care* 28(2):169-173, 1983.

Daily EK, Schroeder LS: *Techniques in bedside hemodynamic monitoring*, ed 4, St Louis, 1989, Mosby–Year Book.

Darovic GO: *Hemodynamic monitoring: invasive and noninvasive clinical application*, Philadelphia, 1987, WB Saunders.

Davenport HW: *The ABC of acid-base chemistry*, ed 5, Chicago, 1971, University of Chicago Press.

Dettenmeier PA, Johnson TM: The art and science of mechanical ventilator adjustment, *Crit Care Nurs Clin North Am* (in press).

Fahey PJ, Harris K, Vanderwarf C: Clinical experience with continuous monitoring of mixed venous oxygen saturation in respiratory failure, *Chest* 86:748-752, 1984.

Feaster WW, Jost KA, Swedlow DB: *Capnography: a quick reference*, Hayward, CA, 1988, Nellcor.

Fromm G: Using basic laboratory data to evaluate patients with acute respiratory failure, *Crit Care Q* 1(4):43-51, 1979.

Grabenkort WR: A cardiopulmonary physiologic profile for use with the Swan-Ganz catheter, *Resident Staff Physician* 29(7):80-85, 1983.

Harper R: *A guide to respiratory care: physiology and clinical applications*, Philadelphia, 1982, JB Lippincott.

Hatle L, Rokseth R: The arterial to end-expiratory carbon dioxide tension gradient in acute pulmonary embolism and other cardiopulmonary diseases, *Chest* 66(4):352-357, 1974.

Jaquith SM: Continuous measurement of $S\bar{v}o_2$: clinical applications and advantages for critical care nursing, *Crit Care Nurse* 5(2):40-43, 1985.

Jaquith SM: The Oximetrix Opticath: what is it and how can it facilitate nursing management of the critically ill patient? *Crit Care Nurse* 4(3):55-58, 1984.

Keyes JL: Blood gas analysis and assessment of acid-base status, *Heart Lung* 5:247-255, 1976.

Kinasewitz G: Use of end-tidal capnography during mechanical ventilation, *Respir Care* 27(2):169-171, 1982.

Lough ME: Introduction to hemodynamic monitoring, *Nurs Clin North Am* 22(1):89-110, 1987.

Morrison M: *Respiratory intensive care nursing*, ed 2, Boston, 1979, Little, Brown.

Narins R, Emmett M: Simple and mixed acid-base disorders: a practical approach, *Medicine* 59(3):161-187, 1980.

Nellcor, Inc.: *Advanced concepts in capnography*, Clinical Education Nellcor.

O'Quin R, Marini J: Pulmonary artery occlusion pressure: clinical physiology, measurement, and interpretation, *Am Rev Respir Dis* 128(2):319-326, 1983.

Osgood C, Watson M, Slaughter M, MacIntyre N: Hemodynamic monitoring in respiratory care, *Respir Care* 29(1):25-34, 1984.

Palmer P: Advanced hemodynamic assessment, *Dimens Crit Care Nursing* 1(3):139-44, 1982.

Popovich J: PEEP: maximizing the benefits without hampering the heart, *J Respir Dis* 33-38, March 1986.

Riedinger M, Shellock F, Swan H: Reading pulmonary artery and pulmonary capillary wedge pressure waveforms with respiratory variations, *Heart Lung* 10(4):675-678, 1981.

Ruppel G: Manual of pulmonary function testing, St. Louis, 1990, Mosby–Year Book.

Rutherford K: Principles and application of oximetry, *Crit Care Nurs Clin North Am* 1(4):649-657, 1989.

Schnapp LM, Cohen NH: Pulse oximetry: uses and abuses, *Chest* 98(5):1244-50, 1990.

Segal J, Pearl RG, Ford AJ, et al: Instantaneous and continuous cardiac output obtained with a doppler pulmonary artery catheter, *J Am Coll Cardiol* 13(6): 1382-92, 1989.

Shapiro B, Harrison R et al: *Clinical applications of respiratory care,* ed 3, St Louis, 1985, Mosby–Year Book.

Shoemaker WC, Thompson WL, Holbrook PR: *The Society of Critical Care Medicine textbook of critical care,* Philadelphia, 1984, WB Saunders.

Spangler R: Hemodynamic monitoring: using the pulmonary artery catheter, *Cardiothoracic Nurse* 5(3):1-3, 1987.

Stock C: Noninvasive carbon dioxide monitoring, *Crit Care Clin* 4(3):511-526, 1988.

Sue D: Measurement of shunt in respiratory failure, *Chest* 78(6):898-899, 1980.

Szaflarski NL, Cohen NH: Use of pulse oximetry in critically ill adults, *Heart Lung* 18(5):444-454, 1989.

Taylor MB, Whitwam JG: The current status of pulse oximetry: clinical value of continuous noninvasive oxygen saturation monitoring, *Anaesthesia* 41(9):943-949, 1986.

Tremper KK, Hufstedler SM, Barker SJ, et al: Accuracy of a pulse oximeter in critically ill adults: effect of temperature and hemodynamics, *Anesthesiology* 63:A175, 1985.

Vij D, Babcock R, Magilligan DJ: A simplified concept of complete physiological monitoring of the critically ill patient, *Heart Lung* 10(1):75-82, 1981.

Thomas F, Burke J, Parker J, et al: The risk of infection related to radial versus femoral site for arterial catheterization, *Crit Care Med* 11(10):807-812, 1983.

Wade JF: *Comprehensive respiratory care: physiology and technique,* ed 3, St Louis, 1982, Mosby–Year Book.

Watts C: Carbon dioxide elimination and capnography, *Respir Therapy* 10(6):107-112, 1980.

Weil MH, Bisera J, Trevino RP, Rackow EC: Cardiac output and end-tidal carbon dioxide, *Crit Care Med* 13(11):907-909, 1985.

West JB: *Pulmonary pathophysiology: the essentials,* ed 3, Baltimore, 1987, Williams & Wilkins.

West JB: *Respiratory physiology: the essentials,* ed 3, Baltimore, 1985, Williams & Wilkins.

White K: Completing the hemodynamic picture: $S\bar{v}o_2$, *Heart Lung* 14(3):272-280, 1985.

Yamanaka MK, Sue DY: Comparison of arterial-end-tidal Pco_2 difference and dead space/tidal volume ratio in respiratory failure, *Chest* 92(5):832-835, 1987.

U·N·I·T T·H·R·E·E

Diagnosis of Pulmonary Dysfunction

Unit 3 applies previous knowledge in discussing common respiratory diseases. The content includes etiology, pathophysiology, and nursing management. Assessment, a few common nursing diagnoses, and therapeutic interventions are covered under nursing management. Entire texts have been written about almost every kind of lung disease, and it is beyond the scope of this text to provide such depth about every lung disease. Therefore the most common lung diseases are chosen for presentation.

Lung diseases are classified into two groups according to physiology: obstructive or restrictive. Obstructive lung diseases (discussed in Chapter 10) block or obstruct normal ventilation by a combination of airway spasm, mucus secretions, airway edema, or airway/alveolar structural changes. The most common obstructive lung disease is chronic obstructive pulmonary disease (COPD), which is actually a combination of lung diseases that commonly occur together.

Restrictive lung diseases (discussed in Chapter 11) limit or restrict thoracic or lung movement by a variety of mechanisms, involving the pleura, lung parenchyma, or neuromuscular system. Restrictive lung diseases are often less familiar to the nurse and include entities such as sarcoidosis and interstitial pulmonary fibrosis. More familiar restrictive lung diseases are pneumothorax, pleural effusion, and lung cancer.

In Chapter 12 lung diseases that cause acute respiratory failure are discussed. These diseases, as with adult respiratory distress syndrome (ARDS), pulmonary emboli, or chest trauma, acutely impair ventilation or oxygenation and require immediate intervention.

C H·A·P·T·E·R 10

Obstructive Diseases

Objectives:

- Explain the pathophysiology of asthma, emphysema, chronic bronchitis, cystic fibrosis, bronchiolitis, and sleep apnea.
- Specify three main physiological nursing problems common in major obstructive lung diseases.
- Formulate common nursing diagnoses for the patient with obstructive lung disease.
- Differentiate assessment of each of the following disorders: asthma, emphysema, chronic bronchitis, cystic fibrosis, bronchiolitis, and sleep apnea.
- Evaluate the role of bronchodilators in obstructive lung disease.
- Propose interventions for patients with obstructive lung disease.

Obstructive lung diseases block or obstruct the normal flow of air through the respiratory system. The purpose of this chapter is to present the pathophysiology and nursing care of the most common obstructive lung diseases. In discussing the diseases, etiology and pathophysiology are presented first. With these concepts in mind, selected nursing problems, diagnoses, goals, and medical and nursing interventions are discussed. The discussion of medications and other treatments is presented in detail in subsequent chapters. The nurse is encouraged to study other sources for information about diseases not covered in this chapter.

CHRONIC OBSTRUCTIVE PULMONARY DISEASE

Emphysema and chronic bronchitis are diseases commonly referred to as *chronic obstructive pulmonary disease (COPD)*. Many clinicians include asthma in the COPD group when there is a component of airway hyperreactivity. Although emphysema and chronic bronchitis can exist alone, they are usually seen together. Some patients may have predominantly one or the other disease. The most important cause of development of COPD is cigarette smoking. Atmospheric pollution from industry and automobiles also contributes to development of COPD.

ASTHMA

Asthma is defined by the American Thoracic Society as a disease characterized by increased responsiveness of the airways to various stimuli. The response results in widespread narrowing of the airways. The airway diameter changes in severity either spontaneously or as a result of therapy; that is, some patients improve spontaneously, and other patients require therapy. Nonmedical descriptions for asthma include twitchy or hyperirritable airways. Millions of people in the United States and worldwide have asthma. In fact, 3% to 5% of the world's population is estimated to have asthma. Because asthma can be fatal, it should be taken seriously, but sometimes it is not.

Etiology

Derived from the Greek word meaning *pant,* asthma affects both children and adults. Overall, asthma does not have a gender preference. Children are frequently diagnosed with asthma in the preschool years although asthma may be diagnosed in infants. Asthma is the leading cause of absence caused by sickness in school-age children. Some children "grow out of" asthma, but other children continue to have asthma into adulthood. Contrary to popular belief, adults may be diagnosed with asthma at any age.

Asthma is an episodic disease. Many people with asthma have intervals without symptoms followed by exacerbations. The intervals are related to seasons in some patients. In other patients asthma remains dormant for years before reappearing. Allergies are common in patients with asthma. Asthma, especially the allergic type, tends to run in families.

Two asthma classifications are used by physicians: extrinsic and intrinsic. Many asthmatic patients have a mixed disorder with components of both extrinsic and intrinsic asthma. As a result the terms *extrinsic* and *intrinsic* are used less frequently. Instead, asthma is often classified by the precipitating factors, such as exercise-induced asthma. The following discussion explains extrinsic and intrinsic asthma.

Asthma is classified as extrinsic or intrinsic based on association with an identifiable immunologic response. Extrinsic asthma is commonly referred to as *allergic asthma* or *atopic asthma.* When the term *atopy* or *atopic asthma* is used, an increase in serum immunoglobulin E (IgE) levels is understood. An environmental antigen and antibody reaction produces bronchospasm. Allergens trigger the asthmatic episode and an immunologic response. This type of asthma is usually familial. The most common allergens include foods, furry animals, molds, pollens, smoke, pollutants, and dusts. Hay fever, allergic rhinitis, eczema, and allergic dermopathy are frequently present.

Intrinsic asthma is triggered by nonallergic elements, such as infection, cold drinks, stress, weather, and exercise. Sinusitis exacerbates intrinsic asthma in many patients. A familial history is often absent. Aspirin and similar products, such as nonsteroidal antiinflammatory agents, induce asthma in susceptible persons. Nasal polyps and urticaria are also observed in patients with aspirin intolerance.

Pathophysiology

The hyperreactivity of airways affected by asthma may be due to one or more mechanisms. Three factors affect contraction of bronchial smooth muscle: neural mechanisms, humoral mechanisms, and immune mechanisms. The autonomic nervous system controls smooth muscles of the airways. Parasympathetic vagal stimulation contracts bronchial smooth muscle, resulting in bronchoconstriction. Inhibition of parasympathetic vagal nerve fibers results in bronchodilation. Adrenergic receptors present in bronchial smooth muscle also respond to stimulation. Alpha adrenergic receptors cause bronchoconstriction, and beta adrenergic receptors cause bronchodilation. Most beta adrenergic receptors in the lung are Type 2. Irritant stretch receptors may also play a role in asthma (Burki, 1982).

Airway smooth muscle is also affected by humoral mechanisms. When cholinergic or alpha adrenergic receptors are stimulated, cyclic 5'-3' guanosine monophosphate (cGMP) is produced. An increase in cGMP causes bronchoconstriction. Smooth muscle relaxation is mediated by cyclic 5'-3' adenosine monophosphate (cAMP). Adenylcyclase, activated by catecholamines, aids in the breakdown of adenosine triphosphate (ATP) to cAMP. An increase in cAMP results in bronchodilation.

IgE is synthesized by nasal and lung mucosa. In a sensitized allergic patient IgE antibody is bound to mast cells and basophils. Upon exposure to the antigen, mast cells in the airway release various mediators. These mediators cause bronchoconstriction by enhancing cGMP production. Histamine, slow-reacting substance of anaphylaxis, and eosinophil chemotactic factor A are all involved in asthma. Histamine, made by the mast cells and basophils, not only causes bronchoconstriction but also enhances vascular permeability and causes edema. Histamine is potentiated by slow-reacting substance of anaphylaxis. Eosinophil chemotactic factor A draws eosinophils to the lungs after contact with an antigen.

Other mediators of asthma released by the lung include bradykinin and prostaglandins E and F. Bradykinins cause smooth muscle contraction and may be involved in the immune response. Prostaglandin E induces bronchodilation when bronchoconstriction is caused by prostaglandin F.

Pathological changes in asthma are varied. The lungs are hyperinflated and do not collapse when removed from the thorax on autopsy. On gross examination thick mucus plugs occlude the airways. The viscid exudate contains epithelial cells and eosinophils. Bronchial mucosa is also edematous, a factor that contributes to airway narrowing. The basement membrane is thickened with enlarged mucous glands and hypertrophied smooth muscle. Dilated capillaries are also present in the submucosal layer.

Nursing management

Assessment. The diagnosis of asthma begins with a thorough history. Frequent respiratory infections are common. Symptoms depend on the severity and type of asthma, but they correlate poorly with severity of bronchospasm or degree of hyperreactivity. Patients frequently complain of dyspnea, or shortness of breath. Narrowed airways (Fig. 10-1, A) and difficulty exhaling (Fig. 10-1, B) resulting in air trapping are presumed to be the causes of dyspnea. Other common symptoms are complaints of cough and chest tightness.

When asthma is not active, the patient frequently has no signs of disease. During periods of exacerbation clinical examination reveals varying degrees of respiratory distress. Assessment of general appearance shows an anxious patient with tachypnea and tachycardia. Mental confusion is present with hypoxemia and acidemia. During an exacerbation, pulsus paradoxus greater than 10 mm Hg is common. Pulsus paradoxus is assessed serially to determine patient condition and response to therapy. A trend of increasing pulsus

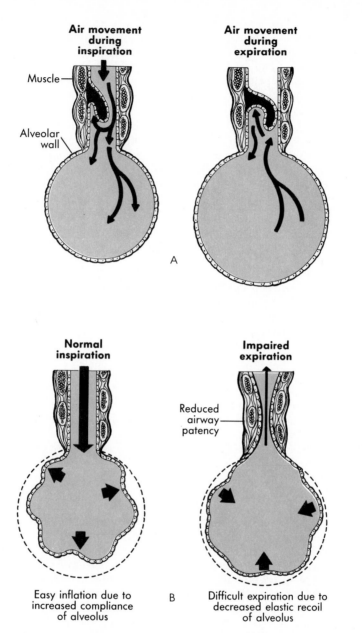

Fig. 10-1. Mechanisms of air trapping in (**A**) asthma or bronchitis and (**B**) emphysema. In asthma, with inhalation, airway diameter widens, and air passes easily by mucus. With exhalation the airway diameter narrows, and mucus traps air in the distal air spaces. This mechanism is often referred to as a ball-valve effect. In emphysema, alveolar walls are destroyed, resulting in loss of support for small airways. On inhalation the alveoli are very compliant, easily inflating. With exhalation, decreased elastic recoil results in early airway closure, and air is trapped in the distal air spaces. (From McCance K, Huether S: *Pathophysiology,* ed 1, St Louis, 1990, Mosby–Year Book.)

paradoxus is associated with increased work of breathing and is analogous to worsening asthma. Conversely, a decreasing pulsus paradoxus may indicate improvement or fatigue. When the asthma improves, the pulsus paradoxus decreases to normal. The pulsus paradoxus also decreases when the patient is unable to generate sufficient intrathoracic pressure to overcome the work of breathing.

Inspection of the chest reveals accessory muscle use. With hyperinflation, anterior-posterior (A-P) diameter is increased, and the diaphragm is lowered. Fremitus may be present on palpation. Percussion elicits hyperresonance in the presence of air trapping. Decreased breath sounds, especially in the lung bases, and wheezes throughout the lung are heard on auscultation. Expiratory wheezing is more common although inspiratory and expiratory wheezes are heard. A reliable test to elicit wheezing is to have the patient forcefully exhale one or several times while the nurse listens in several areas of the chest with the stethoscope. In some patients with severe air-flow reduction, wheezes are absent. Wheezes are not heard because of decreased air flow in the lungs. As the patient's volume and rate of air flow improve, wheezing is heard.

When asthma is suspected, multiple tests are ordered to verify the diagnosis. A pulmonary function test (PFT) confirms the degree of obstruction and responsiveness to bronchodilator therapy. Bronchial provocation PFT, using methacholine or histamine, is the most specific test for diagnosing asthma. In mild asthma, signs of small airway disease are noted: increased residual volume, increased closing volume, and decreased small airway expiratory flow rates, especially the $FEF_{25\%-75\%}$ or maximal midexpiratory flow rate (MMEF). (See Chapter 8 for an explanation of PFTs.) As the degree of bronchoconstriction increases, the FVC, FEV_1, and the FVC/FEV_1 decrease. Flow-volume loops demonstrate an obstructed pattern with a prolonged expiratory phase. Diffusing capacity of the lung, D_L, is usually normal. In asthma, improvement or reversal of obstruction is demonstrated with administration of bronchodilators. Clinically significant improvement is a 15% increase in the FEV_1 or the FVC.

In mild asthma, ABG values are normal or show a decrease in Pa_{CO_2} and respiratory alkalemia because of tachypnea. Some patients may have Pa_{CO_2} as low as 15 to 20 mm Hg during a severe attack. Hypoxemia develops secondary to ventilation-perfusion mismatching. The Pa_{O_2} is frequently as low as 40 mm Hg. As airway resistance intensifies, the Pa_{CO_2} increases to normal or elevated levels. A headache may develop from cerebral vasodilation. Drowsiness also occurs when hypercapnia is present. This is a sign that the patient is no longer able to hyperventilate. The pH falls as the Pa_{CO_2} increases above 40 mm Hg. The patient needs intubation and ventilatory support when the Pa_{CO_2} increases above 40 mm Hg, a sign of respiratory fatigue and inability to compensate. With successful treatment, bronchospasm improves and ABG values normalize.

The chest x-ray film of an asymptomatic patient with asthma is usually normal. Air trapping with low or flat diaphragms is frequently seen during attacks. Pneumothorax (air in the pleural space) or pneumomediastinum (air in the mediastinum) is sometimes present. Bronchial wall thickening and opacities indicative of mucus plugging are observed on some chest x-ray films.

Other, more obscure nonspecific tests used to diagnose asthma include sputum examination, peripheral blood count, ECG, and serum creatinine phosphokinase (CPK). Mucus secreted during an asthma attack adheres to the bronchial walls. The sputum is examined for special formations: Charcot-Leyden crystals released from disintegration of eosinophils, basophils, and mast cells; Curschmann's spirals containing protein, cells, crystals, and debris; and Creola bodies containing clumps of epithelial cells. The peripheral blood count contains increased eosinophils in allergic asthma or increased polymorphonuclear cells in infection. When right heart stress is present, characteristic changes are seen on the ECG. CPK is elevated with increased respiratory muscle activity.

Nursing diagnoses. The main problems in asthma are bronchospasm, edema, and mucus retention (Fig. 10-2, *A*). These problems are present to varying degrees and tend to occur in other obstructive lung diseases also.

Nursing diagnoses are developed based on the patient's condition. Appropriate general nursing diagnoses include alteration in ventilation, alteration in gas exchange, and ineffective airway clearance related to airway obstruction. In specific patients the nursing diagnoses of stress related to a specific irritant or situation, such as job or death of a relative, or ineffective coping related to exacerbation of chronic disease are used.

Interventions. The intent of interventions is to prevent exacerbations of asthma, to promote adequate ventilation and gas exchange, and to enhance secretion removal. Stress reduction and development of alternative coping strategies are needed in some patients.

Management of asthma begins with prevention. Thus education of the patient and significant persons in the patient's life is a primary goal of effective management. The patient learns to avoid precipitating events or triggers. In atopic patients the offending trigger is removed. Sometimes this involves giving a pet away, removing carpeting, curtains, or blinds, avoiding aspirin, or changing occupations. If a pet is given away, there is loss and grieving, which must be included in the nursing care plan. Another aid to reduce asthma attacks is installing an electrostatic air cleaner or purifier to filter dust and other particles. However, the use of these air purifiers is controversial.

The bedroom is often considered a haven in which 8 hours are spent daily, so special care is taken to provide a safe environment. A new mattress and springs may need to be purchased and covered with plastic to avoid dust. Synthetic-fiber pillows aid in control of asthma. The bedroom and all furnishings should be damp-mopped daily. Pictures and other ornamentals that attract dust should be removed. Carpeting, curtains, and cloth-covered chairs should be removed. Nonfabric shades are preferred; blinds, especially horizontal blinds, tend to collect dust. Some patients are able to use nonfabric covered vertical blinds.

Avoidance of triggers is important, but patients may still have symptoms. Desensitization to allergens is appropriate to reduce symptoms in some patients. Pharmacological treatment is used to enhance bronchodilation by controlling bronchospasm, reducing edema, and expectorating mucus (see Chapter 16 for a discussion of the actions, side effects, and nursing considerations of medications).

Bronchodilators (inhaled and oral), mast cell stabilizers, steroids (inhaled and oral), decongestants, antihistamines, and antibiotics are used together to control symptoms. With exercise-induced asthma, pretreatment with an inhaled bronchodilator is effective at reducing or controlling bronchospasm. Depending on the age and health of the patient, the physician may order inhaled or oral bronchodilators. In the infant, nebulized beta-adrenergic agonists are primary treatment. Beta-adrenergic syrups, such as albuterol, or oral theophyllines are also used in children, but they frequently cause hyperreactivity and insomnia. Theophyllines, inhaled beta agonists, and anticholinergics are commonly used in adults. Cromolyn sodium, a mast cell stabilizer, is helpful in treating exercise-induced asthma and antigen-induced asthma. During peak asthma periods, such as certain seasons, inhaled steroids decrease inflammation and edema. Bursts of oral steroids are reserved for uncontrollable bronchospasm.

Adequate hydration enhances secretion clearance. Daily intake of 2 to 4 L of fluids is recommended when cardiac and renal function are intact. Decongestants and antihistamines are used for congestion and excessive drainage. When infection is present, antibiotics are prescribed. Some physicians prescribe antibiotics for use with colds and flus because the patient's immunity is reduced and the patient is susceptible to secondary bacterial infection. Asthmatic patients are encouraged to receive flu and pneumonia vaccinations.

When air trapping is present, the nurse encourages pursed-lip breathing. The goal is to decrease the patient's respiratory rate and allow more time for exchange of gases. It is helpful for the nurse, using pursed lips, to breathe in and out with the patient. At first the nurse breathes at the patient's rate and depth. Gingerly, the nurse changes the rhythm to breathe slower and deeper. Biofeedback and relaxation exercises aid in calming the patient and improving breathing. Instruction in effective coughing techniques prevents paroxysmal coughing episodes and enhances secretion removal with minimal fatigue. Gentle vibration of the lower ribs enhances exhalation and can decrease air trapping. Postural drainage is modified when the patient is unable to lie supine.

Position of the patient is important to facilitate exchange of gases. Most patients breathe easier when sitting in a chair or in high Fowler's position. Supporting the elbows on a table or arms of a chair stabilizes the shoulder girdle. This position, similar to a tripod, permits efficient use of accessory muscles and promotes diaphragmatic breathing.

The patient care environment can aid or impede the patient's recovery. Of utmost importance is the attitude and manner of the nursing and medical personnel. Staff need to approach the patient in a calm, assured manner. Quiet voices are preferred over loud voices. Soft music is calming for certain patients, but the patient should direct use of music. A fan blowing toward the patient decreases feelings of air hunger. The patient usually prefers open curtains to closed curtains and is more comfortable when staff are readily seen or when they respond to call lights rapidly. Dim lighting reduces anxiety and encourages rest. The patient should not expend unnecessary energy, such as in talking or preparing food. Because energy consumption increases after meals, light, easily digested foods are preferred.

Status asthmaticus is a very severe form of asthma that does not respond to conventional therapy. The patient's airway diameter is critically diminished from ongoing bronchospasm, edema, and mucous plugging. The patient with status asthmaticus requires hospitalization. Supplemental O_2 is necessary to correct severe hypoxemia from ventilation-perfusion mismatching. Intubation and mechanical ventilation are required in some patients. Intravenous steroids are needed to control the bronchospasm. Sedation aids in controlling anxiety, but it may contribute to respiratory failure. Status asthmaticus may be fatal.

EMPHYSEMA
Etiology

Emphysema is defined by the American Thoracic Society as an anatomical alteration of the lung characterized by an abnormal enlargement of the air spaces distal to the nonrespiratory bronchioles, accompanied by destructive changes of the alveolar walls. In short, emphysema is a disease with destruction of the gas-exchanging units in the lung parenchyma; the bronchi are not involved as in chronic bronchitis.

The primary cause of emphysema is cigarette smoking although air pollution, heredity, and socioeconomic status also play a role. Not all cigarette smokers develop emphysema, for reasons that are unclear. Because men are more likely to smoke than women (at least before the mid 1980s), emphysema is four times more common in men than in women. The predominance of emphysema in men appears to be lessening with the increase in women smokers. Inhalation of atmospheric pollutants, such as oxidants, dusts, and cadmium vapors, may cause destruction of alveoli. Infection from retained secretions and air trapping may also contribute to the breakdown of alveoli. People of lower economic class have a higher mortality from emphysema than their wealthier counterparts. It is suspected that health care and nutrition are the causes for the higher mortality.

Heredity may affect whether cigarette smokers develop emphysema. Some individuals smoke heavily without developing emphysema; other persons develop emphysema with minimal smoking. There is a type of emphysema called alpha-1 antitrypsin deficiency, which is transmitted genetically and is autosomal and not linked to sex. Alpha-1 antitrypsin is a globulin that is a potent inhibitor of several enzymes, including trypsin and elastase. Lack of alpha-1 antitrypsin allows enzymes, in effect, to digest the alveolar walls. Emphysema caused by alpha-1 antitrypsin deficiency has no gender preference, is more common in people of northern European descent, and occurs regardless of cigarette smoking. Approximately 1% to 2% of patients with emphysema have alpha-1 antitrypsin deficiency emphysema. In alpha-1 antitrypsin deficiency emphysema, symptoms and radiographical evidence usually appear by the second or third decade of life, as opposed to the fourth to sixth decades of life in traditional emphysema.

Three classifications are used to describe the area of emphysema in the lung. Some physicians differentiate the type of emphysema based on historical, clinical, and radiographical findings. These classifications are used less frequently now and are more commonly assigned postmortem. The classifications are centrilobular or centriacinar, panlobular or panacinar, and paraseptal or periacinar emphysema.

Centrilobular emphysema is the most common form and is frequently accompanied by chronic bronchitis. It spares the distal acinus but affects the respiratory bronchioles. Anatomically, centrilobular emphysema occurs in the central portion of the lobule, close to the respiratory bronchioles. Centilobular emphysema is commonly seen in cigarette smokers and is associated with development of bullae.

Panlobular emphysema first affects the distal acinus and then the alveolar ducts and alveoli. Alveoli are fragmented, and air trapping develops. Patients with alpha-1 antitrypsin deficiency develop panlobular emphysema. In later stages centrilobular and panlobular emphysema are indistinguishable. The process of aging produces paraseptal emphysema. The periphery of the lobule develops emphysematous changes.

The term *emphysema* is also applied to other conditions involving hyperinflation, an increase in the RV/TLC ratio, without alveolar destruction. *Congenital lobar emphysema* is a condition of hyperinflation of a lobe, usually the left upper lobe. *Compensatory emphysema* is a term that describes hyperinflation of remaining lung after collapse, destruction, or resection of other lung tissue. *Senile emphysema* is the type resulting from aging.

Pathophysiology

In emphysema, there are pathophysiological problems with ventilation, diffusion, and perfusion. The distal air spaces of the lung are enlarged in emphysema. Alveoli are destroyed with progression of emphysema, producing a lacy pattern made up of thin strands of collagen fibers (see Fig. 10-2, *B*). Alveolar septa and capillaries are destroyed. Physiological dead space (Vd phy) increases. There is loss of lung elasticity, and terminal airways collapse on exhalation. Regional $\dot{V}_A$ is impaired because of decreased elastic recoil, poor support of the small airways, air trapping, and poor gas mixing in the gas-exchanging units. As the distal air spaces enlarge, diffusion is impaired. Impaired diffusion results from increased distance for diffusion, loss of alveolar capillary membrane, and pulmonary vasoconstriction. Adjacent alveoli are often affected by distended alveoli, resulting in reduced capillary blood volume and decreased diffusion capacity. Hypoxemia results in pulmonary artery vasospasm, which shunts blood away from affected alveoli. Even relatively normal areas of lung may be affected by vasospasm (Burton, 1984).

The main complications in emphysema result from loss of pulmonary vasculature. Pulmonary hypertension and cor pulmonale are common sequelae. Symptoms appear with loss of greater than 50% of alveoli and capillaries. The patient also decompensates quickly into acute respiratory failure with minor stresses.

With alpha-1 antitrypsin deficiency, it is postulated that elastase is uninhibited. Elastase is continually released from polymorphonuclear leukocytes and alveolar macrophages. Additional elastase is released in infections of the lower respiratory tract. Elastase digests the lung in the absence of alpha-1 antitrypsin, but it is inhibited in the presence of alpha-1 antitrypsin. The concept of an enzyme and inhibitor balancing each other may apply to traditional emphysema. Research related to this concept is in progress.

Nursing management

Assessment. The patient with emphysema usually seeks medical attention in the fifth decade of life. The first sign of emphysema is exertional dyspnea, which often goes unnoticed until activities of daily living or job performance are affected. It has been estimated that destruction of 20% to 30% of lung tissue occurs before symptoms appear. Over time dyspnea occurs with lesser degrees of activity, until it is present at rest. At first the patient may notice breathing problems with heavy exertion. Then the patient becomes dyspneic while performing less work. Next the patient is symptomatic walking or performing activities of daily living. Finally the patient develops dyspnea even while sitting in a chair.

In examining the general appearance of the patient, the nurse usually notes a thin patient. In advanced stages of emphysema, there is muscle wasting. The patient is frequently positioned in a tripod stance; that is, the elbows rest on the arms of the chair supporting the shoulder girdle. Leaning slightly forward, the patient may be using pursed-lip breathing. Cyanosis and clubbing

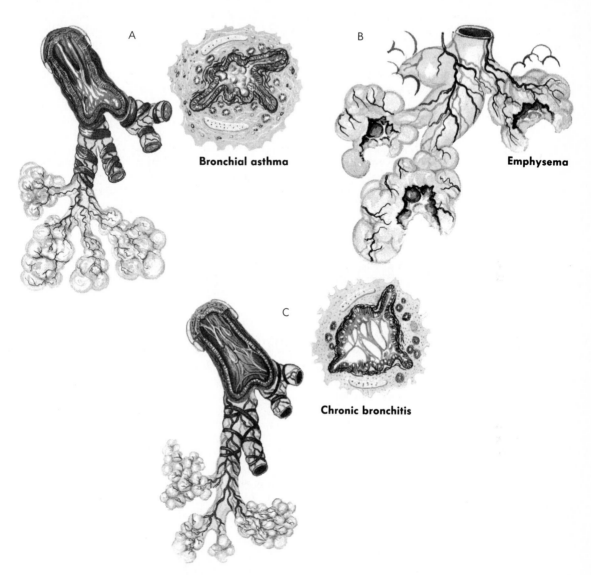

Bronchial asthma

Emphysema

Chronic bronchitis

Fig. 10-2. Airway obstruction caused by COPD (asthma, emphysema, and chronic bronchitis). (**A**) Asthma: bronchospasm, edema, and mucus retention; (**B**) emphysema: enlargement and destruction of distal air spaces with loss of elasticity; and (**C**) chronic bronchitis: inflammation and hypertrophy of mucous membranes with mucus and infection. **A:** Obstruction caused by *edema* of mucous membranes surrounding airways, *bronchospasm* of muscles surrounding airways, and retention of thick *mucus* in airways. **B:** Obstruction results from permanent *destruction of alveolar walls* that allows *small airway collapse*, trapping air in alveoli. Air trapping causes barrel-chested appearance. **C:** Obstruction results from narrowing of airway diameter secondary to *edema, inflammation, hypertrophied mucous membranes,* and chronic *mucus hypersecretion.* (From McCance K, Huether S: *Pathophysiology,* ed 1, St Louis, 1990, Mosby–Year Book.)

are absent in most patients with emphysema.

Assessment of the chest reveals accessory muscle use. Many patients appear to have a sunken supraclavicular fossa. The sternocleidomastoid muscle is frequently hypertrophied. Inspecting the shape of the thorax, the nurse notes an increased AP diameter that is consistent with hyperinflation and air trapping. The patient may have paradoxical diaphragm movement. Upper-chest muscles are usually actively involved in breathing unless the patient is practicing diaphragmatic breathing. Hyperinflation has a hyperresonant tone during percussion. The position of the diaphragm is lower than normal, and diaphragmatic excursion is reduced. When listening to breath sounds, the nurse frequently hears decreased breath sounds, a sign of decreased air movement. Expiration is prolonged. Crackles, wheezes, and other adventitious breath sounds are absent unless an infection is present. Heart sounds are normal. There is usually no cough, even on forced exhalation.

The chest x-ray film of a patient with emphysema is almost normal in mild cases. With progression of the disease the chest x-ray film reveals increased radiolucency with decreased lung markings as alveoli are destroyed (Fig. 10-3). Bullae appear in advanced cases of emphysema and predispose the patient to pneumothorax. Diaphragms flatten as air trapping increases. The heart is of normal size although it sometimes appears small because of the hyperinflated lungs.

PFTs of a patient with emphysema show evidence of hyperinflation; that is, the RV/TLC ratio is increased. Body plethysmography more accurately measures RV, hence air trapping, in patients with emphysema. TLC is increased because of hyperinflated alveoli although VC is decreased because of the increase in RV. Inspiratory flow rates are normal in emphysema. All expiratory flows are reduced consistent with the degree of obstruction. The FEV_1 is also proportionately reduced. A normal person can exhale all air within 3 seconds, but the patient with emphysema may take 15 to 20 seconds. (Some patients perceive that taking so long to exhale is a sign of healthy lungs, that is, lungs containing lots of air.) The expiratory obstruction does not traditionally respond to bronchodilators unless chronic bronchitis is coexistent. Because the capillary bed is diminished, D_L is also reduced in emphysema. Gas exchange is normal as measured by ABG values until emphysema is very advanced even though D_L is decreased. Finally, elastic recoil is low, but compliance is increased.

In emphysema ABG values are normal in the early stages. Because capillaries are destroyed with the alveoli, ventilation-perfusion relationships remain normal. As the disease progresses, relative hypoxemia develops. The Pao_2 ranges from 60 to 80 mm Hg. CO_2 tension is also usually normal unless the patient develops alveolar hypoventilation from impaired mechanics and muscular fatigue. At this point both hypoxemia and hypercapnia occur. The outdated term *pink puffer* is sometimes used to describe the emphysematic patient because he is rarely cyanotic.

Nursing diagnoses. The main physiological problem in emphysema is obstruction of expiratory air flow with air trapping. The patient frequently also engages in risk-factor behaviors, particularly smoking. Nutrition is a problem in advanced emphysema when breathlessness prevents adequate intake of nutrients. Inadequate nutrition results in muscle wasting, including wasting of the diaphragm and other muscles of ventilation. Anxiety about breathlessness is common and worsens as obstruction increases. Performance of activities of

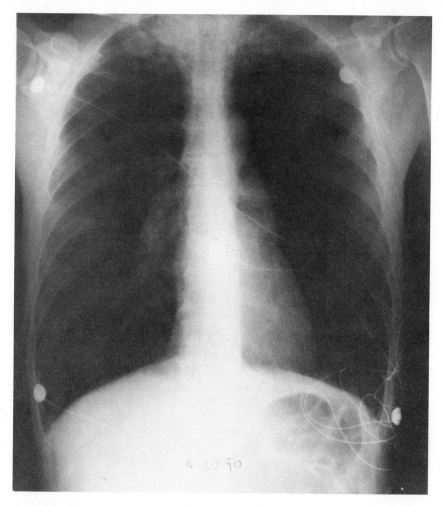

Fig. 10-3. Chest x-ray film of patient with emphysema shows flattened diaphragms from hyperinflation. Bullae may be observed.

daily living is impaired as a result of dyspnea. Increasing inactivity occurs secondary to breathlessness. Inadequately exercised muscles become inefficient at O_2 utilization. A vicious cycle of exertional dyspnea followed by muscle disuse and inefficiency occurs. Pulmonary infections can be devastating in the patient with emphysema because pulmonary reserve is limited.

A variety of nursing diagnoses may be used in the patient with emphysema, depending on the problem list. The most applicable nursing diagnosis is altered ventilation or ineffective breathing pattern related to muscle weakness or decreased $\dot{V}_A$. Ineffective individual or family coping may be considered when the patient is breathless. Anxiety related to breathlessness or to death is a commonly used nursing diagnosis in this population. When ABG values demonstrate hypoxemia, the diagnosis of impaired gas exchange related to ventilation-perfusion mismatching is used. There is always a potential for infection related to vulnerability secondary to malnutrition. Knowledge deficit related to the disease process and its treatments should be considered in all patients with emphysema. Alteration in nutrition (consuming less than body requirements) is applicable when decreased intake results in malnutrition. The patient who is unable to perform activities of daily living related to breathlessness requires a self-care deficit, alteration in body image, or alteration in self-esteem diagnosis. Similarly, activity intolerance is considered for fatigue related to the work of breathing and inability to meet O_2 demands. Finally, because sexual function is often limited by breathlessness, the nursing diagnosis of sexual dysfunction is considered.

Interventions. Interventions are designed to prevent progression of the disease, to prevent exacerbations, including infections, to treat reversible components, such as hypoxemia, to promote nutrition, to foster emotional well being, including coping and self-esteem, to minimize anxiety, and to maintain muscle strength. Some professionals collectively refer to these interventions as pulmonary rehabilitation (see Chapter 19).

The nursing management of a patient with emphysema begins with education about the disease process and methods to prevent exacerbations. Both the patient and close family members are involved in all education. Cigarette smoking is known to be a factor in the development and progression of emphysema; therefore smoking cessation is important in preventing progression of emphysema. Some patients have the attitude that because they already have emphysema, there is no need to quit, but continued smoking places the patient at risk for exacerbation and limits the effectiveness of other treatments. Smoking cessation decreases the level of carboxyhemoglobin so that increased O_2 is available for the tissues and may decrease symptoms. Smoking also places close family members at increased risk for respiratory dysfunction. Encouraging the patient to quit smoking totally is of prime importance. Cessation or continuation of smoking is the patient's decision.

There are many different types of smoking-cessation programs. No program is 100% successful with all patients. Suspicion arises when programs advertise complete success with all patients. Most programs report an immediate high success rate for smoking cessation. However, after 1 year, only about 40% of the people continue nonsmoking behaviors. Patients should choose a smoking-cessation technique that meets their learning and emotional needs. Patients may need to try a variety of programs before finding a compatible one. Failure in one program does not preclude success later in the same program or another program. It often takes several attempts before smoking cessation is complete. For some patients a group program, such as an organized program or group counseling, is successful, but other patients prefer an individualized program, such as going "cold turkey" or self-hypnosis. Self-help booklets aid a select group of motivated patients to quit smoking. Formal programs sponsored by the American Cancer Society or American Lung Association combine a variety of techniques to encourage smoking cessation. Recently, the development of nicotine-containing gum has aided smoking-cessation attempts. Success with nicotine gum is enhanced when the patient is in another smoking-cessation program simultaneously.

Pulmonary infections are the most common cause of exacerbation; therefore prevention of infection is very important in the care of an emphysema patient. Prophylactic vaccinations against pneumococcal pneumonia and influenza are encouraged. Some professionals recommend limited exposure to crowds and children as a means to avoid infection. A difficult recommendation to implement is avoidance of preschool-age children (especially grandchildren or neighbors). Children of these ages seem to be continuously infected with viral syndromes and may expose the patient to increased risk of infection. When contact with children or crowds is unavoidable, a mask or scarf across the patient's face may be helpful in limiting inhalation of microorganisms. In inclement cold weather, a scarf is worn across the nose and mouth. Infection with viral or bacterial microorganisms is usually treated with antibiotics. Although ineffective against viruses, antibiotic therapy prevents secondary bacterial infection in a compromised host.

The maintenance of muscle strength and nutrition is closely linked. Failure to ingest adequate calories, especially proteins, results in catabolism of muscles. Filling the stomach with large meals pushes up on the diaphragm and increases feelings of breathlessness. Shunting of blood to the digestive tract with increased O_2 consumption and CO_2 production increases the work of breathing. Gas-forming foods, such as cabbage, broccoli, beans, and carbonated beverages, also increase gastric distention and breathlessness. Patients should use common sense and sound nutritional principles in choosing foods. Foods that increase breathlessness should be avoided. A balanced diet is essential. Unlike the standard three meals a day that most people eat, a patient with emphysema should eat six or more small, nutritious meals.

Stress and emotional upset also trigger exacerbations. The patient should learn relaxation and stress-reduction techniques. Imagery, video or audio tapes, self-guided relaxation, and diversional activities are used to relax or reduce stress. Pursed-lip and diaphragmatic breathing aid in relaxation and in preventing small airway collapse on exhalation. A support group of patients with similar conditions is helpful. Many local hospitals or the American Lung Association sponsor support groups for patients with COPD.

Medications are not as helpful in treating emphysema as in treating other obstructive lung diseases. There are usually no reversible components, such as bronchospasm, to treat. Some physicians order bronchodilators if the patient's symptoms have improved and if the patient is able to perform better. In patients with alpha-1 antitrypsin deficiency, replacement therapy with Prolastin is helpful in halting progression of the disease. Hypoxemic patients need supplemental O_2 therapy. O_2 is usually required at night and with exertion.

CHRONIC BRONCHITIS
Etiology

Chronic bronchitis is defined by the American Thoracic Society as a clinical syndrome characterized by excessive sputum production manifested by chronic or recurring cough on most days for a minimum of 3 months out of the year for at least 2 consecutive years. The incidence of chronic bronchitis is 10% to 25%. Onset of chronic bronchitis is slow; symptoms appear and worsen over the course of 20 or more years. The most common cause of chronic bronchitis is cigarette smoking. Chronic bronchitis is noted in both the smoker and other persons living in the home. The role of second-hand smoke in causing lung disease is established.

Another cause of chronic bronchitis is air pollution from industry and transportation. Particulates in the air from dusty work environments, such as mining and blasting, contribute to development of chronic bronchitis. Automobiles and other forms of fuel-powered transportation emit gaseous pollutants, such as nitrogen dioxide and sulfur dioxide, into the environment. These gaseous pollutants have been shown experimentally to produce mucus hypersecretion and decreased ciliary function.

Pathophysiology

Chronic bronchitis develops from repeated airway irritation. The pathophysiology of chronic bronchitis includes swelling and hypertrophy of mucosal layers (see Fig. 10-2, C). Inflammation, airway fibrosis and narrowing, and production of thick, tenacious secretions or mucous plugs are also present. Microscopic examination of mucosal tissues reveals an increase in the size and number of submucosal glands in the large airways. In small airways an increased number of goblet cells is found in the epithelial lining layer. The Reid index, or ratio of the thickness of the submucosal gland layer to the bronchial wall, is increased from 0:35 to as high as 0:60 in chronic bronchitis. The basement-membrane thickness is increased, and denuded ciliated areas are noted along the epithelial surface. Without intact cilia, mucociliary clearance is impeded. These changes result in narrowing of the airway lumen. Air-flow resistance is increased or obstructed. Chronic bronchitis is believed to extend from the small to the large airways.

Nursing management

Assessment. The patient with chronic bronchitis usually seeks medical attention between age 40 and 50 and looks very different from the emphysematous patient. Examination of general appearance reveals an overweight, often obese, patient. Cyanosis and overt signs of right heart failure are usually present. These signs include hepatomegaly, peripheral edema, and jugular vein distention. Clubbing is usually absent.

The patient with chronic bronchitis is usually short of breath and produces varying amounts of thick sputum. Sputum production is common in the morning. It often continues throughout the day. The consistency of sputum is usually thick and tenacious. When spit into a container, the sputum adheres to the bottom even when the container is overturned. As fluid intake increases during the day, the sputum may thin although mucus plugs are typical. The color of the sputum is usually white, gray, or tan during normal periods. With an infectious exacerbation, the color changes to green, brown, red, or yellow, depending on the organism. Hemoptysis streaking (versus frank hemoptysis) may also be present.

Inspection of the chest reveals a normal A-P diameter. Accessory muscles may be used. Palpation of the chest may highlight areas of tactile fremitus over congested areas. Percussion of the chest reveals fairly normal diaphragmatic excursion. Resonant lung sounds are elicited with percussion. Auscultation of the chest reveals diffuse early inspiratory and possibly a few expiratory wheezes and crackles suggestive of mucus. The lung bases have more adventitious sounds than the apices. Gurgles may be heard in the large airways. Expiration is prolonged. Heart sounds are significant for accentuated closure of the pulmonary valves and an S_3.

The chest x-ray film of a patient with chronic bronchitis shows increased lung markings (Fig. 10-4). The heart, particularly the right ventricle, is enlarged, as are the pulmonary arteries. When pneumonia is present, an infiltrate appears. Pulmonary edema is absent unless biventricular failure is present.

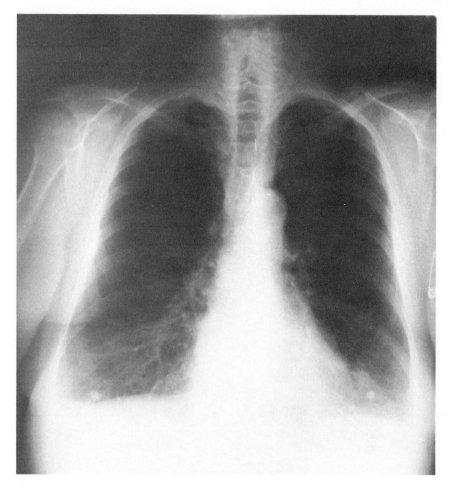

Fig. 10-4. Typical chest x-ray film of patient with chronic bronchitis and cor pulmonale. Note large pulmonary arteries.

PFTs show normal lung volumes although the RV/TLC ratio may be slightly elevated. Because airway narrowing is anatomically fixed, both inspiratory and expiratory flow rates are decreased. Compliance and elastic recoil are normal. The $D_L CO$ is normal. When bronchospasm is present, bronchodilators improve air flow. Bronchodilators cannot improve anatomical obstruction caused by hypertrophy.

ABG values demonstrate hypoxemia that is more severe than that demonstrated by the patient with emphysema. The Pao_2 of the patient with chronic bronchitis is frequently below 55 mm Hg. In an attempt to compensate for hypoxemia, red blood cell production increases, resulting in polycythemia. The hemoglobin is often greater than 16 mg/dl. When the hemoglobin level exceeds 18 mg/dl, the physician considers phlebotomy. Because the elevated hemoglobin is not saturated (reduced), patients with chronic bronchitis are often cyanotic. The outdated term *blue bloater* is sometimes used to describe the edematous, cyanotic, and chronic bronchitic patient.

As chronic bronchitis advances, hypercapnia develops. When renal function is normal, the patient retains HCO_3^- to maintain a near-normal pH. The pH is usually around 7.35 with an elevated HCO_3^-, that is, a compensated respiratory acidosis. The increased $Paco_2$ is often accompanied by a headache because cerebral vasodilation occurs in the presence of hypercapnia. The headache is worse in the morning because of nocturnal hypoventilation. As the patient increases ventilation with arising, the $Paco_2$ decreases, and the headache diminishes or goes away entirely. Hypercapnia may also result in papilledema and dilated conjunctival and facial blood vessels.

The ECG of the patient with chronic bronchitis often reveals "P-pulmonale" from right heart strain. P-pulmonale is a tall (greater than 2.5 mm) peaked P wave in leads 2, 3, and AVF. There is also evidence of right axis deviation and right ventricular hypertrophy.

Nursing diagnoses. The nursing problems of the patient with chronic bronchitis are similar to those of patients with asthma and emphysema. The nurse should refer to the asthma and emphysema nursing problems, nursing diagnoses, and nursing goals sections. Significant differences in patients with chronic bronchitis from patients with asthma and emphysema include airway clearance, fluid volume, and weight management.

Airway clearance is critical in the patient with chronic bronchitis because retained secretions are an ideal media for bacterial growth. The diagnosis of ineffective airway clearance related to the presence of viscous secretions is applicable in patients with chronic bronchitis. Because right ventricular failure is present in the patient with chronic bronchitis, fluid volume excess is a problem. The diagnosis of fluid volume excess related to decreased cardiac output is suggested in the patient with chronic bronchitis. Obesity is a problem in patients with chronic bronchitis not only because it increases cardiac work but also because it may limit diaphragmatic expansion. The nursing diagnosis of alteration in nutrition (consuming more than body requirements) related to obesity from overeating is useful in some patients.

Interventions. Interventions for the patient with chronic bronchitis are designed to maintain a patent airway, promote cardiac output, and control weight. They are often implemented through pulmonary rehabilitation.

Nursing care of the patient with chronic bronchitis is similar to care of the patient with emphysema, with a few changes. Smoking cessation and prevention of infection remain important in care of the patient with chronic bronchitis. Because retained secretions are a common source of infection, clearing the airway of secretions is critical in prevention of infection. Cough is the most important factor in clearing secretions. An effective cough technique is used to clear the secretions without fatiguing the patient. In some patients a huff cough is used; in other patients the controlled cough is effective (see Chapter 13 for an explanation of technique). When cough alone is ineffective at clearing secretions, additional measures are implemented.

Hydration is vital to effective secretion removal. Systemic hydration aids in liquefying secretions for easier expectoration. The goal of hydration is thin, watery secretions that can be expectorated with the first cough. In most patients a minimum of 2 to 4 L of fluids every 24 hours results in adequate hydration. Contraindications to hydration include hyponatremia, renal failure, and some episodes of congestive heart failure. Because congestive heart failure may be produced by the heart working excessively hard in the presence of thickened secretions, hydration is not always contraindicated in the presence of congestive heart failure. The physician determines when to limit hydration. Fluid types are chosen to promote the overall health of the patient. Reduced salt fluids prevent sodium and water retention. Low-calorie fluids are chosen for the overweight patient, and high calorie fluids meet the needs of underweight patients. Water is the best fluid because it is inexpensive, usually contains no salt (except in softened water), and is easily accessible. When hydration therapy is implemented, fluid and electrolyte balance is assessed.

Chest physical therapy, including postural drainage, percussion, and vibration, is useful with many patients to facilitate secretion removal. Indications for use, frequency, and method of chest therapy are controversial in the literature (Rochester and Goldberg, 1980). Patients with more than 30 ml of daily sputum production seem to gain the most benefit from chest physical therapy. In the clinical setting, chest therapy is implemented. If sputum production increases without harming the patient, chest physical therapy is continued. If the patient develops dysrhythmias or hypoxemia, the treatment is altered or discontinued. Patients who do not produce sputum after a series of chest physical therapy treatments should probably not continue to receive them.

Bronchodilator medications are effective in most patients with chronic bronchitis to control bronchospasm and open the airway. A 15% to 20% increase in FVC or FEV_1 demonstrates significant improvement in air flow. Most physicians begin bronchodilator therapy with inhaled bronchodilators alone. Beta adrenergic agonists and anticholinergic inhaled bronchodilators are administered together. Because ciliary function is improved with systemic bronchodilation, theophylline aids in secretion removal. Other systemic benefits of theophylline generally outweigh the risks and side effects. Periodic assessment of theophylline levels indicate the effectiveness of therapy. Depending on the patient and the physician, the theophylline level is usually maintained in the therapeutic range, that is, 10 to 20 mg/dl. Most physicians tend to keep the theophylline level at the lower end of the range to allow for safer increases in theophylline dosage during exacerbations.

Antibiotics are used to treat bacterial infections. As with the asthmatic patient, the patient with chronic bronchitis may take antibiotics with viral illnesses to prevent subsequent bacterial infections in the immune-compromised host. The most common organisms in chronic bronchitis are *Streptococcus pneumoniae* and *Haemophilus influenzae*. Failure to implement prompt antibiotic therapy in acute exacerbations of bronchitis may result in acute respiratory failure. For this reason the patient is taught the signs and symptoms of infection shown in the box on p. 192.

The physician orders steroids to help control edema and inflammation in the airway. When steroids are necessary, inhaled steroids are tried first. Failure of inhaled therapy results in the use of oral prednisone. When no benefit is observed with oral steroid use, the steroid is rapidly tapered and discontinued. A few patients require long-term steroid use.

O_2 therapy is usually required in chronic bronchitis. The goal of O_2 therapy is a minimum Pao_2 of 60 mm Hg or a Sao_2 of 90%. Oxygenation must be preserved in spite of hypercapnia. The patient is allowed to retain HCO_3^- to buffer the pH as long as adequate oxygenation is achieved.

Signs and symptoms of infection

Fever
Chills
Night sweats
Increased cough
Increased or decreased sputum production
Change in color of secretions
Thick secretions
Increased fatigue
Increased dyspnea
Increased chest congestion (crackles, gurgles, or wheezing)

CYSTIC FIBROSIS
Etiology

Cystic fibrosis (CF) is an autosomal recessive genetic disorder that primarily affects the pulmonary and gastrointestinal systems. Sweat glands are also affected. In previous years CF was seen primarily in infants and children. The mortality rate in children with CF was high; thus few of the children lived to adulthood. Now children with CF are living into adulthood. In addition, adults are being diagnosed with CF. Although there is no cure, therapy is much more effective than in the past. CF occurs approximately once in every 2000 Caucasian births and once in every 17,000 black American births (di Sant'Agnese, 1967; Kulczycki and Schauf, 1974). It is extremely rare in Oriental populations.

Pathophysiology

CF affects exocrine glands. Ductal tissues of the pancreas, hepatic biliary tree, and vas deferens are obstructed and fibrose over time. In the upper airway the patient with CF develops chronic rhinosinusitis because of hypertrophied and edematous mucus-secreting cell membranes. Nasal polyps are also common.

In the lower airways, bronchial gland dilation and hypertrophy with goblet cell hyperplasia develop. Lower airway bronchioles appear to be affected first. There is peribronchiolar inflammation, bronchiolar plugging and obliteration, and bronchiolectasis. As CF progresses, large airways are obstructed, and bronchiectasis develops. The airways are filled with degenerating cells, mucus, and other debris. Excessive mucus plugs the airways and provides an ideal environment for bacterial growth. The most common organisms are *Staphylococcus aureus*, *Pseudomonas aeruginosa*, *H. influenzae*, *Klebsiella* species, and *Escherichia coli*. *P. aeruginosa* is ultimately the most prominent organism. As a result of chronic infection the bronchial mucosa undergoes metaplasia, which increases obstruction.

Lung parenchymal changes also occur but at a slower rate than those in the airways. Enlargement of alveolar spaces with air trapping, that is, emphysemalike changes, are seen in CF. Patients also have patchy chronic pneumonitis and septal thickening from pneumonia and hemorrhage. Cysts and abscesses occur throughout the lung, and subpleural blebs appear in the lung. Bronchial and pulmonary arteries become tortuous in CF.

Nursing management

Assessment. In the case of CF in an infant the mother frequently reports difficulty feeding, severe tachypnea and cyanosis. Repeated pulmonary infections require multiple visits to the physician for treatment with antibiotics. As the airways enlarge in childhood, the disease appears to improve because airway clearance is improved. Assessing general appearance reveals a child with a chronic cough, clubbing of the fingers, and cyanosis. Nocturnal cough occurs first because airway clearance is at a minimum and secretions accumulate in the airways. In the early stages of CF the cough is dry and hacking, but it becomes productive as the disease progresses. The cough is usually more productive upon arising and after exercise. Cough increases with exacerbations of infection. A low-grade fever is also common because of the chronic infection.

The child with CF is small for his age and frequently loses weight or remains the same weight while growing in height. Weight loss occurs during acute exacerbations of infection.

Inspection of the chest reveals increased AP diameter with progressive disease. A barrel-shaped chest is seen in advanced CF from hyperinflation and air trapping. Tachypnea is often present. Palpation demonstrates fremitus over areas of increased congestion. Hyperresonance is heard over the chest with percussion. Auscultation of the chest elicits a variety of adventitious sounds. Crackles, wheezes, and gurgles are all assessed.

The chest x-ray film of the patient with CF shows what some radiologists term "dirty" lungs. Bronchial walls are thickened, and bronchiectatic changes are seen. There is evidence of hyperinflation, and in some patients large blebs appear. When pulmonary hypertension exists, enlarged pulmonary artery shadows and right ventricular hypertrophy are observed.

Serial PFTs reflect varying degrees of hyperinflation. RV and FRC are increased because of air trapping. TLC is usually normal when measured by body plethysmography. The RV/TLC ratio is increased. With air-flow obstruction the FEV_1 and MMEF are decreased. The FEV_1/FVC ratio is decreased consistent with the amount of air-flow obstruction.

ABG values in patients with CF usually reflect varying degrees of hypoxemia and hypercapnia. In the early stages of CF ventilation-perfusion mismatching causes hypoxemia. As CF progresses, oxygenation deteriorates, and continuous supplemental O_2 is required. Hypercapnia is a common event in CF, especially in later stages. With each major exacerbation overall hypoxemia and hypercapnia may worsen.

CF also affects the gastrointestinal system. The major problem in the gastrointestinal tract results from pancreatic malfunction. As the pancreatic ducts become obstructed with mucus, they fibrose, producing chemical diabetes with rare ketoacidosis. In the neonate CF manifests as a meconium ileus, causing early bowel obstruction with thick, puttylike stool. A similar problem is seen in older children. Steatorrhea and azotorrhea result in large, frequent, and odoriferous stools. The fatty stools commonly float. Grease may be seen on the surface of the water in the toilet. The patient's inability to absorb fats results in failure to gain weight in spite of adequate appetite. Deficiencies of lipid-soluble vitamins are also caused by inability to digest fats. The most common vitamin deficiency is deficiency of vitamin K, which is necessary for proper blood clotting. Hypoprothrombinemia is seen with vitamin K deficiency. In some patients gallstones, biliary cirrhosis, portal hypertension, hypersplenia, rectal prolapse, and pancreatitis are also observed.

Children with CF often have a salty taste, especially when being kissed. When the mother reports that the child's kisses taste salty, the clinician suspects CF, especially when gastrointestinal abnormalities are present. The most common test to confirm the diagnosis of CF is the sweat test. The sweat test is performed by stimulating a small area of sweat glands with pilocarpine and applying a small electric current (pilocarpine iontophoresis). Sweat, at least 100 mg, is collected on a preweighed piece of filter paper or gauze. The amount of sodium and chloride in the sweat is analyzed. In CF the chloride level exceeds 60 mEq/L and may be as high as 120 mEq/L. When the sweat test reveals a chloride content over 50 mEq/L, CF is suspected, and the test should be repeated. False-positive sweat tests occur with untreated adrenal insufficiency and nephrogenic diabetes insipidus. False-negative tests also occur, usually as a result of technician error. When a positive sweat test is documented, siblings are also tested because CF is hereditary and frequently quiescent (asymptomatic). Genetic counseling is appropriate for siblings.

Most adult males (97%) with CF are sterile but not impotent. Development of secondary sexual characteristics is delayed in males, as is menstruation in females. The causes of delayed female sexual development and menstruation may also be impaired nutrition and pulmonary disease. Adult women have difficulty conceiving because of thick cervical mucus that acts as a barrier to sperm.

Nursing diagnoses. Several problems occur in patients with CF. The most significant problems are respiratory infection and inadequate nutrition. Obviously airway clearance is critical to patients with both of these problems. Other nursing challenges in the patient with CF involve psychosocial family dynamics. The diagnosis of CF is just the beginning of changes within the family structure. The daily-care needs and the prognosis of this disease provide continuing challenges to caregivers.

The most important nursing diagnosis for the patient or family with CF is ineffective airway clearance related to thick, tenacious, and purulent secretions. Nutrition (less than body requirements) related to malabsorption is critical when the patient is unable to absorb sufficient nutrients from food. Failure to ingest adequate nutrition also predisposes the patient to infection and weak muscles. Because family dynamics are altered in the patient with CF, the nursing diagnosis of alterations in family processes related to inability of the patient or family to cope with the diagnosis or lack of support systems is suggested.

Interventions. Interventions for the patient with CF are similar to those for other patients with COPD, such as chronic bronchitis. Preventing infection and minimizing the effects of respiratory infections are very important for the patient with CF because the patient is colonized with pathogens. Therefore mobilization of secretions becomes very important in the patient with CF. Several interventions are appropriate for the nursing diagnosis of alterations in family processes. In some families, overcoming feelings of guilt for producing a child with medical problems requires interventions. In other families there may be feelings of inadequacy or helplessness, tendencies to be overprotective, and sibling resentment. Marital strain and fears about the future are common. The child frequently has an altered body image or altered peer relationships needing improvement. The nurse must help the parents promote normal child development through the stages. Similarly, it is necessary to promote integrity of the family unit.

Having assessed the needs and desires of the patient and family, and having developed nursing diagnoses and goals based on identified problems, the nurse is ready to develop and implement a plan of care. The nurse should realize that many of the interventions have been discussed in previous sections on asthma, emphysema, and chronic bronchitis. Differences are presented below.

There are no curative medications for CF. As with other obstructive lung diseases, treatment is applied to symptoms. One of the most effective treatments is chest physical therapy. Unlike other obstructive lung diseases, CF requires daily chest physical therapy. During "normal" periods treatments once or twice a day are sufficient. When exacerbations occur, chest physical therapy may be needed up to six times daily. Scheduling chest physical therapy more often than two or three times daily is a problem for both the school-age child and the working adult.

Some physicians attempt to suppress the growth of bacteria by prophylactically treating the patient for 7 to 10 days a month with antibiotics. The antibiotic is rotated month to month to prevent development of resistance. When oral antibiotics are not effective at controlling infections, intravenous antibiotics are necessary. Some patients require admission to the hospital, but other patients receive intravenous antibiotics at home.

Because parents are with the child more than the nurse is with the child, the nurse facilitates normal child development through interactions with the parents. Before the diagnosis of CF is made in the infant, parents commonly feel that lack of parenting skills are the cause of inadequate weight gain and frequent respiratory infections. With diagnosis of the disease guilt about producing a genetically "defective" child is a common feeling. By providing knowledge about the disease and about normal growth and development, the nurse aids the parents in caring for the infant. Whenever possible, observing and positively reinforcing proper parenting skills builds parental self-esteem.

As the child grows, autonomy develops. The child enters the toddler years and the "no" stage of development just when the parents have begun to establish a comfortable routine of medications and chest physical therapy. The nurse encourages the parents to set realistic behavior limits for the child. Overprotectiveness, which isolates the child and prevents development of autonomy, is also minimized by the setting of realistic limits. Encouraging the autonomous toddler to participate in chest physical therapy is a challenge to the most experienced parent or nurse. Game playing and special toys, music, or books for use only during chest therapy are techniques that help elicit the child's cooperation. Percussing to a particular musical rhythm is also useful.

The school-age child is usually ready to begin to learn some aspects of self-care. Administration of medications with supervision is one aspect of self-care. Absence from school limits learning, even in bright children. Visits by home-based teachers during periods of illness that interrupt public school attendance keep the child intellectually in line with peers. However, home-based learning does not facilitate development of peer relationships. Encouraging the child to participate in play and other extracurricular activities as he is able is important to normal growth and development.

Problems with peer relationships escalate in the adolescent years when peer relationships are critical. School-age children and teens make cruel comments about physical appearance (barrel chest, productive cough, clubbing, and delayed secondary sexual characteristics). At this stage the adolescent is usually independent in self-care. Rebellion toward treatments and denial of the disease are common expressions of the adolescent's independence. The use of mechanical percussors, versus having parents perform chest physical therapy, and involvement of close friends in care are techniques to get the adolescent safely through this developmental period. Teen-based support groups are helpful in easing the transition into young adulthood. In addition, the adolescent may have concerns about sexual function when secondary sexual characteristics are delayed. Providing information, listening to concerns, and reassuring the adolescent of normal sexual function assist the teen through this rough period.

The young adult with CF and his siblings require information about risks of reproduction. Marriage is not contraindicated; however reproduction carries certain risks. Because CF is genetically transmitted, the risks of an offspring having CF are at least 25% with each birth. Because the chances of pregnancy exist, the use of prophylactic contraceptives or sterilization based on informed decision of the sexual partners is necessary to prevent conception, even in the sexually active teen.

Finally, the parents of the child with CF encounter stressors uncommon in the normal family. There are numerous treatments to schedule. Other children in the family often feel jealous when parents spend extra time with the affected child. Finding babysitters or day care providers that will religiously comply with the treatment regimen is difficult. Because parents spend a significant amount of time with the child, strain develops between the parents. The parental relationship suffers, and divorce is common. Parents must allow time for themselves and each other for the relationship to survive.

Finances are one of the last but not the least areas of concern. The cost of treatments, especially antibiotics, O_2, or hospitalization, is very high. Many children are eligible for assistance from Crippled Childrens Services or the Cystic Fibrosis Foundation. Social Security and Vocational Rehabilitation Services also provide assistance. Many sources only provide assistance until the child is 21 years old. After this time, coverage is very limited. Obtaining insurance coverage with the diagnosis of CF is difficult and very expensive. Many patients qualify for state or federal assistance because employment is limited.

BRONCHIOLITIS
Etiology

Bronchiolitis is an acute viral disease of infancy and early childhood. Males are more frequently and severely affected than females. Most cases of bronchiolitis occur between 2 and 6 months of age although it is seen in children through age 2. Before 2 months of age, placental transfer of maternal antibodies may prevent development of bronchiolitis. Before the child reaches 2 years of age, the small size of lower airways is easily obstructed by a small amount of inflammation. Mortality in patients hospitalized because of bronchiolitis is less than 1%.

Bronchiolitis commonly occurs in late winter and early spring with outbreaks of respiratory syncytial virus (RSV) infection. An extremely contagious virus, RSV is frequently brought home by older children and transmitted to the infant. In older children and adults, RSV infection is associated with prolonged cough and upper respiratory symptoms. When RSV is not prevalent, bronchiolitis is frequently associated with parainfluenza type 3 viruses.

Pathophysiology

Pathophysiology of bronchiolitis is based on findings at autopsy. There is diffuse regional hyperinflation. The bronchioles are plugged with cellular debris and lymphocytes. Edema and inflammation surround the bronchioles. Bronchial epithelium is necrosed; ciliated epithelium is destroyed. Located throughout the lung are patchy areas of atelectasis or pneumonia.

Nursing management

Assessment. Bronchiolitis usually develops very rapidly in an infant 1 to 2 days after a mild upper respiratory infection. During the symptomatic period the child has cough, mild fever, coryza, and irritability. With the development of bronchiolitis, respirations markedly increase, resulting in inability to suck from the bottle or breast and subsequent dehydration. The general appearance of the child is one of respiratory distress, including nasal flaring and cyanosis. The child feels warm to the touch, providing evidence of fever (about 100° F). The fontanels may be depressed in the presence of dehydration.

The symptoms of bronchiolitis usually begin to improve within 3 to 4 days. Within 2 weeks of development of symptoms, the episode is over in most infants although infants with congenital abnormalities often have a prolonged course with residual effects. Asthma may develop in later life. Subsequent viral infections are frequently accompanied by wheezing. Bacterial pneumonia is a common complication for which the nurse must watch.

On inspection the nurse observes use of accessory muscles with intercostal, suprasternal, supraclavicular, and subcostal or substernal abdominal muscle retractions. Expiration is prolonged, and overexpansion of the chest may be assessed. Palpation of the chest may identify areas of increased tactile fremitus over areas of consolidation. Resonance or hyperresonance is elicited with percussion. With auscultation of the lungs the nurse assesses wheezes, crackles, and sometimes gurgles. Expiration is prolonged greatly.

The chest x-ray film of the patient with bronchiolitis shows evidence of hyperinflation. The diaphragm is flattened, and the lungs appear hyperlucent. Because of its pliability, the infant sternum may bow outward from hyperinflation. In many patients patchy perihilar atelectasis and infiltrates are present.

Other assessments include various laboratory tests. PFTs are not performed because the patient cannot cooperate with instructions. White blood cell counts are elevated in some patients but not all of them. Immunofluorescent studies are available in some institutions to identify RSV infection within several hours of admission. Arterial or capillary blood gases reveal hypoxemia in the significantly tachypneic or cyanotic infant. Severe hypoxemia may require intubation and mechanical ventilation.

Nursing diagnoses. The main problems in the patient with bronchiolitis are airway clearance and maintenance of oxygenation. In some infants dehydration and nutrition are problems. Another problem in caring for the child with bronchiolitis is providing emotional support for the parents through the crisis.

Based on identification of the problems, the nurse identifies the nursing diagnoses. A common nursing diagnosis is ineffective airway clearance related to thick, tenacious secretions and/or dehydration. Impaired gas exchange related to ventilation-perfusion mismatching is an appropriate nursing diagnosis when hypoxemia occurs. Nutrition, less than body requirements, related to inability to suck secondary to respiratory distress is appropriate in some infants. Fluid volume deficit related to decreased intake secondary to respiratory distress is used in the dehydrated patient. Altered family dynamics related to the child's hospitalization for an acute life-threatening illness is an important diagnosis in most patients.

Interventions. The main focus of nursing care in the patient with bronchiolitis is promotion of adequate oxygenation. Other interventions are directed at promoting airway clearance and nutrition. Establishing normal hemodynamic volume is necessary in dehydrated patients. Some interventions are needed to promote family integrity during the illness and after hospitalization. The nurse helps the parents to understand what is happening to the child.

Interventions for the child with bronchiolitis are primarily supportive. Supplemental O_2 (40% is usual) corrects hypoxemia in most cases. A few, very severe cases of bronchiolitis require intubation and mechanical ventilation. This is frightening for both the child and the parent. Intravenous fluids with electrolytes remedy fluid volume deficits in the affected child. Hydration with intravenous fluids is continued until the child is able to resume sufficient oral feedings. Gastric feedings via bottle or breast may continue as usual in many patients using supplemental O_2. A few patients may be fed small volumes of formula with a nasogastric tube. Fatigue during or after feedings may lead to respiratory failure requiring ventilatory assistance. Respiratory distress is less common after nasogastric feedings. Antibiotics are used to prevent secondary bacterial infection. Steroids do not affect the course of bronchiolitis and are not recommended. Many parents benefit from being at the child's bedside throughout the hospitalization and are included in the child's care as much as possible.

SLEEP APNEA
Etiology

Sleep apnea is a group of syndromes characterized by periodic cessation of breathing during sleep. The etiology of sleep apnea is unknown although there is decreased drive to breathe, loss of upper airway motor tone, and obstruction of the upper airway. Approximately one third of normal people may have periods of nocturnal apnea. Either children or adults may be affected by sleep apnea. However, the incidence of sleep apnea is highest in middle-age males.

Sleep apnea is often associated with obesity. The obesity hypoventilation syndromes were originally termed *Pickwickian syndrome* named after a Charles Dickens character who was obese and continually falling asleep. The cause of obesity hypoventilation syndromes is also unknown. The mechanical effects of obesity, impaired respiratory drive, and weakened muscles may be factors.

Pathophysiology

Pathophysiologically, there are three types of sleep apnea syndromes: obstructive, central, and mixed. With obstructive sleep apnea, diaphragmatic contractions continue in spite of obstructed oronasal air flow. In other words, there is respiratory effort without air flow. Central sleep apnea is also termed *primary* or *central alveolar hypoventilation syndrome,* or *Ondine's curse.* With central apnea, diaphragmatic and intercostal contractions cease, and there is no respiratory effort. The third form of sleep apnea is a combination of obstructive and central apnea, in which periods of obstructive apnea follow periods of central apnea. Most patients have either obstructive or mixed sleep apnea.

During obstructive sleep apnea the posterior wall of the hypopharynx collapses. The muscles of the neck become hypotonic, obstructing airflow. As the apneic episode continues, CO_2 accumulates in the blood, and O_2 consumption continues. The result is hypercapnia and hypoxemia. With the patient's continued efforts to breathe, negative intrathoracic pressure increases. When the patient arouses from sleep, a loud snort signals the end of the obstructed episode. Breathing rate is increased for a short period, and ABGs return to normal. A normal rate and depth of breathing resume until the next apneic period. Prolonged episodes of sleep apnea result in pulmonary and systemic hypertension, dysrhythmias, and conduction disturbances. Cor pulmonale is a common complication of prolonged sleep apnea. Pulmonary thromboembolism and sudden death may also occur.

Central apnea is usually idiopathic. It is also caused by destructive lesions in the medulla and by central nervous system depressants. With central apnea the patient just stops breathing.

Obesity hypoventilation syndromes have a variety of causes and pathophysiological processes that relate to hypoventilation and to obesity. The pathophysiological consequences of obesity are varied. With obesity hypoventilation syndromes, O_2 consumption and CO_2 production are increased. Chest wall compliance is decreased, thereby increasing work of breathing. The patient has a restrictive ventilatory defect that results in lower lung volumes. Small airways close prematurely, causing ventilation-perfusion mismatching, especially in dependent lung zones. When the patient is supine, gas exchange abnormalities are enhanced because of lower lung volumes and compliance. The diaphragm no longer has the assistance of gravity in ventilation in the supine position.

Nursing management

Assessment. The patient with sleep apnea is generally obese with normal thyroid function. Snoring during sleep is common with obstructive apnea. The snoring worsens as obstruction increases. On arousing from sleep at the end of the apneic period, the patient frequently thrashes about the bed, awakening the sleeping partner or spouse. The partner or spouse is sometimes injured by thrashing arms. In many cases the partner or spouse moves into a separate bed or bedroom. Most patients with sleep apnea report that they cannot sleep at night and that they do not feel rested when rising in the morning. The patient does not recall the reason for insomnia. On awakening, the patient complains of a headache. Hypercarbia resulting in cerebral vasodilation is believed to be the cause of the headache.

Daytime somnolence, that is, frequent naps or hypersomnia, occurs in sleep apnea. Naps are involuntary and do not relieve feelings of sleepiness. The patient with sleep apnea falls asleep anywhere at any time. In severe cases the patient falls asleep in the midst of a sentence. Falling asleep while driving causes accidents, which bring patients to the hospital, resulting in diagnosis. Myocardial infarction can also occur during periods of apnea and result in hospitalization and diagnosis. Patients with diagnosis of central sleep apnea are usually denied medical clearance to drive a car or to operate other machinery.

The diagnosis of sleep apnea is made with a polysomnogram in a sleep laboratory or, less commonly, at home. Multiple electrodes measure electrical brain waves, oral and nasal air flow, ventilatory effort through the esophagus or with chest and abdominal wall leads, heart rate, and SaO_2. The test identifies periods of hypopneas (shallow breaths) and apneas (no breaths). The length and number of the apneas are critical to the diagnosis and treatment of sleep apnea. Significant apneic episodes last longer than 10 seconds, occur at least five times per hour of sleep, and occur during non-rapid eye movement (nonREM) sleep. The time spent with O_2 saturation below 90% is also important.

The PFTs are normal in awake patients with sleep apnea unless there is underlying COPD or a restrictive defect from obesity. Flow-volume loops in some patients have a sawtooth obstructive pattern. If CO_2 response curves are done, the patient may have a normal ventilatory response. With central alveolar hypoventilation CO_2 response curves are diminished or absent.

The chest x-ray film of the patient with sleep apnea is normal unless the patient has underlying COPD. In later stages, when cor pulmonale is present, the heart, particularly the right ventricle, is enlarged.

ABG values in the awake state are normal in some patients although most have hypoxemia and hypercarbia at rest. During sleep all patients have hypercarbia and hypoxemia. Acidemia is usually present from the hypercarbia. With exercise, hypoxemia and hypercarbia worsen in the patient with central apnea because of impaired chemoreceptor response. Over time the patient develops a metabolic alkalosis to compensate for the acidemia. Unexplained metabolic alkalosis is a clue to sleep apnea diagnosis. About half of the patients develop polycythemia from hypoxemia.

Inspection of the chest in an awake patient reveals normal rate and depth of breathing. In the sleeping patient the nurse observes chest wall movements without an increase in lung volume. Retractions are sometimes observed. Palpation and percussion are unremarkable unless the patient has underlying COPD. Auscultation of the lungs during sleep apnea periods reveals no air flow. Applying the stethoscope to the chest during an apneic period usually awakens the patient and ends the apneic period. Leaving the stethoscope on the chest wall for a few minutes allows the patient to fall asleep and repeat the obstructing episode.

Nursing diagnoses. The main problems in sleep apnea are hypoxemia and hypercarbia. Patent airway is another important consideration. Because of obesity or excessive drowsiness the ability to perform adequate hygiene is sometimes impaired. The obesity itself is a problem for the health of the patient.

The most important nursing diagnosis in the patient with sleep apnea is ineffective breathing pattern related to airway obstruction or impaired gas exchange related to inadequate drive to breathe. In the patient with cor pulmonale the nursing diagnosis of altered cardiac output related to decreased right ventricular contraction should be considered. Self-care deficit related to obesity or to sleep deprivation is another important nursing diagnosis. Nutrition in excess of body requirements related to overeating is applicable in the obese patient needing weight reduction.

Interventions. Nursing interventions for a patient with sleep apnea focus on maintaining a patent airway and promoting adequate ABGs. Additional interventions are often directed at improving personal hygiene and reducing total body weight.

The most important nursing intervention is to preserve gas exchange. Therefore O_2 administration during sleep is the first therapy. In patients with obstructive sleep apnea, oral or nasal continuous positive airway pressure

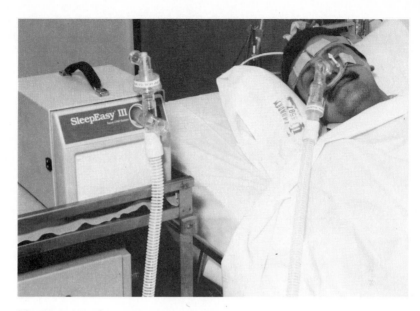

Fig. 10-5. Nasal continuous positive airway pressure system commonly used in treating sleep apnea. (From Beare PG, Myers JL: *Principles and practice of adult health nursing,* ed 1, St Louis, 1990, Mosby–Year Book.)

(CPAP) maintains upper airway patency during sleep (Fig. 10-5). The level of CPAP is determined during the sleep study by trying different levels. Five to ten centimeters of water pressure resolves obstruction in most patients although some patients require as much as 20 cm of water pressure. O_2 is used simultaneously when necessary. When CPAP does not correct the obstruction, a tracheostomy is performed to bypass upper airway obstruction. During the day the tracheostomy tube is plugged, allowing a normal speech and breathing pattern. At night the plug is removed so that air can flow through the tube, bypassing the upper airway obstruction.

Excess weight of 50 to 200 pounds is common in patients with sleep apnea. Weight reduction is critical to reducing obstructive apneic episodes in obese patients. Some patients enroll in liquid-protein diets under medical supervision to rapidly lose weight. However, a balanced, calorie-controlled diet supervised by a professional often has the best results. Weight loss is often tedious and slow.

In some patients respiratory stimulants are effective, but the response is variable. Protriptyline, progesterone, and theophylline can improve nocturnal sleep and decrease daytime somnolence. Rocking beds and nocturnal phrenic nerve pacing are safe and effective in some patients. Sleeping on several pillows or in a reclining chair works for other patients. Surgical removal of excessive postpharyngeal tissue is effective for a select group of patients.

CONCLUSION

The major obstructive lung diseases presented in this chapter are asthma, emphysema, chronic bronchitis, cystic fibrosis, bronchiolitis, and sleep apnea. Obstructive lung diseases diminish air flow into or out of the lung. These ineffective breathing patterns impair gas exchange. In addition to alteration or destruction of normal airway structures, the major problems in obstructive lung diseases are bronchospasm, excessive mucus production, swelling, and inflammation. Common nursing diagnoses for the patient with obstructive lung diseases are ineffective breathing pattern, impaired gas exchange, knowledge deficit, altered nutrition, and altered family dynamics. Caring for the patient with obstructive lung diseases is a challenge requiring multiple assessments and interventions. The assessments vary among the obstructive lung diseases, with hypoxemia being the most common finding. Because there is no cure for obstructive lung diseases, treatments are supportive. Interventions common to the patient with obstructive lung disease include airway clearance measures, bronchodilators, O_2 administration, improved nutrition, and family support and education.

BIBLIOGRAPHY

American Thoracic Society: Cigarette smoking and your health, *Am Rev Resp Dis* 132(5):1133-1138, 1985.

American College of Chest Physicians: Statement on spirometry: a report of the section on respiratory pathophysiology, *Chest* 83(3):547-550, 1983.

American Thoracic Society: Standards for the diagnosis and care of patients with chronic obstructive pulmonary disease (COPD) and asthma, *Am Rev Respir Dis* 136:225-243, 1987.

Barbee R: The medical history in pulmonary disease, *Basics Respir Dis* 11(3), 1983.

Bates B: *A guide to physical examination and history taking,* ed 4, Philadelphia, 1987, J B Lippincott.

Baum GL, Wolinsky E: *Textbook of pulmonary diseases,* ed 3, Boston, 1983, Little, Brown.

Benatar SR: Fatal asthma, *N Engl J Med* 314(7):423-429, 1986.

Burki NK: *Pulmonary diseases: medical outline series,* Garden City, NY, 1982, Medical Examination Publishing.

Burton GC, Hodgkin JE: *Respiratory care: a guide to clinical practice,* ed 2, Philadelphia, 1984, J B Lippincott.

Carrieri VK, Janson-Bjerklie S: Strategies patients use to manage the sensation of dyspnea, *West J Nurs Res* 8(3):284-305, 1986.

Carrieri VK, Janson-Bjerklie S, Jacobs S: The sensation of dyspnea: a review, *Heart Lung* 13(4):436-437, 1984.

Cherniack NS, Widdicombe JG, eds: *Handbook of physiology, section 3: the respiratory system,* vol 3, Baltimore, 1986, Williams & Wilkins.

Cherniack R: Chronic and acute asthma: keys to successful management, *Postgrad Med* 75(2):87-98, 1984.

Chester EH, Fleming GM, Montenegro H: Effect of steroid therapy on gas exchange abnormalities in patients with diffuse lung disease, *Chest* 69(2)(suppl):269-271, 1976.

Chin R, Pesce R: Practical aspects in management of respiratory failure in chronic obstructive pulmonary disease, *Crit Care Q* 6(2):1, 1983.

Cohen CA, Zagelbaum G et al: Clinical manifestations of inspiratory muscle fatigue, *Am J Med* 73(3):308-316, 1982.

Comroe J: *Physiology of respiration: an introductory text,* ed 2, Chicago, 1974, Mosby—Year Book.

Dahms T, Bolin JF, Slavin RG: Passive smoking: effects on bronchial asthma, *Chest* 80(5):530-534, 1981.

Davis P, di SantÁgnese L: Diagnosis and treatment of cystic fibrosis, *Chest* 85(6):802-809, 1984.

Demers R, Irwin R: Management of hypercapnic respiratory failure: a systematic approach, *Respir Care* 24(4):328-335, 1979.

Derrene J, Fleury B, Pariente R: State of the art: acute respiratory failure of chronic obstructive pulmonary disease, *Am Rev Respir Dis* 138:1006-1033, 1988.

di SantÁgnese PA, Talamo RC: Pathogenesis and pathophysiology of cystic fibrosis of the pancreas, *N Engl J Med* 277:1287, 1967.

Felson B: The chest roentgenologic workup: what and why? Conventional methods, *Basics Respir Dis* 8(5):1-5, 1980.

Felson B, Weinstein AS, Spitz HB: *Principles of chest roentgenology: a programmed text,* Philadelphia, 1965, W B Saunders.

Felson B: *Chest roentgenology,* Philadelphia, 1973, W B Saunders.

Fishman A: *Pulmonary diseases and disorders,* New York, 1980, McGraw-Hill.

Fishman A: *Assessment of pulmonary function,* New York, 1980, McGraw-Hill.

Forster RE: *The lung: clinical physiology and pulmonary function tests,* ed 3, Chicago, 1986, Mosby—Year Book.

Fraser R, Paré J: *Diagnosis of diseases of the chest,* vol 3, ed 2, Philadelphia, 1979, W B Saunders.

Fraser R, Paré J: *Diagnosis of diseases of the chest,* vol 1-3, ed 2, Philadelphia, 1977-1979, W B Saunders.

Gold WM: *Cholinergic pharmacology in asthma.* In Austen KF, Lichtenstein LM, eds: *Asthma,* New York, 1973, Academic Press.

Guenter C, Welch M: *Pulmonary medicine,* ed 2, Philadelphia, 1982, J B Lippincott.

Guyton AC: *Textbook of medical physiology,* ed 6, Philadelphia, 1981, W B Saunders.

Harper R: *A guide to respiratory care: physiology and clinical applications,* Philadelphia, 1982, J B Lippincott.

Hinshaw H, Murray J: *Diseases of the chest,* ed 4, Philadelphia, 1980, W B Saunders.

Hogg JC: The pathology of asthma, *Chest* 87:152S, 1985.

Janoff A: Elastases and emphysema: current assessment of the protease-antiprotease hypothesis, *Am Rev Respir Dis* 132:417-433, 1985.

Kanner R, Renzetti A: Predictors of spirometric changes and mortality in obstructive airway disorders, *Chest* 85(6):15S-19S, 1984.

Kulczycki LL, Schauf V: Cystic fibrosis in blacks in Washington, DC: incidence and characteristics, *Am J Dis Child* 127(1):64-67, 1974.

Loudon RG: Cough: a symptom and a sign, *Basics Respir Dis* 9:4, 1981.

Luce J, Culver B: Respiratory muscle function in health and disease, *Chest* 81(1):82-90, 1982.

Malasanos L et al: *Health assessment,* ed 2, St Louis, 1981, Mosby—Year Book.

Morgan WKC: Pulmonary disability and impairment: can't work? won't work? *Basics Respir Dis* 10(5), 1982.

Morrison M: *Respiratory intensive care nursing,* ed 2, Boston, 1979, Little, Brown.

Mountcastle VB, ed: *Medical physiology,* St Louis, 1980, Mosby—Year Book.

Murray JF, Nadel JA, eds: *Textbook of respiratory medicine,* Philadelphia, 1988, W B Saunders.

Netter F: *The CIBA collection of medical illustrations, vol 7, respiratory system,* New York, 1979, CIBA Pharmaceutical Co.

Paré JAP, Fraser RG: *Synopsis of diseases of the chest,* Philadelphia, 1983, W B Saunders.

Petty T: Clinical evaluation of patients with chronic respiratory insufficiency, *Semin Respir Med* 1(1):1-8, 1979.

Plymat KR, Bunn C: Monitoring asthma with a mini-wright peak flow meter, *Nurse Pract* 10:25, 1988.

Prior J, Silberstein J, Stang J: *Physical diagnosis: the history and examination of the patient,* ed 6, St Louis, 1981, Mosby—Year Book.

Rochester DF, Goldberg SK: Techniques of respiratory physical therapy, *Am Rev Respir Dis* 122(5pt 2):133-146, 1980.

Ruppel G: *Manual of pulmonary function testing,* St Louis, 1990, Mosby—Year Book.

Schwartz JL: *Review and evaluation of smoking cessation methods: the United States and Canada 1978-1985,* Bethesda, Md, 1987, Division of Cancer Prevention and Control, National Cancer Institute.

Shapiro B, Harrison R et al: *Clinical applications of respiratory care,* ed 3, St Louis, 1985, Mosby—Year Book.

Shoemaker WC, Thompson WL, Holbrook PR: *The Society of Critical Care Medicine textbook of critical care,* Philadelphia, 1984, W B Saunders.

Simmons DH, ed: *Current pulmonology,* vol 7, St Louis, 1986, Mosby—Year Book.

Slonim N, Hamilton L: *Respiratory physiology,* ed 5, St Louis, 1987, Mosby—Year Book.

Strohl KP, Cherniack N, Gothe B: Physiologic basis of therapy for sleep apnea, *Am Rev Respir Dis* 134:791-802, 1986.

Swearingen PL, Sommers MS, Miller K: *Manual of critical care: applying nursing diagnoses to adult critical illness,* St Louis, 1988, Mosby—Year Book.

Wade JF: *Comprehensive respiratory care: physiology and technique,* ed 3, St Louis, 1982, Mosby—Year Book.

Wanner A, Sackner MA: *Pulmonary diseases: mechanisms of altered structure and function,* Boston, 1983, Little, Brown.

Wanner A: Bronchial provocation testing in clinical practice, *Respir Care* 31(3):207-212, 1986.

West J: *Respiratory physiology: the essentials,* ed 3, Baltimore, 1985, Williams & Wilkins.

West JB: *Pulmonary pathophysiology: the essentials,* ed 3, Baltimore, 1987, Williams & Wilkins.

Williams MH, ed: Disturbance of respiratory control, *Clin Chest Med,* vol 1, Philadelphia, 1980, W B Saunders.

Wood R, Boat T, Doershuk C: State of the art: cystic fibrosis, *Am Rev Respir Dis* 113:833-878, 1976.

C·H·A·P·T·E·R 11

Restrictive Diseases

Objectives

- Identify the mechanism for restrictive lung disease induced by neuromuscular disease.
- Discuss assessment and nursing care of the patient with neuromuscular disease and identify interventions.
- Differentiate types of pleural disease and nursing interventions.
- Discuss interstitial lung disease with regard to assessment, nursing diagnoses, and interventions.
- Discuss the TNM classification of lung tumors.
- Discuss assessment and nursing care of the patient with sarcoidosis.
- Examine role of skin testing and sputum analysis in diagnosis of tuberculosis.

Restrictive lung diseases alter respiratory function and result in a decrease of lung volumes and compliance. Mechanisms of restrictive lung disease include impaired neuromuscular contraction, impaired lung expansion, thoracic deformities, and pleural-based diseases. Not all restrictive lung diseases are presented in this chapter. The etiology, pathophysiology, and nursing assessment for the most common restrictive lung diseases are discussed in detail. Some nursing diagnoses are suggested based on the assessment. Interventions for each type of disease are reviewed. Specific interventions, such as medications and breathing exercises, are discussed in subsequent chapters.

NEUROMUSCULAR DISEASES
Etiology

A variety of lung diseases are categorized as neuromuscular diseases. Included in this category are diseases that involve skeletal muscle, peripheral nerves, neuromuscular junction, and spinal cord (see the box on p. 205 for a list of the common diseases by group).

Pathophysiology

In neuromuscular diseases the primary pathophysiology is respiratory muscle weakness from dysfunction of the chest wall, including the rib cage, diaphragm, and abdominal muscles. The exception is tetanus, which causes muscle spasm. With skeletal muscle and neuromuscular junction disorders and

---

Neuromuscular diseases

Skeletal muscle disorders

Muscular dystrophy (Duchenne, fascioscapulohumeral (FSH), and limb girdle, inflammatory myopathy (polymyositis and dermatomyositis), and myotonic dystrophy

Peripheral nerve disorders

Polyneuritis, metabolic (uremia and hepatic failure), endocrine (diabetes and thyroid), toxic (lead, arsenic, and vincristine), and hereditary (Charcot-Marie-Tooth)

Neuromuscular junction disorders

Myasthenia gravis, botulism, Eaton-Lambert syndrome, and tick paralysis

Spinal cord disorders

Amyotrophic lateral sclerosis, Guillain-Barré syndrome, traumatic spinal cord injuries, poliomyelitis, and tetanus

---

with some spinal cord and peripheral nerve disorders, the patient develops generalized muscle weakness. Both inspiratory and expiratory muscles are weakened. With traumatic spinal cord injuries below L1, there is usually no respiratory impairment. As the trauma ascends the spinal cord, progressive respiratory dysfunction occurs. Lesions between T6 and L1 result in limited ability to exhale forcibly because of impaired abdominal contraction. Thoracic spine injuries paralyze the internal and external intercostal muscles, limiting both inspiration and expiration. As the injury approaches C5, only the diaphragm and accessory muscles continue to function. Between C3-C5, the diaphragm is partially functional or totally denervated. Above C3 the patient requires total ventilatory support because phrenic nerve stimulation of the diaphragm is eliminated.

Nursing management

Assessment. The physician uses multiple tests to distinguish neuromuscular diseases. Depending on the extent and acuity of the disease, the patient may have evidence of respiratory distress. The patient often appears anxious. In the acute stage the patient looks well nourished and has normal musculature. As the disease progresses or in time, muscle groups waste from disuse.

On inspection the nurse observes decreased depth of breathing. The patient with a high spinal cord injury may be moving a V_T of 100 ml or less. When accessory muscle groups are intact, they are used to increase V_T. Palpation and percussion of the chest sometimes demonstrate an elevated diaphragm. (Diaphragmatic elevation is also seen on the chest x-ray film.) Auscultation is usually unrevealing unless the patient has a concomitant problem.

The most frequently assessed tests of respiratory muscle strength are vital capacity (VC), peak inspiratory pressure (PIP) or maximum inspiratory pressure (MIP), and peak expiratory pressure (PEP) or maximum expiratory pressure (MEP). Serial measurements are made at appropriate intervals. In the acute patient measurements are made daily (or more frequently as indicated by patient condition). In the critical care unit, strength is assessed every 1 to 4 hours. As the patient stabilizes, assessments are made every 4 to 12 hours. In the chronic patient measurements are made at each visit or change in therapy or symptomatology. The nurse assesses for signs of impending respiratory failure. A decrease in VC, especially to less than three times V_T, a MIP less than 30 cm of water pressure (cwp), or a falling MIP or VC indicates impending respiratory failure.

ABG values are usually normal in the patient with neuromuscular disease. When inspiratory volumes fall significantly, the $Paco_2$ begins to elevate from inadequate minute ventilation ($\dot{V}_E$). Oxygenation is generally unaffected although the Pao_2 can decrease if hypoventilation is significant.

Nursing diagnoses. The primary nursing problem is inadequate alveolar ventilation ($\dot{V}_A$). The patient frequently also has difficulty expectorating sputum and protecting the airway because of weakened muscle strength that results in an inadequate cough.

The nursing diagnoses specific to the patient with neuromuscular diseases affecting the pulmonary system include ineffective breathing pattern related to respiratory muscle weakness, ineffective airway clearance related to abnormal fatigue or paralysis of respiratory muscles, impaired gas exchange related to respiratory muscle weakness or paralysis, grieving related to changes in body image, potential for infection related to ineffective cough, knowledge deficit related to disease process and therapies, and impaired physical mobility related to muscle weakness or paralysis.

Interventions. Many interventions for the patient with neuromuscular disease focus on maintaining adequate $\dot{V}_A$. Improving the patient's knowledge about his disease and treatments is also important. Other interventions are directed at improving airway clearance to prevent infection and accepting changing body image. Maintaining intact skin and muscle strength and preventing contractures are other important therapies.

There are no cures for most neuromuscular diseases. Over time some patients with neuromuscular diseases recover from acute episodes. Other patients are left with permanent disabilities. Therefore most of the therapies for patients with neuromuscular diseases are supportive. In specific patients bronchodilators are useful to decrease airway resistance and obstruction.

Some patients require the institution of mechanical ventilation. It is important to note that some patients with progressive neuromuscular diseases, such as amyotrophic lateral sclerosis, prefer to die than to be mechanically ventilated. The patient should give informed consent, whenever possible, for the institution of mechanical ventilation. It is important to discuss the patient's wishes for various treatments throughout the course of the disease because, as his condition changes, the patient may choose an alternative treatment to one previously stated.

Initially, when muscle fatigue is progressive, an artificial airway may be inserted, and positive pressure ventilation may be started. As the patient improves, he is weaned from positive pressure ventilation. Most patients with neuromuscular diseases respond very well to noninvasive negative pressure ventilation although spinal cord injury patients continue to need positive pressure ventilation. (Methods of mechanical ventilation are discussed in Chapter 15.) When available and appropriate, negative pressure ventilation replaces positive pressure ventilation.

PLEURAL DISEASES
Etiology

Pleural diseases limit chest expansion by the accumulation of fluid, air, or solid masses in the pleural space. The three types of pleural disease discussed in this chapter are pleural effusion, pneumothorax, and mesothelioma. The pathophysiology of these three pleural diseases is discussed separately, but the nursing care is combined.

Pathophysiology

The nurse should recall from physiology that the pleura is a single layer of mesothelial cells lying on a layer of connective tissue. The visceral pleura adheres to the lung, and the parietal pleura covers the chest wall, diaphragm, and mediastinum. The visceral pleura has a rich vascular supply, lacks a nerve supply, and shares lymphatic drainage with the lung. In direct contrast the parietal pleura is innervated by the intercostal nerves and drains into the internal mammary nodes and intercostal nodes. The potential space between the visceral and parietal pleurae is called the *pleural space*. It contains no air and approximately 25 ml of low-protein fluid. A dynamic equilibrium exists between pleural fluid production and absorption. As fluid is produced, it is reabsorbed.

A *pleural effusion* is the accumulation of fluid in the pleural space (Fig. 11-1, *B*). A bloody pleural effusion is termed a *hemothorax*, and a fatty or lymphatic pleural effusion is called a *chylothorax*. Several possible mechanisms interrupt the dynamic equilibrium, allowing fluid accumulation in the pleural space. An increase in hydrostatic pressure (as in congestive heart failure) or a decrease in colloid osmotic pressure (as in hypoalbuminemia) favors the development of a pleural effusion. Another mechanism, inflammation of the pleura, generates an excess of pleural fluid. With inflammation capillary membrane permeability is altered, or lymphatic drainage is impaired. Pleural effusions are also caused by increased negative intrapleural pressure (as in atelectasis), increased microvascular permeability (as in pneumonia), and extravasation of blood (as in traumatic hemorrhage). Table 11-1 lists common causes of pleural effusion and divides them into transudates and exudates, which are discussed below.

When a pleural effusion develops, it compresses lung tissue. Lung volumes are reduced. Ventilation to the affected area is decreased, but perfusion remains fairly normal. This results in a ventilation-perfusion mismatch and hypoxemia.

Pleural effusions are characterized as either transudates or exudates according to specific criteria. Table 11-2 lists criteria to differentiate transudative from exudative pleural effusions. In general a transudate is produced by edematous states. The nurse should recall that edema is caused by an increase in hydrostatic pressure (fluid overload) or decrease in colloid osmotic pressure (low albumin). An exudate is produced by infection, inflammation, or malignancy.

Most pleural effusions are free flowing in the pleural space. This means that the fluid moves to dependent areas of the lung. For example, in the upright patient fluid flows to the bases, and in the supine patient the fluid displaces to the posterior lung fields. When a pleural effusion does not move freely in the pleural space, the term *loculated* is used. Loculated areas are associated more often with exudative pleural effusions.

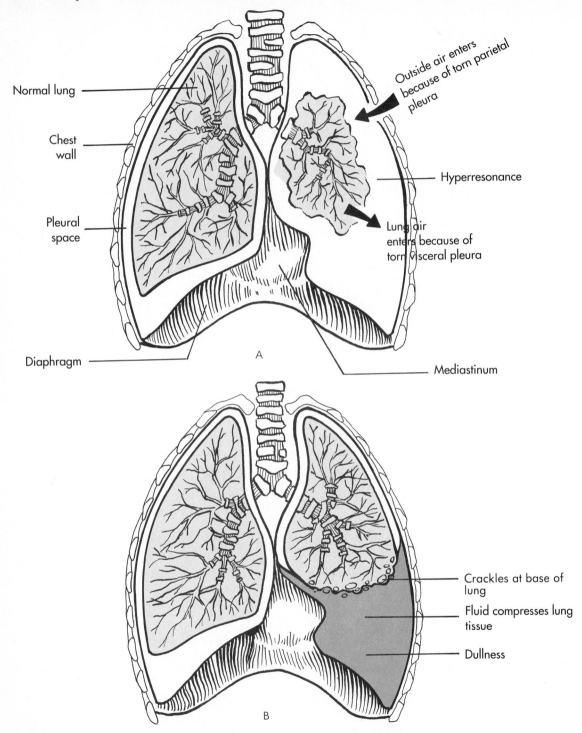

Normal lung

Chest wall

Pleural space

Diaphragm

Outside air enters because of torn parietal pleura

Hyperresonance

Lung air enters because of torn visceral pleura

A

Mediastinum

Crackles at base of lung

Fluid compresses lung tissue

Dullness

B

Fig. 11-1. Pleural diseases limit lung expansion: pneumothorax (**A**), which causes the lung to collapse toward the hilum and which can displace mediastinal contents, and pleural effusion (**B**), which compresses lung tissue.

Table 11-1. Etiology of pleural effusions

Transudate	Exudate
Atelectasis, cirrhosis, congestive heart failure, hypoalbuminemia, nephrotic syndrome	Asbestosis, chylothorax, collagen vascular disease, empyema, fungal diseases, hemothorax, hypersensitivity, malignancy, pancreatitis, pneumonia, pulmonary embolism, tuberculosis

Table 11-2. Characteristics of pleural effusions

	Protein*	Lactate dehydrogenase (LDH)*	White blood cells†	Pleural LDH	Glucose*	pH
Transudate	<0.5	<0.6	<1000/mm^3	>200	>0.6	>7.30
Exudate	>0.5	>0.6	>1000/mm^3	—	<0.6	<7.30

*Pleural to serum ratio.

.†Lymphocyte predominance usual in tuberculous, malignant, and transudative effusions; polymorphonuclear leukocyte predominance usual in inflammatory and infectious effusions.

The second major type of pleural disease is *pneumothorax*. Any process that tears either pleura can cause a pneumothorax (Fig. 11-1, *A*). When the parietal pleura is torn, as occurs with penetrating chest trauma or a pleural biopsy, air enters from the atmosphere. If the visceral pleura is torn, as occurs with barotrauma from mechanical ventilation or with rupture of a bleb, air enters from the lung.

Processes that tear the pleura are either spontaneous, iatrogenic, or traumatic. A spontaneous pneumothorax that results from a tear in the visceral pleura is caused by rupture of a subpleural bleb or erosion by a parenchymal process (Fig. 11-2). In some instances obstruction in the bronchial tree acts as a check valve, allowing air in but not out. Progressive hyperinflation of the distal air spaces then causes rupture. The air dissects into either the fascial planes of the neck, as evidenced by subcutaneous emphysema, or the pleural space, that is, a pneumothorax. A spontaneous pneumothorax is more common in young males age 20 to 30 who are characteristically tall and thin. Spontaneous pneumothorax also occurs during periods of rapid growth in teens. Asthma and other obstructive lung diseases may also produce spontaneous pneumothorax. Mechanisms include rupture of blebs and hyperinflation.

Iatrogenic pneumothorax occurs after invasive thoracic procedures. These procedures include central vein catheterization, thoracentesis, pleural biopsy, and transbronchial lung biopsy. Insertion of a pointed object lacerates the parietal or visceral pleura. Positive pressure mechanical ventilation, especially with the use of high levels of positive end-expiratory pressure (PEEP), also results in iatrogenic pneumothorax. The mechanism is either excessive pressure, called *barotrauma*, or check-valve obstruction.

Traumatic pneumothorax occurs after blunt or penetrating chest trauma. Rapid deceleration in motor vehicle accidents ruptures bronchi, the trachea,

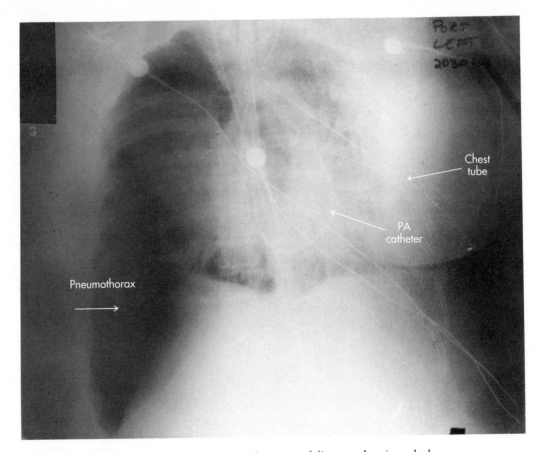

Fig. 11-2. Left spontaneous pneumothorax. The arrow delineates the visceral pleura line. Note the small left lung volume and beginning displacement of mediastinal structures.

or esophagus. Rib or sternal fractures puncture the pleura and lung parenchyma, causing pneumothorax. Tears in the diaphragm from stab or bullet wounds also can result in traumatic pneumothorax. Penetrating stab or bullet wounds directly tear the pleura. Pneumothorax occurs when air enters the pleural space from a hole in the lung or from the atmosphere through the tear.

As a result of a pneumothorax, when air at atmospheric pressure enters the pleural space (which is normally under negative pressure), the lung collapses toward the mediastinum. Both ventilation and perfusion decrease in the affected lung. However, ventilation decreases much more than perfusion. Hypoxemia usually results, depending on the degree of pneumothorax and the amount of lung collapse. As a pneumothorax enlarges, it compresses lung tissue. An entire lung may collapse and push mediastinal structures to the opposite side. This occurrence is termed *tension pneumothorax* and is life threatening.

The third major pleural disease is *mesothelioma*. Mesothelioma is classified as benign (25%) or malignant (75%). Benign mesothelioma has no sex predominance and usually occurs in the fourth to sixth decades of life. The prognosis is good with benign mesothelioma. Malignant mesothelioma has a 3:1 male predominance with peak incidence between the ages of 50 and 60. Malignant mesothelioma has also been diagnosed in children although it is rare. Malignant mesothelioma is strongly associated with asbestos exposure. The mesothelioma appears initially as multiple small gray or white patches on the pleura. As the tumor grows it encases the lung in a thick sheath. Mortality from respiratory failure, infection, or cardiac failure is high.

Nursing management

Assessment. Assessment of the patient with pleural disease varies with the type of disease. There is no characteristic posture or muscle structure as with other diseases. The patient may be in acute distress, depending on the extent of the disease.

Pleural effusion. In general a small pleural effusion is approximately 500 ml, and 1500 ml is considered a large pleural effusion. With small pleural effusions the respiratory rate and depth are normal. When a pleural effusion sufficiently compresses the lung, creating a ventilation-perfusion mismatch, inspection frequently reveals tachypnea. Intercostal spaces bulge with very large pleural effusions function is impaired. When right ventricular function is impaired, the nurse may also observe pedal edema or distended neck veins, which suggest congestive heart failure. When listening to the heart tones, an S_3 gallop may also indicate congestive heart failure.

With palpation, reduced tactile and vocal fremitus are present over the pleural effusion. A pleural effusion must usually be large to assess fremitus.

Percussion is significant for dullness over the area of fluid accumulation, depending on the size of the pleural effusion. In an upright patient, dullness occurs at the base of the lung. In the side-lying patient, fluid flows to the dependent lung, causing dullness there. When the pleural effusion is loculated, dullness is heard over the effusion.

With auscultation, diminished breath sounds are heard over the area of the pleural effusion. Crackles are heard just above the effusion. Egophony and bronchial breath sounds indicate atelectasis.

The chest x-ray film of the patient with a pleural effusion classically shows blunting of the costophrenic angle on an upright film (see Fig. 7-6). A pleural effusion is frequently bilateral. With a subpulmonic pleural effusion the diaphragm appears elevated. The nurse should recall that accumulation of 300 ml is required to blunt the costophrenic angle. Larger effusions obliterate the diaphragm, and the affected hemithorax appears opacified. The pleural effusion is higher laterally than medially. In a supine patient a ground glass, or homogenous hazy opaque appearance, is noted over the affected lung. A lateral decubitus chest x-ray examination is performed to identify layering or loculation of the pleural fluid. With a free-flowing pleural effusion, fluid accumulates in dependent areas. With the affected lung on the top the costophrenic angle clears; with the affected lung on the bottom the fluid accumulates along the lower edge of the lung. A loculated pleural effusion does not move with position changes. With large pleural effusions the mediastinum can shift to the opposite side.

The ABG values of a patient with pleural effusion are frequently normal. With large pleural effusions hypoxemia occurs.

Pneumothorax. The patient with a pneumothorax is usually in acute distress. The patient complains of rapid onset of pleuritic pain or sharp chest pain and dyspnea. The nurse observes rapid, shallow breathing with splinting. Sometimes coughing is observed.

Fremitus is decreased with palpation. The trachea shifts to the opposite side with a tension pneumothorax.

Percussion is usually the most revealing assessment method to detect a pneumothorax. A tympanic or hyperresonant note is heard, especially with a large pneumothorax.

With auscultation the nurse notes decreased breath sounds on the affected side. Heart sounds are normal or muffled. When heart tones are not heard in their normal position, mediastinal shift should be suspected.

The chest x-ray film demonstrates a pneumothorax that is best visualized on an expiratory exposure when the lungs are smaller. When a pleural effusion is concomitantly seen with a pneumothorax, blood (hemothorax) is usually the cause. The term *hemopneumothorax* is used to describe blood and air in the pleural space.

The ABG values of the patient with a pneumothorax encompass a wide range. With a small pneumothorax the ABG values are normal or demonstrate respiratory alkalosis from tachypnea. ABG values deteriorate as the size of the pneumothorax increases. With a larger pneumothorax, hypoxemia develops. Severe hypoxemia, hypercarbia, and acidemia are observed with a tension pneumothorax.

Mesothelioma. The most common patient complaint with mesothelioma is gnawing chest pain. Dyspnea, cough, and fever are sometimes present. As with other malignancies, weight loss occurs with mesothelioma.

Inspection of the patient with mesothelioma occasionally reveals clubbing. The patient's respiratory rate and depth are normal except in very advanced stages. Restriction of the lung by mesothelioma limits lung volumes, producing shallow, rapid respirations. Palpation of the chest is nonspecific except when rib destruction has occurred. Percussion commonly elicits dullness or flatness, especially with a concomitant pleural effusion. Assessment of breath sounds demonstrates basilar crackles and pleural friction rubs in most patients with mesothelioma. The pleural friction rub is usually absent when a pleural effusion is present.

The chest x-ray film of a patient with mesothelioma is variable. A unilateral pleural effusion occurs in many patients. The radiologist may note presence of pleural thickening or nodularity. In some instances a localized mass is observed. In very advanced stages ribs are destroyed by the malignancy. Within the lung itself fibrotic changes suggest asbestos exposure, especially when diaphragmatic pleural plaques are also present. Computed tomography (CT) scan aids in the diagnosis of mesothelioma because it provides three-dimensional reproduction of structures.

If done, PFTs show a restrictive pattern with decreases in all volumes. The FEV_1/FVC ratio is normal.

ABGs are frequently normal. Depending on the size of the pleural effusion, ABG values may change as previously indicated.

The best methods for identifying mesothelioma are thoracentesis and pleural biopsy. Serial thoracentesis and pleural biopsy assessments improve the ability for positive diagnosis. With malignant mesothelioma, pleural fluid is often bloody and usually exudative. White blood cell counts are low, with a lymphocyte predominance. Cytology is frequently positive though open-lung biopsy or thoracotomy is sometimes required for diagnosis.

Unlike many carcinomas in the lung, sputum cytology is not positive in mesothelioma because the pleura are not in contact with the airway. Similarly, bronchoscopy demonstrates no endobronchial lesions, although external compression of the airways may be seen occasionally.

Nursing diagnoses. The main problems in pleural disease are compression of lung tissue and limited lung expansion from air, fluid, or tumor. These problems result in ventilation-perfusion mismatching and hypoxemia. Because invasive therapies, such as thoracentesis or chest tubes, are often used in caring for patients with pleural disease, infection may be a problem. Also, patients are usually concerned about the cause and complications of their disease.

The nursing diagnoses common to the diagnosis of pleural diseases are impaired gas exchange related to lung collapse or compression, potential for infection related to invasive procedures, knowledge deficit related to disease process, and anticipatory grieving related to terminal illness (particularly mesothelioma). Patients also have pain and limited mobility.

Interventions. General interventions focus on promoting lung expansion and adequate gas exchange. The nurse also strives to prevent infection or to efficiently recognize it and to relieve pain from procedures and the disease. Because patients usually have a need to identify the cause and sequelae of the disease process, the nurse attempts to increase the patient's knowledge of the disease process and treatments.

Pleural effusion. The treatment for a pleural effusion is initiated by the physician and usually involves either observing the pleural effusion or removing pleural fluid. Thoracentesis, that is, acute removal of the fluid through a needle or thin catheter, is often the first step for diagnostic purposes. Multiple serial thoracenteses are performed when pleural fluid reaccumulates. In some instances a large bore chest tube is inserted to drain pleural fluid. Sclerosing agents may be inserted to eliminate malignant pleural effusions. This procedure is termed *pleurodesis.* When a chest tube is inserted, specific nursing care is indicated. This care is discussed in Chapter 14.

Positioning and breathing exercises are two areas of specific nursing care. **Patients are positioned with the "good," or less diseased, lung down and the "bad," or more diseased, lung up to improve ventilation-perfusion matching.** The nurse should recall from physiology that dependent areas of the lung have better ventilation and perfusion than nondependent lung zones; this means improved gas exchange in dependent lung areas. In patients with unilateral lung disease the decision for positioning the good lung down is obvious. When bilateral disease is present, the nurse uses assessment skills and the patient's subjective feelings to choose appropriate positioning. The chest x-ray film may aid in determining which lung is more affected. In any event the patient's position (alternate between supine, prone, and "good" lung down) is changed frequently. Breathing exercises, such as deep breathing and coughing, promote lung expansion and prevent atelectasis. Deep breathing aids in removal of lung mucus and helps prevent pneumonia.

Pneumothorax. The treatment for a pneumothorax depends on the size of the pneumothorax. A small pneumothorax, usually estimated to be 5% or

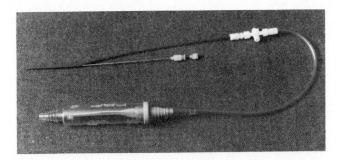

Fig. 11-3. Cook catheter with Heimlich valve. (From Perry A, Potter P: *Clinical nursing skills and techniques,* ed 2, St Louis, 1990, Mosby—Year Book.)

less, is frequently observed for growth or absorption unless the patient's gas exchange is compromised. Larger pneumothoraces require insertion of a chest tube. Depending on the institution a trocar and small chest tube, a pneumothorax catheter with Heimlich valve, or a regular chest tube is inserted to remove air from the pleural space (Fig. 11-3). In an emergency, such as when a tension pneumothorax is suspected, an 18-gauge needle is inserted in the second or third intercostal space anteriorly to release air. Insertion of the needle is usually done in the emergency area or intensive care unit to relieve the pressure from a tension pneumothorax until a chest tube can be inserted. In the case of recurrent spontaneous pneumothorax a pleurodesis is sometimes implemented.

Mesothelioma. Treatment of mesothelioma involves surgical resection, chemotherapy, and radiation therapy. The prognosis is poor. In most cases the lung becomes completely entrapped within 2 years, and the patient dies.

INTERSTITIAL LUNG DISEASES
Etiology

There are a variety of interstitial lung diseases (ILD), the causes of which are unknown in many cases. Onset is gradual or rapid. These diseases are usually classed as *idiopathic interstitial pneumonitis (IIP)* and commonly occur in the fifth to seventh decade of life. There is also a variety of known causes of ILD. Antineoplastic agents, including bleomycin and methotrexate, antibiotics such as nitrofurantoin, and other drugs, such as amiodarone, cause interstitial pulmonary pneumonitis or fibrosis. Occupational irritants, such as asbestos and silica, damage the lung and produce ILD when inhaled over long periods. Inhalation of bird droppings (bird breeder's lung), iron dust (siderosis), moldy sugar cane (bagassosis), coal dust (coal worker's disease, or black lung), germinating barley (malt worker's lung), or moldy straw (farmer's lung) also cause interstitial lung disease. The term *pneumoconiosis* is used to describe the chronic interstitial lung diseases that result from long-term exposure to dusts. Pneumoconiosis usually develops 20 or more years after substantial exposure to the irritant.

Pathophysiology

The pathophysiology of IIP is unknown, although the patient develops interstitial infiltrates of mononuclear and polymorphonuclear cells with or without eosinophils and plasma cells. Interstitial fibrosis develops. Some small airways are compressed, and other airways are obliterated or develop tortuosity. When airways are alternately compressed or stretched by the fibrosis, honeycombing appears.

The size of inhaled particles is important in the development of some forms of interstitial fibrosis. Particle size in asbestos varies from 5 to 200 μm, and in silicosis and coal dust the particles range from 1 to 2 μm. The smaller particles are inhaled into the lower airways, where alveolar macrophages engulf the fibers. Lysis of the macrophages results in hyaline membrane formation and fibrosis.

Other characteristics of the particles are also important in pathophysiology and diagnosis. Asbestos fibers are rod-shaped with clubbed ends. They are yellow to brown in color and may be coated or free. Ferritin (ferruginous bodies) is contained in the coat and seen on lung resection. Asbestosis involves the lung parenchyma and/or the pleura. When the pleura is involved, an exudative pleural effusion or calcified pleural plaques develop. Development of asbestosis carries an increased risk for malignant mesothelioma and bronchogenic lung cancer, and tuberculosis and hemoptysis can occur with silicosis.

Nursing management

Assessment. Assessment of the patient with ILD begins with accurate history taking in an attempt to identify the irritant. Because development of ILD occurs 20 or more years after exposure, obtaining an accurate history is often difficult. In general the patient with ILD is not in acute distress until very late in the course of the disease. The first signs of disease are insidious. Dyspnea on exertion and easy fatigue are the most common presenting symptoms. In some cases the patient attributes the changes to "just getting older." Dry, hacking cough and chest pain are also sometimes present. As the disease progresses, dyspnea occurs at lower levels of exertion and ultimately at rest. Weight loss is frequent.

On inspection the nurse observes accessory muscle use as work of breathing increases. Respiratory rate is frequently more shallow and rapid than normal, especially in later stages. In most patients clubbing and cyanosis are late signs. Palpation and percussion are usually unremarkable. Auscultation of the lungs is normal at first but then demonstrates late inspiratory crackles, especially at the bases.

PFTs are normal for many years, especially with pneumoconiosis. Over time all lung volumes decrease, consistent with a restrictive pattern. Expiratory flow rates remain normal unless concomitant obstruction is present. Compliance measurements are reduced; this is consistent with stiff lungs. Also reduced is the diffusing capacity of the lungs for carbon monoxide (D_{LCO}).

ABG values follow the pattern of the PFTs. In the early stages ABG values are normal. With progression of the disease exertion-induced arterial hypoxemia develops. In the later stages hypoxemia is present at rest. Hypercapnia is seen in some patients with advanced disease.

The chest x-ray film of the patient with ILD varies with the cause. In idiopathic interstitial pneumonitis, generalized interstitial fibrosis with diffuse reticulonodular infiltrates or honeycombing is common. Pleural or diaphragmatic plaques and interstitial fibrosis beginning at the base of the lungs are commonly present with asbestosis. As asbestosis advances, the pleural plaques are seen in upper lung fields. In silicosis, multiple rounded bilateral nodules and calcified lymph nodes are found. The nodules in silicosis have an upper lobe predominance. In selected patients, evidence of congestive heart failure or pulmonary hypertension are noted.

Nursing diagnoses. The main problem in ILD is hypoxemia. Selected patients may also smoke cigarettes and be at increased risk for lung cancer and more hypoxemia. Uncertainty about the disease, its cause, and its treatment are common in patients with ILD.

The most important nursing diagnoses are impaired gas exchange and knowledge deficit, both related to the primary disease. Because of hypoxemia, exercise tolerance and mobility are reduced. Dyspnea affects a patient's comfort. Particular patients may also require a nursing diagnosis directed toward effective coping or grieving.

Interventions. The primary focus of nursing care is to promote adequate gas exchange for activities of daily living. The patient should also have basic knowledge about the pathophysiology, progression, and treatment of the particular lung disease. When the patient is in the diagnosis phase, knowledge about the testing procedures is essential for informed consent and cooperation.

Diagnosis of ILD involves multiple tests. ABG samples, PFTs, blood tests, sputum analysis, nuclear medicine or CT scans of the chest, and bronchoscopy are among the diagnostic tools of the physician. The nurse coordinates scheduling of the various tests and prepares the patient for each test. For instance the patient cannot eat or drink for 4 or more hours before a bronchoscopy and should receive inhaled bronchodilators. However, the patient undergoing PFTs can eat a light meal and can drink but should not receive inhaled bronchodilators for at least 6 hours before the test. The patient could potentially have both tests in the same day if the PFT were performed early in the morning after the patient had a light breakfast and the bronchoscopy were performed in the afternoon (no lunch for the patient).

For ILD there is no specific treatment other than limiting exposure; there is no cure. Bronchodilators are useful in patients with ILD who have hyperreactive airways. Corticosteroids or other immunosuppressive agents are used to treat some types of ILDs. Patients, especially those with asbestos exposure, should stop smoking because of the increased risk of lung cancer. When hypoxemia occurs, supplemental O_2 is initiated.

TUMORS
Etiology

Cigarette smoking, occupation, and heredity are three important factors that contribute to the development of primary malignant tumors, that is, lung cancer. Cigarettes contain more than 2000 chemicals, some of which are known carcinogens in animals. The incidence of lung cancer is at least 10 times higher in cigarette smokers and 2 times higher in cigar and pipe smokers than in nonsmokers. Factors important in the development of lung cancer from smoking include the number of cigarettes smoked daily (more is worse), the number of years as a smoker (longer is associated with greater damage), the use of nonfiltered versus filtered cigarettes (more particles are inhaled with nonfiltered cigarettes), and the depth of inhalation (shallow inhalation damages mainly the upper airway, but deeper inhalation also injures the lower airway).

The risk of lung cancer is also increased with some occupations, including metallurgy, mining, pharmaceutical and soap production, and manufacture of paints, synthetic rubber, and inorganic pigments. Excessive exposure to radiation increases the risk of lung cancer. Air pollution in urban areas is associated with a slightly increased incidence of lung cancer.

Some studies suggest increased incidence of cancer in families, especially those who have other risk factors. Heredity and environment are factors. Passive, or side-stream, smoke is dangerous to the nonsmoker. Family members of a smoker may develop cancer from passive smoke, inhalation of which is potentially more dangerous than actually smoking a cigarette.

There are three types of pulmonary neoplasms: benign tumors, primary malignant tumors, and metastatic malignant tumors. Less than 10% of lung tumors are benign. Lung tumors cause air-flow obstruction and may be confused with obstructive airways disease. Included in the category of benign tumors are bronchial adenomas, bronchial cystadenomas, bronchial carcinoid tumors, mucoepidermoid tumors, and pulmonary hamartomas.

Primary malignant tumors currently occur more frequently in men than women, presumably because of increased smoking in the male population. The incidence of lung cancer is unfortunately rising in women. In men the incidence of lung cancer is highest in the sixth decade of life; in women the diagnosis usually occurs in the seventh decade of life.

There are four main types of primary lung cancer: squamous cell or epidermoid carcinoma, adenocarcinoma, small (oat) cell carcinoma, and large cell carcinoma (Fig. 11-4). Squamous cell carcinomas account for 40% to 50% of all lung cancer. Small cell carcinomas represent about 25% to 35% of lung cancer cases, and adenocarcinoma is responsible for about 20%. About 10% of lung cancer cases are due to large cell carcinoma (Baum and Wolinsky, 1983).

Malignant tumors elsewhere in the body metastasize to the lung in about 30% to 40% of patients. Breast cancer is one that commonly metastasizes to the lung. Other common sites of primary tumors that metastasize to the lung are the pancreas, kidney, and colon.

Pathophysiology

The pathophysiology of the primary lung carcinoma varies with the cell type. Characteristics of each cell type are discussed below (see Fig. 11-6 for pictorial comparison).

Squamous cell carcinomas usually arise from altered segmental or subsegmental bronchial epithelium and are usually centrally located. In the early stages of growth the tumor appears as a red granular or white plaque. As the tumor grows it appears as a gray-white or yellow endobronchial lesion. Analysis of the cellular structure reveals intercellular bridges and keratin formation. Some squamous cell carcinomas cause cavitation. Squamous cell carcinomas grow slowly. They usually metastasize first to hilar and mediastinal lymph nodes, then to liver, adrenals, bones, and brain.

Adenocarcinoma usually arises in the periphery of the lungs from the submucosal glands. It forms poorly to well-developed glandular or acinar structures and usually produces mucin. Adenocarcinoma rarely cavitates. The tumor is usually described as a well-circumscribed, gray-white, subpleural mass. Although usually slow to moderate in growth, adenocarcinoma quickly invades lymph and blood systems to produce distant metastases.

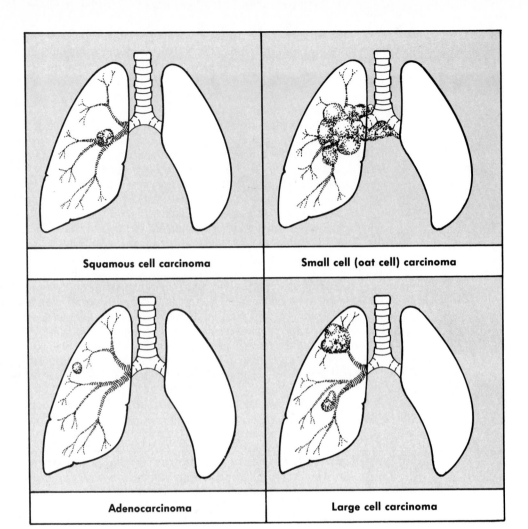

Fig. 11-4. Predominant sites and extension of primary lung cancer. (From McCance K, Huether S: *Pathophysiology: the biologic basis for disease in adults and children,* ed 1, St Louis, 1990, Mosby – Year Book.)

Small cell carcinomas develop proximally and are the most aggressive and rapidly growing of all lung carcinomas. They appear as large, gray-white, soft tumors. Small cell carcinomas are composed microscopically of neoplastic cells surrounded by dark, round to spindle-shaped nuclei. Cytoplasm is scanty. On biopsy the cells appear crushed. Small cell carcinoma rapidly metastasizes through lymphatic and blood systems to near and distant sites.

Large cell carcinomas are usually located in the periphery. The tumors form large necrotic masses that result in cavity formation. The nuclei and cytoplasm of large cell carcinomas are, as the name implies, quite large. Large cell carcinomas grow rapidly and metastasize early and throughout a widespread area.

Nursing management

Assessment. The assessment of the patient with lung cancer begins with diagnosis and staging. Unfortunately for most patients, discovery of the lung mass usually occurs late in the course of the disease. In a few patients the diagnosis of lung cancer is initiated by an abnormal finding on a routine chest x-ray film. Most patients come to the physician with complaints of dyspnea, cough, chest pain, or weight loss. In some instances the patient may experience an episode of hemoptysis with the cough. Clubbing is not a frequent initial symptom of lung cancer, but it is often observed in later stages. In others obstructive pneumonia is the presenting symptom. When obstructive pneumonia occurs, the patient usually also has fever, chills, night sweats, purulent sputum, and wheezing. Nonspecific signs of lung cancer include hypercalcemia, nausea, vomiting, weakness, dysphagia (esophageal involvement), upper body edema and redness (obstruction of superior vena cava), rib pain (metastases), hoarseness (recurrent laryngeal nerve affected), and headache (brain metastases).

Assessment of the chest may reveal the presence of a pleural effusion. However, in most cases chest assessment is unrevealing. Localized wheezing signals localized airway obstruction that may be caused by tumor. The wheezing is more pronounced with forced exhalation. A paralyzed diaphragm is noted when the phrenic nerve is involved.

The first step in diagnosing lung cancer after seeing a mass on a chest x-ray film is obtaining tissue for study. However, some physicians perform additional radiographical studies, such as polytomes or CT scans. The purpose of early CT scanning is to more accurately position the tumor in preparation for procedures and to identify presence of enlarged lymph nodes and metastases.

When pleural effusions are present, thoracentesis is performed first. This procedure removes fluid, which allows the lung to expand fully so that anatomy and extent of disease are more easily assessed radiographically and bronchoscopically. Thoracentesis fluid is studied in the laboratory. The pleural fluid is sent for cytological examination and other laboratory studies, including those to differentiate transudative from exudative pleural effusions. A biopsy is performed on accessible lymph nodes, such as supraclavicular or axillary nodes, when available.

All patients with a suspected diagnosis of lung cancer undergo bronchoscopy with endobronchial or transbronchial biopsy, Wang needle aspiration at the carina, bronchoalveolar lavage, and brushings of the bronchial mucosa. The purpose of bronchoscopy is to identify lung anatomy, presence of endobronchial lesions, and extrinsic compression of airways. Specimens from the bronchoscopy are sent for diagnosis. With a peripheral tumor close to the chest wall a closed-chest fine-needle biopsy (directed by ultrasound, fluoroscopy, or CT scan) is done to obtain a tissue sample for diagnosis. If these techniques do not yield a diagnosis, the patient may undergo mediastinoscopy, or open-lung biopsy. In some instances diagnosis is made at the time of thoracotomy.

Staging of the tumor proceeds after diagnosis. Treatment (discussed later) is based on staging. The tumor, node, metastases (TNM) classification and staging of lung cancer is shown in Table 11-3. T refers to primary tumor, N refers to regional lymph nodes, and M refers to distant metastases. A chest x-ray film and bronchoscopical examination usually aid in providing the T

Table 11-3. TNM classification and staging of lung cancer

Designation	Parameters			
Tumor				
T_X	Tumor cells present in cytology, but not visualized by x-ray film or bronchoscopy			
T_{IS}	Carcinoma in situ			
T_0	No evidence of primary tumor			
	Diameter	Distance from carina	Extension into extrapulmonary structures	Pleural invasion
T_1	<3 cm	Lobar bronchus	Absent	Absent
T_2	>3 cm	>2 cm	Absent	Present
T_3	Any size	<2 cm	Present	Present
T_4	Any size	Involves carina	Present	Present
Regional lymph nodes	Peribronchial or hilar		Mediastinal or subcarinal	
N_0	Absent		Absent	
N_1	Present (ipsilateral)		Absent	
N_2	Present (ipsilateral)		Present (ipsilateral)	
N_3	Present (contralateral)		Present (contralateral)	
Distant metastases				
M_0	Absent			
M_1	Present			

designation, and CT scanning or radionuclide scanning are often necessary for determining N and M.

PFTs are necessary to identify lung function if a patient is a surgical candidate, based on TNM classification. Depending on the condition and wishes of the patient, results of the PFTs, and sometimes results of ventilation-perfusion studies, the surgeon determines how much lung the patient can afford to have resected. In general the surgeon needs to resect affected lung but leave the patient a minimum FEV_1 of 1 L.

Nursing diagnoses. With the suspected diagnosis of lung cancer comes fear of many unknowns. Early unknowns concern the testing procedures. The ultimate unknown is whether the cancer is curable. Therefore, during diagnosis, the main nursing problems are keeping the patient educated and providing emotional support. As the disease and treatment progress, other problems include maintaining comfort, nutritional status, activity level, and airway patency (the latter to prevent infection and promote gas exchange).

The nursing diagnoses for the patient with a lung tumor vary with the stage of cancer and the patient. Nursing diagnoses in the diagnosis stage may be similar or different from those in the treatment stage. Knowledge deficit related to tests, procedures, and therapies is perhaps the most general and the most-used diagnosis when caring for a patient with lung cancer. Activity intolerance, alteration in nutrition, or alteration in bowel elimination related to the effects of chemotherapy are used in patients undergoing chemotherapy. Ineffective airway clearance related to a tumor obstructing the airway is useful in patients with obstructive pneumonia. Anxiety related to diagnosis or fear of death is a common nursing diagnosis for patients with lung cancer and their families. Similarly, alteration in comfort or pain related to metastases, surgical procedures, or chemotherapy should also be considered in patients with lung cancer.

Interventions. Many general interventions focus on increasing the patient's

Table 11-4. Staging and prognosis of TNM lung cancer

Stage	T	N	M	5-year survival rate*
Occult cancer	T_X	N_0	M_0	
0	T_{IS}	N_0	M_0	
I	T_{1-2}	N_0	M_0	45%-50%
II	T_{1-2}	N_1	M_0	25%-30%
IIIa	T_3	N_{0-1}	M_0	15%-20%
	T_{1-3}	N_2		
IIIb	T_{1-4}	N_3	M_0	5%
	T_4	N_{0-3}		
IV	T_{1-4}	N_{0-3}	M_1	2%

* From Mitchell, Petty, Schwartz: Synopsis of clinical diseases, ed 4, 1989, Mosby–Year Book. Data are based on clinical staging, which typically underestimates the extent of disease; survival based on surgical staging is better.

knowledge about the diagnosis and the treatment of lung cancer. Specific interventions focus on increasing caloric intake to approximately 2500 calories or more per day because metabolic needs are increased and appetite is usually decreased; controlling nausea, vomiting, and diarrhea in patients with altered bowel function; maintaining muscle strength in patients with activity intolerance; clearing retained secretions to prevent infection and promote gas exchange; and helping the patient verbalize fears and anxieties. Controlling pain without impairing the patient's cognitive or motor function is important in the care of patients with terminal lung cancer or metastases.

The treatment of lung cancer depends on staging and type of lung cancer. In general, unless the tumor is very small without metastasis or nodes when discovered, it is often not curable. In noncurable lung cancer, the 5-year survival rate is 2% to 20%, depending on stage (see Table 11-4). In general 33% of patients with localized disease and 13% of all lung cancer patients survive 5 years after diagnosis (American Cancer Society, 1988).

Surgery is considered the ultimate cure for lung cancer. Patients with T_1 or T_2, N_0 or N_1, that is, Stage I or Stage II disease, usually have operable cancer, and patients with T_3, N_2, and M_1, that is, Stage III or Stage IV disease, are generally not resectable. Patients who are not candidates for operative intervention include those with small cell carcinoma; distant metastasis; vena caval obstruction; carinal, tracheal, mediastinal, vocal cord, or esophageal involvement; and malignant pleural effusion. Presence of nodes may exclude surgery, depending on number, character, and location. Surgery is attempted when the patient meets established criteria. A segment (wedge), lobe (lobectomy), or entire lung (pneumonectomy) are removed. The surgeon removes the smallest portion of lung, leaving the margins free from tumor.

Chemotherapy protocols are ineffective for most types of lung cancer. Chemotherapy is the treatment of choice for small cell carcinoma. Chemotherapy is often combined with radiation. Palliative or nondurable comfort-enhancing interventions for lung cancer are radiation applied externally or endobronchially (brachytherapy). Laser therapy is useful in decreasing the size of obstructing endobronchial tumors. Some protocols institute immunotherapy as an adjunct. In patients with reaccumulating pleural effusions, serial thoracentesis or chest tube insertion with pleurodesis is instituted.

Specific nursing care of the patient with lung cancer involves education and physical care through all phases. When therapeutic surgery is performed, the patient usually has fluid and air draining from chest tubes for several days. The exception is the pneumonectomy patient, who may have no chest tubes, allowing fluid in the empty chest cavity to consolidate. Throughout radiation and chemotherapy sessions the nurse educates the patient and family about techniques to improve the quality of life. These interventions are directed at improving caloric intake, preventing skin breakdown, preventing or treating oral yeast infections, and caring for central venous catheters.

Lung cancer greatly affects the quality of life. Patients undergo major lifestyle changes, including physical side effects of cancer and treatments, role changes with spouse and other family members, and psychological readjustment to a chronic disease that frequently results in death. Emotional support by physicians, nurses, support groups, and significant others is critical to patients and their families. Patients benefit from psychosocial interventions directed at aiding acceptance of the diagnosis of cancer and the prognosis. The nurse offers hope when appropriate but is realistic in her comments to patients and does not offer false hope. Visiting nurses, physician's office nurses, and hospital nurses develop rapport with the patient and family. They assist the family through the stages of death and dying. In the terminal stages of cancer, hospice nurses are integral in providing support for the patient and the family. They continue to provide support to the family after the patient has died.

SARCOIDOSIS
Etiology

Sarcoidosis is the most common multisystem noninfectious granulomatous disease. The etiology is unknown. The noncaseating granuloma develops in any organ although the lungs, eyes, kidney, skin, lymph nodes, liver, and spleen are the most affected. In the United States, blacks are affected 12 to 15 times more frequently than whites. Women are affected more often than men. The incidence of sarcoidosis peaks between the ages of 20 and 40.

Pathophysiology

The lesion in sarcoidosis is a noncaseating granuloma that usually measures 3 to 4 cm in diameter. *Noncaseating* means that the lesion does not form necrotic tissue that develops into a granular amorphous mass. Microscopical examination of the cells shows clusters of epithelioid cells with giant cells and lymphocytic infiltration. In the lungs, focal or diffuse interstitial fibrosis or inflammation of the alveolar septa is noted on biopsy. These conditions restrict alveolar expansion. Sarcoidosis is also associated with abnormal humoral and cellular hypersensitivity responses.

Nursing management

Assessment. In the early stages the patient is typically in no acute distress, except for dyspnea on exertion. As the disease progresses, other symptoms appear. The patient usually comes to the physician because of one or more symptoms, including arthralgia, fatigue and malaise, weakness, weight loss, low-grade fever, nonproductive cough, or cough with minimal sputum production, hemoptysis, and dyspnea. Chest pain is possible but fairly uncommon and is usually located substernally in the area of the hilar nodes. Club-

Table 11-5. Staging for sarcoidosis

Stage 0	Normal chest x-ray film with positive tissue biopsy
Stage I	Bilateral hilar adenopathy
Stage II	Bilateral hilar adenopathy with infiltrates
Stage III	Normal hilar lymph nodes with infiltrates and positive tissue biopsy
Stage IV	Parenchymal destruction including blebs

bing is usually not seen in sarcoidosis. Depending on the other organs involved, there may be splenomegaly, hypercalcemia, hypercalcuria, elevated liver enzymes, elevated angiotensin-converting enzyme level, and increased immunoglobulin A, G, and E. The physician may perform a Kveim test (intradermal injection of a minute amount of ground sarcoid tissue suspended in saline) to confirm diagnosis of sarcoidosis.

Assessment of the chest is generally unremarkable and provides few clues to the problem. Some patients with endobronchial sarcoidosis wheeze. Occasionally, crackles are heard in patients with extensive pulmonary involvement.

PFTs demonstrate a typical restrictive pattern with decreased volumes. D_{LCO} and lung compliance are reduced.

The chest x-ray is often the most useful examination because bilateral hilar adenopathy and right paratracheal adenopathy are frequently present. Pulmonary interstitial or alveolar infiltrates are usually bilateral and spare both the bases and the apices. In some cases, evidence of pulmonary fibrosis is seen on the chest x-ray film. With long-term sarcoidosis, bullae and thick-walled cysts form in the lung. Patients also develop pulmonary hypertension and cor pulmonale secondary to pulmonary fibrosis. Staging for sarcoidosis is based on findings in chest x-ray films and is shown in Table 11-5.

The diagnosis of sarcoidosis is made by skin biopsy (when lesions are present) or by bronchoscopy. At bronchoscopy both transbronchial biopsy and bronchoalveolar lavage are performed. The biopsy shows noncaseating granuloma with giant cells and lymphocytic infiltrates. There is also fibrosis and inflammation of the alveolar walls. A high lymphocyte/polymorphonuclear granulocyte ratio in bronchoalveolar lavage fluid suggests active granuloma formation. Serial bronchoalveolar lavages are used to follow course of disease and treatment. Some physicians use gallium scintigraphy to assess active disease and response to therapy.

Nursing diagnoses. The disease, sarcoidosis, is not one generally known (like pneumonia) by the patient. Therefore he not only does not know what it is but also does not know what its treatments and complications are. The patient and family members have a knowledge deficit. The main problem in sarcoidosis is development of complications from the disease or treatments. These problems include muscle wasting from inactivity, weight loss, complications of steroid use, and pulmonary hypertension.

The main nursing diagnoses for the patient with sarcoidosis are impaired gas exchange and knowledge deficit related to disease process. Because of impaired gas exchange, the patient often has activity intolerance and fatigue. In some patients, mobility is altered.

Interventions. The main focus of therapy is to improve gas exchange by halting the progression of the disease. By improving gas exchange, the patient's fatigue level decreases and activity level increases. In addition the patient must have some understanding of the disease and its treatments, especially the potential complications of steroids.

The majority of patients with sarcoidosis require frequent follow-up but no treatment. When needed, the primary treatment for pulmonary sarcoidosis is corticosteroids, especially for Stage II or III disease. Treatment does not usually begin until the patient is symptomatic. Once begun, steroids are usually continued for at least 6 to 12 months. Some symptomatic patients require longer use of steroids, often for several years. With prolonged steroid use comes complications, including osteoporosis, vision disturbances, cataracts, diabetes, peptic ulcers, fluid and electrolyte imbalances, psychoses, increased appetite, capillary fragility, and immunosuppression (impaired ability of the immune system to recognize and fight infections). Many physicians also prophylactically administer isoniazid (a drug used to treat tuberculosis) to patients receiving prolonged steroid therapy because patients with sarcoidosis are anergic. Educating the patient about the complications of steroids is important. Some patients with hypoxemia require supplemental O_2.

TUBERCULOSIS
Etiology

Tuberculosis (TB) is a fungal airborne disease that primarily manifests in the lung although other organs may also be involved. Unlike sarcoidosis, TB is a disease of caseating granuloma, meaning there is necrotic tissue. The kidney, skeletal system, and central nervous system are frequent additional sites of infection.

Typical TB, an infectious disease caused by *Mycobacterium tuberculosis*, was formerly known as consumption. Atypical pulmonary cases of TB are caused by bacteria such as *M. kansasii, M. simiae, M. szulgai, M. intracellulare-avium, M. xenopi, and M. fortuitum*. A worldwide health problem with no age or sex preference, TB was declining in the United States until very recently, when a slight increase occurred in some states. Two areas of increase are among immigrants and patients with acquired immunodeficiency syndrome (AIDS). Areas of limited access to health care, including low socioeconomic neighborhoods, tend to be exposed to TB and infected with it more often. Migrant workers on the southwest border of the United States, American Indians, and Eskimos are among those affected. Some people think of TB as a disease of the poor, but this is untrue; TB also infects individuals in wealthy neighborhoods.

Although a single exposure can cause TB, repeated exposure is usually necessary. People living in the home of an infected individual are at greatest risk for contracting TB. Risk factors for contracting or reactivating TB include malnutrition; alcoholism; immunosuppression, including AIDS; gastrectomy or jejunoileal bypass surgery; postpartum period; diabetes; residence in a prison or nursing home; and renal dialysis.

Pathophysiology

The initial port of entry for the tubercle bacillus is the lung. When actively infected (cavitary tuberculosis) individuals talk, cough, or sneeze, they spray very small particles (1 to 5 μm). The infected individuals may not feel sick or know that they have TB. Only airborne tubercles have the potential to cause infection when they are unsuspectingly inhaled by others. These particles are small enough to deposit in the terminal bronchioles. Some of these particles are cleared by macrophage ingestion. Larger particles are deposited on mucus-laden cilia for transport out of the lung or remain airborne in the lung. The particles that land on inanimate objects, such as tables or clothing, are not involved in the spread of TB. They die from drying, heat, or ultraviolet light. Therefore hand washing is very effective at removing tubercle bacteria.

The tubercle usually lodges in the apices, where, unnoticed, it begins growing. In most cases there is dilation of the capillaries, swelling of endothelial and alveolar lining cells, and an increase in fibrin, macrophages, and polymorphonuclear leukocytes into the alveoli (exudative phase). In effect an undetected localized pneumonia develops as the tubercles grow. Caseation (necrosis of the center of the lesion) occurs, and healing begins as a result of invasion by fibroblasts. There is progressive hyaline membrane formation and calcification. Drainage to regional and hilar lymph nodes causes adenopathy, also usually undetected. From the lymph nodes systemic transmission may occur. Within 6 weeks of infection, most individuals develop cellular immunity to the tubercle, which is demonstrated as a positive skin test. The infection is controlled without the individual's knowledge.

The tubercle may remain in the lung as a calcified granuloma (Ghon lesion) or calcified hilar lymph nodes (Ranke complexes), or it may caseate with tissue necrosis. In most individuals the initial infection is walled off and does not progress to active tuberculosis. Months to years after initial infection, TB can reactivate. Those patients most prone to TB reactivation include elderly persons, alcoholics, and diabetics. Other patients at risk for reactivation tuberculosis are those with malignant tumors, silicosis, prolonged corticosteroid use, and recent gastrectomy (within 3 to 4 years).

Nursing management

Assessment. A skin test for TB, using purified protein derivative (PPD), is routinely performed in 1-year-old infants and before enrollment in the first, fifth, and ninth grades. In individuals suspected of exposure to TB, an intradermal PPD skin test is administered 6 weeks and 3 months later. The skin test may convert to positive between 2 and 10 weeks after exposure. The TB skin test tells whether the individual has developed antibodies to the tubercle bacillus, but it does not indicate whether the infection is active or quiescent. A positive test means that the individual has been exposed to tuberculosis and has mounted a cellular response to the bacteria. It does not necessarily mean that the patient has active infection. However, a positive test is seen in most patients with active TB.

The intradermal Mantoux test applies five tuberculin units of PPD under the skin to determine cell-mediated immunity to the tubercle bacillus. A Mantoux skin test is positive, according to the American Thoracic Society, if there is a 10 mm or greater area of induration and erythema at the site when observed at 24, 48, or 72 hours after administration. There must be edema; erythema alone is not a positive skin test. An easy way to determine the area of induration is to draw a line toward it with a felt-tip or ball-point pen. The pen deviates at the point of induration. Areas of induration and erythema 4 mm or less are negative. Between 5 and 9 mm the test is indeterminate, except in housemates of infected individuals. In the latter the test is considered positive.

When tests are indeterminate, a second dose of PPD is applied within 7 days to determine booster effect. This is particularly helpful in elderly patients and other patients who may have a waning or lack of reactivity with time. A reaction of 10 mm or more or a 6 mm increase in the size of induration and erythema indicates a positive test. Even with the second dose, anergic-infected individuals and noninfected individuals have a negative skin test response.

A negative skin test does not necessarily mean that the patient does not have TB. Some patients, especially elderly and immunocompromised patients, have altered cellular immunity. It is essential at the time of PPD skin testing to determine anergic status of the patient. For this reason skin test controls are commonly used. In most areas, *Candida* and/or mumps skin tests are used as controls for the PPD (some areas may apply histoplasmosis skin testing controls). If the control demonstrates a positive response (erythema and induration) and the PPD is negative, the likelihood of the patient having TB is minimal unless exposure was very recent. The PPD is repeated in 3 months. If the controls are negative, the patient is said to be anergic. Further testing is necessary to confirm or deny the diagnosis of TB.

In patients suspected of having TB, sputum is obtained for histological examination (caseating granuloma), smear, and culture. The best time to obtain sputum is early morning immediately after the patient awakens, when bacteria counts are presumably highest. Aerosols with hypertonic saline or a bronchodilator are helpful in obtaining sputum. Sputum specimens are initially stained by Ziehl-Neelsen or fluorescent techniques or both. Acid-fast bacilli are not observed all the time, and not all acid-fast bacilli are *M. tuberculosis*. Therefore the sputum specimen is also cultured on special media. The tubercle bacillus grows very slowly and may take 6 to 8 weeks to appear. Identification of the bacteria is essential to proper treatment, which starts as soon as a culture is obtained and before the results are available.

In patients with nonproductive coughs analysis of early-morning gastric fluid may reveal the presence of acid-fast bacilli, although its use is diminishing. Bronchoscopy with brushings, transbronchial biopsies, and washings replaces the use of gastric lavage. In some cases fine-needle aspiration of lung tissue yields specimens for culture.

The chest x-ray film in TB frequently reveals infiltrates in the upper lobes, usually in the apical and posterior segments. Alternately, the superior segments of the lower lobes may contain the fluffy or fibronodular infiltrates. Cavities are sometimes seen on the chest x-ray film; they rarely have fluid levels. Apical scarring, fibrosis, or volume loss are changes characteristic of a TB infection.

ABG values are usually normal with TB infections, but PFTs sometimes are abnormal. However, with extensive alveolar involvement hypoxemia develops from ventilation-perfusion mismatching.

The PFT shows a restrictive pattern when there is fibrosis of lung parenchyma; otherwise the PFT is normal. There is a decrease in VC, TLC, and other lung volumes. Some patients, especially those with endobronchial involvement, demonstrate an obstructive pattern in addition to restriction. The FEV_1 and FEV_1/FVC ratio are decreased with obstruction (see Chapter 8).

Other assessment findings in the patient with TB are nonspecific. They include anorexia, chest pain, cough, fatigue, flulike symptoms, hemoptysis, indigestion, low-grade fever (especially in the afternoon), malaise, myalgia, night sweats, and weight loss. Some patients develop inappropriate antidiuretic hormone secretion (low sodium) or hypercalcemia. Unilateral or bilateral pleural effusions may occur. Analysis of pleural fluid reveals a predominantly lymphocytic exudative pleural effusion. Patients with pericardial tuberculosis often present with symptoms of pericardial tamponade or constrictive pericarditis. Calcifications in the pericardium suggest pericardial TB. When TB invades the central nervous system, meningitis with changes in mental status occurs. TB meningitis is more common in the very young patient. Some patients complain of (or their parents notice) a headache, confusion, and lethargy. Cerebrospinal fluid analysis shows lymphocyte predominance, low glucose level, and elevated protein level.

Examination of the chest does not usually correlate with findings on the chest x-ray film. Percussion demonstrates slight dullness or flatness, but auscultation reveals crackles. Bronchial breath sounds may be heard.

Nursing diagnoses. The main nursing problems are spread of TB and lack of knowledge about the disease and its treatment. Because treatment for TB often spans several months to a year or more, noncompliance may be a problem. Also, anti-TB medications commonly cause nausea and other side effects, which can contribute to poor eating habits and malnutrition.

Therefore common nursing diagnoses include infection or potential for infection related to TB or risk of transmitting TB to other persons; knowledge deficit related to the disease, its transmission, and treatment (side effects of drugs); and noncompliance related to prolonged medication administration and its side effects. In patients with weight loss, less than body requirements of nutrition related to nausea is an appropriate nursing diagnosis.

Interventions. Interventions are necessary to prevent the spread of TB, to improve the patient and caregivers' knowledge about the disease and its treatments, and to improve patient compliance in medication administration. The nurse also strives to maintain normal patient weight or to aid the underweight patient to gain weight.

Treatment for TB has changed drastically over the past several decades. Before the development of chemotherapeutic agents, patients with TB were treated in hospitals or sanitariums for months or years. Now they are treated at home, and most are allowed to return to work a few days after chemotherapy is initiated.

In patients who have converted their PPD from negative to positive, 1 year of isoniazid (INH) is prescribed unless it is contraindicated. Care and additional monitoring are needed in administering INH to patients over the age of 35 because of the increased risk for hepatitis.

The treatment for smear-positive or culture-positive TB involves the use of two or more antituberculous medications, which are summarized in Table 11-6. The basis for multiple drug therapy was devised several decades ago by Canetti (1965). He calculated the bacterial populations in cavitary (10^7 to 10^8 organisms) and "hard caseous" foci (10^2 to 10^3 organisms). Resistance of tuberculous bacteria to single-drug therapy occurs in 10^5 to 10^6 organisms. In cavitary TB, 10^3 organisms may be resistant to one drug. According to Canetti's theory, resistance to two or more drugs requires more bacteria than are usually present.

The duration of TB treatment has varied over the years. Extended therapy, that is, 18 to 24 months of multiple drugs, has produced relapse rates of 2% or less. In the past the most common TB prescriptions for extended therapy used INH and ethambutol. Most physicians added a third drug (pyrazinamide or streptomycin) for the first 6 to 8 weeks to decrease the chance of

Table 11-6. Antituberculous drugs

Drug	Adult dosage	Route	Adverse reactions
Primary			
Isoniazid (INH) (bacterio-cidal)	300 mg qd	PO	Anemia, hepatitis, hypersensi-tivity, peripheral neuritis, seizures, systemic lupus erythematosus
Rifampin (RFP) (bacterio-cidal)	600 mg qd	PO	Decreased effectiveness of oral contraceptive, hemolysis, hepatic toxicity, increased metabolism of hepatically excreted drugs, induction of methadone withdrawal, re-nal failure, thrombocytope-nia
Secondary			
Ethambutol (EMB) (bacterio-static)	15-25 mg/kg qd	PO	Reversible optic neuritis
Paraamino salicylic acid (PAS) (bacteriostatic)	12-15 g qd	PO	Gastrointestinal upset, hepati-tis, hypersensitivity rash, interferes with absorption of RFP (separate doses by 4+ hours)
Pyrazinamide (PZA) (bacterio-cidal with streptomycin)	20-35 mg/kg up to 3 g qd	PO	Anorexia, arthralgia, gout (rare), hepatitis, hyperurice-mia, nausea, renal failure (rare), vomiting
Streptomycin (bacteriocidal with PZA)*	0.75-1 g qd	IM	Eighth cranial nerve damage, paresthesias, renal toxicity (rare), tinnitus, vertigo
Tertiary			
Capreomycin (bacteriostatic)*	1 g (2-3 times a week)	IM	Hepatotoxicity, hypersensitiv-ity, hypokalemia, ototoxic-ity, renal toxicity, vestibular toxicity
Cycloserine (bacteriostatic)	0.75 g qd-tid	PO	Personality changes, psycho-sis, rash, seizures
Ethionamide (bacteriocidal)	0.5-1 g qd-tid	PO	Depression, gastrointestinal upset, hepatitis, peripheral neuropathy, rash
Kanamycin (bacteriostatic)*	0.5-1 g qd	IM	Same as streptomycin with greater renal toxicity

*aminoglycoside.

drug resistance and to prevent having only one effective drug if drug resistance occurs. With newer drugs the treatment interval is lessened. The current recommendation by the American Thoracic Society (1983) is 9 months of therapy with both isoniazid and rifampin in noncomplicated cases of TB. Inability to use either drug increases the treatment interval to 18 months. When resistance is suspected (as in patients who have received previous treatment), three or more drugs are used until bacterial sensitivities are available. Intermittent treatment programs have also been studied. These intermittent programs are used when compliance is a problem, and they involve administration of higher drug doses given under direct supervision of health care personnel. Initial dosing is daily for up to 4 months followed by therapy twice a week for up to 24 months.

Patients become noninfectious very rapidly. Within 2 weeks the number of acid-fast bacilli on smears is markedly reduced. Smears and cultures become negative after 2 months of treatment in half the patients. After 4 months of treatment, 75% of patients have negative smears and cultures. Only 5% of patients have positive cultures after 6 months of treatment.

The best method of prevention is containing spread of aerosolized bacteria. When a patient has active TB and is contagious, it is important to contain aerosolized bacteria. Hospitalized contagious patients need to wear masks when out of the room or when other persons enter the room to prevent contamination. The patient must be alert and must be able to effectively clear his airway. If the patient is unable to contain his own secretions, hospital personnel must wear masks. If O_2 is used (as for severe, advanced cases), the patient does not wear a mask. In the home, masks are occasionally used for a few days to protect noninfected members and visitors. Nurses wear masks when unable to avoid face-to-face contact with the infected patient. Soiled tissues are promptly disposed of in a wastebasket or closed paper bag.

Respiratory isolation is only indicated for actively infected patients who are unable to contain their secretions and for patients who are in the diagnosis period. Ideally, air from the patient's room does not recirculate within the hospital. Rooms with one-way air conditioning or laminar-flow rooms effectively isolate contaminated air. Because TB bacteria die when in contact with ultraviolet light, these lights are sometimes used to kill TB bacteria in areas where exposure occurs unknowingly, such as emergency rooms. Ultraviolet lights are also used in rooms without adequate ventilation.

One of the main problems in achieving adequate control of TB is ensuring adequate drug levels for an extended period. Lack of compliance with long-term therapy is a problem. The medication must be taken every day. Patients at risk for taking medication improperly are homeless, mentally incompetent, alcoholic, and confused elderly persons. Supervised intermittent therapy in a home, shelter, or clinic is beneficial for these patients.

Noncompliance is also a problem when patients experience adverse reactions to one or more of the drugs. The patient is essential in identifying problems. Patients are taught to recognize early symptoms of adverse drug reactions, especially hepatic injury. Nausea and vomiting are two signs of acute hepatitis. Liver function tests are assessed regularly to help prevent hepatic injury. Educating the patient about transmission of the disease and the need for prolonged therapy aids in achieving patient compliance.

CONCLUSION

A variety of restrictive lung diseases limit expansion of the lungs by impairing chest wall movement, encasing the lung, or invading the alveolar space. Multiple nursing problems are seen in patients with restrictive lung diseases. Many of the problems are similar to those seen in patients with obstructive lung diseases. The most common problems are knowledge deficit, impaired gas exchange, comfort, dyspnea, impaired nutrition, ineffective breathing patterns, and anxiety. The nursing care for the patient with restrictive lung disease is a challenge. It encompasses caring for the patient and family through diagnosis, treatment, rehabilitation, and sometimes death. Close follow-up is required to assess the patient's health and response to treatment because many complications are possible. Teaching is very important in the care of patients with restrictive lung diseases. It helps to lessen anxiety and dyspnea and encourages cooperation and participation in the treatment plan.

BIBLIOGRAPHY

American Cancer society: *Cancer facts and figures: 1988,* New York, 1988, The Society.

American Thoracic Society: Diagnostic standards and classification of tuberculosis and other mycobacterial diseases, *Am Rev Respir Dis* 123:343-358, 1981.

American Thoracic Society: Treatment of tuberculosis and other mycobacterial diseases, *Am Rev Respir Dis* 127:790-796, 1983.

American Thoracic Society: Treatment of tuberculosis and tuberculosis infection in adults and children, *Am Rev Respir Dis* 134:355-363, 1986.

American Thoracic Society and Centers for Disease Control: Guidelines for short-course tuberculosis chemotherapy, *Am Rev Respir Dis* 121:611-614, 1980.

Baum GL, Wolinsky E: *Textbook of pulmonary diseases,* ed 3, Boston, 1983, Little, Brown.

Burki NK: *Pulmonary diseases: medical outline series,* Garden City, NY, 1982, Medical Examination Publishing.

Burton GC, Hodgkin JE: *Respiratory care: a guide to clinical practice,* ed 2, Philadelphia, 1984, JB Lippincott.

Canetti G: Present aspects of bacterial resistance in tuberculosis, *Am Rev Respir Dis* 92:687-703, 1965.

Canobbio M: Chest x-ray film interpretation, *Focus Crit Care* 11(2):18-24, 1984.

Chester EH, Fleming GM, Montenegro H: Effect of steroid therapy on gas exchange abnormalities in patients with diffuse lung disease, *Chest* 69(2suppl):269-271, 1976.

Cohen C, Zagelbaum G et al: Clinical manifestations of inspiratory muscle fatigue, *Am J Med* 73(3):308-316, 1982.

Costello HD, Caras GJ, Snider DE, Jr: Drug resistance among previously treated tuberculosis patients: a brief report, *Am Rev Respir Dis* 121:313-316, 1980.

Crystal R, Gadek J: Interstitial lung disease: current concepts of pathogenesis, staging and therapy, *Am J Med* 70:542-568, 1981.

Doll NJ, Stankus R, Barkman W: Immunopathogenesis of asbestosis, silicosis, and coal worker's pneumoconiosis, *Clin Chest Med* 4(1):3-14, 1983.

Felson B: The chest roentgenologic workup: what and why? Conventional methods, *Basics Respir Dis* 8(5):1-5, 1980.

Felson B: *Chest roentgenology,* Philadelphia, 1973, W B Saunders.

Felson B, Weinstein AS, Spitz HB: *Principles of chest roentgenology: a programmed text,* Philadelphia, 1965, W B Saunders.

Fishman A: *Pulmonary diseases and disorders,* New York, 1980, McGraw-Hill.

Fishman A: *Assessment of pulmonary function,* New York, 1980, McGraw-Hill.

Fraser R, Paré J: *Diagnosis of diseases of the chest,* vol 1-3, ed 2, Philadelphia, 1977-1979, W B Saunders.

Fulmer J: The interstitial lung diseases, *Chest* 82(2):172-178, 1982.

Glassroth J: Tuberculosis: a review for clinicians, *Clinical Notes on Respiratory Disease* 20(2):5-13, 1981.

Guenter C, Welch M: *Pulmonary medicine,* ed 2, Philadelphia, 1982, J B Lippincott.

Guyton AC: *Textbook of medical physiology,* ed 6, Philadelphia, 1981, W B Saunders.

Harper R: *A guide to respiratory care: physiology and clinical applications,* Philadelphia, 1982, J B Lippincott.

Haskell CM, ed: *Cancer treatment,* ed 2, Philadelphia, 1985, W B Saunders.

Hillerdal G, Nöu E et al: Sarcoidosis: epidemiology and prognosis, *Am Rev Respir Dis* 130(1):29-32, 1984.

Hinshaw H, Murray J: *Diseases of the chest,* ed 4, Philadelphia, 1980, W B Saunders.

Iannuzzi MC, Scoggin CH: Small cell lung cancer, *Am Rev Respir Dis* 134(3):593-608, 1986.

Israel HL, Atkinson GW: Sarcoidosis, *Basics Respir Dis* 7(1):1-6, 1978.

Israel HL, Goldstein RA: Relation of Kveim-antigen reaction to lymphadenopathy: study of sarcoidosis and other diseases, *N Engl J Med* 284(7):345-349, 1971.

Johnston RF, Wildrick KH: State of the art review: the impact of chemotherapy on the care of patients with tuberculosis, *Am Rev Respir Dis* 109:636-664, 1974.

Jones LA: Superior vena cava syndrome: an oncologic complication, *Semin Oncol Nurs* 3(3):211, 1987.

Luce J, Culver B: Respiratory muscle function in health and disease, *Chest* 81(1):82-90, 1982.

Lyons H: Differential diagnosis of hemoptysis and its treatment, *Basics Respir Dis* 5:2, 1976.

Malasanos L et al: *Health assessment,* ed 2, St Louis, 1981, Mosby–Year Book.

Matthews MJ, Mackay B, Lukeman J: The pathology of non-small cell carcinoma of the lung, *Semin Oncol* 10(1):34-55, 1983.

Morrison M: *Respiratory intensive care nursing,* ed 2, Boston, 1979, Little, Brown.

Mountcastle VB, ed: *Medical physiology,* St Louis, 1980, Mosby–Year Book.

Murray JF, Nadel JA, eds: *Textbook of respiratory medicine,* Philadelphia, 1988, W B Saunders.

Netter F: *The CIBA collection of medical illustrations, vol 7, respiratory system,* New York, 1979, CIBA Pharmaceutical Co.

Paré JAP, Fraser RG: *Synopsis of diseases of the chest,* Philadelphia, 1983, W B Saunders.

Pearson FG: Lung cancer: the past twenty-five years, *Chest,* 89:200S-205S, 1986.

Prior J, Silberstein J, Stang J: *Physical diagnosis: the history and examination of the patient,* ed 6, St Louis, 1981, Mosby–Year Book.

Ruppel G: *Manual of pulmonary function testing,* St Louis, 1990, Mosby–Year Book.

Sanderson DR: Lung cancer screening: the Mayo study, *Chest* 89:324S, 1986.

Schwartz JL: Review and evaluation of smoking cessation methods: the United States and Canada 1978-1985, Bethesda, Md, Division of Cancer Prevention and Control, National Cancer Institute, 1987.

Shapiro B, Harrison R et al: *Clinical applications of respiratory care,* ed 3, St Louis, 1985, Mosby–Year Book.

Shoemaker WC, Thompson WL, Holbrook PR: *The Society of Critical Care Medicine textbook of critical care,* Philadelphia, 1984, W B Saunders.

Simmons DH, ed: *Current pulmonology,* vol 7, St Louis, 1986, Mosby–Year Book.

Slonim N, Hamilton L: *Respiratory physiology,* ed 5, St Louis, 1987, Mosby–Year Book.

Snukst-Torbeck G, Werhane MJ, Schraufnagel DE: Treatment of tuberculosis in a nurse-managed clinic, *Heart Lung* 16(1):30-33, 1987.

Swearingen PL, Sommers MS, Miller K: *Manual of critical care: applying nursing diagnoses to adult critical illness,* St Louis, 1988, Mosby–Year Book.

Tinker JH: Understanding chest x-rays, *Am J Nurs* 76(1):54-58, 1976.

Wade JF: *Comprehensive respiratory care: physiology and technique,* ed 3, St Louis, 1982, Mosby–Year Book.

Wanner A, Sackner MA: *Pulmonary diseases: mechanisms of altered structure and function,* Boston, 1983, Little, Brown.

West JB: *Pulmonary pathophysiology: the essentials,* ed 2, Baltimore, 1982, Williams & Wilkins.

West JB: *Respiratory physiology: the essentials,* ed 3, Baltimore, 1985, Williams & Wilkins.

Williams MH, ed: Disturbance of respiratory control, *Clinics in Chest Medicine,* vol 1, Philadelphia, 1980, W B Saunders.

Wolinsky E: State of the art: nontuberculous mycobacteria and associated diseases, *Am Rev Respir Dis* 119:107-159, 1979.

Yancik R, Yates JW: Quality of life assessment of cancer patients: conceptual and methodologic challenges and constraints, *Cancer Bulletin* 38(5):217, 1986.

C·H·A·P·T·E·R — 12

Respiratory Failure

*O*bjectives

- Differentiate etiology and pathophysiology of hypoxemia and hypercapnia.
- Discuss assessment and treatment of both hypoxemia and hypercapnia.
- Differentiate assessment of and interventions for cardiogenic and noncardiogenic pulmonary edema (ARDS).
- Evaluate a patient with chest trauma.
- Differentiate assessment and treatment of various types of pneumonia.
- List risk factors for and sources of pulmonary embolism.
- Discuss treatment considerations for pulmonary embolism.

Any obstructive or restrictive lung disease may cause acute respiratory failure. Either failure of oxygenation or failure of ventilation may occur, and some patients develop total respiratory failure with insufficient oxygenation and ventilation. This chapter differentiates assessment and interventions for failure of oxygenation from failure of ventilation. Specific treatments, including medications, pulmonary hygiene measures, and mechanical ventilation, are discussed in detail in subsequent chapters. Special cases of common causes of respiratory failure, namely adult respiratory distress syndrome (ARDS), pulmonary edema, pulmonary emboli, chest trauma, and pneumonia, are discussed here.

HYPOXEMIA
Etiology

Hypoxemia is low blood oxygen tension, whereas *hypoxia* is inadequate oxygen at the tissue level. Hypoxemia and hypoxia are distinctly separate conditions. Tissue hypoxia may occur despite normal blood oxygen tension. For example, in carbon monoxide poisoning, the arterial oxygen tension (Pao_2) is normal, whereas the oxygen bound to hemoglobin (arterial oxygen saturation) is abnormally low. This is because carbon monoxide has a greater affinity for hemoglobin than oxygen. Because little oxygen is bound to hemoglobin, tissue may become hypoxic even though Pao_2 is normal.

There are five causes of hypoxemia: decreased inspired oxygen (Pio_2), hypoventilation, ventilation-perfusion mismatching, anatomical shunt, and impaired diffusion.

Decreased Pio_2 is an unusual problem in most areas of the United States. At higher elevations, the air contains less oxygen, or is "thinner." Although the percentage of oxygen remains the same, about 21%, the barometric pressure is lower, resulting in lower Pio_2. (Review concepts of the alveolar air equation in Chapter 9.) Individuals living at higher altitudes adapt to the lower level of inspired oxygen by increasing the number of red blood cells. More red blood cells are able to carry more oxygen through the body. Problems with oxygenation can arise when individuals used to living at sea level or anemic individuals travel to higher altitudes, because they do not have extra red blood cells to carry oxygen to the tissues. For example, people with normal lung function have limited oxygen reserves when climbing Mount Everest; they need supplemental oxygen. The same is true when hypoxemia-susceptible patients travel by airplane or to higher altitudes. Airplanes are generally pressurized at 5000 to 8000 feet, roughly the altitude of Denver or higher. The patients most at risk for hypoxemia when traveling at higher altitudes are those using supplemental oxygen, those with hypercapnia, and those with marginal oxygenation (Pao_2 just above 60 mm Hg).

Hypoventilation, or hypercapnia, is a state of decreased alveolar ventilation, which is caused by a decrease in tidal volume, respiratory rate, or both. Using the alveolar air equation (refer to Chapter 9), it is easy to see how an increase in arterial carbon dioxide tension ($Paco_2$) results in a lower Pao_2. For each increase of 10 mm Hg in the $Paco_2$, there is a decrease of approximately 12 mm Hg in the Pao_2. The main causes of hypoventilation are drug overdose, excessive sedation or analgesia, head injury, sleep apnea, some neuromuscular diseases, and some thoracic deformities.

Ventilation-perfusion mismatching usually is the most common cause of hypoxemia. Pneumonia, pulmonary edema, atelectasis, chronic bronchitis, emphysema, and asthma are examples of diseases with ventilation-perfusion mismatching. When affected alveoli receive less ventilation than perfusion, blood leaving the area is poorly oxygenated; this results in hypoxemia. The most severe form of ventilation-perfusion mismatching is clinical, or physiological, shunt. With clinical shunt, there is no ventilation in a perfused area of the lung. One example of clinical shunt is noncardiogenic pulmonary edema, in which the alveoli are filled with fluid and perfusion is normal.

Anatomical shunt is another form of hypoxemia. With anatomical shunt, blood bypasses the lungs and never participates in gas exchange. The classic anatomical shunts are ventricular septal defect in adults and tetralogy of Fallot in children. In these disorders, blood passes through the heart without ever reaching the lungs. Another fairly infrequent example is pulmonary arteriovenous fistula or anastomosis. In the latter case, blood bypasses the pulmonary capillary bed because it flows directly from the pulmonary artery to the pulmonary vein.

Impaired diffusion is an unusual form of hypoxemia that results when the alveolar-capillary membrane becomes sufficiently thickened to impair oxygen transport. Since the blood normally is fully oxygenated before it is one third of the way through the lung, the alveolar-capillary membrane can be somewhat thickened without impairing oxygen transport. Some clinicians feel that diffusion defects are present in severe forms of interstitial lung disease or collagen-vascular diseases, although ventilation-perfusion mismatching also may be responsible for hypoxemia in these cases.

Nursing management

Assessment. The early signs of hypoxemia are very subtle. As hypoxemia worsens, the signs and symptoms become apparent. The respiratory, neurological, and cardiovascular systems display most of the symptoms. The patient's respiratory rate or depth increases slightly, resulting in increased minute ventilation. The pulmonary circulation response to hypoxemia is increased pulmonary vascular resistance and pulmonary hypertension.

Most patients with hypoxemia have difficulty thinking clearly, and both impaired judgment and confusion occur. Some patients have vision disturbances, especially diplopia. These patients usually are irritable or anxious, although depression and lethargy also occur. With severe hypoxemia, convulsions and permanent brain damage occur.

The cardiovascular system responds to hypoxemia by increasing the heart rate and blood pressure in an attempt to increase cardiac output and oxygen delivery. Some patients develop cardiac dysrhythmias. Cyanosis is a late sign of hypoxemia, since approximately one third of the hemoglobin (5 g of the normal 15 g/dl) is not saturated before cyanosis is detectable. In addition, the presence of cyanosis does not necessarily imply inadequate oxygenation, as in patients with polycythemia. Similarly, the absence of cyanosis does not imply adequate oxygenation, as in anemic patients who have severely decreased Pao_2.

The only way to truly identify hypoxemia is by arterial blood gas analysis. Relative hypoxemia is a Pao_2 between 60 and 80 mm Hg; Absolute hypoxemia is a Pao_2 below 60 mm Hg. The latter is true even for patients with obstructive lung disease and chronic hypoxemia.

Nursing diagnoses. The problem is hypoxemia, which may be related to low Pao_2, hypoventilation, ventilation-perfusion mismatching, anatomical shunt, or impaired diffusion. Common nursing diagnoses include ineffective breathing pattern, impaired gas exchange, ineffective airway clearance, or fluid volume excess.

Interventions. The goal is to reestablish normal oxygenation, and interventions are directed at immediately reversing the hypoxemia and treating the cause. The first treatment for hypoxemia is applying oxygen. Depending on the level of hypoxemia, a nasal cannula or face mask is used first. Progressive hypoxemia sometimes responds to the use of partial or non–rebreather masks. If these fail, continuous positive airway pressure masks are tried, or the patient is intubated. In severe cases, intubation and mechanical ventilation are instituted with a higher concentration of inspired oxygen (Fio_2) and increased positive end-expiratory pressure (PEEP). Hypoxemia caused by hypoventilation often responds to increased minute ventilation through the mechanical ventilator and no or low levels of supplemental oxygen. To improve oxygenation when ventilation is normal, Fio_2 and PEEP are adjusted. (Note: Intubation and mechanical ventilation are instituted earlier in patients with acute rather than chronic hypoxemia.) Ventilation-perfusion mismatching and diffusion defects require institution of higher levels of oxygen and PEEP. Shunt is the only cause of hypoxemia that does not respond to oxygen therapy.

A common misconception is to limit the amount of oxygen administered to patients with chronic carbon dioxide retention (hypoxemia is drive to breathe). When the Pao_2 falls below 60 mm Hg and the oxygen saturation of arterial blood (Sao_2) falls below 90%, the patient is on the steep portion of the oxyhemoglobin dissociation curve. Oxygen levels decelerate rapidly. Never deprive the patient of necessary oxygen because of hypercapnia. When higher levels of oxygen are administered to patients with hypercapnia, the patient must be assessed more frequently. Oxygen is used with caution. If the patient hypoventilates excessively, resulting in lower Pao_2, intubation and mechanical ventilation are necessary. Sometimes the physician uses noninvasive types of mechanical ventilation. If the patient refuses intubation and mechanical ventilation, the physician and patient choose an alternative plan. In some instances, they accept a certain degree of hypoxemia, which possibly results in organ injury; in other cases, they make the patient as comfortable as possible and allow nature to determine the course.

Once the immediate hypoxemia is corrected, the cause is treated. In many instances oxygen and other treatments are started simultaneously. However, other treatments generally take longer to work. In the case of anatomical shunt, surgery is required. Bronchodilators and pulmonary hygiene measures aid in clearing excessive secretions, which can cause ventilation-perfusion mismatching. Antibiotics also aid in secretion removal by limiting debris in mucus when bronchitis or pneumonia is the cause of hypoxemia. Thrombolytic therapy is instituted for pulmonary emboli. Diuresis or dialysis improves fluid imbalance caused by congestive heart failure or renal failure.

HYPERCAPNIA
Etiology

Hypercapnia is caused by acute or chronic hypoventilation and ventilation-perfusion mismatching. There are many causes of hypoventilation, including decreased drive to breathe, decreased ability to respond to ventilatory needs, increased dead space, and increased carbon dioxide production. Neuromuscular diseases and drug-induced central nervous system depression are the primary causes of hypoventilation. Other causes include diseases of the medulla resulting from trauma, hemorrhage, or encephalitis; spinal cord defects; strokes; brain tumors or infections; and some obstructive and restrictive lung diseases (especially chest wall defects such as kyphoscoliosis).

Pathophysiology

Inadequate exchange of fresh alveolar air with blood results in retention of carbon dioxide. A significant rise in $Paco_2$ is always associated with a concomitant decrease in Pao_2. The increase in $Paco_2$ is also associated with a decrease in pH. The degree of change in pH depends on the rapidity with which the hypercapnia evolves. With acute hypercapnia, the pH falls sharply. With chronic hypercapnia, the kidneys retain bicarbonate to buffer the pH change. Chronic hypercapnia has a small pH decrease for a greater increase in $Paco_2$. In most instances the pH is nearly normal or normal. Some clinicians believe that ventilation-perfusion mismatching does not interfere with carbon dioxide elimination. The belief is that overventilated areas compensate for underventilated areas, which West (1987) disputes. Some patients with ventilation-perfusion mismatching have an abnormal $Paco_2$; others have a normal $Paco_2$. Central neurogenic control of ventilation may be different in the two groups.

Nursing management

Assessment. The clinical signs and symptoms of hypercapnia are vague. Many of the symptoms occur simultaneously with hypoxemia and are difficult to differentiate. All of the signs and symptoms associated with hypoxemia may be found in the patient with hypercapnia. Lethargy, somnolence, and headaches, especially upon awakening, are common symptoms of hypercapnia. On examining the eyes, the clinician may note papilledema from cerebral vasodilation. Facial and conjunctival blood vessels are often dilated, and patients generally complain of dyspnea. Asterixis is also often elicited by the clinician. In severe cases of hypercapnia, coma develops.

The patient's general appearance usually is that of a sleepy individual. Because these patients have dilated facial vessels, their faces often look reddened or ruddy. The nurse notes decreased rate or depth of breathing (or both) on physical examination. Some patients with low tidal volumes are tachypneic, a compensatory response.

Arterial blood gases (ABGs) are analyzed to define the extent of hypercapnia and the success of treatment. With hypercapnia, the $Paco_2$ is elevated above 45 mm Hg. With acute hypercapnia, the pH is below 7.35. With chronic hypercapnia, the pH is in the range of 7.35 to 7.4.

Nursing diagnoses. The main problem is hypercapnia from inadequate ventilation. Because of this, the most appropriate nursing diagnosis is impaired gas exchange related to the cause (for example, increased dead space and oversedation).

Interventions. The focus of care is to reestablish a normal $Paco_2$ and pH. In the patient with acute hypercapnia, the goal is a pH near 7.4 with a $Paco_2$ of approximately 40 mm Hg. In the patient with chronic hypercapnia, the goal is slightly different: interventions are geared to obtain a pH near 7.35 regardless of the elevated $Paco_2$ value; bicarbonate elevates to buffer the pH.

The basic treatment for hypercapnia is to increase the patient's minute ventilation acutely while treating the cause of hypoventilation. In many instances the physician chooses to observe the patient and administer conservative treatment. This is especially true with patients with chronic hypercapnia. Bronchodilators, antibiotics, narcotic antagonists, chest physical therapy, hydration, and breathing exercises are among the treatments. Respiratory stimulants are prescribed for some patients.

If the patient's condition worsens, intubation and mechanical ventilation are necessary. It is important to discuss intubation and mechanical ventilation with the *stable* patient, before a crisis of hypoxemia and acidemia, to obtain informed consent for intubation. The primary adjustments on the mechanical ventilator that correct **hypercapnia** are **rate and tidal volume.** In some instances changing from intermittent mandatory ventilation to assist control corrects hypoventilation. When assist control is instituted, caution is exercised to prevent alkalemia. Remember that the goal of treatment is a normal pH, especially in the patient with chronic hypercapnia. The patient is allowed to retain bicarbonate to buffer the $Paco_2$ and obtain a nearly normal to normal pH.

CARDIOGENIC PULMONARY EDEMA
Etiology

Pulmonary edema, the abnormal collection of fluid in the extravascular spaces and tissues of the lungs, has many causes. Pulmonary edema caused by increased capillary hydrostatic pressure (cardiogenic pulmonary edema), the most common type, is caused by myocardial infarction, mitral stenosis, decreased myocardial contractility, left ventricular failure, or fluid overload. With this type of pulmonary edema, the left ventricle is unable to pump blood efficiently from the heart. Fluid backs up into the lungs, and oxygen delivery to the tissues is impaired. Pulmonary edema may also be caused by increased capillary permeability, a condition known as noncardiogenic pulmonary edema or adult respiratory distress syndrome (ARDS); lymphatic insufficiency (lymphangitis carcinomatosa); decreased interstitial pressure (rapid reexpansion of the lung after removal of air or fluid); and decreased colloid osmotic pressure (hypoproteinemia).

Pathophysiology

The capillary endothelium is very permeable to water, small molecules, and ions, although protein movement is restricted. In contrast, the alveolar epithelium is not very permeable to even large molecules or proteins. According to Starling's law, opposing factors control the movement of fluid across the alveolar-capillary membrane; that is, interstitial colloid osmotic pressure versus hydrostatic colloid osmotic pressure and interstitial hydrostatic pressure versus capillary hydrostatic pressure. The equation also contains a permeability coefficient and a reflection coefficient, which control the transfer of protein and other large molecules. In the normal individual, there is a small net flow of fluid out of the capillary and into the interstitial spaces. The fluid moves through the interstitial spaces of the alveoli to the perivascular and peribronchial interstitium. The lymphatics are located in these areas and actively move the lymph toward bronchial and hilar nodes.

There are two stages of pulmonary edema. The first stage, called *interstitial edema,* is characterized by engorgement of the perivascular and peribronchial interstitial tissues as fluid backs up into the lungs from the left heart. The second stage, *alveolar edema,* is traditional pulmonary edema. Surface tension increases, causing edematous alveoli to shrink in size. The lungs become stiff and noncompliant, increasing the work of breathing. Ventilation is limited, creating a ventilation-perfusion mismatch and hypoxemia. In fulminant pulmonary edema, the fluid moves into the smaller and then larger airways, where it is coughed out as pink, frothy sputum. The pink color comes from red blood cells that have crossed the alveolar-capillary membrane.

Nursing management

Assessment. The signs and symptoms of cardiogenic pulmonary edema involve several systems and vary according to the degree of failure (see box on p. 238). The patient with cardiogenic pulmonary edema is usually dyspneic. Orthopnea (increased dyspnea when lying flat) and paroxysmal nocturnal dyspnea (awakening with severe dyspnea and wheezing) are common. In the early stages, the patient complains of a dry, hacking cough; as the pulmonary edema progresses, pink, frothy sputum develops.

On inspection, the nurse notes an elevated respiratory rate and shallow respirations. Cheyne-Stokes breathing pattern may occur. Palpation sometimes reveals fremitus. Percussion can elicit dullness in dependent regions of the lung secondary to fluid. Auscultation is the most revealing. The nurse frequently assesses crackles in dependent areas of the lung. As the patient changes position, so do the crackles. Heart sounds are often consistent with congestive heart failure. S_3 gallop rhythm or S_4 and murmurs often are present with cardiogenic pulmonary edema. The blood pressure is frequently abnormally low.

The chest x-ray film of the patient with cardiogenic pulmonary edema reveals an enlarged heart and prominent pulmonary arteries and veins (Fig. 12-1). Cuffing may be observed. When interstitial edema is present, Kerley lines appear. Alveolar infiltrates emerge with alveolar filling, and the infiltrates gravitate to dependent areas of the lung.

Signs and symptoms of cardiogenic pulmonary edema

Vital signs
Tachycardia with S_3, S_4 or murmurs and weak pulse
Hypotension with narrow pulse pressure
Tachypnea with dyspnea, orthopnea, nocturnal dyspnea, and increased work
   of breathing

Hemodynamics
Decreased cardiac output
Increased pulmonary artery wedge pressure (PAWP) greater than 18 mm Hg
   and often 25 to 30 mm Hg
Increased right heart pressures with biventricular failure

Laboratory values
Decreased Pao_2, Sao_2, and saturation of mixed venous blood (Svo_2)
Decreased pH (sometimes)

Other indicators
Apprehension or restlessness
Cardiomegaly, pulmonary hypertension
Coma (sometimes)
Coughing, sometimes with hemoptysis
Crackles, fremitus, dullness to percussion, especially in bases
Decreased level of consciousness, drowsiness, confusion, or lethargy
Decreased urine output
Diaphoresis

Hydrostatic pressure or cardiogenic pulmonary edema usually is diagnosed during cardiac catheterization or insertion of a pulmonary artery catheter. When measuring the pulmonary artery wedge pressure (PAWP) or pulmonary artery occlusion pressure (PAOP), the nurse notes an increase in the PAWP above 18 mm Hg. Many patients have a PAWP of 30 mm Hg or more. Right-sided heart pressures also are elevated in some patients, and in many patients cardiac output is decreased.

The arterial blood gases of a patient with cardiogenic pulmonary edema indicate hypoxemia from ventilation-perfusion mismatching. Hypoxemia worsens with increased alveolar filling. When cardiac failure worsens, the pH may fall from increased fixed acids, especially lactic acid.

Nursing diagnoses. There are several difficulties in caring for the patient with cardiogenic pulmonary edema. Hypervolemia, impaired cardiac contractility, hypoxemia, and skin breakdown are important problems. Many patients also experience anxiety, discomfort, dyspnea, impaired cognition, and a decreased activity level.

The primary nursing diagnoses for the patient with cardiogenic pulmonary edema include fluid volume excess related to fluid overload or decreased contractility, impaired gas exchange related to ventilation-perfusion mismatching, and potential impairment of skin and tissue integrity related to edema from hypervolemia or impaired perfusion from decreased contractility or hy-

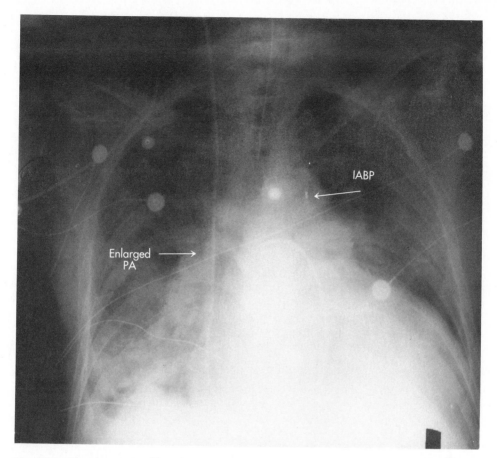

Fig. 12-1. The chest x-ray film of a patient with cardiogenic pulmonary edema shows an enlarged heart and enlarged pulmonary veins. Fluid accumulates in dependent alveoli, resulting in dependent (basilar) infiltrates.

potension. The nurse may also choose, as appropriate, altered comfort related to dyspnea or chest pain, anxiety related to hypoxemia or hospitalization, altered cerebral and renal tissue perfusion related to low cardiac output, and decreased activity level secondary to impaired cardiovascular function or bed rest.

Interventions. The focus of care is to induce normovolemia with adequate urine output and normal vital signs, to reestablish normal ABGs, and to keep the patient's skin intact and free of sores or ulcerations (which may result from decreased perfusion with heart failure). It is also necessary to ease the patient's anxiety and promote comfort, to promote muscle strength, and to prevent proximal vein thrombi. These goals are accomplished through frequent observation, often in the intensive care unit.

Blood gases (or pulse oximetry), hemodynamics, and urine output are assessed frequently. Normal Pa_{O_2}, pH, PAWP, and cardiac output are the goals. The interventions for cardiogenic edema begin with application of oxygen and administration of diuretics. Many patients are more comfortable with the head of the bed elevated. Usually a nasal cannula suffices to improve Pa_{O_2}. Sometimes mask oxygen or, in rare cases, intubation and mechanical ventilation with PEEP are needed. Fluids and sodium are restricted, as indicated. Vasodilators, inotropic drugs, afterload or preload agents, contractility agents, and other cardiac medications may also be administered. Patients who do not respond to conservative measures may require intraaortic balloon pumping for diastolic augmentation of the left ventricle. Many patients require morphine to control pain and improve cardiovascular function. Frequent position changes and pressure-minimizing devices help prevent skin breakdown.

NONCARDIOGENIC PULMONARY EDEMA (ADULT RESPIRATORY DISTRESS SYNDROME)
Etiology

Adult respiratory distress syndrome (ARDS) is defined as pulmonary edema with normal cardiac function. ARDS is a severe form of respiratory failure that results from local or systemic lung injury. Other names have been used to describe ARDS since it was first described in 1967, including shock lung, Da Nang lung, adult hyaline membrane disease, wet lung, pump lung, and congestive atelectasis.

The cause of ARDS is unknown, although there are several risk factors. The site of injury in ARDS is the alveolar-capillary membrane. Some of the factors implicated in the cause are neutrophils; platelets; complement; tumor necrosis factor; proteases; surfactant inactivation, dilution, or loss; arachidonic acid metabolites; and oxygen radicals. Some risk factors are associated with direct injury to the lung. These include pneumonia, aspiration of gastric contents, pulmonary contusion, near drowning, and smoke inhalation. Lung injury also occurs from indirect contact; that is, through the blood. These risk factors include sepsis (especially gram-negative rod) or sepsis syndrome (no positive blood culture), hemorrhagic or hypovolemic shock, multiple blood transfusions, multiple long bone fractures, pancreatitis, uremia, cardiopulmonary bypass, and drug overdose. (One form of ARDS is caused by neurological trauma.) The risk of developing ARDS varies with each risk factor and the number of risk factors involved (see Table 12-1). The most common predispositions for development of ARDS are sepsis, aspiration, sepsis syndrome, and trauma. Overall the mortality of ARDS averages 50%.

Pathophysiology

With ARDS the permeability coefficient in Starling's law is altered, allowing efflux of water and plasma from the capillary. The capillaries become more permeable and leak. Hydrostatic and colloid osmotic pressures are normal in ARDS, as is cardiac function. Early in ARDS interstitial edema develops, followed by alveolar edema. Alveoli are flooded with red blood cells, cellular debris, and protein-rich plasma fluid. The type II cells are damaged, resulting in inactivation or destruction of surfactant. Loss of surfactant results in patchy atelectasis and ventilation-perfusion mismatching. In areas of alveolar collapse and alveolar filling, ventilation is minimal or absent, resulting in a physiological shunt (perfusion without ventilation). There are also wide-

Table 12-1. Risk factors for developing adult respiratory distress syndrome (ARDS)

Thoracic predispositions (Local)	Nonthoracic predispositions (Systemic)
Aspiration of gastric contents	Cardiopulmonary bypass
Near drowning	Drug overdose
Pneumonia	Fat embolism
Pulmonary contusion	Multiple long bone fractures
Smoke inhalation	Multiple blood transfusions
	Pancreatitis
	Sepsis syndrome
	Sepsis
	Shock
	Uremia

spread areas of very low ventilation that are still perfused by capillaries; these areas contribute to hypoxemia.

Lung mechanics are also altered with ARDS. Elastic recoil is increased. Compliance and functional residual capacity (FRC) are decreased as a result of increased lung water, increased alveolar surface tension, and atelectasis. The lungs become stiff, requiring high ventilating pressures to attain an adequate tidal volume. In the patient who is not being mechanically ventilated, the work of breathing is markedly increased.

Nursing management

Assessment. Assessment begins with identifying which patients are at risk for ARDS (see Table 12-1). In some instances ARDS may be prevented by meticulous care, such as stabilizing fractures, controlling bleeding, maintaining blood pressure, and preventing infection or treating it promptly. Assessing the patient's clinical condition frequently helps identify early onset of ARDS. Patients with ARDS generally have worsening dyspnea with deterioration in arterial blood gases. They appear to be in acute distress and are restless or sometimes obtunded.

Inspection of the patient with ARDS reveals tachypnea with normal to small tidal volumes. Grunting, diaphoresis, and intercostal retractions are observed in some patients; some have cyanosis. Palpation and percussion are not revealing. In the early stages of ARDS, the lungs are clear. Later crackles develop throughout the lung.

The chest x-ray film reveals a normal cardiac shadow. (In contrast, cardiogenic pulmonary edema demonstrates an enlarged heart). Infiltrates are fluffy and bilateral (Fig. 12-2), diffuse, and not located primarily at the bases. The infiltrates affect both the apices and the bases. The patient's position does not grossly alter the position of the infiltrates.

Analysis of arterial blood gases is essential to the diagnosis of ARDS and classically demonstrates severe hypoxemia that is partly or totally refractory (shunt) to supplemental oxygen. In assessing serial blood gases, the nurse observes progressive hypoxemia on the same or higher Fio_2. Increasing the Fio_2 does not result in a significant increase in Pao_2 (shunt). In patients receiving mechanical ventilation with PEEP, the Pao_2 is usually equal to or less than

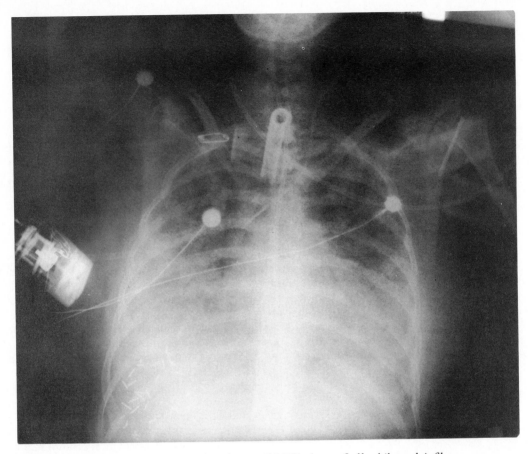

Fig. 12-2. Adult respiratory distress syndrome (ARDS) shows fluffy, bilateral infiltrates. These infiltrates affect all five lobes and are not dependent.

double the Fio_2 (for example, Pao_2 below 100 mm Hg on Fio_2 of 50% or Pao_2 below 200 mm Hg on Fio_2 of 100%). In other words, the Pao_2 to Fio_2 ratio is less than 200. Some sources use an arterial/alveolar ratio (a/AO_2) below 0.2 as an indicator of hypoxemia. Others measure intrapulmonary shunt or oxygen consumption. In ARDS, physiological shunt increases above 20%. The pH is generally normal or increased (tachypnea results in alkalosis) in the early stages of ARDS. In severe cases of ARDS, the pH decreases; this is a very late and often ominous sign. The acidosis has either a respiratory or metabolic cause. Respiratory acidosis is caused by retention of carbon dioxide. Metabolic acidosis results from endotoxin- or hypoxia-induced anaerobic metabolism.

A pulmonary artery catheter is inserted to evaluate heart function for response to institution of high levels of PEEP and for possible fluid overload.

Pulmonary artery catheterization reveals normal filling pressures for both the right and the left heart. The PAWP is classically normal but may be slightly elevated to 17 mm Hg because of other treatments. When the PAWP is above 18 mm Hg, cardiogenic pulmonary edema is also present. ARDS and cardiogenic pulmonary edema can coexist.

The ratio of tracheal protein to plasma protein is a relatively new assessment tool for differentiating cardiogenic from noncardiogenic (ARDS) pulmonary edema. The ratio of protein in tracheal aspirates to plasma is less than 0.5 in cardiogenic pulmonary edema. In ARDS, the ratio is increased because of the amount of proteins in the pulmonary edema fluid. The tracheal protein to plasma ratio is generally over 0.7 in ARDS.

Nursing diagnoses. The chief problems in ARDS are hypoxemia and stiff, noncompliant lungs. Pulmonary infection is also a problem in the protein-rich pulmonary edema fluid. Also, nutrition frequently is impaired because the patient is generally unable to eat and must be given supplements. There are other complications of immobility from prolonged bed rest.

A wide variety of nursing diagnoses are useful in caring for the patient with ARDS. The most important is impaired gas exchange related to ventilation-perfusion mismatching and shunt. Other useful nursing diagnoses are potential for ineffective breathing pattern related to increased work of breathing or anxiety, potential for infection related to compromised defense mechanisms, potential for ineffective airway clearance related to intubation and mechanical ventilation, alteration in nutrition related to intubation, altered comfort related to intubation and increased work of breathing, potential for impaired physical mobility or activity intolerance related to deconditioning and prolonged bed rest.

Interventions. Many interventions are designed to restore adequate oxygenation, prevent pulmonary infection, and maintain nutritional stores and muscle function. Other interventions focus on easing anxiety and improving comfort.

All interventions for ARDS are supportive; there is no cure. Several agents (for example, prostaglandin E_1 and steroids) have been studied to treat ARDS, but none has been successful. In fact, steroids may actually predispose the patient to worse complications (Bones, 1987). Potential ARDS treatments on the horizon are ibuprofen and surfactant repletion. Surfactant has been used successfully to treat infant respiratory distress syndrome.

Oxygen therapy is the first treatment initiated. The goal of care is to achieve a Pao_2 of at least 60 mm Hg on 50% oxygen or less. High levels of oxygen contribute to the development of oxygen toxicity. When oxygen alone is insufficient to improve the Pao_2, continuous positive airway pressure (CPAP) is sometimes attempted. Failure of the latter requires intubation and mechanical ventilation to restore oxygenation and ventilation.

When the patient is unable to overcome the work of breathing of noncompliant lungs, mechanical ventilation is needed. Using mechanical ventilation improves alveolar gas exchange and often improves oxygenation. Most patients with ARDS require mechanical ventilation with positive end-expiratory pressure (PEEP) to increase FRC. PEEP is useful in expanding alveoli in ARDS because of diffuse alveolar involvement, resulting in homogenous PEEP distribution. (PEEP is not as effective in diseases with focal involvement, such as pneumonia, because the PEEP goes first to areas of least resistance, such as normal lung.) Five to 20 cwp PEEP is usually needed to keep alveoli open for participation in gas exchange. Use of PEEP frequently allows a decrease in the Fio_2. Sometimes patients develop bronchopleural fistulas from barotrauma as a result of mechanical ventilation. Jet ventilation is an approved therapy for bronchopleural fistulas.

It is important to remember other techniques that improve oxygen delivery to the tissues. Instituting pharmacological paralysis with heavy sedation decreases oxygen consumption. It is also helpful to maintain a normal hemoglobin level, pH, $Paco_2$, cardiac output, and body temperature.

Airway care is an important consideration in the patient with ARDS. Because the patient usually is intubated, secretion clearance mechanisms are altered. Sterile suctioning techniques are necessary to prevent bacterial contamination of the protein-rich lower airway. A change in the color, consistency, or amount of secretions indicates a possible pulmonary infection. Chest physical therapy is not usually effective, especially in early ARDS, because the fluid is not in the airways but in the interstitium. If the patient has retained secretions or pneumonia, chest physical therapy is useful in moving the secretions to the large airways. Positioning of the patient is always important. Unlike unilateral lung diseases, bilateral lung diseases such as ARDS do not usually have a position that improves ventilation-perfusion matching and gas exchange. Routine frequent repositioning aids in preventing complications of immobility and in mobilizing secretions.

Fluids are administered conservatively to the patient with ARDS. The goal is to prevent fluid overload but to provide adequate intravascular volume for body functions. It is often difficult to assess fluid volume in a patient receiving large amounts of PEEP, since intrathoracic volume is increased. Maintaining the patient in a too-dry state can cause renal damage and imposes other body stresses.

Nutrition is maintained with the institution of enteral or parenteral feedings. Parenteral feedings are more common, since intestinal absorption may be impaired. Caloric needs vary with the patient's status; because the patient with ARDS often has many other problems such as wound healing, infection, or bleeding, caloric needs may be greatly increased. In general, adult patients with ARDS usually require about 2500 calories. However, nutritional assessment using a metabolic cart is suggested.

CHEST TRAUMA
Etiology

Health care workers in emergency rooms and intensive care units are seeing many patients with numerous chest injuries caused primarily by motor vehicle accidents (automobile and motorcycle) and homicide attempts. Other causes of chest trauma include blasts or explosions, falls from great heights, and gunshots or stabbings. Chest injuries result from blunt or penetrating trauma and range from mild to severe. The injuries may involve the chest wall (rib fractures, flail chest), pleura (pneumothorax, hemothorax, tension pneumothorax), parenchyma (pulmonary contusion, ruptured trachea or bronchus), or heart and great vessels (cardiac tamponade, cardiac contusion, ruptured aorta). Surrounding structures (perforated diaphragm, esophageal tear) are also affected at times. Because of the number of vital structures contained within the chest, trauma to this area is particularly hazardous and often life threatening. Table 12-2 presents the pathophysiology, nursing assessment, and interventions for patients with chest trauma.

Table 12-2. Chest trauma

Disorder	Pathophysiology	Nursing assessment	Interventions
Rib fractures	Fracture of rib at point of impact by blunt or penetrating trauma	Pain on palpation Pain on inspiration Suspect vascular injury with fracture of ribs 1 and 2 Suspect underlying lung injury with fracture of ribs 3-9 Suspect abdominal or liver injury with fracture of lower ribs Ineffective ventilation Secretion retention ABGs: normal, low Pao_2, low $Paco_2$ Chest x-ray film: vertical fracture line or nonunion of rib	Analgesia Intercostal nerve block with local anesthetic Epidural catheter with analgesia or anesthetic No constrictive appliances Incentive spirometry Chest physical therapy
Flail chest	Fracture of two or more ribs on both sides of the point of impact produces unstable rib cage Prevents full lung expansion, leading to atelectasis and hypoxemia Flail segment responds to changes in intrapleural pressure Heals in 6 weeks	Pain on palpation Pain on inspiration Paradoxical movement of flail segment; moves in on inspiration and out on expiration Lowered tidal volumes Increased respiratory effort Shortness of breath (dyspnea) ABGs: low Pao_2, high $Paco_2$ Chest x-ray film: multiple adjacent rib fractures	Patent airway Analgesia: intravenous Patient controlled analgesia (PCA), transcutaneous electric nerve stimulation (TENS) Intercostal nerve block External splinting Oxygen Mechanical ventilation PEEP Surgical fixation Chest physical therapy Incentive spirometry
Pneumothorax	Perforation of lung by fractured rib or penetrating trauma Air collects in pleural cavity, preventing lung expansion and compromising gas exchange Normal negative intrathoracic pressure is lost All or part of the lung collapses	Chest pain Shortness of breath (dyspnea) Asymmetrical lung expansion Diminished or absent breath sounds on affected side Hyperresonance Crepitus (subcutaneous emphysema) ABGs: normal, low Pao_2, high $Paco_2$ Chest x-ray film: air in pleural space, decreased lung volume	Cook catheter with Heimlich valve Small-bore chest tube second intercostal space midclavicular line to water seal or suction Watch for tension pneumothorax Oxygen Analgesia

Continued.

Table 12-2. Chest trauma—cont'd

Disorder	Pathophysiology	Nursing assessment	Interventions
Hemothorax	Perforation of blood vessel Internal mammary artery—(IMA; chest wall vessels; intercostal, systemic, and pulmonary arteries and veins) by rib fracture or penetrating trauma causes collection of blood between pleural layers Part of lung tissue on affected side is compressed, compromising gas exchange Hemothorax may also result from lacerated liver or perforated diaphragm	Chest pain Shortness of breath (dyspnea) Asymmetrical lung expansion Diminished or absent breath sounds on affected side Dullness or flatness over blood collection ABGs: normal, low Pao_2, high $Paco_2$ Chest x-ray film: pleural effusion on upright film, 300 ml blunts costophrenic angle, 1000 ml extends 5 cm above diaphragm	Large-bore chest tube fifth intercostal space midaxillary line to water seal or suction Oxygen Excessive blood loss (1000 ml immediate or 200-500 ml/hr) is an indication for surgery Analgesia
Perforated diaphragm	Blunt or, more commonly, penetrating trauma as high as T4 tears diaphragm Predominant incidence involves left hemidiaphragm because most assailants are right handed, right side is protected by liver, and left-sided heart is usual target	Decreased breath sounds Decreased respiratory excursion Decreased diaphragmatic excursion Shortness of breath Chest pain (may be referred to shoulder or abdomen) Persistent air leak in chest tube Tachypnea Bowel sounds in chest cavity Tympany to percussion Difficulty in passing nasogastric tube with herniated bowel Mediastinal shift to opposite side Chest x-ray film: normal, bowel herniated into chest cavity, or elevated hemidiaphragm	Surgical repair

Disorder	Pathophysiology	Nursing assessment	Interventions
Tension pneumothorax	Air in pleural cavity trapped without exit (one-way valve effect) may result from primary traumatic injury or be delayed Pressure collapses lung, pushes mediastinum to opposite side, compromising contralateral lung Venous return is impaired as mediastinal shift distorts vena cava and air increases intrathoracic pressure	Severe respiratory distress Trachea deviated to opposite side Asymmetrical chest movement Distended neck veins Absent or diminished breath sounds on affected side Chest pain Hyperresonance or tympany to percussion Tachycardia Hypotension Cyanosis Extreme agitation Decreased cardiac output ABGs: low Pao_2 and Sao_2, high $Paco_2$ Chest x-ray film: collapsed lung on affected side, mediastinum and trachea shifted to opposite side	Oxygen Needle decompression (16 to 18 gauge), second intercostal space midclavicular line Small-bore chest tube to water seal or suction
Cardiac contusion	Myocardial contusion is similar to myocardial infarction and frequently results from blunt chest wall injuries, including fracture of ribs and sternum	Dysrhythmias, especially for 48-72 hours ECG: similar to ischemia (elevated ST and inverted T wave), premature atrial and ventricular contractions, ventricular tachycardia Decreased or normal cardiac output Chest pain Elevated cardiac enzymes	Continuous assessment of rhythm and hemodynamics Normal fluid balance Inotropic agents Decrease stressors Decrease oxygen consumption
Cardiac tamponade	Life-threatening accumulation of blood in the pericardial sac Usually the result of blunt injury or puncture wound to heart Patient develops cardiogenic shock as cardiac output falls with increased intrapericardial pressure Volume of fluid varies, usually is greater than 50-100 ml Symptoms and treatment depend on rapidity of accumulation	Midthoracic pain, especially in second to seventh intercostal spaces left of sternum Distant, muffled heart sounds Hypotension Dyspnea Tachycardia Elevated central venous pressure (CVP) Decreased cardiac output Narrow pulse pressure Distended neck veins Pulsus paradoxus greater than 15 mm Hg	Pericardiocentesis with large-bore long needle below or along left xiphoid process Aspirated blood should not clot, since it is defibrinated by cardiac motion in pericardium Pericardial catheter Surgery Observe for recurrence

Continued.

Table 12-2. Chest trauma—cont'd

Disorder	Pathophysiology	Nursing assessment	Interventions
Ruptured aorta	Complete or partial dissection of aorta, usually from deceleration injury Tears occur at points of anatomical fixation Most common site is distal to left subclavian artery on descending thoracic aorta Other sites include ascending aorta at pericardial sac and at diaphragm On deceleration, intima and media tear and adventitia balloons into pseudoaneurysm Long-term survival is 6%-8%, 90% die at scene of injury First or second rib fractured; high sternal fracture, or left clavicular fracture is often associated with aortic injury	Sternal or interscapular back pain Upper extremity hypertension Absent or delayed femoral or radial pulse Hypovolemic shock Dyspnea Hypotension Precordial or interscapular murmur caused by turbulence across disrupted area Hoarseness caused by hematoma pressure around aortic arch Lower extremity neuromuscular or sensory deficit Tachypnea Cyanosis Cardiopulmonary arrest Low hemoglobin and hematocrit ABGs: low Pao_2, low Sao_2, low or high $Paco_2$ Chest x-ray film: widened mediastinum on upright film. Massive pleural effusion more commonly on left, entire left side may be opacified; tracheal and esophageal deviation to the right Aortogram confirms	Fluid resuscitation Large-bore chest tube to gravity or suction drainage with blood salvaging device, although this may provide route for exsanguination by eliminating tamponade effect; chest tube may be clamped Reparative surgery Sedatives Antihypertensives Antibiotics Surgery for bowel ischemia Cardiopulmonary resuscitation (CPR)
Ruptured trachea or bronchus	Usually caused by blunt forces Suspect with fracture of first to fifth ribs Typical site within 1 inch of carina Frequently incomplete and circumferential May result in tracheal stenosis or tracheal malacia	Shortness of breath (dyspnea) Hemoptysis Difficulty intubating Persistent pneumothorax Early atelectasis from secretions or blood clot Subcutaneous emphysema (crepitus) Signs of air embolus	Patent airway Careful suctioning Careful neck positioning Double lumen endotracheal tube (such as Carlens or Bronchocath) Chest tube Bronchoscopy Surgical repair

Disorder	Pathophysiology	Nursing assessment	Interventions
Ruptured esophagus	Deceleration injury tears esophagus at one of three areas of narrowing: cricoid cartilage, arch of aorta, or diaphragm Penetrating trauma more frequently associated with ruptured esophagus Corrosion of mediastinal structures by digestive juices and bacterial contamination are major concerns Most common complications are mediastinitis, periesophageal abscess, empyema, esophageal fistula, or peritonitis Mortality is reported to be 19%-27%	Pain (may radiate to neck, chest, shoulders, or abdomen) Resistance of neck to passive range of motion (ROM) Peritoneal signs Dyspnea Hoarseness Cough Stridor Bleeding from mouth or nasogastric tube Fever Dysphagia Subcutaneous emphysema Pneumothorax Chest x-ray film: normal, mediastinal or pleural air; esophagoscopy or esophagogram to confirm	Surgical repair may include closure of esophagus and mucous fistula Gastric decompression Antibiotics Wound drainage Skin care Nutritional support
Pulmonary contusion	Compression or decompression injury that ruptures lung tissue, small airways, and alveoli Interstitial and alveolar edema accompanied by inflammation Bruising may be accompanied by pulmonary laceration or tear More common in thin chest walls and young people with compliant chest walls; older individuals usually have more fractures but fewer contusions May be unilateral or bilateral Ventilation-perfusion abnormalities and shunt present in damaged or collapsed gas exchanging units. Atelectasis and secretion retention problems	Tachypnea Crackles and wheezes Dyspnea Hemoptysis Increased peak ventilating pressures Decreased lung compliance ABGs: low Pao_2 and Sao_2, low $Paco_2$ Chest x-ray film: focal area of infiltrate usually within 6-24 hours	Oxygen Intubation and mechanical ventilation with PEEP Jet ventilation Suctioning with lavage Chest physical therapy Rotokinetic therapy Analgesia Sedation Pharmacological paralysis Normal fluid balance Observe for barotrauma and infection

Nursing diagnoses

The main problems in chest trauma vary with the type and the severity of the injury. Generally the patient has difficulty ventilating or oxygenating. Most patients have pain or anxiety and limited activity, and some patients have impaired cardiac output; also, the potential for infection is great.

Based on these problems, the nurse may choose one or more nursing diagnoses from the following nonexclusive list: ineffective breathing pattern related to specific chest trauma disorder, pain, or lung compression; activity intolerance related to fatigue secondary to increased work of breathing; anxiety related to dyspnea; alteration in cardiac output secondary to specific chest injury, mediastinal shift, hemorrhage, or hypovolemia; alteration in comfort related to specific chest injury; impaired verbal communication related to intubation or tracheostomy; fluid volume deficit related to hemorrhage from ruptured aorta; impaired gas exchange related to atelectasis, specific chest injury, or sepsis; and potential for infection related to mechanical ventilation, invasive monitoring, or disruption in tissue integrity.

PNEUMONIA
Etiology

Pneumonia, also called *pneumonitis,* is an inflammatory response in the lungs, usually caused by an infectious agent. Infection enters the lung either by inhalation of bacteria or by seeding of the lung with bacteria from the blood. Infectious organisms are viral or bacterial, and some organisms are more infectious than others. Most inhaled organisms never enter the lungs, because they are blocked by effective upper airway defense mechanisms. Once organisms enter a normal lung, the mucociliary escalator, macrophages, and lymph system remove them and prevent infection. Bypassing the upper airway, such as with endotracheal intubation or tracheostomy, alters the lungs' ability to defend themselves from organism invasion. Other factors that predispose the patient to the development of pneumonia are dehydration, drugs that impair mucociliary clearance, coma, weakness, sedation, malnutrition, chronic lung diseases, and immunosuppression.

Pathophysiology and assessment

There is a variety of common pneumonia-producing organisms, and the pathophysiology varies slightly among them. In general, a pneumonia produces an area of low ventilation with fairly normal perfusion. Because the alveoli fill with exudate, ventilation to affected lung segments is decreased. Perfusion usually is fairly normal, although hypoxic vasoconstriction reduces blood flow to the affected area. The net effect is an area of low ventilation to perfusion ratio ($\dot{V}/\dot{Q}$) and hypoxemia. In some patients a shuntlike effect is seen. When pleural effusions occur, ventilation is further decreased because lung expansion is further restricted; hypoxemia is more severe. Pneumonia commonly causes tracheobronchial edema and increased secretions. The combined effect of edema and secretions increases both airway resistance and work of breathing.

Pneumococcus pneumonia. Pneumococcal pneumonia is a common community acquired pneumonia that is usually seen in the winter and spring. The incidence of pneumococcal pneumona is decreasing in many parts of the world. This is believed to be the result of improved living conditions and earlier treatment of upper respiratory tract infections. There are 82 types of

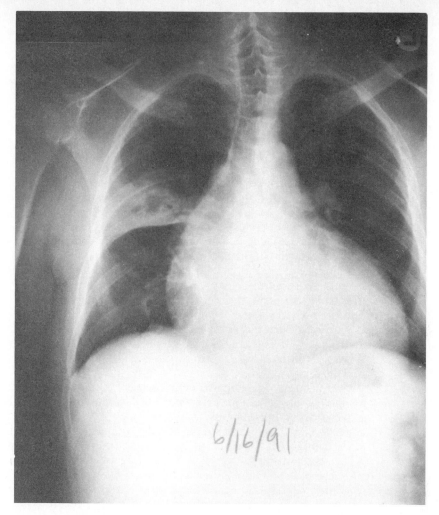

Fig. 12-3. Pneumonia in the right mid lung.

pneumococci, but only nine cause pneumonia. These nine have a characteristic capsular swelling that may protect the bacteria from phagocytosis. Pneumococcal pneumonia classically appears 2 to 14 days after a viral upper respiratory illness. The patient has a high fever, shaking chills, pleuritic chest pain, and a cough that produces rusty-colored or green purulent sputum. The chest pain usually is worse on inspiration or when coughing. Hemoptysis and myalgia may occur, and the white blood cell count is elevated. The patient looks acutely ill. If a pleural effusion is present and tapped, thoracentesis demonstrates an exudative parapneumonic pleural effusion.

On inspection, the patient is diaphoretic and tachypneic. Unilateral splinting is sometimes observed. Fremitus and tenderness are often palpated. Percussion elicits dullness or flatness over areas of consolidation and pleural effusion. Crackles and occasionally a pleural rub are assessed by auscultation. Egophony, bronchophony, or whispered pectoriloquy are heard over areas of consolidation.

The chest x-ray film traditionally reveals lobar alveolar filling; that is, pneumonia (Fig. 12-3). An ipsilateral (same side) pleural effusion is commonly observed around the affected lung.

Sputum analysis is useful in identifying the causative organism. A deep cough produces a good sputum sample for diagnosis. Pneumococcal organisms are round, ovoid, or lancet-shaped gram-positive cocci that usually occur in pairs (diplococci) or possibly short chains. They are sometimes indistinguishable from staphylococci and streptococci. Blood cultures are also positive in about 25% of cases.

Arterial hypoxemia is present in most patients with pneumococcal pneumonia; some patients develop hypotension and sepsis.

Staphylococcus **pneumonia.** Staphylococcal pneumonia usually is nosocomial, or institution acquired, rather than community acquired, and it has a mortality rate of about 35%. Among children, the incidence of staphylococcal pneumonia is greatest under 2 years of age. The patients who develop nosocomial staphylococcal pneumonia are those who are immunocompromised, debilitated, mechanically ventilated, or being treated with broad-spectrum antibiotics. Hospital epidemics occur in nurseries and intensive care units and on surgical, orthopedic, and obstetric floors. With community-acquired staphylococcal pneumonia, the patient typically seeks treatment 2 weeks after a viral illness, complaining of a high fever, shaking chills, dyspnea, dull or pleuritic chest pain, and productive cough. This pneumonia is hemorrhagic. Airways are denuded of mucosa and ulcerated. There is also necrosis of bronchial walls, peribronchial abscesses, and alveoli filled with bloody exudate.

On inspection, the patient is tachypneic. Infants frequently have cyanosis. The findings on palpation, percussion, and auscultation are similar to those for pneumococcal pneumonia.

On the chest x-ray film, the nurse observes segmental consolidation that usually is bilateral. There are no air bronchograms, which is consistent with copious secretions in the airways. Infiltrates with consolidation are frequently multisegmental or multilobar and bilateral. Fluid is sometimes observed in the fissures. Abscesses, pneumatoceles (thin-walled cavities), and pleural effusions (empyema) are seen in about half of adult patients. The cavities may have fluid levels.

The purulent sputum in staphylococcal pneumonia is usually odorless and yellow-green to salmon pink in color. *Staphylococcus aureus* is usually the causative organism. Sputum analysis for *S. aureus* reveals encapsulated gram-positive cocci in pairs, triads, or clusters.

Laboratory tests in staphylococcal pneumonia reveal leukocytosis in most patients. Patients without leukocytosis or with leukopenia, as in elderly or immunocompromised patients, have a poor prognosis. Arterial blood gas analysis indicates hypoxemia.

Streptococcus **pneumonia.** Streptococcal pneumonia accounts for up to 5% of all pneumonias and has an overall mortality rate of 5% or less. In children it may occur after measles or chickenpox. Streptococci lodge in the alveoli, especially in the lower lobes. Lymphatics become occluded with mucus and exudate early in the disease process, and this may explain the high incidence of pleural effusions in streptococcal pneumonia.

Symptoms are usually abrupt and rapidly progressive. The patient complains of high fever, shaking chills, cough, and pleuritic chest pain. About half of the patients also complain of pharyngitis. Inspection reveals tachypnea and sometimes accessory muscle use. Fremitus can occur with palpation. Percussion often locates a pleural effusion. Auscultation demonstrates crackles and in rare cases friction rubs. There are no signs of consolidation.

Sputum is purulent and frequently blood tinged. Streptococci are gram-positive cocci usually appearing in chains on Gram stain and are cultured on blood agar plates. In culture, alpha streptococci produce a zone of incomplete hemolysis, whereas beta streptococci produce complete hemolysis and gamma streptococci produce no hemolysis.

Laboratory tests are significant for an elevated white blood cell count with left shift (elevated bands) in most patients. Antistreptolysin O (ASO) titers are usually elevated. Blood cultures are negative.

The chest x-ray film shows infiltrates indicative of pneumonia. Pleural effusion commonly is present.

Haemophilus **pneumonia.** *Haemophilus influenzae* pneumonia is commonly seen in children and in adults with chronic conditions such as alcoholism, chronic obstructive pulmonary disease (COPD), and lung cancer. (*H. influenzae* also causes epiglottitis in children.) The clinical presentation is similar to that seen in pneumococcal pneumonia.

The chest x-ray film shows various patterns. Focal lobar, lobular, or multilobular infiltrate usually involves the lower lobes. Pleural effusions are frequently observed.

Sputum cultures do not always grow *H. influenzae,* which grows best on chocolate agar. On Gram stain, pleomorphic gram-negative rods indicate possible *Haemophilus* infection.

Klebsiella **pneumonia.** *Klebsiella* pneumonia usually is considered a community-acquired disorder, although nosocomial cases also occur. Patients with *Klebsiella* pneumonia have rapid onset of rigors, fever, a productive cough, severe dyspnea, pleuritic chest pain, and fatigue to the point of prostration. The mortality rate may be as high as 50%.

On inspection, the patient appears acutely ill and in acute respiratory distress. Cyanosis and hypotension are present in severe forms of the disease. Patients may use accessory muscles. The nurse commonly assesses signs of consolidation, including dullness to percussion and egophony, bronchophony, whispered pectoriloquy, and fremitus by auscultation.

Sputum in *Klebsiella* pneumonia is usually grossly purulent. Sometimes it is thick, gelatinous, and red. There may be blood streaking in the sputum or frank hemoptysis. The Gram stain shows many pleomorphic, encapsulated, fat gram-negative rods.

The chest x-ray film usually reveals a pattern of lobar consolidation. Multiple lobes are involved, more commonly the upper lobes. Fissures bulge as a result of excessive inflammatory exudates in the parenchyma. Many chest x-ray films show loss of volume and abscess formation. Pleural effusions and empyema are not common. In severe cases of *Klebsiella* pneumonia, x-ray films show pulmonary necrosis with fibrosis, cavity formation, and bronchiectasis.

Laboratory tests are significant for anemia and an elevated white blood cell count or, less commonly, leukopenia. Hypoxemia may occur, especially in debilitated and anemic patients.

Other gram-negative rod nosocomial pneumonias. A variety of other gram-negative rod pneumonias are considered nosocomial, including those caused by *Pseudomonas, Escherichia, Proteus, Serratia,* and *Enterobacter* species.

Pseudomonas organisms grow and multiply in tap water and are spread by direct contact. Soap dispensers, nebulizers, and other hospital equipment may harbor these organisms. *Pseudomonas aeruginosa* is a common pathogen that colonizes or infects tracheostomy sites, burns, wounds, and the urinary tract. It is also commonly seen in patients with cystic fibrosis and bronchiectasis. Aspiration is a common initiating event for this type of pneumonia. *Pseudomonas* pneumonia differs from other types in that a morning fever is common, and pleuritic chest pain is rare. There is lower lobe predominance for infiltrates and consolidation. Infiltrates may be focal or diffuse, and small abscesses and pleural effusions may be assessed.

Escherichia coli pneumonia commonly occurs from aspiration. It may also develop from urinary or gastrointestinal tract infections. In patients with transient hypotension, bowel integrity is altered and may be involved in the seeding of *E. coli* into the blood and lung. Patients with *E. coli* pneumonia are in acute respiratory failure. They have fever, dyspnea, a productive cough, and pleuritic chest pain. There are no signs of consolidation. The chest x-ray film reveals patchy bronchopneumonia, often in the lower lobes, and sometimes a pleural effusion.

Proteus pneumonia is fairly uncommon and results from aspiration following an altered level of consciousness. Patients with *Proteus* pneumonia are acutely ill with chills, fever, dyspnea, a productive cough, and pleuritic chest pain. A physical examination reveals decreased breath sounds on the affected side, and signs of volume loss and consolidation are common. Tracheal shift to the affected side is a sign of volume loss. Chest x-ray films show that *Proteus* pneumonia commonly involves the upper lobes and in rare cases the pleura. Infiltrates are dense in the posterior segments of the upper lobes and in the superior segments of the lower lobes.

Serratia pneumonia is fairly rare and is frequently associated with contaminated respiratory therapy equipment. Clinically, the patient has fever, chills, and a productive cough. Some strains of *Serratia* have a red-orange color. Sputum may appear orangish and reddish in color and is sometimes confused with hemoptysis. The chest x-ray film shows diffuse bronchopneumonia. Occasionally pleural effusion and empyema are observed.

Enterobacter pneumonia commonly produces yellow sputum. The signs and symptoms are similar to those for *Klebsiella* pneumonia.

Viral **pneumonia.** More than 75% of all acute respiratory illnesses are thought to be caused by viral infections. Most of these disorders involve the upper respiratory tract. Viral pneumonia may result from upper respiratory tract infection, or the lungs may be the primary site. Patients with a viral syndrome are susceptible to secondary bacterial infection. Viral pneumonia usually is community acquired, although it may be nosocomial. It is transmitted by airborne droplets.

Many different viruses cause pneumonia. (The following technical discussion aids in understanding the influenza vaccine, which is discussed in Chapter 16.) The pneumonia viruses are categorized into types A, B, and C, based on complement fixation and immunoprecipitation tests. Types A and B undergo hemagglutination inhibition tests for further subdivision; that is, H0, H1, H2, or H3. In addition, type A contains antigenically distinct neurominidases (N1, N2). Complete classification of viruses includes the strain, geographical location of discovery, strain number, year, and H and N designations. The viruses mutate as immunity results in the common population. About every 10 years, major mutations occur in the viral envelope. Influenza virus type A is commonly associated with epidemics every 2 to 3 years. Late fall and winter are times of peak incidence.

Type A virus is responsible for most viral pneumonia. In immunosuppressed patients, cytomegalovirus (CMV) is common. In children, most viral pneumonia is caused by respiratory syncytial virus (RSV), which usually causes bronchiolitis, and by parainfluenza virus, which usually causes croup. Children and military recruits also commonly develop pneumonia from adenovirus. Rhinoviruses and enteroviruses are rarely associated with pneumonia. Varicella pneumonia may follow chickenpox, whereas measles pneumonia (giant cell interstitial pneumonia) follows measles, especially in immunocompromised patients.

Patients with uncomplicated viral pneumonia have a sudden onset of fever, dry cough, myalgia, headache, and prostration. Occasionally bronchiolitis or peribronchial pneumonitis develops within 48 hours. These patients also have chest pain that usually is retrosternal, worse on coughing, and unaffected by respiration. Varying degrees of dyspnea and a cough that produces mucoid or blood-tinged sputum are seen. Patients with bronchiolitis or peribronchial pneumonitis may develop ARDS.

Chest assessment is nonspecific in viral pneumonia. Some patients use accessory muscles; most do not. Cyanosis is rare, unless ARDS develops. Since consolidation is rare, palpation and percussion usually demonstrate normal findings. With auscultation, the nurse may hear crackles or wheezes.

Sputum analysis in viral pneumonia usually reveals few or no bacteria on Gram stain, although white blood cells are present.

Pulmonary function tests are rarely done in patients with infections. However, if performed, they reveal both mild restriction and mild obstruction in uncomplicated influenza. Diffusing capacity for carbon monoxide usually is reduced.

The chest x-ray film in early viral pneumonia is unremarkable. Some x-ray films may show prominent peribronchial markings. When bronchiolitis or peribronchial pneumonitis occurs, subsegmental or segmental infiltrates appear. With the onset of ARDS, diffuse alveolar infiltrates develop.

Mycoplasma **pneumonia.** *Mycoplasma* pneumonia, formerly called walking pneumonia, is an atypical pneumonia acquired through inhalation. The onset of this illness is insidious or acute, and the incubation period averages 21 days after exposure. *Mycoplasma* pneumonia commonly occurs in children and teenagers in the winter, although older individuals are also affected. Patients have a persistent, racking, nonproductive cough, fever, a pounding frontal or generalized headache, and myalgia. Some patients also have coryza, pharyngitis, pleuritic chest pain, and shaking chills.

On inspection, the nurse usually observes a moderately ill patient. Cyanosis is sometimes present. In the early phase of the disease, the chest examination is unremarkable, although a few crackles may be heard in the bases. As the disease progresses, percussion elicits dullness and auscultation reveals increased crackles and wheezes.

The chest x-ray film is fairly normal. Nodular, patchy, or perihilar infiltrates involving one or two lobes are commonly observed.

Laboratory tests are not diagnostic for *Mycoplasma* pneumonia, although cold agglutinins are helpful in establishing the diagnosis of this disorder. Viral titers rise between 2 and 6 weeks and may persist for several months. Sputum analysis, when available, reveals normal flora and polymorphonuclear leukocytes. When cultured, *Mycoplasma* organisms are slow growing.

Nursing management

Nursing diagnoses. The primary problems in pneumonia are infection, secretions, and hypoxemia. Appropriate nursing diagnoses include infection, ineffective airway clearance, and impaired gas exchange related to the infectious process. In certain patients, activity intolerance related to dyspnea or hypoxemia, anxiety or altered comfort related to dyspnea and chest pain, or knowledge deficit related to the disease process may apply.

Interventions. Treatment focuses on curing existing infection, preventing the spread of infection, auscultating clear lung sounds, and obtaining a normal Pao_2. The treatment for pneumonia begins with administration of intravenous (or sometimes oral or intramuscular) antibiotics after a sputum culture (and usually a Gram stain) is obtained. The antibiotic regimen is later altered based on reports of culture and sensitivity. Penicillin G is the drug of choice for pneumococcal pneumonia and streptococcal pneumonia, whereas semisynthetic penicillins or first-generation cephalosporins are the drugs of choice for staphylococcal pneumonia. When drug resistance is present in staphylococcal pneumonia (methicillin-resistent staphylococci), vancomycin is indicated. *Haemophilus* infections are treated with ampicillin, chloramphenicol, cefamandole, trimethoprim-sulfamethoxazole, and third-generation cephalosporins. *Klebsiella* pneumonia responds fairly well to cephalosporin and aminoglycoside antibiotics, although resistance to both has been reported. Antibiotic treatment of a gram-negative pneumonia usually requires two drugs, one being an aminoglycoside; in *Pseudomonas* pneumonia, the second drug is a semisynthetic penicillin. Amantadine can ease the symptoms of viral pneumonia. Adenine arabinoside and acyclovir are beneficial in patients with *herpes* and *varicella* infections. *Mycoplasma* pneumonia is treated with erythromycin or tetracycline.

Vaccines are available for pneumococcal pneumonia and some strains of viral pneumonia. The 23-valent pneumococcal vaccine protects against 90% of pneumococcal organisms. It is recommended for individuals with chronic lung and heart disease, the elderly, asplenic individuals, those with sickle cell disease, and other high-risk patients. Current studies recommend one dose for a lifetime of prevention against pneumococcal infections. Developed each year, the flu vaccine is effective against the most common virulent viruses in a given year. The vaccine is administered annually to the elderly, to residents of long-term care facilities, and to individuals with chronic disease of the lungs, heart, and endocrine systems, as well as to health care providers involved in the care of susceptible patients.

To prevent the spread of infection, hand washing and containment of contaminated secretions are essential. Nursing personnel must wash their hands before leaving the patient's room and before caring for another patient. Materials contaminated with secretions are contained in a trash receptacle or linen bag.

Airway clearance adjuncts include bronchodilators, chest physical therapy, augmented coughing techniques, deep-breathing exercises, and hydration. Aerosolized and systemic bronchodilators are frequently used to improve removal of secretions. Specific chest physical therapy positions are applied when infiltrates are localized. General side-lying positions are used in other cases. Unless coughing is preventing adequate rest, a cough suppressant is not used, since coughing is needed to expel secretions. Augmented coughing techniques and deep-breathing exercises are additional nursing measures to improve airway clearance. Secretion removal is also enhanced by adequate hydration, which thins and liquefies secretions. Dehydration thickens secretions, making them more difficult to expectorate.

Education is important for all patients. Patients' anxiety eases and they tend to participate more fully in their care when they understand the disease and the treatment plan. For instance, if a patient is sent home with oral antibiotics, he must understand that he must take them exactly as prescribed, without skipping doses or failing to complete the prescribed interval of 10 to 14 days. Another important component of the education plan is how to avoid recurrent pneumonia.

Most patients with pneumonia need to take longer rest periods. Since oxygen exchange is impaired in the lungs, most patients must limit physical activity to reduce oxygen consumption. Some patients require supplemental oxygen to improve the Pao_2. A few very ill patients need intubation and mechanical ventilation with PEEP and supplemental oxygen. The recovery period after pneumonia is long, often at least 6 weeks.

PULMONARY EMBOLISM
Etiology

Pulmonary embolism is an obstruction to blood flow in a pulmonary artery or capillary. The usual obstruction is a thrombus that begins in the deep veins, but the blockage may also be lipid. Pulmonary emboli are a major source of morbidity and mortality. In 1986, the National Institutes of Health reported that at least 50,000 people die annually from pulmonary embolism, although most people survive a pulmonary embolism.

Three factors contribute to the development of venous thrombosis: stasis of blood flow, injury to the intima of the vein, and alterations in the coagulation-fibrinolytic system, predisposing the blood to clot. The risk factors for pulmonary thromboembolism are listed in the box below. Most pulmonary emboli arise in the deep veins of the legs. Other sites of origin include the pelvic, prostatic, uterine, and renal veins, as well as the right side of the heart with right ventricular failure or atrial fibrillation. Other forms of pulmonary

---

Risk factors for pulmonary embolism

Age over 55 years
Atrial fibrillation
Birth control pills
Burns
Cancer of chest or abdomen
Congestive heart failure
Chronic pulmonary disease
Extreme dehydration
Immobility
Lower extremity or pelvic trauma
Multiple long bone fractures
Obesity
Pregnancy
Prior thromboembolic disease
Prolonged immobility
Thoracic, pelvic, or abdominal surgery
Varicose veins

Table 12-3. Types of pulmonary emboli

Type	Source
Air	Intravenous catheter or needle insertion; oral sex; gas decompression (the "bends")
Amniotic fluid	Difficult or complicated labor, especially in an older or multiparous woman; cesarean section
Fat	Multiple fractures in the pelvis, lower extremities, or other long bones; sickle cell crisis; osteomyelitis; burns
Foreign body	Fragmented indwelling catheter tips, especially through-the-needle types; illegal intravenous drug use (fillers or filters)
Parasitic	Uncommon in the United States; worldwide, especially schistosomiasis
Septic	Infected or contaminated tissues, substances, or foreign bodies; illegal intravenous drug use
Thrombotic	Deep veins of leg; pelvic, renal, uterine, or prostatic veins; right side of heart
Tumor	Fragmented malignant tissue

emboli are fat emboli, amniotic fluid emboli, air emboli, tumor emboli, septic emboli, and foreign body emboli. Table 12-3 lists common types of pulmonary emboli and their sources.

Pathophysiology

Thrombi are formed by aggregation of platelets, often near a venous valve. Layers of fibrin and platelets (lines of Zahn) accumulate to produce the clot. After a thrombus is formed, it undergoes resolution, either by fibrinolysis or by organization; some thrombi undergo both. With fibrinolysis, the thrombus is dissolved over a period of hours to days. Sometimes the thrombus is dissolved completely. In other cases, remaining thrombus is incorporated into the venous wall. This small zone of fibrotic tissue is then reendothelialized, also called organized. With organization, one or more venous valves become incompetent as the thrombus is incorporated. A pulmonary embolism occurs when the clot breaks loose and travels to the lungs before fibrinolysis or resolution has been completed; this is more likely to occur early in the cycle.

Once the thrombus has lodged in the lung, it reduces the size of the pulmonary vascular bed. Pulmonary vascular resistance and pulmonary artery pressure rise, increasing right ventricular work and possibly causing failure. The pulmonary effects of pulmonary emboli include an increase in alveolar dead space (ventilation without perfusion). Hypoxemia results from the ventilation-perfusion imbalance. Surfactant is lost in embolized zones, resulting in atelectasis and increased permeability of the alveolar-capillary membrane. Pulmonary infarction occurs in fewer than 10% of cases of pulmonary emboli. With pulmonary infarction, an area of lung is destroyed.

Nursing management

Assessment. Clinical assessment of deep vein thrombosis includes tenderness, redness, warmth, and edema of the lower extremity involved. Other diagnostic tests may be performed to verify clinical suspicion. The most common tests are impedance plethysmography, Doppler ultrasound, leg scanning after injection of radiolabeled fibrinogen, and contrast venography. The first

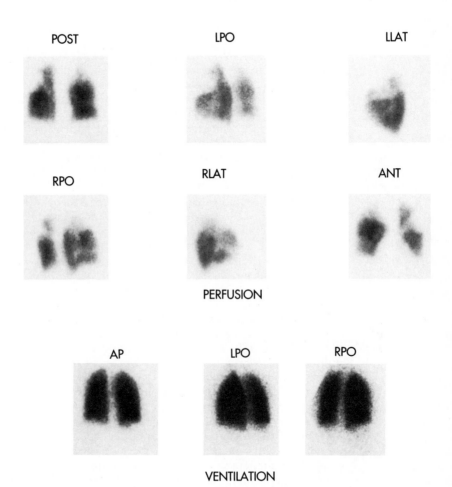

Fig. 12-4. Multiple segmental ventilation-perfusion defects, suggesting pulmonary embolism.

two procedures are noninvasive, whereas the latter two require venous cannulation and injection. Leg scanning is sensitive for calf and lower thigh clots, whereas impedance plethysmography is sensitive for thigh but not calf clots. Doppler ultrasound is more reliable in identifying thigh clots. Only venography identifies clots in both the calf and thigh and is absolutely diagnostic; it is considered the gold standard against which all other tests are measured. Most clinicians believe calf clots are fairly insignificant for pulmonary emboli.

When pulmonary emboli are suspected, ventilation-perfusion lung scanning is the first diagnostic test performed (Fig. 12-4). Unfortunately, many ventilation-perfusion scans are of indeterminate diagnostic value. Ventilation-perfusion scans are more difficult to interpret in patients with lung diseases because of altered ventilation or perfusion. Segmental or larger perfusion defects with normal ventilation, with a clear chest x-ray film, indicate high probability for embolism. When a lung scan is not diagnostic, pulmonary angiography confirms the diagnosis.

A pulmonary angiogram is performed in patients with a high index of suspicion for pulmonary embolism who have an indeterminate ventilation-perfusion lung scan. Pulmonary angiography is the gold standard for pulmonary embolism, although it carries many risks. The risks of the procedure are weighed against confirmation of the diagnosis and prolonged systemic anticoagulation. Because of the radiopaque dye load involved patients with renal disease may not be eligible for venography or pulmonary angiography. A positive pulmonary angiogram shows filling defects or an abrupt vessel cut off.

The most common symptom with pulmonary emboli is dyspnea. Other symptoms include pleuritic chest pain, acute anxiety, diaphoresis, a cough, nausea, and hemoptysis. With fat emboli, the nurse observes a triad of symptoms: petechiae (especially in the chest and axilla areas), dyspnea, and mental confusion. Fever is present with septic emboli and with infarction. Patients with hemodynamically significant pulmonary emboli develop hypotension.

On physical examination the patient frequently appears to be in acute distress. Other signs and symptoms vary from minor to significant. A few patients may be cyanotic. Most patients are tachycardiac. Palpation and percussion are not revealing. Upon auscultation, the nurse may hear a few wheezes or crackles. With infarction a pleural friction rub and sometimes dullness to percussion (pleural effusion) are heard. At this point the patient generally appears very ill. Massive pulmonary emboli are associated with increased pulmonic closure, S_3, and right ventricular tap.

In early thrombotic pulmonary embolism, the chest x-ray film is normal. With destruction of surfactant, a small area of atelectasis or infiltrate develops. Septic emboli appear as several small, round or irregularly shaped, shaggy densities. Older septic densities usually develop cavities after several days. When infarction occurs, a pleural effusion and wedge-shaped infiltrate are common (see Fig. 12-4).

Laboratory tests in patients with pulmonary embolism include an electrocardiogram (ECG) and arterial blood gas analysis. The ECG shows signs of pulmonary hypertension (right axis deviation, tall and peaked P waves, ST segment changes, and T wave inversion in V_{1-4}) when pulmonary embolism is significant. Arterial blood gases in pulmonary embolism vary with the severity of vascular obstruction. Most patients have a slight respiratory alkalosis from hyperventilation (tachypnea) and anxiety. Hypoxemia is fairly common, especially when large or several pulmonary emboli are present.

Nursing diagnoses. The primary problems with pulmonary embolism are hypoxemia, chest pain, and recurrent pulmonary emboli. Appropriate nursing diagnoses include impaired gas exchange related to ventilation-perfusion mismatching, chest pain related to pulmonary embolism, potential for injury related to anticoagulant therapy, and knowledge deficit related to disease process and treatment.

Interventions. Therapy focuses on reestablishing a normal Pao_2, relieving chest pain, preventing complications, and improving patient knowledge. The first intervention for pulmonary embolism is preventing development and migration of a deep vein thrombus. Measures to achieve this include applying mechanical leg compression devices (such as pneumatic stockings); stabilizing fractures; removing intravenous catheters properly; early mobilization, when possible; careful positioning of injured extremities; and administering prophylactic anticoagulants. The most common prophylactic anticoagulants are subcutaneous minidose heparin and oral warfarin.

Once a pulmonary embolism (or deep vein thrombus) has occurred, treatment is supportive. The patient is given a bolus of 5000 to 10,000 units of heparin, and a continuous infusion is started. The dosage of heparin is adjusted to maintain the activated partial thromboplastin time (APTT) 1.5 to 2 times the control. Heparin inhibits further thrombus growth, but it does not enhance thrombus resolution. It usually prevents further embolization by inhibiting clot formation and allows the body to dissolve or organize the existing clots. The effect of heparin is decreased by digitalis, tetracycline, nicotine (smoking), and antihistamines.

Oral warfarin is started at the same time as the heparin. Since these drugs act at different points in the clotting cascade, several days of heparin-warfarin overlap are necessary. After a 7- to 10-day course of therapy, heparin is discontinued and the patient continues oral warfarin for 6 months. The goal is to maintain the prothrombin time (PT) about 2.5 seconds above control (or 1.25 to 1.5 times control). The patient's PT is assessed at least every 2 weeks while he is on warfarin, and the dosage is adjusted as needed. Aspirin and nonsteroidal antiinflammatory medications (such as ibuprofen) interfere with platelet function and are avoided, because they can cause or prolong bleeding. Antacids, diuretics, oral contraceptives, and barbiturates decrease the effectiveness of warfarin. Vitamin K (20 mg) reverses the effects (within 24 to 36 hours) of excessive anticoagulation with warfarin; protamine sulfate (1 mg per 100 units) counteracts heparin.

In some instances the physician may choose to perform thrombolytic therapy. The most common reason for use of thrombolytic therapy is hemodynamic compromise (life threatening), although it may be the standard of care in the near future. Urokinase and streptokinase are the most common thrombolytic agents. They are given within the first 72 hours of pulmonary embolism to speed clot lysis. Heparin is withheld while thrombolytic agents are administered. Investigations are currently assessing the role of tissue plasminogen activator (TPA) in the treatment of pulmonary embolism and deep vein thrombosis.

The major complication of anticoagulation is hemorrhage. Certain patients are at increased risk for hemorrhage and cannot be given anticoagulants. These individuals include the very elderly (because of the risk of falls) and patients with internal bleeding, uremia, malignancies, strokes, brain tumors, recent urological or orthopedic manipulations, recent head injury or neurosurgery, and thrombocytopenia. Vena caval filters (such as a Greenfield filter) are inserted in these patients and in patients who develop clots while taking anticoagulants. The filter, which looks like a wire umbrella, is inserted through the femoral vein and positioned in the inferior vena cava. Because collateral circulation occurs, the risk of thromboembolism is not excluded but it is diminished.

Other interventions for care of the patient with pulmonary thromboembolism include oxygen and in rare cases mechanical ventilation to reverse hypoxemia, steroids and diuretics (fat emboli only), antibiotics (septic emboli), and antidysrhythmic agents. Some patients require sedation. It is important to avoid positioning the immobilized patient with deeply bent knees, since this can impede venous return from the legs and predispose the patient to deep vein thrombosis.

Special discharge instructions are needed for the patient taking oral anticoagulants. The nurse recommends that the patient obtain a medical bracelet indicating his condition and anticoagulation therapy. The patient should consult a pharmacist or physician before taking any over-the-counter medications, since many such medications, especially cold remedies, contain agents that could alter the effects of warfarin. Patients taking anticoagulants require vitamin K–controlled diets to prevent swings in PT levels. Foods high in vitamin K include green leafy vegetables, tomatoes, cauliflower, and fish. Avoiding injuries that involve bruising (falls) and cutting (shaving, cooking) prevents excessive bleeding. Electric razors are preferable to blade razors. Patients prone to bleeding gums need to alter their toothbrushing techniques. A soft, foam brush (such as toothettes) or cotton swabs can be used as substitutes for a regular toothbrush. The patient should assess each bowel movement for evidence of gastrointestinal bleeding (frank blood, maroon or black tarry stools). The home should also be assessed to identify hazards for falls and bruises. Also, the patient must learn the importance of promoting venous return by not crossing the legs at the knees, by not sitting for prolonged periods (position should be changed frequently), and by not wearing constrictive clothing. Some patients may need to wear antiembolism stockings daily.

CONCLUSION

This chapter has reviewed the common types of lung diseases associated with acute respiratory failure. Although not inclusive, it has provided a basis for general nursing practice on the general floor or in the intensive care unit. Many diseases can cause acute respiratory failure. In some instances, ventilation is primarily affected. Hypoventilation ultimately decreases oxygenation. The primary treatment for ineffective ventilation is mechanical ventilation. In other cases, oxygenation is predominantly affected. When oxygenation is impaired, ventilation may be normal. The primary treatment for inadequate oxygenation is supplemental oxygen. Some types of acute respiratory failure greatly affect both oxygenation (Pao_2) and ventilation ($Paco_2$). These patients usually require intubation and mechanical ventilation with PEEP.

BIBLIOGRAPHY

Ayres SM: Mechanisms and consequences of pulmonary edema: cardiac lung, shock lung, and principles of ventilatory therapy in adult respiratory distress syndrome, *Am Heart J* 103(1):97-112, 1982.

Baum GL, Wolinsky E: *Textbook of pulmonary diseases,* ed 3, Boston, 1983, Little, Brown.

Bell RC, Coalson JJ, Smith JD, Johanson WG: Multiple organ system failure and infection in adult respiratory distress syndrome, *Ann Intern Med* 99(3):293-298, 1983.

Bernard GR, Bradley RB: Adult respiratory distress syndrome: diagnosis, management, *Heart Lung* 15(3):250-255, 1986.

Bernard GR, Brigham KL: Pulmonary edema: pathophysiologic mechanisms and new approaches to therapy, *Chest* 89(4):594-600, 1986.

Bone RC, Clemmer TP, Slotman GJ, Metz CA: Early methylprednisolone treatment for septic syndrome and the adult respiratory distress syndrome, *Chest* 92(6):1032-1036, 1987.

Bradley RB: Adult respiratory distress syndrome, *Focus Crit Care* 14(5):48-59, 1987.

Brigham KL, Meyrick B: State of the art: endotoxin and lung injury, *Am Rev Respir Dis* 133(5):913-927, 1986.

Burki NK: *Pulmonary diseases: medical outline series,* Garden City, NY, 1982, Medical Examination Publishing.

Burton GC, Hodgkin JE: *Respiratory care: a guide to clinical practice,* ed 2, Philadelphia, 1984, JB Lippincott.

Cardona VD, Hurn PD, Mason PJB, et al: *Trauma nursing: from resuscitation through rehabilitation,* Philadelphia, 1988, WB Saunders.

Carroll PF: The ins and outs of chest drainage systems, *Nursing 86* 16(12):26-34, 1986.

Cella G, Palla A, Sasahara AA: Controversies of different regimens of thrombolytic therapy in acute pulmonary embolism, *Semin Thromb Hemost* 13(2):163-170, 1987.

Dantzker DR: Gas exchange in the adult respiratory distress syndrome, *Clin Chest Med* 3(1):57-67, 1982.

Daugherty D: *Thoracic trauma,* Boston, 1980, Little, Brown.

Drazen JM, Austen KF: State of the art: leukotrienes and airway responses, *Am Rev Respir Dis* 136(4):985-998, 1987.

Fishman A: *Pulmonary diseases and disorders,* New York, 1980, McGraw-Hill.

Fowler AA, Hamman RF, Good JT, et al: Adult respiratory distress syndrome: risk with common predispositions, *Ann Intern Med* 98(5pt1):593-597, 1983.

Fraser R, Paré J: *Diagnosis of diseases of the chest,* ed 2, vols 1-3, Philadelphia, 1977, WB Saunders.

Fulkerson WJ, Coleman RE, Ravin CE, Saltzman HA: Diagnosis of pulmonary embolism, *Arch Intern Med* 146(5):961-967, 1986.

Glenny RW: Pulmonary embolism: complications of therapy, *South Med J* 80(10):1266-1276, 1987.

Guenter C, Welch M: *Pulmonary medicine,* ed 2, Philadelphia, 1982, JB Lippincott.

Guyton AC: *Textbook of medical physiology,* ed 6, Philadelphia, 1981, WB Saunders.

Harper R: *A guide to respiratory care: physiology and clinical applications,* Philadelphia, 1982, JB Lippincott.

Heim CR, Des Prez RM: Pulmonary embolism: a review, *Adv Intern Med* 31:187-212, 1986.

Hinshaw H, Murray J: *Diseases of the chest,* ed 4, Philadelphia, 1980, WB Saunders.

Hopewell PC: Basics of RD: adult respiratory distress syndrome, New York, NY 1979, American Lung Association.

Hyers TM: Venous thromboembolic disease: diagnosis and use of thrombotic therapy, *Clin Cardiol* 13(4, suppl 6):vi 23-28, 1990.

Jobe A, Ikegami M: State of the art: surfactant for the treatment of respiratory distress syndrome, *Am Rev Respir Dis* 136(5):1256-1275, 1987.

Kessler CM, Druy E, Goldhaber SZ: Acute pulmonary embolism treated with thrombolytic agents: current status of tPA and future implications for emergency medicine, *Ann Emerg Med* 17(11):1216-1220, 1988.

Kramer FL, Teitelbaum G, Merli GJ: Pan-venography and pulmonary angiography in the diagnosis of deep venous thrombosis and pulmonary thromboembolism, *Radiol Clin North Am* 24(3):397-418, 1986.

Luce JM, Montgomery AB, Marks JD, et al: Ineffectiveness of high-dose methylprednisolone in preventing parenchymal lung injury and improving mortality in patients with septic shock, *Am Rev Respir Dis* 138(1):62-68, 1988.

Marks JD, Marks CB, Luce JM, et al: Plasma tumor necrosis factor in patients with septic shock: mortality rate, incidence of adult respiratory distress syndrome, and effects of methylprednisolone administration, *Am Rev Respir Dis* 141(1):94-97, 1990.

Merlotti G: Penetrating thoracic trauma, *Trauma Q* 1:42-53, 1985.

Morrison M: *Respiratory intensive care nursing,* ed 2, Boston, 1979, Little, Brown.

Murray JF, Nadel JA, eds: *Textbook of respiratory medicine,* Philadelphia, 1988, WB Saunders.

Naclerio EA: *Chest injuries,* Orlando, Fla, 1971, Grune & Stratton.

Netter F: *The CIBA collection of medical illustrations,* vol 7, *Respiratory system,* New York, 1979, CIBA Pharmaceutical Co.

Paré JAP, Fraser RG: *Synopsis of diseases of the chest,* Philadelphia, 1983, WB Saunders.

Popovich J: PEEP: Maximizing the benefits without hampering the heart, The Journal of Respiratory Diseases, pp. 33-38, March, 1986.

Popovsky J: Perforation of the esophagus from gunshot wounds, *J Trauma* 24(4):337-339, 1984.

Propp DA, Cline D, Hennenfent BR: Catheter embolism, *J Emerg Med* 6(1):17-21, 1988.

Richardson JD, Adams L, Flint LM: Selective management of flail chest and pulmonary contusion, *Ann Surg* 196(4):481-487, 1982.

Shapiro B, Harrison R, et al: *Clinical applications of respiratory care,* ed 3, Chicago, 1985, Mosby–Year Book.

Shapiro B, Harrison R, et al: *Clinical applications of respiratory care,* ed 3, Chicago, 1985, Mosby–Year Book.

Shoemaker WC, Thompson WL, Holbrook PR: *The Society of Critical Care Medicine textbook of critical care,* Philadelphia, 1984, WB Saunders.

Simmons DH, ed: *Current pulmonology,* vol 7, Chicago, 1986, Mosby–Year Book.

Sons HU: Pulmonary embolism and cancer: predisposition to venous thrombosis and embolism as a paraneoplastic syndrome, *J Surg Oncol* 40(2):100-106, 1989.

Swearingen PL, Sommers MS, Miller K: *Manual of critical care: applying nursing diagnoses to adult critical illness,* St Louis, 1988, Mosby–Year Book.

Wade JF: *Comprehensive respiratory care: physiology and technique,* ed 3, St Louis, 1982, Mosby–Year Book.

Wanner A, Sackner MA: *Pulmonary diseases: mechanisms of altered structure and function,* Boston, 1983, Little, Brown.

Weir EK, Archer SL, Edwards JE: Chronic primary and secondary thromboembolic pulmonary hypertension, *Chest* 93(3 suppl): 149S-154S, 1988.

West JB: *Pulmonary pathophysiology: the essentials,* ed 3, Baltimore, 1987, Williams & Wilkins.

Wright JR, Clements JA: State of the art: metabolism and turnover of lung surfactant, *Am Rev Respir Dis* 136(2):426-444, 1987.

Methods of Intervention

Unit 4 discusses interventions introduced in Unit 3 to improve ventilation and oxygenation. The chapters in this section cover noninvasive techniques, invasive techniques, mechanical ventilation, and medications.

Noninvasive techniques are initiated by the nurse, often without the physician's orders in some institutions. These noninvasive techniques include administration of oxygen, use of aerosols, deep-breathing and coughing techniques, positioning considerations, and chest physical therapy.

Unfortunately, noninvasive techniques are inadequate for many patients. The most common invasive techniques are resuscitation with an artificial airway and insertion of a chest tube. The nurse does not commonly initiate invasive therapy, but the nurse is responsible for assisting the physician during insertion and then for maintaining the airway or chest tube. These skills, along with bronchoscopy, are discussed in Chapter 14.

Mechanical ventilation and weaning are discussed separately. Chapter 15 discusses conventional mechanical ventilation with reference to many newer modes of such ventilation, including jet ventilation.

The final interventions discussed in Unit 4 are medications, which are covered in Chapter 16. Bronchodilators, the primary medications used in obstructive lung diseases, are emphasized. The actions and side effects of these medications, as well as of steroids, mast cell stabilizers, decongestants, antihistamines, expectorants, mucolytics, and diuretics, are reviewed. Because inhalers are commonly prescribed and commonly misused, a special section on using inhalers properly, alone or with spacer devices, is included at the end of Chapter 16.

C·H·A·P·T·E·R — *13*—

Noninvasive Techniques for Improving Oxygenation and Ventilation

*O*bjectives:

- Identify indications for oxygen therapy.
- Differentiate high-flow oxygen systems from low-flow systems.
- Discuss the complications of oxygen therapy.
- Discuss types of aerosol equipment.
- List the components of a normal cough.
- Identify causes of an ineffective cough.
- Differentiate cascade cough, huff cough, end-expiratory cough, and augmented cough.
- Describe techniques to improve deep inhalations.
- Identify the importance of inspiratory hold in incentive spirometry.
- Identify the positions for chest physical therapy.
- Differentiate the techniques of postural drainage, percussion, vibration, and rib shaking.

Techniques for improving oxygenation or ventilation may be invasive or non-invasive. This chapter focuses on noninvasive techniques, including oxygen therapy, humidification and nebulization therapy, chest physical therapy, effective coughing, augmented coughing, incentive breathing exercises, and positioning. Noninvasive mechanical ventilation is discussed in Chapter 15.

OXYGEN THERAPY

Oxygen has been used as therapy for almost two centuries. The primary indication for using the drug oxygen is hypoxemia, either acute or chronic. Oxygen therapy is also used to treat several conditions, even without hypoxemia, to enhance oxygen delivery to the tissues and to prevent hypoxia. These conditions include severe anemia before and during blood transfusions, carbon monoxide poisoning, hypotension, and congestive heart failure. Hypoxemia, or low blood oxygen, is determined by an arterial oxygen tension (Pao_2) below 60 mm Hg or by an arterial oxygen saturation (Sa_{O_2}) below 90%. (*Note:* The clinician uses these parameters as guidelines for therapy. For purposes of current Medicare reimbursement, oxygen is not reimbursed unless the Pa_{O_2} is below 55 mm Hg or the Sa_{O_2} below 88%, unless there is evidence of right heart failure. This is discussed in Chapter 17.)

Administering oxygen can reverse or prevent complications of hypoxemia, including activity intolerance, dyspnea, erythrocytosis, heart failure, pulmonary hypertension, and some mental abnormalities. The goals of oxygen therapy are to relieve hypoxemia and to prevent tissue hypoxia by boosting the Pa_{O_2} above 60 mm Hg and the Sa_{O_2} above 90%. Remember, however, that Pa_{O_2} is only one parameter determining adequate tissue oxygenation; also important are hemoglobin, cardiac output, the oxygen-hemoglobin dissociation curve, and cellular metabolic factors.

Oxygen delivery systems

There are many oxygen delivery devices, but they can be divided into two types, low-flow or high-flow systems, depending on whether they partly or completely meet the patient's inspiratory demands. Low-flow and high-flow oxygen delivery systems have nothing to do with low or high oxygen concentrations; low flow is not synonymous with a low concentration of inspired oxygen (Fi_{O_2}). A high-flow system may deliver low concentrations of oxygen, just as a low-flow system can deliver high levels of inspired oxygen.

A low-flow oxygen delivery system does not meet all the patient's inspiratory needs, whereas a high-flow system does. A nasal cannula is an example of a low-flow system. With a low-flow system, room air in varying amounts is breathed in with the oxygen. The Fi_{O_2} depends on the capacity of the reservoir (usually the nasal and oral pharynx), oxygen flow, size of the tidal volume, and breathing frequency. Smaller tidal volumes and slower respiratory rates increase the Fi_{O_2}, whereas rapid, shallow breathing decreases the Fi_{O_2}. A low-flow system is used primarily because of patient comfort, cost, and availability, not for precision in delivering a given Fi_{O_2}.

The variability in Fi_{O_2} is demonstrated by the following example. The anatomical reservoir is estimated to be 50 ml, or one third of anatomical dead space. A nasal cannula is placed at 6 liter's per minute (LPM); or 100 ml per second for a normal adult breathing a 500 ml tidal volume 20 times a minute. If the inspiration to expiration ratio (I:E) is normal, about 1:2, then inspiration takes 1 second and expiration takes 2 seconds. With each inspiration, the patient receives 50 ml of 100% oxygen (O_2) from the anatomical reservoir, 100 ml of 100% O_2 from the cannula (100 ml per second), and 350 ml of 21% O_2 (equals 70 ml O_2) for a total of 223.5 ml of 100% oxygen. The Fi_{O_2} of each similar breath is

$$\frac{223.5 \text{ ml O}_2}{500 \text{ ml V}_t} = 44.7\% \text{ O}_2$$

If the tidal volume is decreased by half, to 250 ml, then the patient receives the same 150 ml of 100% oxygen from the cannula. Only 100 ml of 21% O_2 (or 21 ml) is inhaled from room air. The Fi_{O_2} for this breath is 171/250, or 68.4% oxygen.

The nasal cannula is the most popular low-flow oxygen delivery system, and many manufacturers make the inexpensive device. Most nasal cannulas are lightweight green or white plastic with two prongs, 1 cm long or smaller,

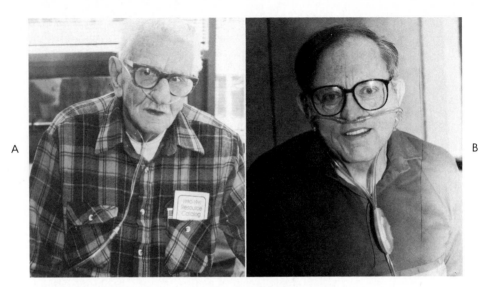

Fig. 13-1. Examples of a nasal cannula, a low-flow oxygen delivery system. **A,** A standard nasal cannula. **B,** The Oxymizer cannula, which enlarges the anatomical reservoir, increasing the Fio_2.

Correct application of a nasal cannula

1. Connect the nasal cannula to an oxygen source.
2. With the curve pointing downward, gently insert the nasal prongs into the patient's nose.
3. Being careful not to pull on the prongs, loop the tubing over the patient's ears and under the chin.
4. Slide the fastener snugly under the patient's chin.
5. Turn on the oxygen to the correct flow.

---

that fit into the patient's nose (Fig. 13-1, *A*). Compared with other oxygen delivery systems, a nasal cannula is inexpensive, comfortable, and easy to apply (see box above). Contrary to popular belief, mouth breathing does not generally interfere with oxygen flow unless the nares are obstructed. Patients may wear a nasal cannula continuously, without needing to remove it during eating, toothbrushing, drinking, or coughing. The disadvantages of using a nasal cannula are nasal stuffiness, dryness, or rhinitis and the development of irritated areas over the ears, under the chin, or under the nose. Another disadvantage is that patients who *hypoventilate* receive *higher* concentrations of oxygen, whereas patients who *hyperventilate* receive a *lower* Fio_2 because of dilution with room air. Some nasal cannulas have built-in reservoirs to increase the Fio_2, such as the Oxymizer cannula and pendant (Fig. 13-1, *B*).

Another low-flow oxygen delivery system is the simple open mask, which

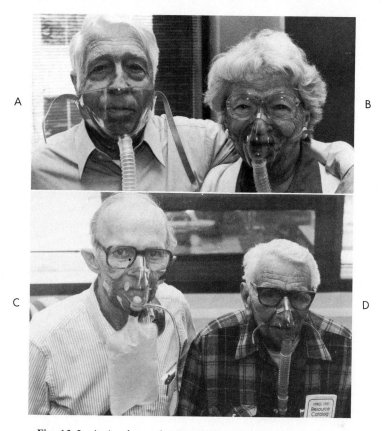

Fig. 13-2. A simple mask (**A**) and face tent (**B**) are low-flow oxygen delivery systems. The Venti mask (**C**) and non–rebreather mask (**D**) are examples of a high-flow system.

covers the nose and mouth. A simple mask is lightweight and has numerous holes that allow air to enter and exit (Fig. 13-2, *A*). There are neither valves to direct gas flow nor reservoir bags. As with the nasal cannula, when the patient breathes at high volumes or high rates (increased $\dot{V}E$), the FiO_2 is lower than when breathing at low volumes or low rates (decreased $\dot{V}E$). Oxygen concentrations are difficult to control with the simple face mask. An oxygen concentration of up to about 60% is available with the simple mask. Minimum flow rates of 5 to 6 LPM, or equal to the patient's minute ventilation, are necessary to prevent carbon dioxide (CO_2) from accumulating in the mask. More precise FiO_2 is obtained with a secure rather than loose-fitting mask. A main reason for switching from nasal cannula to simple face mask is the addition of humidity or aerosol therapy. One disadvantage is that the mask must be removed for such activities as eating, drinking, expectorating, and taking medications. Also, masks commonly are found on the patient's forehead, chin, or ear, limiting oxygen delivery. In addition, patients often complain of claustrophobia and heat buildup when wearing face masks. Some patients develop pressure areas where the elastic strap rubs the tops of the ears.

A face tent is similar to a simple mask, although it is less confining (Fig. 13-2, *B*). Usually used in patients with extensive facial injuries or sutures, a face tent fits securely under the patient's jaw and is open at the top. Oxygen concentration is less controlled in a face tent than in a mask. In most instances 8 to 10 LPM delivers an approximate FiO_2 of 40%.

A partial rebreathing mask is another form of low-flow oxygen. Fairly high concentrations of oxygen are possible with this mask. A partial rebreathing mask is a simple face mask with the addition of a bag, but there are no valves controlling air flow. The bag serves as an additional oxygen reservoir, not as a carbon dioxide reservoir, making the term "partial rebreather" confusing. With inhalation, the patient draws most oxygen-rich air from the bag and some air through the holes in the mask. With exhalation, a small portion of air, mostly from anatomical dead space, enters the bag. Recall that anatomical dead space contains little CO_2. As with the simple mask, an oxygen flow of at least 5 to 6 LPM is necessary to prevent excessive carbon dioxide buildup. Oxygen flow is increased to reinflate the bag rapidly after inhalation. This mask is ideal for patients who require short-term, high FiO_2 oxygen supplementation. (See box for correct application of mask.)

A high-flow oxygen delivery system has a reservoir and a gas flow that totally meet the patient's inspiratory needs. A Venturi mask, non-rebreathing mask, or mechanical ventilator are three examples of a high-flow oxygen system. With these devices the patient's respiratory rate and pattern of breathing do not affect the FiO_2; it is controlled by the device. The patient does not breathe in room air separately from oxygen. In a high-flow system, room air and supplemental oxygen are mixed by the device.

One of the most accurate ways to supply a given amount of oxygen to a patient is a Venturi or Venti mask (Fig. 13-2, *C*). A Venti mask applies the Bernoulli principle by infusing 100% oxygen through a narrow orifice. The high-velocity stream of oxygen creates subatmospheric pressure after leaving the orifice, entraining room air through ports at the base of the mask. By altering the size of the orifice, various concentrations of oxygen are achieved. A minimum amount of oxygen flow is required to achieve a given concentration of oxygen. Flow rates above this level do not result in a significant change in FiO_2. The maximum FiO_2 with a Venti mask is 55%. The patient's respiratory rate and pattern do not affect the concentration of oxygen. The Venti mask is used when fairly exact concentrations of oxygen are needed, such as with hy-

---

Correct application of mask

1. Connect the mask to an oxygen source.
2. Turn on the oxygen to the correct flow, especially with a reservoir bag.
3. Place the mask under the chin and then up and on the nose.
4. Mold the flexible metal device over the bridge of the nose.
5. Holding the mask in place with one hand, pull the elastic strap over the head so that it rests above ears.
6. Snug the ends of the elastic strap.
7. Adjust the oxygen flow to meet the patient's needs, if necessary.

Note: Choose an appropriate-sized mask for the patient. Various sizes are available, including special sizes for adults and children.

percapnic hypoxemic patients. Patients with obstructive lung disease commonly use a Venti mask when a nasal cannula is inadequate and exact concentrations of oxygen are needed. Home use of the Venti mask is limited by inconvenience and expense (high-flow rates). The disadvantages are the same as those previously discussed for other masks.

Non-rebreather masks are similar to partial rebreather masks with two exceptions: the non-rebreather mask has a one-way valve that prevents exhaled air from entering the reservoir bag (Fig. 13-2, *D*), and one or more valves covering the air holes on the face mask, to prevent inhalation of room air but allow exhalation of air. When a tight seal over the nose and chin is achieved, a non-rebreather mask delivers up to 100% oxygen. In most instances, the FIO_2 is about 80% to 90%.

When choosing an oxygen delivery device, the amount of oxygen delivered is an important factor; other considerations are the accuracy of the oxygen concentration, patient comfort, and patient expense. Table 13-1 identifies

Table 13-1. Oxygen delivery systems

System	Type	O_2 flow rate	FIO_2
Nasal cannula	Low flow	1 LPM	24%
		2 LPM	28%
		3 LPM	32%
		4 LPM	36%
		5 LPM	40%
		6 LPM	44%
Simple mask	Low flow	5-6 LPM	40%
		6-7 LPM	50%
		7-8 LPM	60%
Partial rebreathing mask	Low flow	6 LPM	60%
		7 LPM	70%
		8 LPM	80%
		9 LPM	90%
		10 LPM	99+%
Venturi mask*	High flow	2 LPM	24%
		3 LPM	28%
		4 LPM	30%
		6 LPM	35%
		8 LPM	40%
		10 LPM	45%
		12 LPM	50%
		14 LPM	55%
Non—rebreathing mask	High flow	4 LPM	40%
		5 LPM	50%
		6 LPM	60%
		7 LPM	70%
		8 LPM	80%
		9 LPM	90%
		10 LPM	100%

*Information is based on Baxter Venti mask; other products may vary.

flow and Fio_2 limitations of various devices. In general, the severity of the oxygenation deficit and the patient's overall acid-base status determine which system to use. In a patient with normal acid-base status and mild hypoxemia, a few liters of oxygen by nasal cannula usually reverses the hypoxemia. When the hypoxemia is moderate, a mask is used. Worsening hypoxemia with normal acid-base status requires institution of a mask with a reservoir bag, either a partial or a non-rebreather mask. For patients with alveolar hypoventilation (elevated $Paco_2$) and hypoxemia, a Venturi mask is applied so that actual Fio_2 is controlled. Although high concentrations of oxygen can be achieved with mask systems, the mask usually does not fit tightly and allows entrainment of room air. When hypoxemia is not reversed with cannula or mask, nasal continuous positive airway pressure (CPAP) or intubation with mechanical ventilation and positive end-expiratory pressure (PEEP) are instituted.

Specific concerns related to home oxygen administration are discussed in a subsequent chapter.

Adverse effects

Like any drug, oxygen has several undesirable effects. Major adverse effects include hypoventilation, absorption atelectasis, and oxygen toxicity. Hypoventilation with resultant hypercapnia is of prime concern in administering oxygen to patients with blunted carbon dioxide stimulation of the respiratory centers. Patients in this category include not only those with severe chronic obstructive pulmonary disease (COPD) and hypercapnia, but also patients with acute drug overdoses, especially barbiturates, narcotics, and heroin. Hypoventilation is such a concern because the drive to breathe results from hypoxemic stimulation of carotid and aortic bodies. When the hypoxemic drive to breathe is reduced or eliminated by supplemental oxygen, the patient hypoventilates, resulting in worsening hypercapnia. Although oxygen is administered cautiously in these patients, the Pao_2 and Sao_2 are never compromised because of increasing $Paco_2$. When hypoxemia exists, supplemental oxygen is necessary. Some clinicians talk of patients belonging to the 50-50 club, when the Pao_2 and $Paco_2$ are each about 50 mm Hg. Supplemental oxygen to increase the Pao_2 to 60 mm Hg is recommended, even though the $Paco_2$ will probably also increase. As long as the patient's renal function is intact, bicarbonate is retained to buffer the change in pH caused by the increased $Paco_2$. Continued hypoventilation and increased $Paco_2$ that is developing into CO_2 narcosis are not treated by inducing hypoxemia but by instituting mechanical ventilation.

Absorption atelectasis is seen in patients receiving high concentrations of oxygen. During administration of high concentrations of oxygen, nitrogen, an inert gas relatively insoluble in blood, is washed from the alveoli. The nitrogen, which is responsible for much of the residual volume in alveoli, is replaced by oxygen. Readily soluble in blood, oxygen is rapidly absorbed. With little or no nitrogen to keep them open, the alveoli collapse. This is particularly true in areas where ventilation is low in relation to perfusion. Oxygen is absorbed from the alveoli faster than fresh air can replace it. Areas of mucus plugging are notorious for developing absorption atelectasis.

Oxygen toxicity. Oxygen toxicity is seen in patients receiving high levels of oxygen therapy for an extended period. It complicates the course in patients with adult respiratory distress syndrome (ARDS) and other diseases requiring high FiO_2. Most cases of oxygen toxicity occur in mechanically ventilated patients because there is little chance for dilution of oxygen by room air. Patients receiving high concentrations of oxygen by mask have less exposure because the mask is removed frequently, and air leaks around it.

With administration of 90% oxygen or higher concentrations, bronchoscopy identified decreased mucociliary clearance within 3 hours of exposure. In normal individuals, administration of 100% oxygen for 6 hours irritated the tracheobronchial tree, producing a cough and substernal chest pain. Signs of oxygen toxicity occur in patients after administration of 100% oxygen for 24 hours, although pulmonary function is unchanged until after this point. Frank pulmonary edema requires exposure of 48 to 72 hours to an O_2 concentration of 50% or higher. With hyperbaric oxygen, signs of oxygen toxicity may occur as soon as 6 to 12 hours.

Research in oxygen toxicity implicates free oxygen radicals in the development of oxygen toxicity. Both direct and indirect cellular injury occur as a result of high FiO_2. Direct cytotoxic effects result from incomplete reduction of oxygen, which leads to generation of toxic oxygen radicals. Superoxide anion, hydrogen peroxide, hydroxyl radical, and singlet oxygen are a few types of oxygen radicals that cause structural and functional derangements. Indirect cytotoxic effects include damage of the alveolar macrophage, destruction of type I alveolar cells, and injury of the pulmonary-capillary endothelium. When alveolar macrophages are injured, neutrophils rush to the area and release other injurious agents, including prostaglandins.

Early in oxygen toxicity there is an exudative phase that causes alveolar and interstitial pulmonary edema. Surfactant production is reduced, causing atelectasis. Progression of the disease causes hyaline membrane formation and focal hemorrhage. The exudative phase is followed by a subacute proliferative phase, which involves hyperplasia of type II pneumocytes and interstitial cells. In some patients the injury resolves; in others, interstitial fibrosis and focal emphysema occur. Oxygen toxicity is difficult to differentiate from ARDS.

Symptoms of oxygen toxicity develop after 48 hours of exposure to FiO_2 of 50% or higher. Patients have tracheobronchial irritation, a dry cough, and chest tightness. Progression of oxygen toxicity gives rise to progressive breathlessness and sometimes hemoptysis. Chest assessment often identifies crackles and wheezes but no findings of consolidation. Arterial blood gas analysis reveals progressive hypoxemia despite oxygen therapy. The $A\text{-}aO_2$ widens; similar changes indicating worsening oxygenation are noted in the decreased arterial/alveolar ratio (a/AO_2) (see Chapter 9). The chest x-ray film shows patchy atelectasis and alveolar and interstitial infiltrates. Signs of volume loss may appear, and pleural effusions are present in many patients. Pulmonary function tests demonstrate restriction with decreases in lung volumes and capacities. Compliance and diffusing capacity (D_{LCO}) are also reduced.

The amount of oxygen and the length of exposure determine the risk of lung injury. Although the FiO_2 is important in determining the risk for oxygen toxicity, partial pressure is also notable. For instance, astronauts breathe 100% oxygen for days to weeks without developing oxygen toxicity. The difference is that they breathe the high concentration at one third atm (approximately 250 mm Hg) instead of 1 atm (760 mm Hg). (Using the alveolar air equation, the FiO_2 at one third atm is about 30%).

The following guidelines can help reduce the risk of oxygen toxicity:

- Use the least amount of oxygen required to normalize Pa_{O_2} and Sa_{O_2}; if Sa_{O_2} is above 90% and Pa_{O_2} is above 60 to 80 mm Hg, decrease Fi_{O_2}. A Pa_{O_2} above 100 mm Hg is unnecessary.
- Use intermittent exposure to high Fi_{O_2}.
- Use 50% Fi_{O_2} or less whenever possible, since it is associated with much less risk.
- Use PEEP for mechanically ventilated patients to decrease high Fi_{O_2}.
- Decrease the Fi_{O_2} as soon as the patient's condition permits.
- Avoid factors that increase the patient's susceptibility to oxygen toxicity, including corticosteroids, hyperthyroidism, vitamin E deficiency, hyperthermia, adrenergic stimulation, and the weed killer paraquat.

In infants excessive oxygen administration often results in the development of retrolental fibroplasia. In premature newborns, exposure to high levels of oxygen causes constriction of retinal vessels and damage to endothelial cells. The Fi_{O_2} is not as critical as the Pa_{O_2} in these infants. Progression of the injury causes retinal detachment and blindness. Development of retrolental fibroplasia depends on the infant's degree of prematurity, the Pa_{O_2}, and the length of exposure. Maintaining the Pa_{O_2} in a normal range decreases the likelihood of retrolental fibroplasia. Similar problems are seen in adults with previous retinal disease.

HUMIDIFICATION AND AEROSOLIZATION

One of the functions of the respiratory system is humidification. Air is breathed into the body at different temperatures and different humidities. By the time inspired air reaches the lungs, it is warmed to body temperature (37° C) and fully saturated with water (100% relative humidity). Most of this is achieved by the upper respiratory system. When this system is bypassed, as with endotracheal intubation or tracheostomy, warming and humidifying inspired air is a necessary therapy in most patients. Failure to provide adequate humidity in inspired air predisposes the patient to thickened secretions and infection, because the mucociliary clearance system requires warmth and moisture to function properly.

A thin layer of fluid supports the mucus layer that covers the cilia. Drying of the fluid or mucus layers can damage cilia, dry mucous membranes, and promote infection. Aerosol therapy supplies additional humidity to the respiratory system, but it is *not* a substitute for adequate systemic hydration; neither is normal saline lavage through an artificial airway.

Recall that goblet cells produce mucus, which the ciliated, pseudostratified columnar cells propel up to the epiglottis. Innervated by the autonomic nervous system, goblet cells respond to nervous activity or to drugs that affect the autonomic nervous system. These cells are also affected by direct irritation and chronic pulmonary conditions. In some chronic lung diseases, goblet cells undergo metaplasia or hyperplasia, which increases the amount of mucus and impairs the lungs' ability to expel excessive mucus. Lung mucus is relatively insoluble in water and has properties of both a fluid and a solid. Like a fluid, mucus flows when stressed; like a solid, it has properties of elasticity (that is, it can stretch and relax). Mucus also has properties of viscosity, which can impede or promote mucus flow from the lung.

In the hospital humidity is usually supplied by bubblers or nebulizers, whereas in the home a simple centrifugal humidifier or vaporizer usually is used. Bubblers are commonly used to humidify low-flow oxygen systems and are rarely heated. Current recommendations suggest limiting the use of bubblers in patients receiving less than 4 LPM of supplemental oxygen.

Bubblers work by breaking gas into small particles as it passes through the water. A porous stone on a long stem accomplishes this task. Bubblers provide up to 5 LPM of gas with 38% to 48% relative humidity at 37° C and typically have high airflow resistance. Efficiency is improved as bubbles are made smaller, because a larger total gas surface contacts water for maximum vaporization. At higher flow rates, efficiency and humidity are decreased. Many bubbler devices are prefilled and disposable, although reusable devices are available.

Bubble humidifiers of the diffuser-bubbler type are also used. They are less flow dependent than plain bubble humidifiers, and airflow resistance is lessened. More and smaller bubbles are produced at higher gas flows. Diffuser-bubbler humidifiers can provide 100% humidity to the airway. Diffuser-bubbler humidifiers are used in high-flow oxygen systems, high humidity masks and tents, and ventilator circuits. Heated water commonly is used in the lower airway, but cool water is usually used to supply humidity in the upper airway. In practice, a ventilator cascade is a diffuser-bubbler-type humidifier. Bennett Cascade is a common brand of diffuser-bubbler humidifier.

The humidifiers just described, which supply only water vapor to the airway, are often classified as true humidifiers. Other humidifiers, such as nebulizers, can add water vapor and particulate water or aerosols, such as medications or saline, to the airway. The most common aerosols used for inhalation are sterile distilled water and physiological or weak saline (less than 0.9% sodium chloride [NaCl]).

A nebulizer is a baffled device that produces a relatively stable aerosol. Also called a jet atomizer or jet nebulizer, the nebulizer is pneumatically powered and delivered through a mask or mouthpiece. In the nebulizer reservoir, liquid is sheared by a high-velocity stream of air. Droplets of liquid are formed, varying in size from a few micrometers to 50 μm or more. Larger droplets of liquid impact and are either subjected to subsequent renebulization or are deposited. In general, particles smaller than 30 μm are deposited in the lower airway, whereas larger particles impact in the tubing or upper airway. The inhaled aerosolized particles are relatively uniform in size and remain stable in suspension. Heating nebulized aerosols increases the humidity.

Either large or small reservoirs are used with this type of nebulizer. When small reservoirs are used intermittently, the process usually is called *sidestream nebulization,* indicating that nebulized particles are injected into a main gas flow. The alternative is *mainstream nebulization,* in which the aerosol is part of the main gas flow. Large reservoirs are used with mainstream nebulization because it usually is continuous therapy. Many of the mainstream jet nebulizers can also deliver variable oxygen concentrations through a Venturi device called a dilution control valve.

Nebulizers also generate aerosols with ultrasonic energy converted from electricity. These devices use ultrasonic pressure waves to break liquids in a special chamber into small particles. At higher frequencies smaller particles are produced, often as small as 5 μm. The aerosolized particles are suspended in air and transported to the patient. Ultrasonic aerosols are naturally high in humidity and do not require heating. In addition, particle size is more uniform than with nebulizers.

Centrifugal humidifiers use a rotating set of radially oriented blades to produce an area of low pressure in the center and high pressure at the periphery of the container. Water, drawn through an immersed tube, is flung centrifugally against a screen, where it is broken into small particles. A mist containing gas flows from the periphery of the rotating unit to be channeled through a tube or blown into a room. DeVilbiss and Hankscraft, among others, produce cool spray versions of centrifugal humidifiers.

The primary indication for aerosol therapy is improving mucus expulsion from the lung, although there is disagreement over whether bland aerosols actually thin mucus to aid in expectoration. Aerosols may deliver water, saline, or medications. When water or saline are used, the term *bland aerosol* is applied. Bland aerosols may increase airway resistance, especially in patients with hyperreactive airways (such as with asthma). Because of this bland aerosol sputum induction often is preceded by inhaled bronchodilator therapy. Bland aerosols may also cause weight gain, increased respiratory rate, and lowered serum osmolalities suggestive of fluid overload; they also have caused atelectasis and pulmonary edema in animal studies. Antibiotics, bronchodilators, and corticosteroids are among inhaled medications administered by nebulizer. Normal airway functioning causes much of inhaled humidity and medications to be deposited in the upper airway. To enhance deposition of aerosols in the lower airway, the nurse should encourage the patient to take slow, deep breaths through the mouth.

Another indication for aerosol therapy is inducing a cough for sputum production. Sputum is induced by this method when the patient is unable to produce sputum for laboratory analysis, especially microbiological or cytological tests. Usually performed very early in the morning, before the patient has been up and moving, sputum induction involves inhalation of aerosolized water or hypertonic saline using a jet nebulizer or ultrasonic nebulizer. Water is used first, since it usually is effective in inducing a cough. Failure of water to achieve sputum results in administration of hypertonic saline (usually 3% to 10% NaCl). It is believed that hypertonic saline produces bronchorrhea from irritation of the tracheobronchial mucosa or that it changes the viscosity of the sputum. Hypertonic saline sputum induction is not performed in patients with hyperreactive airways, such as with asthma, because severe bronchospasm can result.

One of the biggest problems with aerosol equipment is that when improperly handled or inadequately cleaned or disinfected, it can introduce bacteria or mold into the patient's airway. This is true whether the device is a handheld nebulizer or a floor centrifugal humidifier. Preventing aerosolization of bacteria and mold is very important. It is essential that the equipment be rinsed with water after each use and cleaned with soap and water at least daily. In hospitalized patients, use of disposable equipment or daily disinfection is important.

EFFECTIVE COUGHING

One of the most important components of airway clearance is effective coughing. Encouraging effective coughing is a primary nursing responsibility that cannot be overemphasized. Clearing secretions improves air exchange and ultimately gas exchange. A cough is elicited in a normal individual when the mucociliary clearance system is unable to clear secretions effectively. The primary stimulants for a cough are irritant receptors in the lower airways.

The larynx and carina are more sensitive to irritants, and coughs originate there more frequently.

Effective coughing requires a deep inspiration followed by closure of the glottis (epiglottis and vocal cords) and active contraction of the expiratory muscles, especially abdominal muscles. Deep inspiration not only increases lung volume but also widens the airway to allow air to pass distal to obstructing mucus. Air must be behind mucus to propel it forward. Contraction of the expiratory muscles against a closed glottis results in increased intrathoracic pressure. Upon opening of the glottis, air is expelled at high flow and speed to enhance movement of mucus out of the lungs. Since higher flows are achieved when lung volumes are high and recoil is greatest, a large breath is necessary for effective coughing.

The disadvantage to coughing from high lung volumes is that only large airways will be cleared of secretions, because of the point of equalization of pressures between the alveoli and the environment. Coughing from smaller lung volumes moves the point of equal pressure more distal, resulting in airway clearance from smaller airways. It is important to remember that coughing from lower lung volumes also decreases the expiratory flow rate and lessens the effectiveness of the cough. The most effective coughing techniques encourage one large breath followed by several "coughs" at successively smaller lung volumes to clear secretions from all airways.

Patients have ineffective coughs for many reasons. Some patients have altered irritant receptors, perhaps from prolonged intubation or neurological trauma. Other patients are unable to initiate a deep breath because of pain or neuromuscular or musculoskeletal abnormalities. Muscles weakened or dysfunctional from prolonged immobility, inflammation, surgery, trauma, or sedation cannot generate sufficient volume or intrathoracic pressure to produce an effective cough. Also, intubated patients cannot close the glottis and increase intrathoracic pressure. Patients with obstructive lung diseases cannot generate high expiratory flows, and those with spinal cord injuries cannot actively contract abdominal muscles. In addition, other structural abnormalities such as bronchiectasis or tracheal malacia can impair the patient's ability to clear secretions effectively.

Posture is important in effective coughing. Lying supine in bed is not conducive to effective coughing. The preferred position is sitting upright with feet on the floor and leaning slightly forward to compress abdominal contents against the diaphragm. Alternately, a side-lying position with the hips and knees flexed improves muscular contraction and the effectiveness of the cough.

Distinguishing an effective cough from an ineffective one is fairly easy, based on the sound of the cough and whether sputum is produced. A normal effective cough has a deep, hollow sound and occurs at various lung volumes from total lung capacity (TLC) through functional residual capacity (FRC) to expel mucus from both large and small airways. It generally produces sputum. Conversely, an ineffective, nonproductive cough usually is high pitched. It commonly originates in the throat or high in the chest and is accompanied by low volumes and inadequate contraction of abdominal muscles. An ineffective cough does not usually produce sputum. Some patients have an annoying hacking or tickling cough, especially after extubation. This cough also occurs with the initiation of chest physical therapy. Sipping warm or room-temperature water reduces irritation that induces a hacking cough from these causes.

Table 13-2. Types of effective coughs

Cascade cough

1. Take a deep breath and hold it for 1-3 seconds.
2. Cough out forcefully several times until all air is exhaled (usually two to six coughs).
3. Inhale slowly through the nose.
4. Repeat once, if necessary.
5. Rest.
6. Repeat as needed.

Huff cough

1. Take a deep breath and hold it for 1-3 seconds.
2. Keeping glottis open, cough out several times until all air is exhaled (usually two to six huff coughs). Sometimes it helps to say the word "huff" while coughing.
3. Inhale slowly through the nose.
4. Repeat as necessary.

End-expiratory cough

1. Take a deep breath and hold it for 1-3 seconds.
2. Exhale slowly.
3. At the end of the exhalation, cough once.
4. Inhale slowly through the nose.
5. Repeat as necessary.
6. Follow with a cascade or huff cough, in which secretions are moved from small to larger airways.

Augmented cough

1. Take a deep breath and hold it for 1-3 seconds.
2. Perform one or more of the following maneuvers:
    a. Tighten knees and buttocks to increase intraabdominal pressure
    b. Bend forward at the waist to increase intraabdominal pressure
    c. Place the hand flat on the upper abdomen just under the xiphoid process and press in and up abruptly during the cough or exhalation, *or* place hands on the lateral rib cage and quickly press in and release with each cough (called rib springing).
    d. Keep hands on the chest wall and press inward with each cough.
3. Inhale slowly through the nose.
4. Rest, if necessary.
5. Repeat as needed.

The error that most nurses make in attempting to induce sputum by coughing is that they try only one method. This method, the "take a deep breath and cough" technique, clears only large airways. It also increases intracranial pressure and causes pain in patients who have thoracic injuries or are recovering from surgery. Table 13-2 gives instructions for several different types of effective coughs that can clear secretions.

The first step in any effective cough maneuver is a deep breath. Breathing in slowly promotes recruitment of alveoli without overinflating patent alveoli. Holding the full breath for 1 second or longer allows some previously collapsed alveoli to open. Getting the patient to take a deep breath often is challenging, especially with patients who have had surgery. Techniques such as asking the patient to yell or to blow up a balloon encourage deep breathing. However, actually blowing up the balloon can cause small airways to collapse; the important part of blowing up a balloon (or using blow bottles) is the deep breath taken before blowing out. For this reason blow bottles are rarely used today. The nurse may also encourage lateral chest expansion by placing her hands on the patient's chest wall and asking the patient to focus on moving the hands out. Changing the focus from taking a deep breath to moving the hands works with some patients. Incentive spirometers are useful visual aids for how deep a breath the patient is taking. They are discussed later in this chapter.

Critical to every cough is breathing in through the nose after coughing. This prevents mucus that has been moved higher in the airways but not expelled from being sucked back down into the airways by a too-rapid, open mouth inhalation. Paroxysmal coughing is also prevented or minimized by breathing in through the nose instead of the mouth after a cough. Another important consideration is pain control, both systemically and locally. Systemic pain control with analgesics often improves the patient's efforts to maintain a patent airway. In addition, local counterpressure with a firm pillow or folded pad against broken ribs, chest tubes, thoracic and abdominal incisions, and other pain-inducing points helps assists the patient initiate a more effective cough. Ideally, with surgical patients the techniques of effective coughing are taught and practiced before surgery.

The goal of coughing is to produce mucus. The cascade cough, or controlled cough, is performed by taking a deep breath and coughing several times, until all air has been exhaled. The cough occurs at various lung volumes and is generally effective in producing sputum. Modifying the cascade cough by maintaining an open glottis produces the huff cough. A huff cough does not have the characteristic hollow sound of the cascade cough; rather, it sounds like exaggerated or forced exhalations. Some explain the huff cough as more like clearing the throat, only from the lungs. Huff coughing is useful in patients with hyperreactive airways. In patients with secretions in the distal airways, an end-expiratory cough aids in moving secretions more proximally. The end-expiratory cough is initiated from functional residual capacity. The augmented cough, also called the manual or diaphragmatic cough, involves augmenting expiratory movements by increasing intrathoracic or intraabdominal pressure during coughing.

DEEP BREATHING AND INCENTIVE THERAPY

Deep breathing is a very important technique for preventing secretions from accumulating in the lungs. It helps loosen secretions for coughing and maintains the patency of alveoli. Without deep breathing, atelectasis and pneumonia occur. Other beneficial effects of deep breathing are improved venous return of blood to the heart, improved muscle relaxation, and improved control of anxiety and dyspnea. The best position for deep breathing is sitting with the feet firmly placed on the floor. The head is upright, and the shoulders are relaxed. For patients unable to assume an upright position, semi-Fowler position with the head and arms supported by pillows facilitates deep breathing. Knees are flexed on pillows to relax abdominal muscles for maximum diaphragmatic movement.

Deep breathing begins with a slow, deep inhalation. A slow breath pre-

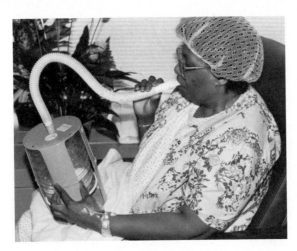

Fig. 13-3. Patient using a volume incentive spirometer to prevent postoperative atelectasis.

vents or minimizes pain from sudden pressure changes in the chest. The number of breaths should not exceed 10 to 12 per minute. At the end of inspiration, the patient holds his breath for a few seconds to promote alveolar expansion. Exhalation is passive. Some patients may prefer to yawn instead of deep breathing.

Incentive breathing therapy, also called incentive spirometry, is a method of providing visual feedback for inspiratory efforts. The primary indication for incentive spirometry is prevention of postoperative atelectasis. It is also useful for patients with signs of mucus retention in the lungs, shallow breathing, and chronic lung disease, and for those confined to complete bed rest. Incentive spirometry is useful for patients with reduced vital capacity or for those who cannot deep breathe without visual cues. For postoperative incentive spirometry to be most effective, it should be practiced before surgery to demonstrate the patient's ability to deep breathe *to the patient*. This serves as a potent reminder of loss of lung function compared to the patient's own normal and not to a nebulous graph of normal people of the same age, sex, and height.

Incentive spirometers work by increasing negative intrathoracic pressure. Transient increases in negative intrathoracic pressure, such as periodic sighs, maintain airway patency, especially postoperatively, when analgesics and pain decrease normal sighing.

There are two types of incentive spirometers: volume spirometers and flow spirometers. Volume incentive spirometers are the better of the two types. With this spirometer, the patient places a mouthpiece firmly between the teeth and takes in a deep breath through the mouth while watching a volume gauge (Fig. 13-3). The patient is encouraged to take as deep a breath as possible to achieve a goal based on the patient's age, sex, and height or preoperative performance. At the end of inspiration, the patient ideally holds his breath for up to 10 seconds for maximum alveolar opening. For optimum benefit, especially with atelectasis, an inspiratory hold is necessary; once collapsed, alveoli require more pressure to open. The patient then removes the mouthpiece and exhales normally.

Volume incentive spirometers are available in nondisposable and disposable models. The nondisposable type functions as a pneumotachometer. It usually has lights or a tone to indicate that the patient has achieved a given volume. Some are geared specifically to children. Mouthpieces are changed between patients to control infection. Nondisposable incentive spirometers are generally reserved for institutional use.

With disposable models the nurse or therapist moves an indicator or pointer to the desired predicted or preoperative volume. The disposable incentive spirometer contains a piston or bellows to register volumes as the patient inhales. Because disposable incentive spirometers are made of light-weight plastic, they are reasonably inexpensive and can easily be used in the home.

The flow incentive spirometer depends on inspiratory flow to elevate one or more balls in a chamber. Upon elevating the balls, the patient holds his breath for as long as possible to maximize alveolar opening. With a flow incentive spirometer it is difficult to sustain inspiratory flow and to keep the balls elevated for longer than 1 to 2 seconds. Tidal volume is unknown with flow incentive spirometers, although it may be estimated by multiplying the flow rate by the length of time the balls are suspended in the air. Errors in assessment of lung function can occur, however, because the balls can be elevated with a brisk but relatively low-volume breath. In addition, patients who breathe in slowly but deeply may not elevate the balls, even though they inspire to total lung capacity.

The most important component of successful deep breathing or incentive spirometry, after mastering the technique, is repetition. With acutely ill patients, incentive spirometry is performed hourly while the patient is awake for at least 10 deep breaths or 5 minutes. As the patient's condition improves, the interval between treatments is increased. Most patients continue to perform incentive spirometry at least every 4 hours while hospitalized. Upon discharge, if the patient is still producing sputum, incentive spirometry is performed soon after awakening and throughout the day as needed to enhance sputum production. Incentive spirometry is performed before coughing and chest physical therapy to enhance secretion removal.

CHEST PHYSICAL THERAPY

A major complication of immobility and illness is the development of retained secretions, which predisposes the patient to atelectasis or pneumonia. Some patients, such as those with chronic bronchitis, bronchiectasis, cystic fibrosis, or a lung abscess, have hypersecretion of mucus and retention of sputum from chronic lung diseases. Chest physical therapy (also called chest PT or CPT) uses one or more techniques to enhance removal of secretions from the airways when deep breathing (including incentive spirometry) and coughing are ineffective.

Traditionally, chest physical therapy includes postural drainage, chest percussion, vibration, and rib shaking. Deep breathing and coughing remain important when chest physical therapy is used. Review the pulmonary rehabilitation techniques of pursed-lip and diaphragm breathing before initiating chest physical therapy. Throughout chest physical therapy, the patient performs pursed-lip and diaphragm breathing to enhance relaxation, to promote gas exchange, and to prevent alveolar collapse.

The nurse works with the respiratory and physical therapists in performing chest physical therapy. In some institutions the respiratory therapist is responsible for administering CPT; in others the physical therapist, the nurse, or both perform CPT. Nurses may perform CPT or may coordinate it with additional treatments by other therapists. Especially with patients fed by gastric tube, the nurse works with the therapist to schedule feedings and treatments. Chest physical therapy also must be scheduled with regard to sitting in the chair, weaning trials, rest periods, and other treatments. When a physical therapist performs CPT but a respiratory therapist administers inhaled bronchodilator treatments, efforts must be coordinated to optimize both treatments.

Postural drainage

Postural drainage (also called PD) refers to positioning of the patient to facilitate gravitational drainage of secretions from various segments of the lung (Fig. 13-4). The rationale for positioning is that secretions will move by gravity, instead of against it, from distal to proximal areas of the lung, where they can be coughed out. This is analogous to pouring ketchup from a bottle: the ketchup flows when the bottle is turned upside down to allow gravity drainage. In general, the area being drained is uppermost, usually facing the ceiling. This allows the bronchus to be at a vertical or near vertical position to maximize gravitational drainage.

The positions used for PD are determined by the patient's clinical status. Before performing postural drainage, the nurse must know the following:

The patient's diagnosis and clinical status, as well as his neurological status, cardiac status, and activity level

The lung areas involved (as indicated by auscultation and chest x-ray film)

The history of previous thoracic operations

Whether the patient has osteoporosis or any structural abnormalities, such as fractured ribs

The patient's diagnosis often identifies the area to receive percussion, such as "right lower lobe pneumonia." Most patients do not need every postural drainage position. A common exception is patients with cystic fibrosis or some other homogenous disease. When a specific segment or lobe is involved, chest physical therapy is directed to that area, saving the nurse and the patient time and energy.

Secretions usually pool in the lower and middle lung fields. In hospitalized or bedridden patients, the posterior areas of the lung are often involved. Unless the patient is positioned prone, the right middle lobe is rarely involved because of its anterior position. Some patients are dyspneic even when sitting upright. Positioning the patient in a head-down position often is not possible with severely dyspneic patients, because the shortness of breath worsens when the diaphragm is pushed up by the abdominal contents. CPT positions are modified according to the patient's clinical condition. Realize that altering the chest physical therapy position may decrease the effectiveness of the treatment.

The type and amount of sputum produced sometimes can be predicted on the basis of the patient's diagnosis. Sputum production is usually minimal with atelectasis. Patients with bronchiectasis have copious, thick, viscid sputum that often is hard to expectorate. With lung abscesses, secretions are foul smelling, purulent, and thick. Thick mucous plugs usually accompany pneumonia. Longer periods of gravitational drainage are necessary to allow thicker secretions to move.

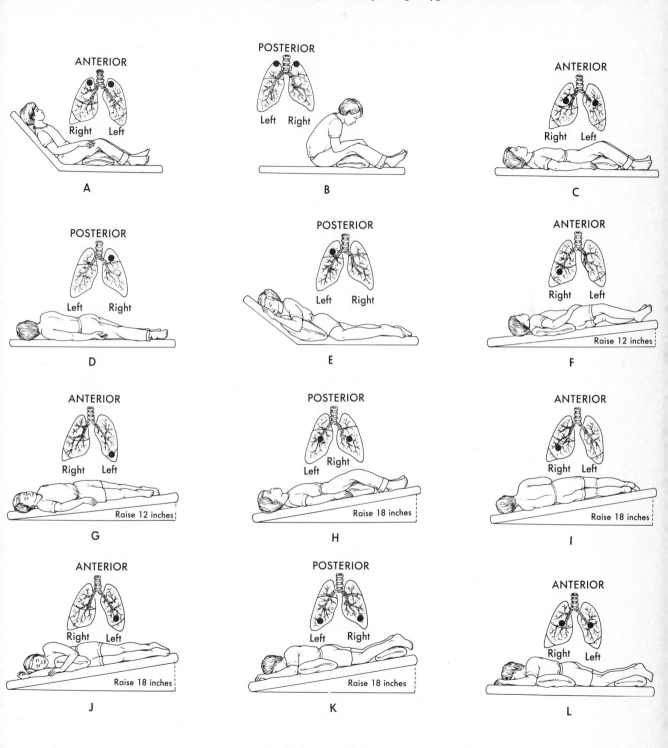

Fig. 13-4. Chest physical therapy positions. (From Thompson J, et al: *Mosby's manual of clinical nursing*, ed 2, St Louis, 1989, Mosby–Year Book.)

The patient's neurological and cardiovascular status are two important factors to consider when administering chest physical therapy. Gravitational drainage can aggravate the condition of patients with certain conditions, such as a cervical spine injury, a closed head injury, or a subarachnoid hemorrhage. Head-down positions are not used with patients with increased intracranial pressure, because the increased blood flow to the brain elevates the intracranial pressure further. The same is true for patients who have had eye surgery or who have various types of cardiac disease. Congestive heart failure and some dysrhythmias are exacerbated by head down positions.

In mobile patients the upper lobes frequently do not require gravitational drainage unless certain segments are involved, since the upper lobes drain in upright individuals. The exception is the patient with upper lobe tuberculosis who requires postural drainage, usually in conjunction with percussion. In addition, patients confined to bed and lying with the head of the bed flat are apt to aspirate or accumulate secretions throughout the lung fields. Frequently changing the patient's position (side lying, supine, or prone with head flat and at various elevations) helps to prevent secretions from accumulating in a particular area.

In patients who have had previous thoracic surgery involving lung resection or a severe lung abscess, the normal anatomy of the lung is altered, and the postural drainage positions are adapted to the changed anatomy. The posterior-anterior, portable anterior-posterior, and lateral chest x-ray films provide clues to proper positioning. Sometimes trial- and-error positioning is necessary to find the most appropriate position for producing secretions.

The patient may have other conditions that affect chest physical therapy. Osteoporosis, for example, is not a contraindication to PD, but positioning may need to be altered for patients with thoracic compression fractures. Also, percussion is painful for patients with thoracic compression fractures. Fractured ribs rarely require special positioning, but they usually require care during administration of percussion. Precautions to consider with postural drainage are highlighted in Table 13-3.

Percussion

Percussion is an adjunct to postural drainage. In some patients postural drainage alone moves secretions from smaller to larger airways, where they can be coughed out. In other patients mucus requires the assistance of percussion (also called cupping, tapping, or clapping) to facilitate the flow of mucus out of the lungs. Percussion is most useful in patients who produce at least 30 ml of sputum daily. The best analogy is again the ketchup bottle. Some brands of ketchup do not flow well unless one pounds on (percussion) the bottom of the bottle. Some brands require shaking (vibration or rib shaking) in addition to pounding. After a few shakes and some pounding on the bottle, the ketchup suddenly comes out. This is how postural drainage, percussion, vibration, and rib shaking work, although they are done more gently than with a ketchup bottle.

To perform percussion, the hand must be cupped as if to swim, cover the mouth, or scoop up a handful of water (Fig. 13-5). The fingers and thumb are held together tightly so that air cannot escape. The wrists rhythmically flex and extend as the hands alternately strike the chest. The arms are extended without locking the elbows, and the shoulders are relaxed. The whole rim of the hand touches the chest at the same time. As the hands contact the chest,

Table 13-3. Precautions with chest physical therapy

Cardiac precautions

Acute myocardial infarction	Head-down positions may aggravate ischemia and extend infarct.

Gastrointestinal precautions

Gastric reflux	Use caution and perform CPT before meals; head-down positions promote gastric reflux.
Gastric tube feedings	Use caution. Continuous feedings should be stopped 1 hour before PD, which can greatly reduce caloric intake. PD is performed before administration of intermittent feedings. Duodenal or jejunal tube feedings may continue if there is no retrograde reflux.

Neurological precautions

Increased intracranial pressure	Head-down positions increase intracranial blood volume and intracranial pressure.
Cervical spinal cord injury with patient in tongs	Altering the incline of the neck changes alignment and may aggravate injury. However, in some cases the head of the bed can be kept at its ordered level and Trendelenburg positioning of the entire bed can be used to alter the position of the lower lungs relative to the head.
Subarachnoid hemorrhage	Head-down positions increase cerebral blood pressure and may exacerbate bleeding.

Pulmonary precautions

Severe dyspnea and anxiety	Head-down positions exacerbate dyspnea and anxiety; abdominal contents push up against the diaphragm, making inhalation difficult, and the patient enters a vicious circle of increased anxiety and increased dyspnea.
Bronchopulmonary fistula	Chest tubes are not an absolute contraindication to CPT; however, percussion may prevent sealing or enlarge the fistula.
Frank hemoptysis	Percussion may disrupt clots and exacerbate bleeding, resulting in pulmonary hemorrhage. Also, head-down positions increase blood return to the chest and may cause recruitment or distention of capillaries.
Flail chest	Percussion over the flail area exacerbates bruising or bleeding and may cause additional lung punctures.
Pulmonary embolism	Local consolidation is due to pulmonary embolism. Other clots, especially in the heart and central veins, may dislodge.

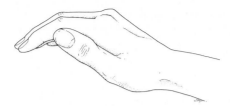

Fig. 13-5. Hand position for percussion. (From Beare P, Myers J: *Principles and practice of adult health nursing,* St Louis, 1990, Mosby–Year Book.)

an air pocket is created that sends vibrations through the chest. Percussion creates a hollow sound and is not painful when performed properly. Some clinicians liken the sound to a horse's hooves on pavement. Flattened hands produce a slapping sound, and percussion performed with flat hands usually is painful for the patient. Some families become upset when they first see percussion, because they think the patient is being beaten. Percussing the chest of the family member for a few seconds demonstrates that CPT is not painful, but actually feels good.

Percussion is performed over a single thin layer of clothing such as a T-shirt or pajamas. Using thick clothing or towels dampens the vibrations, making the nurse work harder and the treatment less effective. After percussion the skin should not be reddened or bruised. The nurse should also note the following points when performing postural drainage and percussion:

Before

- Encourage fluids to promote hydration for thinner secretions.
- Perform chest physical therapy 30 to 60 minutes after use of inhaled bronchodilators.
- Use pillows to support the patient and to promote relaxation in postural drainage positions; knees and hips are flexed to prevent back strain.
- Help the patient into the PD position at least 5 minutes before percussion, as able.
- Avoid percussion for 2 hours after a meal to lessen the danger of vomiting. Schedule chest physical therapy at least 30 to 60 minutes before meals or bolus (intermittent) tube feedings. With continuous feedings through a gastric feeding tube, stop feedings at least 1 hour before CPT. With duodenal or jejunal continuous infusion feedings, continue feedings.

During

- Perform chest physical therapy, alternating percussion and vibration, for at least 3 to 5 minutes in each position, longer if tolerated and time permits.
- Auscultate the chest before and after CPT to evaluate the effectiveness of the treatment.
- Encourage pursed lip and diaphragm breathing during chest physical therapy. Slow, deep inhalations and exhalations are important. Air must get behind the mucus before it can be expectorated.
- Do not perform percussion over bony prominences such as the scapula, spine, or clavicles.

- Do not perform percussion over vital organs and sensitive tissue (for example, the breasts, kidneys, liver, and spleen).
- Provide rest periods and coughing breaks as needed.
- Rinse the patient's mouth after sputum has been expectorated.
- Chest physical therapy is usually performed every 2 to 4 hours in acutely ill patients. When several positions are used and bilateral disease is involved, the nurse's time is precious. To effectively drain each lung, the nurse completely performs CPT on one lung and 2 hours later on the opposite lung. In this manner CPT is being performed on each lung every 4 hours with a treatment every 2 hours.
- At home patients usually perform CPT two to four times daily. When CPT is performed twice daily, the best times are early in the morning and before bed. If CPT is performed four times daily, it should be done before meals and at bedtime. Some patients perform CPT only once a day when they are feeling well and sputum production is minimal.

Vibration and rib shaking

Vibration is another technique for enhancing gravitational drainage of secretions. Gentler than percussion, vibration is thought to increase the velocity and turbulence of exhaled air, aiding in the movement of secretions. To perform vibration, the hands are placed on the chest over the area being drained. Some clinicians fan their hands around the chest wall, whereas others place them side by side or on top of each other. The wrists are kept stiff, and the elbows are also kept stiff but not locked. Vibration is generated from the shoulder and upper arm muscles, causing a fine tremulous movement in the hands. During vibration the chest wall is gently compressed. Compression increases throughout exhalation. *Performed only during a slow, controlled exhalation,* vibration does not involve gross shaking of the patient. Rib shaking, on the other hand, is very vigorous. During rib shaking the chest wall is shaken or alternately compressed and released. Vibration and rib shaking are performed three to four times, at 1-minute intervals, during percussion. Performing vibration or rib shaking during percussion aids in preventing fatigue of the nurse.

Although CPT is used in many patients, its effectiveness is controversial. Various studies have demonstrated effectiveness, no effect, and detrimental effects. Also, the role of other therapies clouds the effectiveness of chest physical therapy alone. In general, the literature agrees that CPT benefits patients who produce sputum, especially large volumes of sputum. Some patients expectorate sputum during or immediately after CPT. Other patients do not expectorate sputum until 1 to 2 hours after the procedure, when secretions move up into larger airways. CPT seems to be more beneficial in patients who move around after the treatment. In addition, chest physical therapy is as effective as bronchoscopy in atelectasis. Since chest physical therapy is noninvasive, it is usually instituted before bronchoscopy to promote removal of secretions. The nurse must be sure to confer with the physician or radiologist to identify involved segments so as to use appropriate positions that enhance gravitational drainage. If chest physical therapy is ineffective, the physician may perform bronchoscopy. Contrary to popular belief, bronchoscopy is effective at clearing only the larger airways of mucus plugs.

The possible hazards of CPT are listed in the box below. Some patients

---

Hazards of CPT

Increase in airway resistance
Bruising
Fluctuations in cardiac output
Dysrhythmias
Fatigue
Hypoxemia or a decrease in Pao_2
Pain
Rib fractures
Wheezing

---

develop dyspnea during the procedure or fatigue afterward. Fatigue is more common when the treatment is prolonged and when several positions are used. Other patients develop wheezing and increased airway resistance. The most common side effect of CPT is a decrease in the Pao_2 immediately after a treatment. This fall is presumably due to changes in ventilation-perfusion matching as the patient is placed in various positions. It is well known that the Pao_2 decreases when a patient is placed with the worse lung down, especially with unilateral lung disease. Some patients develop fluctuations in cardiac output or dysrhythmias as a result of CPT. If the nurse's hands are positioned improperly, rib fractures, bruising, and pain can occur.

CONCLUSION

This chapter has reviewed noninvasive techniques to improve oxygenation and ventilation. Most of the techniques, such as coughing, are simple and can be initiated by the nurse. Timely implementation of these noninvasive techniques often can prevent the use of more aggressive invasive measures by the physician. It is important to remember that the basic nursing acts, such as teaching a patient how to deep breathe and cough effectively, learned early in nursing education, are very important in maintaining or restoring the patient's normal state of wellness.

BIBLIOGRAPHY

Bartlett RH: Respiratory therapy to prevent pulmonary complications of surgery, *Respir Care*, 29(6): 667-679, 1984.

Brown LH: Pulmonary oxygen toxicity, *Focus Crit Care* 17(1):68-75, 1990.

Burton GC, Hodgkin JE: *Respiratory care: a guide to clinical practice,* ed 2, Philadelphia, 1984, JB Lippincott.

Campbell EJ, Baker MD, Crites-Silver P: Subjective effects of humidification of oxygen for delivery by nasal cannula: a prospective study, *Chest* 93(2):289-293, 1988.

Christopher KL, Spofford BT, Petrun MD, et al: A program for transtracheal oxygen delivery: assessment of safety and efficacy, *Ann Intern Med* 107(6):802-808, 1987.

Fedorovich C, Littleton MT: Chest physiotherapy: evaluating the effectiveness, *Dimens Crit Care Nurs* 9(2):68-74, 1990.

Georgopoulos D, Anthonisen NR: Continuous oxygen therapy for the chronically hypoxemic patient, *Annu Rev Med* 41:223-230, 1990.

Harper R: *A guide to respiratory care: physiology and clinical applications,* Philadelphia, 1982, JB Lippincott.

Kirilloff LH, Owens GR, Rogers RM, Mazzocco MC: Does chest physical therapy work? *Chest* 88:436-444, 1985.

Mazzocco MC, Owens GR, Kirilloff LH, Rogers RM: Chest percussion and postural drainage in patients with bronchiectasis, *Chest* 88(3):360-363, 1985.

McHugh J: Perfecting the three steps of chest physiotherapy, *Nursing 87* 17(11):54-57, 1987.

McPherson SP: *Respiratory therapy equipment*, St Louis, 1985, Mosby–Year Book.

Mims BC: The risks of oxygen therapy, *RN* 50(7):20-26, 1987.

Moore-Gillon J: Oxygen-conserving delivery devices, *Respir Med* 83(4):263-264, 1989.

Netter F: *The CIBA collection of medical illustrations*, vol 7, *Respiratory system*, New York, 1979, CIBA Pharmaceutical Co.

Nocturnal Oxygen Therapy Trial Group: Continuous or nocturnal oxygen therapy in hypoxemic chronic obstructive lung disease: a clinical trial, *Ann Intern Med* 93(3):391, 1980.

Norton LC, Conforti CG: The effects of body position on oxygenation, *Heart Lung* 14(1):42-52, 1985.

Petty TL: Practical tips on prescribing home oxygen therapy, *Postgrad Med* 84(6): 83-85, 88-90, 1988.

Shapiro B, Harrison R, et al: *Clinical applications of respiratory care*, Chicago, 1985, Mosby–Year Book.

Shigeoka JW, Bonekat HW: The current status of oxygen-conserving devices, *Respir Care* 30(10):833-836, 1985.

Shoemaker WC, Thompson WL, Holbrook PR: *The Society of Critical Care Medicine Textbook of Critical Care*, Philadelphia, 1984, WB Saunders.

Stehlin CS, Schare BC: Systemic and pulmonary changes in rabbits exposed to long-term nebulization of various therapeutic agents, *Heart Lung* 9(2): 311-315, 1980.

Tiep BL, Christopher KL, Spofford BT, et al: Pulsed nasal and transtracheal oxygen delivery, *Chest* 97(2):364-368, 1990.

Tiep BL, Lewis MI: Oxygen conservation and oxygen-conserving devices in chronic lung disease: a review, *Chest* 92(2):263-272, 1987.

Tyler ML: Complications of positioning and chest physical therapy, *Respir Care* 27(4):458, 1982.

Villeneuve MJ, Hodnett ED: Cerebrovascular status and Trendelenburg position in severe head injury, *Axone* 11(3):64-67, 1990.

Wade JF: *Comprehensive respiratory care: physiology and technique*, ed 3, St Louis, 1982, Mosby–Year Book.

Wanner A: Does chest physical therapy move airway secretions? *Am Rev Respir Dis* 130(5):701-702, 1984.

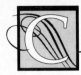

C H·A·P·T·E·R 14

Invasive Techniques for Improving Oxygenation and Ventilation

Objectives:

- Describe the indications, complications, and techniques for inserting nasal and oral airways.
- Identify the indications and procedure for intubation.
- Identify complications of artificial airways.
- Discuss proper cuff care.
- Describe the procedure for extubation.
- Differentiate types of tracheostomy tubes.
- Discuss tracheostomy care and the complications of tracheostomy.
- Describe the technique and complications of suctioning.
- Describe the nurse's role in bronchoscopy.
- Describe the setup and assessment of a chest tube.
- Differentiate milking and stripping of a chest tube.
- Discuss the indications and procedure for pleurodesis (pleurosclerotherapy).

Noninvasive techniques for improving oxygenation and ventilation (discussed in Chapter 13) are fairly basic and thus do not meet the needs of all patients. Many patients also need invasive, technologically advanced treatments that usually require additional nursing interventions. The patients who need invasive respiratory care frequently are in the intensive care unit, but not always. The trend increasingly is toward caring for more acutely ill patients, including those receiving mechanical ventilation, on general nursing floors rather than in the intensive care unit. Also, patients frequently are sent home with a mechanical ventilator; therefore the home also is becoming a place of high technology. This chapter reviews invasive methods of improving oxygenation and ventilation: airways, intubation, tracheostomy, suctioning, bronchoscopy, chest tubes, and pleurodesis.

AIRWAYS

Artificial airways frequently are inserted to maintain airway patency or to prevent trauma from other procedures. The airways discussed in this section are the nasal airway, the oral airway, and the esophageal obturator. A discussion of intubation and tracheostomy follows.

A *nasal pharyngeal airway* or trumpet is inserted to relieve nasal obstruction. Nasal airways are made of flexible plastic or rubber and are available in many sizes. A nasal airway also is used to prevent damage to nasal mucosa when the patient requires frequent nasal tracheal suctioning. Table 14-1 lists the appropriate sizes of nasal pharyngeal airways for adults and children. A nasal airway is inserted in much the same way as a nasogastric tube. The tip of the nasal airway is lubricated and then slid medially and downward along the floor of the nose and through the turbinates. When properly positioned, the nasal airway extends into the posterior nasal pharynx. With slight hyperextension of the neck, a catheter inserted through the nasal airway is positioned in the hypopharynx, just above the epiglottis.

It is common nursing practice to secure the nasal pharyngeal airway in the same way as a nasogastric tube. Alternately, some clinicians insert a large safety pin crosswise in the nasal pharyngeal airway to prevent internal migration. Nasal airways are routinely removed at least every 8 hours for cleaning. To promote sinus drainage, which is obstructed by insertion of a nasal airway, placement of the airway is rotated from one naris to the other, if possible. If the sinuses are not allowed to drain periodically, obstructive sinusitis frequently results. Other complications include epistaxis, ulceration of the nasal mucosa, and otitis media. Contraindications to nasal pharyngeal airways include a basilar skull fracture or nasal fracture.

An *oral airway* is used primarily to relieve upper airway obstruction by a flaccid tongue. In some instances, it is used as a bite block. An oral airway is shaped like a comma or an S and is made of rigid plastic or rubber. The outer flange is flat so as to fit against the lips and allow artificial ventilation without obstruction. The inside of an oral airway has either one central channel or two smaller side channels. Many oral airways do not allow suctioning through them, but around them.

The oral airway is inserted with the curved side down, up, or sideways (according to personal preference and the patient's condition) after the distal end is lubricated with a water-soluble jelly. The more common technique is to insert the oral airway with the curved side down, following the natural curve of the tongue. When an alternate technique is used, the airway is inserted with the curve up or sideways for about one third of its length and then turned curved side down to follow the tongue. In proper position, the oral airway extends just past the base of the tongue in the posterior oral pharynx. It holds the tongue up and away from the posterior pharynx, maintaining a patent hypopharynx. Frequently the oral airway is secured by placing two pieces of tape, ½ to 1 inch wide, from cheek to cheek across the top and bottom flange of the oral airway; however, this arrangement makes it difficult for the nurse to perform mouth care.

During a seizure, the oral airway is useful for preventing mucosal injury of the tongue and cheek from teeth clenching or grinding, as well as for keeping the airway patent. It may not prevent broken teeth from the powerful jaw spasms that accompany seizures. In orally intubated patients, the oral airway prevents damage to the endotracheal tube from biting. With patients who do

Table 14-1. Artificial airway sizes

	Nasal pharyngeal airway	Oral pharyngeal airway	Endotracheal tube or tracheostomy tube* (internal diameter in mm)	Suction catheter (FR†)
Adult male	7-10	3+	7.5-9	14+
Adult female	5-8	3+	7-8.5	12+
Children				
16 years	5+	3+	7	10-12
12 years	4-5+	3	6.5	10
8 years	3-4+	3	6	10
6 years	3+	2	5.5	10
5 years	2	2	5	10
3 years	2	2	4.5	8
Infants				
18 months	x	2	4	8
6 months	x	1	3.5	8
Newborns	x	00	3	6
Preterm infants	x	000	2.5	6

*The size of the endotracheal tube in children is usually the same as the size of the child's little finger. Because of variations in the external diameter of tracheostomy tubes, it is impossible to identify a specific size; see Table 14-3, p. 311, which compares sizes of tracheostomy tubes by manufacturer.
†Denotes French sizes, which are three times the size in millimeters.

not voluntarily open their mouths for oral hygiene, an oral airway facilitates nursing care. When coupled with an endotracheal tube, however, an oral airway also impedes oral hygiene because of its fairly large size. As with nasal airways, oral airways are removed at least every 8 hours for cleaning.

Oral airways have few complications. If the airway inserted is too large for the patient's mouth, it causes gagging from excessive stimulation of the posterior pharynx. (Table 14-1 lists the appropriate sizes of oral airways for adults and children.) Gagging can lead to emesis and aspiration. Improperly positioned airways may cause ulcerations of the patient's mouth, and oral infections result from improper hygiene.

An *esophageal obturator airway* (EOA) is used primarily by emergency personnel to establish an airway for assisting ventilations in an adult. An EOA can be passed easily and requires minimal training for insertion, but it is not available in pediatric sizes. An EOA, which contains a removable transparent mask, is inserted into the esophagus rather than the trachea. An EOA is similar to an endotracheal tube except that the distal end is closed to prevent air from entering and vomitus from leaving the stomach. After the cuff is inflated, occluding the esophagus, mouth-to-mask artificial ventilations are instituted. There are approximately 16 holes in the upper third of the EOA that distribute air from the pharynx into the lungs. The major complications of the EOA are esophageal perforation, inadvertent tracheal intubation, and vomiting on removal of the tube.

An EOA is never removed until an endotracheal tube has been inserted. After the endotracheal tube has been placed, the cuff on the EOA is temporarily deflated to allow passage of a nasogastric tube into the stomach. The cuff is reinflated while the stomach is decompressed. When gastric drainage has been controlled, the EOA cuff is again deflated and the tube removed. Oral suction frequently is necessary when the EOA is removed before gastric decompression. Newer models of the EOA allow gastric suctioning through a one-way valve at the distal end of the tube.

AIR-MASK-BAG UNIT (AMBU)

The first air-mask-bag unit, or ambu, was developed almost 40 years ago. Since that time several ambus of various sizes, shapes, and capabilities have been developed. Other terms used to describe an ambu are resuscitator bag, bag valve mask, manual resuscitator, and hand ventilator. In emergency situations, an ambu is used to manually ventilate patients who have not been intubated. With intubated patients, the mask is removed, allowing the ambu to be connected to the endotracheal tube. Ambus are not restricted to emergency resuscitation. They also are used before and after suctioning to promote hyperinflation in mechanically ventilated patients and in spontaneously breathing patients. An ambu is used during ventilator malfunctions or ventilator circuit changes and when an intubated patient is transported between service areas (for example, to and from the emergency room, operating room, and radiology). When an ambu is used to provide or assist ventilations, the term *bagging* is used.

The ideal ambu rapidly refills after delivery of a breath and does not allow rebreathing. This is accomplished with diaphragms or spring-loaded, leaf, or duckbill valves. Available in both pediatric and adult sizes, the ambu has a standard universal connector with a 22-mm outside diameter and a 15-mm inside diameter. The 22-mm size fits standard anesthesia masks, and the 15-mm size adapts to endotracheal and tracheostomy tubes. An ambu should be capable of delivering high concentrations of oxygen and positive end-expiratory pressure (PEEP). Contrary to popular belief, an ambu does not always deliver 100% oxygen. Most bags achieve an inspired oxygen concentration (Fio_2) between 30% and 95%. The actual percentage of oxygen varies, depending on the construction of the bag, including the presence and length of oxygen reservoir tubing, and the patient's respiratory pattern. Higher concentrations of oxygen require the addition of oxygen reservoir tubing at the end of the bag. With oxygen reservoir tubing, less room air is entrained with reinflation of the bag after delivery of a breath.

The procedure for using an ambu begins with attaching the bag to a source of oxygen. The oxygen is turned on to at least 10 to 15 LPM. Lower oxygen flow rates result in a lower Fio_2. In emergency situations, or to deliver high Fio_2 at high rates, the flowmeter is completely opened, or "turned flush." With a few models, high flow causes the valve to chatter and stick open. In patients who have not been intubated, the mask is attached to the unit. The neck is hyperextended, using the head-tilt/chin-lift or jaw-thrust maneuvers described in Chapter 15. The mask is applied from the chin up over the nose. It helps to hook the thumb and first finger around the center of the mask and the three outer fingers under the jaw to keep the mask in good position. A good seal is necessary for adequate ventilation. The bag is squeezed with the remaining hand. The nurse watches the chest rise and fall as an indicator of adequate positioning of the neck and bag. In some instances one nurse holds the mask on the patient and another squeezes the bag. With two people, ventilations are larger in the adult and more effective.

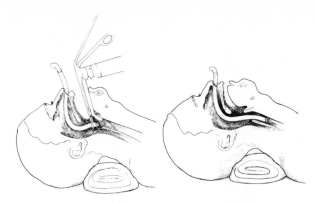

Fig. 14-1. Endotracheal tubes are placed through the nose or mouth into the trachea. (From Abels LF: *Mosby's manual of critical care,* St Louis, 1979, Mosby–Year Book.)

After use the mask and elbow are removed and cleaned with soap and water. They are immediately reconnected to the bag (for rapid access) and allowed to air dry.

Bagging an intubated patient is much easier. The nurse removes the mask from the ambu after connecting the unit to the oxygen source. The elbow adapter on the ambu is connected to the endotracheal or tracheostomy tube. The nurse squeezes the bag to deliver a breath. With an intubated patient, the nurse can squeeze the ambu with both hands and deliver higher volumes. The elbow routinely is removed and cleaned of secretions after each use to prevent the growth of bacteria and nebulization of bacteria into the patient's lungs.

Complications of using an ambu include either underventilating or overventilating the patient. The patient may also be underoxygenated or overoxygenated, depending on the bag, the oxygen flow, and the volume of breaths. When a patient is ventilated with a mask, the chance of air entering the stomach is great. Patients may vomit and aspirate when excessive air enters the stomach. When bags are improperly cleaned, the patient can become infected by nebulization of bacteria into the lungs as the bag is compressed.

INTUBATION

Endotracheal intubation is the insertion of an artificial airway through the nose or mouth into the trachea (Fig. 14-1). An endotracheal tube is inserted because of lower airway obstruction, inability to clear secretions, inadequate minute ventilation, or because adequate oxygenation cannot be achieved with noninvasive methods. A physician, specially trained nurse, paramedic, or respiratory therapist performs the intubation. In most instances the patient is intubated through the mouth, although some patients are intubated through one naris.

Nasal intubation is technically more difficult than oral intubation, because it usually is blind. Nasal intubation is discouraged with patients with bleeding disorders, because insertion of the tube irritates the nasal mucosa and may cause bleeding. Nasal intubation reportedly is more comfortable for the patient. It also allows easier oral hygiene and prevents the patient from biting the tube. With nasal intubation, the tongue cannot manipulate the tube as easily. Thus the nasal tracheal tube is considered more stable than its oral

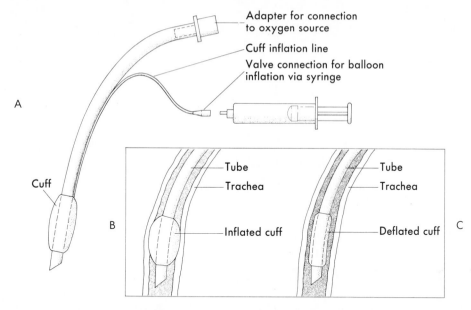

Fig. 14-2. **A,** Parts of a cuffed endotracheal tube. **B,** Cuff inflated in the trachea. **C,** Cuff deflated in the trachea. (From Beare P, Myers J: *Principles and practice of adult health nursing,* St Louis, 1990, Mosby–Year Book.)

counterpart. Better stabilization of the endotracheal tube may prevent damage to the lower airway, especially the larynx, from movement of the tube. With an endotracheal tube in place, the patient should not eat or drink fluids because the epiglottis is being held open by the tube; some physicians do allow eating with a nasal endotracheal tube.

A nasal or oral endotracheal tube is an artificial airway made of permanently curved, flexible plastic. Many manufacturers produce tubes suitable for either oral or nasal intubation. The main difference between an oral and a nasal endotracheal tube is length. Sizing is the same; the physician usually places one size smaller in the nose than in the mouth. An adult endotracheal tube is approximately 30 to 35 cm long; a pediatric tube can be as short as 10 cm.

The size of the endotracheal tube is based on internal diameter (Table 14-1 lists the appropriate sizes for children and adults). The intubationist chooses the correct size tube for the size of the patient. With a child, the size of the child's little finger often is used to approximate the size of the tube. Some sources recommend choosing a pediatric size based on the formula 4.5 + age in years/4 = size in mm, *or* 18 + age in years = French size. (Note: The outcome is about the same with either method. Remember that French sizes are three times the size in mm; that is, a 7-mm tube is equivalent to a 21-mm FR.) In adults, a 7- to 8.5-mm tube is used in women, and a 7.5- to 9-mm tube is used in men.

An endotracheal tube has several features (Fig. 14-2). Adult endotracheal tubes are equipped with cuffs, which usually inflate symmetrically, evenly distributing pressure on the trachea. Cuffs currently in use are high volume and low pressure (soft cuffs), a combination that causes less damage to tracheal walls than the low-volume, high-pressure cuffs (hard cuffs) used formerly. The difference in the two types of cuffs is how much of the cuff is in contact with the tracheal mucosa. The places where the cuff contacts the trachea are points where pressure is exerted. In low-volume (hard) cuffs, all the pressure is exerted against a small area (low compliance, high pressure), whereas high-volume (soft) cuffs spread the pressure over a larger area. The high-volume cuff is better able to conform to the trachea.

The cuff is inflated by means of an inflating tube, which is fused to approximately the lower two thirds of the endotrachael tube. The upper third of the inflating tube is free, so that the tube can be shortened as needed. At the end of the inflating tube is a pilot balloon. The pilot balloon contains a Luer one-way valve, which allows air to be infused and removed with a syringe. This valve also prevents air from escaping from the cuff when the syringe is removed. Some models contain a rubber cap to protect the valve from additional manipulation after the syringe is removed.

The endotracheal tube has depth markings at 1- or 2-cm intervals, extending from about half way up the tube to the 15-mm adapter (machine or proximal end). A radiopaque line extends the entire length of the tube. The distal (or patient) end of the tube is beveled; most tubes have a Murphy eye at the tip.

Procedure

The cuff of the endotracheal tube is assessed for patency by instilling air into the cuff and observing for air leak. (Sometimes patency is also assessed by withdrawing all air from the cuff and watching to see if the cuff reinflates, even slightly, indicating a leak; this is normal procedure for a foam cuff.) The cuff is then completely deflated and lubricated with a water-soluble jelly. Tapering the cuff away from the tip during deflation is desirable, because the bulk of the cuff will be away from the tip of the tube.

The procedure is explained to the patient. Hyperextension of the neck and placing a rolled towel between the patient's shoulder blades, unless contraindicated, aids in placement of the tube in the trachea. After sedating the patient, as indicated, the intubationist inserts a laryngoscope with either a straight or curved blade over the tongue and into the posterior pharynx. The end of the blade is placed in the vallecula. Without using the patient's teeth as a fulcrum, the intubationist lifts up on the blade to visualize the larynx. With the vocal cords in view, the lubricated endotracheal tube is inserted past the epiglottis and between the vocal cords. Care is taken to avoid the arytenoid cartilages, which can tear the cuff.

Some intubations are more difficult than others. Patients with short necks and obese patients are harder to intubate. When an intubation is difficult, the patient is bagged for several minutes between attempts. This restores oxygen and eliminates carbon dioxide. With apneic patients, intubation is attempted at 30-second intervals. A fiberoptic bronchoscope or laryngoscope is sometimes used by a specially trained physician to visualize the vocal cords. The endotracheal tube is inserted over the bronchoscope before it is inserted into the mouth (or nose). The bronchoscope is positioned just below the vocal cords, and the endotracheal tube is slid into place. Use of a bronchoscope ensures correct placement.

Most nasal intubations omit use of a laryngoscopic blade. The tube is blindly inserted through the nose and down into the trachea. The intubationist times insertion of the tube with inspiration. As the patient inhales, the tube is inserted further. A vapor column is seen in the endotracheal tube as the patient exhales. If a vapor column is not seen, this usually means that the tube has entered the esophagus; it is then withdrawn slightly and reinserted with the next inhalation. A carbon dioxide detector is used in some institutions to verify correct placement. In intubations where a blade is used, a Magill forceps is used to guide the tube through the posterior pharynx and between the vocal cords (see Fig. 14-1). Care must be taken so that the teeth of the forceps do not tear the cuff.

Nursing care

Immediately after the endotracheal tube has been inserted, the nurse grossly observes the chest for rise and fall with each breath from the ambu. A stethoscope is used to auscultate the chest. Because breath sounds are transmitted across the mediastinum, bilateral breath sounds may be present on auscultation with intubation of a main stem bronchus. Equal bilateral breath sounds indicate that the tube probably is in the trachea and not in one main stem bronchus. Improved color is another sign that the patient has been intubated correctly, although poor color is not necessarily a sign that the esophagus has been intubated. Inadequate cardiac output causes cyanosis, even with adequate ventilation. Intubation of the esophagus usually is ruled out by auscultation over the stomach. If air sounds are louder over the stomach than the lungs, the endotracheal tube is in the esophagus and must be replaced. Distention of the stomach is another sign that the esophagus has been intubated instead of the lungs. However, since most patients are bagged with a mask before intubation, air is usually in the stomach. Remember that, except for apneic patients, the patient can still breathe when either the trachea or the esophagus has been intubated. Seeing the previously mentioned vapor column rising and falling in the endotracheal tube with each breath is a very good indication that the tube is in the trachea and not the esophagus.

Accurate placement of an endotracheal tube is verified by fluoroscopy, bronchoscopy, or a chest x-ray film; chest x-ray verification is the most common means. The best position for the tip of an endotracheal tube is *2 to 3 cm above the carina*. Higher positioning predisposes the patient to injury of the vocal cords or extubation. Positioning the tube closer to the carina can result in accidental intubation of a main stem bronchus. Because its angle is less sharp, the right main stem usually is intubated. Once correct position has been verified, the nurse notes the depth marking on the tube at the teeth or lips. Since the teeth are not prone to swelling, they are the preferred marker. A notation of correct position (for example, 24 cm at teeth) is made on the Kardex. (Sometimes the depth marking is enhanced with tape or a permanent marking pen.) In some institutions, a sign is placed at the bedside or on the ventilator indicating correct depth of the endotracheal tube.

Table 14-2 shows the general guidelines used by the intubationist for correct depth placement of an endotracheal tube in an adult. Remember that these are just guidelines to position the tube below the vocal cords and above the carina. Chest x-ray confirmation is still necessary, since patients vary in size and anatomy.

Table 14-2. Guidelines for correct depth placement of an endotracheal tube

Oral		Nasal	
Men	Women	Men	Women
25-27 cm	23-25 cm	27-29 cm	25-27 cm

Cuffs

Inflation. After a patient has been intubated and physical assessment shows that the tube has been positioned correctly, the cuff is inflated. Ideal cuff inflation is the lowest possible pressure that allows delivery of adequate tidal volumes and prevents major pulmonary aspiration. Several techniques can be used to assess proper cuff inflation, including minimal leak, minimal occlusive pressure, and cuff pressure manometry.

The best technique for cuff inflation is the minimal leak method: The nurse slowly and carefully inflates the cuff, using 0.5 ml increments of air, while auscultating for air leak in the sternal notch or cricothyroid area. The nurse listens for the point where no air leak is heard at end-inspiration. When no air is heard at end-inspiration, the term *minimal occlusive pressure, minimal occlusive volume,* or *no-leak technique* is used. The nurse slowly withdraws air in 0.1 ml increments until air is heard only at end-inspiration. This point, at which a **small air leak is heard only at end-inspiration, is minimal leak.**

Assessing exhaled tidal volumes usually reveals escape of 25 to 50 ml of tidal volume using the minimal leak technique. In general, the patient's lips don't move, and there are no visible signs of a tiny air leak. As noted above, with minimal occlusive pressure, there is no air leak; the trachea is in constant contact with the cuff. With minimal leak technique, the trachea is in contact with the cuff only during exhalation. When the airway diameter increases with inhalation, a cushion of air separates the cuff and the trachea. Mucosal injury from pressure is reduced. In addition, the intermittent flow of air past the cuff allows secretions either to move up and out of the epiglottis or to drain into the trachea to be expelled by coughing. The chance for secretions to accumulate between the cuff and the epiglottis (and cause infection and stenosis) is reduced, because they are allowed to drain.

The third technique for cuff inflation involves the use of a cuff pressure manometer. A mercury or aneroid manometer is connected to the pilot balloon with a three-way stopcock. The cuff is inflated with air to achieve a predesignated pressure, usually 20 to 25 centimeters of water pressure (cwp). In healthy individuals, capillary flow is obstructed at 32 mm Hg. Venous flow may be obstructed at a lesser value in hospitalized patients who have altered homeostasis. Depending on the size of the endotracheal tube and the size of the patient's airway, the cuff may be overinflated or underinflated. If the same size tube is inserted into a patient with a narrow airway (120 pound woman) and a large airway (180 pound man), and the same volume of air is inserted into both tubes, the patient with the smaller airway may have greater pressure exerted against the mucosa.

Some cuffs, such as the Lanz cuff, have built-in valves that regulate cuff pressure. Cuff pressure controllers can be attached to the endotracheal tube and pilot balloon for continuous automatic assessment and adjustment of cuff pressure. One such model is the Pressure Easy by Respironics. This device maintains the intracuff pressure between 18 and 27 cwp. Although useful, these devices do not eliminate the need to assess cuff pressure. The only cuff that does not require special inflation techniques is the Fome cuff by Bivona; its insertion technique varies, however. This cuff has no pilot balloon. The port connecting the cuff to the atmosphere is left open and inflates under ambient pressure. As the patient's airway diameter increases, air enters the cuff. When the diameter decreases, air is squeezed from the cuff. Cuff pressure is continuously maintained at or below 25 cwp.

Cuff pressure is assessed at least every 8 hours. Some institutions recommend removal of air and reinflation every 4 hours. Although this policy may be a holdover from low-volume, high-pressure cuffs, it does allow secretions to drain into the lungs for expectoration and reduces complications caused by accumulation of secretions and cuff inflation. According to institution policy, the volume of air instilled in the cuff is recorded separately on the Kardex, in the nursing progress notes, or on a flow sheet. The volume of air instilled in the cuff fluctuates with changes in airway diameter (for example, with edema or bronchospasm) and cuff pliability, and therefore is not usually helpful. The exception is with patients being sent home with a cuffed tracheostomy tube, when instilling a given volume is easier than assessing pressure.

It is especially important to assess intracuff pressure after anesthesia has been administered. Because nitrous oxide diffuses into the cuff during surgery, cuff pressure may increase. After the patient returns to the room, air is removed from the cuff and it is then reinflated.

Deflation. Some institutions routinely deflate the cuff, a practice that originated with the low-volume, high-pressure cuff. The cuff was deflated for 5 minutes every hour to minimize injury to the tracheal walls. However, this practice predisposes the patient to aspiration, hypoxemia, and hypoventilation and probably was not that effective at preventing necrosis. This routine generally is not necessary with high-volume, low-pressure cuffs. In fact, deflating the cuff in selected patients receiving continuous mechanical ventilation may promote hypoxemia, overinflation, and aspiration while the cuff is totally deflated. Current practice encourages use of the minimal leak technique to inflate the cuff. The cuff is deflated only when problems arise that require reinflation. Some institutions routinely deflate the cuff temporarily every 48 to 72 hours.

Other times when the cuff is systematically deflated and reinflated include meals and weaning trials. In some patients, the cuff of a tracheostomy tube is actually deflated for eating; in others, it is inflated. A modified barium swallow with the cuff deflated is usually performed to confirm ability to prevent aspiration during swallowing. The patient who requires cuff inflation for eating or drinking aspirates when swallowing. The cuff is inflated during meals and for 1 hour afterward, including gastric tube feedings. Patients in whom cuff deflation during eating or drinking is encouraged do not aspirate food or fluids with the cuff deflated. An inflated cuff, especially an overinflated cuff, impinges on the esophagus. Since the anterior cartilaginous rings are fixed and the posterior tracheal membrane is flexible, inflation of the cuff pushes the normally D-shaped trachea into an O shape. The posterior wall bulges out into the esophagus, which can impair swallowing.

In some patients the cuff is deflated during weaning trials; this allows air to pass through the vocal cords, facilitating speech. It also encourages the patient to assume more responsibility for inhaling tidal volumes through the normal nasal-oral route. The work of breathing is decreased because of increased airway diameter. Turbulent flow may also be decreased. Deflating the cuff allows secretions to be coughed out through the mouth. In patients receiving mechanical ventilation at home, use of a noncuffed tracheostomy tube is best, because the patient and family do not have to worry about cuff-related problems such as leaks.

Leaks. One of the more challenging areas of cuff management, after proper cuff inflation, is cuff leaks. Management of cuff leaks begins with identifying the origin. Most cuff leaks are caused by patient position changes. Turning the patient from side to center to back or sitting the patient up in bed or in a chair changes the diameter of the trachea and the position of the tracheostomy tube, and air leaks around the cuff. The nurse assesses that there is an air leak because air is heard coming up through the mouth or lips or around the tracheostomy stoma. The patient often loses a significant amount of tidal volume, up to several hundred milliliters, depending on the circumstances. Some patients develop dyspnea or hypoxemia. Slightly changing the position of the patient's head or neck usually resolves the problem. If this does not resolve the difficulty, and if the patient is symptomatic and is going to remain in the position for a while, the cuff is deflated and reinflated with the patient in the new position. The nurse is cautioned to remember to reassess cuff inflation when the patient's position is changed later.

When position changes are not the cause, the nurse assesses each part of the endotracheal or tracheostomy tube involved in cuff patency. Assessment begins with the one-way valve. A syringe of air is attached to the Luer pilot balloon. A small amount of air is inserted into the cuff to minimal leak or minimal occlusive pressure. Leaving the syringe in place, the nurse waits a few moments for the leak to reappear. If the leak does not reappear, the cuff is intact. If the leak reappears, the problem is between the one-way valve and the cuff. Another test of a patent cuff is to assess the volume of air in the cuff and to compare it to the previous inflation volume. If the volumes are equal, the cuff is patent and the problem is usually positional. If the deflation volume is less, there is a leak in the system.

If the nurse assesses that the cuff is intact, the most common cause of air leak is damage to the one-way valve. This is the most common cause for leaks after position changes. Removing the syringe from the one-way valve, the nurse again assesses for air leak. If air leak occurs, the one-way valve has been damaged, causing it to stick open and allow air to escape. Damage to the one-way valve is frequently caused by pushing too hard against the valve, breaking it, or by leaving a syringe in the valve port.

If the nurse assesses a problem between the cuff and the one-way valve, the nurse applies a padded clamp on the pilot tubing, just below the pilot balloon, immediately after reinflating the cuff. If the air leak recurs, the problem is a ruptured cuff or the pilot balloon tubing has broken, usually at the site of attachment to the endotracheal or tracheostomy tube. If the air leak does not recur, the pilot balloon has been damaged. If the latter is the case, the nurse can cut off the pilot balloon and insert a *blunt* needle attached to a stopcock. After the cuff has been inflated, the stopcock is turned off to prevent air leak. This is temporary fix; the tube should be replaced as soon as possible and as soon as it is safe for the patient. (If a patient is being given high levels of supplemental oxygen and PEEP, the tube is not changed until the patient is more stable.) If the pilot balloon tubing is broken or the cuff has a hole or tear, the tube must be replaced, if the patient is in distress. A physician or specially trained nurse or respiratory therapist changes the tube.

Stabilization. After the cuff has been inflated, the tube is secured with adhesive, cloth, or waterproof tape. (*Note:* After the chest x-ray film, the endotracheal tube may need to be repositioned slightly.) For long-term intubation, waterproof tape, although more expensive, is preferred, because it adheres well, even in patients with copious oral secretions, and prevents movement of the tube. Paper tape is not used because it tears easily and does not adhere well in a moist environment. Depending on the institution, silk tape is not used because it is easily lifted by saliva, and many patients are sensitive to transparent micropore tape.

Other methods can be used to secure endotracheal tubes. In some institutions Velcro ties are used. In other institutions a mouth guard and head gear similar to that used with nasal continuous positive airway pressure (CPAP) secures the endotracheal tube. Several manufacturers make endotracheal tube holders. Preliminary studies suggest that these holders may decrease internal and external tube movement. However, some patients and nurses feel that tube holders are bulky and visually unappealing, and mouth care is difficult with some models. Nurses may observe excessive gagging, pressure necrosis, and inadequate tube stabilization, depending on the design.

Securing an endotracheal tube usually requires two people (physician, nurse, nurse's aide, student, respiratory therapist, unit technician). One individual holds the endotracheal tube in a stable position while the other secures it. The procedure for securing an endotracheal tube correctly with tape is highlighted in the box on p. 302.

After the endotracheal tube has been secured, the nurse assesses the patient every 15 to 30 minutes until stable. Complete assessment includes taking vital signs and observing for signs of hypoxemia or air hunger, epistaxis, tooth avulsion, biting the tube, and fighting the ventilator. In many institutions soft wrist restraints are required for intubated patients to prevent self-extubation.

EXTUBATION

When a patient no longer requires mechanical ventilation or protection of the airway, the physician usually orders extubation. The decision to extubate a patient is based on criteria for adequate muscle strength, inspiratory effort, and airway protection mechanisms. Depending on the institution, extubation is performed by the physician, nurse, or respiratory therapist. The procedure for extubating a patient is given in the box below. The patient is assessed frequently after extubation for signs of hypoxemia, inadequate ventilation, cardiopulmonary arrest, laryngospasm, bronchospasm, stridor, and other potential problems. Equipment for reintubation is kept nearby.

TRACHEOSTOMY

The terms *tracheostomy* and *tracheotomy* are often confused and used interchangeably. The tracheotomy is the surgical incision made in the trachea, and the tracheostomy is the opening or stoma created. A tracheostomy tube or artificial airway is inserted into the trachea through the tracheostomy. The horizontal or lateral external incision in an adult patient's neck is about 2 to 3 cm long at about the level of the third cartilaginous ring of the trachea.

Tape method for securing an endotracheal tube

1. Tell the patient what you intend to do, and enlist his cooperation (that is, he must hold his head still and try not to cough for approximately 5 minutes).
2. Suction the patient to reduce the need to cough. While he is recovering, prepare the tape. Also get a wet washcloth to clean the patient's face and other supplies for oral hygiene.
3. For a child, ½-inch wide tape is used; for an adult, 1- to 1½-inch tape is needed. Cut a strip of tape long enough to go around the patient's head plus 6 to 8 inches (24 to 30 inches for adults). Cut a second piece of tape long enough to extend from ear to ear around the back of the head (about 6 inches for adults).
4. Lay the long piece of tape sticky side up on a clean, dry surface such as a bedside table. Position the second piece of tape sticky side down in the center of the first piece.
5. Position the tape under the patient's head, centering the double-faced tape between the ears. The double-faced tape prevents hair on the patient's neck from adhering and being pulled.
6. Remove the old tape from the endotracheal tube and the patient's face. Do not use scissors, since you may cut the pilot balloon. Have the assistant hold the tube securely as close as possible to the patient's nose or mouth to prevent the tube from moving.
7. Clean the patient's face, and provide oral hygiene. Inspect the face and mouth for irritation or sores. Move the oral tube to another position. Ideally, the tube is moved from side to side or side to center to side each time the tape is changed.
8. Apply tincture of benzoin or a protective dressing swabstick, according to institution policy, to the patient's face from ear to nose or mouth and across the upper lip or nose to protect the skin. Allow the tincture of benzoin or protective dressing to dry. Fan the area to quicken drying, if necessary. Do not apply tincture of benzoin to broken skin.

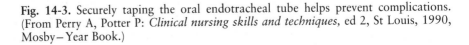

9. Secure the tape on one side of the face from the ear to the corner of the mouth or nose (Fig. 14-3). Tear the remaining tape lengthwise. (*Note:* Some clinicians do not split the length of tape.)
10. Wrap one piece of the split tape around the tube as close to the mouth or nose as possible. Usually this is the upper tape. The tape should encircle the tube two or three times. Cut or tear off excess tape. Fold a ¼-inch piece of tape back on itself to make a tab that facilitates later removal of the tape. Secure the other piece across the upper lip or over the nose. (*Note:* Some clinicians prefer to wrap both pieces around the tube.)
11. Repeat the last two steps on the other side of the face. The tube is now secured.

Fig. 14-3. Securely taping the oral endotracheal tube helps prevent complications. (From Perry A, Potter P: *Clinical nursing skills and techniques,* ed 2, St Louis, 1990, Mosby–Year Book.)

Procedure for extubation

1. Administer an inhaled bronchodilator, if ordered, and obtain a supplemental oxygen source for use after extubation (that is, a nasal cannula or mask to connect to high-humidity, large-bore tubing *or* a partial rebreather mask).
2. Suction the patient. Deflate the cuff, and suction the patient again.
3. While the patient recovers, loosen and remove the tape or securing device.
4. Ask the patient to take in a deep breath and cough. The airway is wider during inhalation and coughing.
5. Gently but quickly remove the endotracheal tube at the peak of inhalation.
6. Apply the oxygen source; encourage a cough if indicated.
7. Assess for stridor (inspiratory crowing sounds), indicating severely decreased airway size. Anticipate an order for racemic epinephrine or steroids. (Cool mist is preferred over warm mist when laryngospasm or edema is present; think of the patient with croup who improves in the cool evening air.)
8. Withhold fluids for at least 2 hours. The patient may have glottic incompetence secondary to edema and may be unable to control the flow of fluids or solids away from the lungs. Acute aspiration may occur. (*Note:* Some patients develop chronic glottic incompetence and aspirate unless they use special techniques to eat and drink.) Room-temperature or warm liquids are administered first, then iced or cool liquids.

(Some physicians make a vertical incision in the skin.) A much smaller, horizontal, T-shaped or U-shaped internal incision, usually about 1 cm long, is made through the cartilaginous rings for insertion of the tracheostomy tube. The actual placement of the tube depends on the patient's anatomy.

A tracheostomy tube is inserted to relieve upper airway obstruction, to provide a long-term route for effective secretion removal, to prevent massive aspiration, or for long-term mechanical ventilation. In a patient with massive facial injuries, a tracheotomy frequently is performed at the scene of an accident or in the emergency room, when swelling or injury prevents intubation. Percutaneous cricothyroid puncture or cricothyroidotomy is often performed in emergency situations instead of a full tracheotomy.

Ideally, a tracheotomy is performed in the operating room with optimal asepsis, lighting, anesthesia, and resuscitation equipment. In some critically ill patients, the tracheotomy is performed in the intensive care unit, where conditions are less optimal but ultimately safer for the patient. With this type of patient, several of the following factors usually are involved: a pulmonary artery catheter, arterial line, vasoactive drugs, several chest tubes, cervical spine or skeletal traction, intraaortic balloon pump or ventricular assist device, or hemodynamic instability.

Some patients can be successfully weaned from mechanical ventilation but are unable to clear their secretions. The physician recommends tracheotomy to enhance secretion removal. Depending on the patient, the tracheostomy tube is temporary or permanent. The figure on p. 304 contains a decision tree to help in choosing the most appropriate tracheostomy device for a particular patient.

In patients unable to protect the airway from aspiration, tracheotomy is performed when conservative swallowing techniques are unsuccessful. Alter-

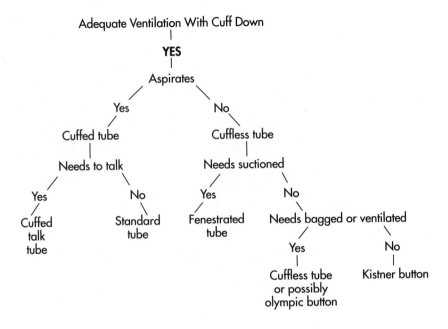

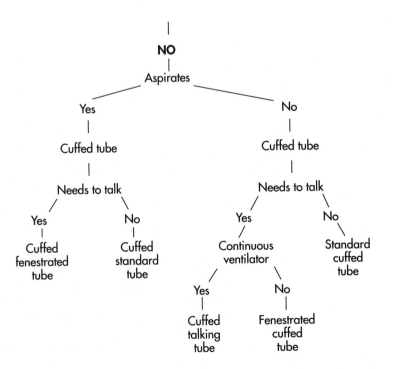

ing the consistency of food and fluids and using different swallowing techniques are tried before deciding to perform a tracheotomy.

The decision to perform a tracheotomy in long-term mechanically ventilated patients is made at different intervals, depending on the patient and the physician. In some patients a tracheotomy is performed to decrease anatomical (in this case, mechanical) dead space, which facilitates weaning and clearance of secretions. Many physicians choose to perform a tracheotomy after a week of intubation, whereas others wait 4 to 6 weeks before performing a tracheotomy. A few physicians leave the patient intubated indefinitely.

There are disadvantages to a tracheostomy versus an endotracheal tube; for example, morbidity and mortality are increased with a tracheostomy. Some differences between an endotracheal tube and a tracheostomy tube are related to oral hygiene, ability to eat food, and improved communication. The complications are about the same, except that they are more severe with the tracheostomy tube, and the patient has a surgical wound, which leaves a permanent scar.

Features

A tracheostomy tube has many parts, some of which are similar to those of an endotracheal tube. A tracheostomy tube is approximately 2 to 6 inches long (Portex makes an extra-long size). and is made of plastic or metal (Fig. 14-4). There are polyvinyl chloride, nylon, and silicone tubes. Metal tubes are made of stainless steel or silver. All tracheostomy tubes contain an outer cannula, or main shaft, and a faceplate or flange, which rests on the neck between the clavicles. The Shiley neckplate is made of rigid plastic and is approximately 2 inches long; the Portex model is made of soft plastic and is about 4 inches long. Some neckplates, such as the Shiley version, swivel up and down slightly to accommodate neck position, but most models do not. The neckplate contains small holes on the outer edge, which are used to secure tracheostomy ties. The tip of the tube is dissimilar to an endotracheal tube in that it is not beveled but straight cut, to maximize air flow and prevent occlusion of the tip by the tracheal wall.

Most tracheostomy tubes contain an inner cannula, although some do not, such as the Bivona Fome cuff and some Portex tubes. Most pediatric tubes do not have an inner cannula because of the small diameter. An inner cannula is removed from the outer cannula for cleaning; the outer cannula is left in place. An inner cannula is necessary for the patient who does not require suctioning to clear crusted secretions, which can occlude the airway. With patients who receive routine or intermittent suctioning, the suction catheter removes most if not all of the crusted secretions. When inhaled air is not humidified, crusting secretions are more of a problem. Especially with the Shiley tracheostomy tube, removal of the inner cannula prevents connection of respiratory equipment, including the mechanical ventilator, because the outer cannula does not have a standard 15- or 22-mm connection. When the inner cannula is optional, as in the Portex line of tracheostomy tubes, use of the inner cannula decreases the internal diameter of the tracheostomy tube by about 1 mm.

The means of securing the inner cannula to the outer cannula varies with the manufacturer. Some inner cannulas have a twisting or snapping locking mechanism (Shiley model), whereas others simply slide into place (Portex model) or secure with a hinge (Jackson model). The nurse must know which

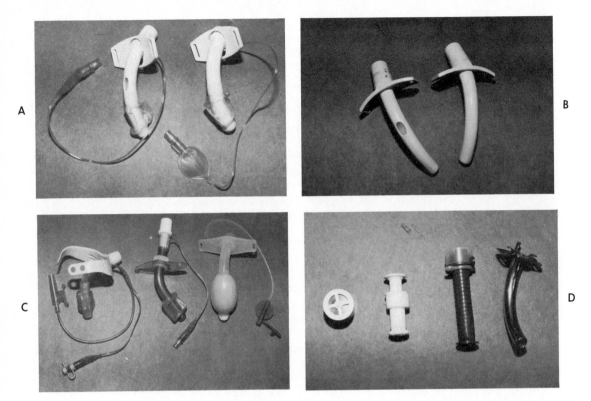

Fig. 14-4. Tracheostomy tubes. **A,** Shiley cuff, left tube is fenestrated. **B,** Shiley cuffless, left tube is fenestrated. **C,** Left to right: Portex trach-talk, Rusche, Bivona Fome cuff. **D,** Left to right: Passy-Muir speaking valve, Olympic button, Kistner button, Jackson metal trach.

kind of technique secures the inner cannula into the outer cannula. The inner cannula is routinely removed every 8 hours, cleaned, if reusable, and replaced. Depending on the institution, reusable or disposable inner cannulas are used. Aseptic procedure is used in the hospital. In the home, clean technique is used more often.

Most tracheostomy tubes have an external cuff for use when aspiration is a problem. Mechanical ventilation may be another indication for cuffed tracheostomy tubes but isn't automatically. Many mechanically ventilated patients have a cuffless tracheostomy tube. Cuffed tubes have a pilot balloon similar to that for an endotracheal tube. The pilot balloon connects to the outer cannula at the neckplate.

Pediatric tubes, those smaller than a Shiley size 4, do not have cuffs, because the airway diameter is so small, and a cuff would reduce it further. Most tracheostomy tubes, especially those with cuffs, contain a standard 15-mm adapter for connection to an ambu or other respiratory equipment. Other tubes, particularly the Jackson model and some other cuffless tubes, have an adapter that, when inserted, provides for connection of respiratory therapy equipment. The adapter is easily removed or dislodged.

Another feature of tracheostomy tubes that makes them different from endotracheal tubes is a fenestration, or straw-sized hole, in the outer cannula (see Fig. 14-4). Pediatric tubes do not have a fenestration. A fenestration is available on cuffed and cuffless tracheostomy tubes. With the inner cannula in place, the fenestration is occluded and respiratory treatments, especially mechanical ventilation, are uninterrupted. Speech is also inhibited, except with cuffless tracheostomy tubes that allow some air flow over the vocal cords. When the inner cannula is removed, the cuff is deflated, and the outer cannula is occluded, more air flows past the vocal cords, permitting voice. Deflation of the cuff allows greater air flow over the vocal cords. Failure to deflate the cuff, especially when the outer cannula is occluded, can increase the work of breathing as the patient tries to draw air through a straw-sized opening.

Speech is enhanced by occlusion of the outer cannula with a finger, cork, or specially fitted short, closed-lumen cannula, also called a *decannulation cannula.* (*Note:* Finger occlusion is a source of contamination. The patient is taught to use a tissue or gauze to occlude the outer cannula instead of an uncovered finger.) When the patient requires suctioning or reconnection to the mechanical ventilator, the decannulation plug is easily removed.

Because tissue can granulate around the fenestration, a fenestrated tracheostomy tube is inserted when the patient is off the mechanical ventilator for at least 30 minute intervals. Insertion before this time can result in development of granulation tissue around the fenestration. When a fenestrated tracheostomy tube is finally warranted, granulation tissue obstructs the opening, prohibiting or limiting speech. A mechanically ventilated patient with a cuffed (inflated), fenestrated tracheostomy tube can talk only when the ventilator is disconnected.

Mechanically ventilated patients, who require inflation of the cuff, usually cannot speak while using the ventilator, even with a fenestrated tracheostomy tube. For these individuals, there is a special type of tracheostomy tube called a talking trach, such as Communitrach (Implant Technologies, Inc.), Pitt Trach Speaking Tube (National Catheter Co.), and Portex Trach-talk Tube, and Bivona fome-cuff with sideport airway connector (see Fig. 14-4). These special tubes have an additional piece of hollow tubing that extends from just above the cuff to past the neckplate. Air is blown through the tube and exits over the vocal cords through one or more openings. The Pitt Trach Speaking Tube has eight holes in the outer cannula through which air flows; the Portex Trach-talk Tube has two holes.

When connected to an air source at 1 to 10 LPM (average 4 to 6 LPM), the patient can talk by occlusion of a port much like that of a suction catheter. A fair amount of manual dexterity and minimal strength are needed to occlude the port. The voice varies from an audible whisper to clear but coarse speech. Use of the talking port does not interfere with mechanical ventilation. The patient receives the same minute ventilation, with extra ventilation over the vocal cords. To keep the line patent and to prevent the vocal cords from drying, 5 ml of normal saline is instilled at least every 8 hours. The air source is disconnected when not in use.

Other devices for enhancing speaking in mechanically ventilated patients and spontaneously breathing patients with a tracheostomy tube and in those receiving nonmechanical forms are the Olympic Trach-talk (Olympic Medical Corp.), the Passy-Muir Speaking Valve (Passy & Passy, Inc.), the Olympic button (Olympic Medical Corp.) and the Kistner tracheostomy tube (Pilling Co.). The multipiece Olympic Trach-talk is composed of a spring-loaded one-way valve attached to a T piece that allows spontaneously breathing patients to talk. The one-way valve closes on exhalation, forcing air through the vocal cords. When a cuffed tracheostomy tube is used, the cuff is deflated. Secretions are cleared through the mouth as well.

The Passy-Muir Speaking Valve is different from the Olympic Trach-talk in that it is simpler and essentially of one-piece construction. Containing a silastic, one-way–valved membrane, the Passy-Muir Speaking Valve automatically closes after the patient inhales and begins to exhale. It is used either in mechanically ventilated patients or in those spontaneously breathing and receiving nonmechanical forms who cannot tolerate decannulation plugs. Whereas a decannulation plug forces all inhaled *and* exhaled air to originate from the mouth or nose, the Passy-Muir Speaking Valve permits inhalation through the valve with exhalation through the mouth or nose.

The Passy-Muir Speaking Valve is sometimes used in mechanically ventilated patients who tolerate cuff deflation. The valve is placed in the expiratory line, forcing air through the vocal cords. In spontaneously breathing patients the valve is placed directly on the exposed high-profile, 15-mm adapter of the inner or outer cannula. The Passy-Muir device and other one-way valve talking devices are not useful in patients with severe tracheal or laryngeal stenosis; in unconscious patients, who can't protect the airway from aspiration (and can't speak anyway); in critically ill or unstable patients; or in patients who need cuff inflation.

The Olympic button and Kistner tracheostomy tube (also referred to as the Kistner button) are actually tracheostomy tubes, whose only purpose is to keep the stoma open. These devices provide an additional step between a tracheostomy tube and decannulation. When the patient receiving nonmechanical ventilation is thought to clear secretions adequately but the physician is not sure, an Olympic or Kistner button is inserted to maintain a patent stoma. The device is also used to maintain the stoma when a subsequent surgical procedure requiring intubation and mechanical ventilation is planned in the near future. Use of the button prevents subsequent oral intubation or tracheotomy for the procedure.

The Olympic and Kistner buttons are designed differently. The Olympic button is made of rigid plastic (Teflon) of various lengths and diameters. The size of the tube is determined by the distance between the skin and the anterior tracheal wall and by the width of the tracheal opening. The length of the button is determined by inserting a probe to measure the distance between the skin and the anterior tracheal wall. The diameter of the button is judged by measuring the tracheal opening or by the external diameter of the tracheostomy tube it replaces. Spacers or rings are inserted on the outside of the button to assure that the tip does not extend into the trachea. A plug is inserted to occlude the lumen of the tube and to force normal inhalation and exhalation. Some models contain an inner canula for delivering respiratory therapy treatments, bagging, or mechanical ventilation.

The Olympic button is inserted like a standard tracheostomy tube. Once the tip is in the trachea, the button is pulled slightly back to place the flange against the anterior tracheal wall.

The Kistner button is made of flexible plastic. It is made in two diameters, junior and adult. The junior size is roughly equivalent to a size 4 or smaller Shiley tracheostomy tube and the adult to a size 8 Shiley tracheostomy tube.

When a size 6 or smaller Shiley tracheostomy tube is replaced, it is difficult to insert the adult Kistner button; however, the junior Kistner button is too small and usually will fall out.

The length of the adult button varies. The size of the Kistner button is determined by the distance in millimeters between the skin and the anterior wall of the trachea. Care is taken to determine the proper size, because a button that is too short allows the tract to granulate and occlude ventilation. A button that is too long occludes the trachea, limiting ventilation and removal of secretions.

The Kistner button contains a plastic cap with a floppy plastic one-way valve. Inhalation opens the valve and exhalation closes the valve. The valve is removed frequently for cleaning, since occlusion of the valve with mucus impairs inhalation. The cap can be removed for suctioning, but this is discouraged; when suctioning through the Kistner or Olympic button, insertion and removal of the suction catheter causes it to slide along and irritate the posterior wall of the trachea.

To insert the Kistner button, the plastic is folded in fourths lengthwise. After lubrication, the tip is inserted into the stoma and pushed in full length. The tube is then pulled back until the flange settles against the anterior tracheal wall. Inspection of the lumen of the Kistner button with a flashlight reveals pink tissue; the tube should not be invaginated. When the correct position has been verified, the external white ring is positioned against the neck and the button is secured. Umbilical tape is needed to secure the button because of the device's small eyelets. When Velcro ties are used, the Velcro is cut to fit the tiny eyelets. After the button has been secured, the cap is positioned. Care is taken when changing ties, or providing tracheostomy care, not to change the position of the white ring and green button, which can inadvertently dislodge the Kistner button.

Insertion

Tracheostomy tubes usually are inserted and removed under controlled conditions by a physician or specially trained nurse or therapist. Accidental removal of a tracheostomy tube should never happen with good airway management techniques. A tracheostomy tube is inserted with the aid of an obturator, which is a round-tip plug that fits inside the outer cannula. In proper position, the obturator extends just past the tip of the tracheostomy tube. Because the tip of the obturator is rounded and gradually increases to the size of the tracheostomy tube, it facilitates insertion and prevents mucosal injury from the blunt-ended tracheostomy tube. The procedure for changing a tracheostomy tube is discussed in the Box on p. 310.

How often a tracheostomy tube is changed varies among institutions. In some institutions the tube is changed weekly; in others, monthly or when a problem arises. A physician usually performs the first changing of the tracheostomy tube, especially if the stoma is not mature. The stoma usually matures by 7 days, unless the patient has poor nutritional status and has impaired healing.

Sometimes it is necessary to use a tracheostomy tube from a different manufacturer. This is particularly true when a talking tracheostomy tube is needed. Unfortunately a size 7 does not mean the same to all manufacturers. Some manufacturers, such as Shiley, do not make a size 7. When a different manufacturer must be used, the more important number to consider is the external diameter. Since the surgeon usually has inserted a tracheostomy tube

---

Changing a tracheostomy tube

1. Obtain the same size and kind of tracheostomy tube. It should be at the bedside at all times.
2. Suction the patient. Keep gloves on.
3. While the patient is recovering, prepare the tracheostomy tube:
   a. Check the cuff by inflating it according to the manufacturer's recommendations. Regular cuffs are filled with air and assessed for air leaking from the cuff. With the foam-filled cuff, patency is tested by removing all air from the cuff and observing for air leaking into the cuff.
   b. Fully deflate the cuff, tapering cuff bulk away from the tip. Remove the inner cannula, and insert the obturator.
   c. Lubricate the tip of the tube and obturator with water-soluble jelly.
4. Position the patient so that he is sitting upright or lying supine in the bed with a towel roll under his neck.
5. Deflate the cuff, and remove the tracheostomy ties.
6. Quickly remove the tracheostomy tube with an upward and outward movement with the nondominant hand. (The surgeon usually changes the tracheostomy tube the first time, especially if the incision is less than 7 days old or the patient is healing poorly. If unsure of the condition of the tracheostomy tract, change the tracheostomy tube over a suction catheter, sterile nasogastric or feeding tube, or tube changer.)
7. With the tracheostomy tube in the dominant hand, insert the tracheostomy with an inward and downward movement.
8. Remove the obturator quickly, since it occludes ventilation. Hold the tube in place with one or two fingers on the neckplate. Assess for air movement through the outer cannula. (*Note:* If there is no air movement, the tracheostomy tube may be in the pretracheal tissues. Remove the tube, and reinsert it.)
9. Reattach the oxygen or ventilator supply tubing, as needed.
10. Secure the tracheostomy tube with ties.
11. Suction the patient as needed.
12. Clean the peristomal skin, as needed, and apply a clean dressing to the stoma.

---

of the proper external diameter in the patient, it is necessary to find a tracheostomy tube of approximately the same external diameter. Table 14-3 lists the size, internal diameter, and external diameter of several models of tracheostomy tubes. If in doubt, try to determine from the packaging of the existing tube either the French equivalent or the Jackson equivalent to choose the proper size.

Once the tracheostomy tube has been placed, it is secured with twill tape or Velcro ties. In the home, grosgrain ribbon, bias tape, or shoelaces are sometimes used to secure the tracheostomy tube. When using twill tape, a double square knot is tied at the side of the neck. Although bows are attractive and easy to retie, they do not adequately secure the tracheostomy tube. To prevent excessive movement of the tube, the ties should allow only one finger to be inserted snugly under them. Here is an easy technique for tying twill tape that keeps the ends out of the stoma: cut a piece of the twill tape long enough to go around the patient's neck twice plus a few inches (about 30 inches for adults); bring one end through the eyelets, and pull the ends even; draw both ends under the head around the back of the neck; bring one end through the second eyelet; knot the two ends securely.

Table 14-3. Tracheostomy tube conversion*

	Jackson		Bivona Fome cuff		Portex		Shiley		French
Size	Internal diameter	External diameter	Internal diameter	External diameter	Internal diameter	External diameter	Internal diameter	External diameter	Size
00	2.5	4.3	x	x	x	x	3.1	4.5	13
0	3	5	x	x	3	5	3.4	5	15
1	3.5	5.5	x	x	3.5	5.5	3.7	5.5	16.5
2	4	6	x	x	4	6	4.1	6	18
	x	x	x	x	4.5	6.5	x	x	x
3	4.5-5	7	x	x	5	7	4.8	7	21
4	5.5	8	x	x	6	8.1	5.5	8	24
5	6-6.5	9	6	8.7	x	x	5	8.5	26-27
6	7	10	7	10	7	9.7	7	10	30
7	7.5-8	11	8	11	8	11	x	x	33
8	8.5	12	9	12.3	9	12.1	8.5	12	36
9	9-9.5	13	9.5	13.3	10	13.5	9	13	39
10	10	14	x	x	x	x	x	x	42
11	10.5-11	15	x	x	x	x	x	x	45
12	11.5	16	x	x	x	x	x	x	48

*Sizes are approximate in millimeters from product label or enclosure.

An alternative method uses less twill tape: insert the twill tape through one eyelet; bring the twill tape across the top of the neckplate, and insert the same end through the second eyelet; the long piece of tape is drawn behind the head and secured in a double knot at the side of the neck.

Velcro ties have been used for years in institutions and homes. They are made of 1-inch wide piece of lightweight foam that has Velcro straps attached to the ends. Dale tracheotomy tube holder is covered with a thin piece of cloth, whereas the Posey Velcro ties are not. When Velcro ties are used, they also should allow only one finger to fit snugly between the skin and the ties. Depending on the manufacturer, excessive foam is cut off at the back of the neck for a proper fit. The ties are brought around the back of the neck, inserted through the eyelet, and fastened to the foam.

Removing a tracheostomy tube (decannulation)

Removing a tracheostomy tube is both a science and an art. No magic formula determines how to decannulate a patient, although there are guidelines. In general, decannulation is considered when the patient no longer needs mechanical ventilation and can adequately clear secretions from the airway. Secretion clearance through the tracheostomy tube is the first step in decannulation. When the patient can cough secretions out of the tracheostomy tube, it is sometimes removed. In other instances, the physician inserts the next smaller size of tracheostomy tube to evaluate the patient's ability to clear secretions orally. If the patient cannot clear the secretions orally, the next smaller tracheostomy tube or a Kistner or Olympic button is inserted. Some patients have difficulty clearing secretions even when a small tracheostomy tube is in the trachea. Removing the obstruction facilitates removal of secretions; this is frequently evaluated with one of the buttons. If the patient clears secretions with the smaller tracheostomy tube or button, the tracheostomy tube is removed.

After the tracheostomy tube has been removed, the stoma is covered with a dry dressing. Some physicians prefer to use butterfly tape to approximate the edges of the wound, and others cover the area with petrolatum-impregnated gauze (Vaseline or Xeroform gauze). The patient's voice is raspy or gravelly for several days, until the stoma is completely closed. Applying an occlusive dressing enhances voice. During this time the dressing is changed at least daily to assess and clean the stoma.

COMPLICATIONS OF ENDOTRACHEAL AND TRACHEOSTOMY TUBES

Complications of endotracheal and tracheostomy tubes are divided into those that accompany the actual procedure, those that occur while the tube is in place, and those that follow removal of the tube. Table 14-4 highlights all three types of complications. Many of the complications can be prevented with good airway management. The nurse cannot alter procedural complications unless personally inserting or changing the endotracheal or tracheostomy tube. Aspiration and dysrhythmias are the most common serious complications during endotracheal intubation and insertion of a tracheostomy tube. Using suction during intubation and application of supplemental oxygen minimizes their risks. Whenever possible, a nasogastric tube is inserted or the esophageal obturator airway is left in place to prevent aspiration.

Using aseptic techniques in stoma care and suctioning prevents some infections that occur while the tube is in place. Proper cuff inflation techniques and securing the tube adequately prevent many of the cuff-related problems such as migration of the tube into the main stem bronchus, obstruction of the tube with secretions, tracheal esophageal fistula, tracheal malacia, and tracheal stenosis. Because of the tracheostomy's position below the larynx, laryngeal complications are fewer in patients with a tracheostomy; however, localized stoma infections occur frequently. It is important to observe the color, quantity, and consistency not only of pulmonary secretions but also of peristomal secretions. When coughing, laryngospasm, or bronchospasm is a problem, instillation of bronchodilators or anesthetics (a few milliliters of 1% lidocaine) lessens symptoms.

SUCTIONING

Suctioning is one technique for maintaining patency of the upper or lower airway. Performed both in patients who are intubated and those who are not, suctioning is used when the patient cannot expectorate oral or pulmonary secretions. In some patients 5 to 10 ml of sterile normal saline is instilled through an artificial airway to stimulate a cough. Administering saline through an artificial airway does not necessarily thin secretions and is not a substitute for adequate systemic or local humidity.

Table 14-4. Complications of endotracheal and tracheostomy tubes

Procedural	Durational	Postextubation
Aspiration*	Aspiration*	Aspiration*
Barotrauma*	Atelectasis*	Bronchospasm*
Bronchospasm*	Chondritis*	Cardiac arrest*
Cardiopulmonary ar- rest*	Cuff leak*	Chondritis*
Cuff laceration	Cuff herniation*	Dysphagia*
Discomfort*	Disconnection from ox- ygen source	Glottic injury
Dental accidents	Ineffective cough*	Hoarseness
Dysrhythmias*	Infection of wound	Keloid
Edema*	Innominate artery ero- sion*	Laryngeal edema
Epistaxis		Laryngeal stenosis
Esophageal intubation	Laryngeal dysfunction, web formation, or granuloma	Laryngospasm
Hemorrhage*		Nasal stricture
Hypoxemia*		Permanent scar
Intubation of main stem bronchus	Malnutrition*	Sore throat
	Mucosal injury*	Tracheal stenosis*
Laceration	Obstruction of tube*	Tracheal malacia*
Laryngeal trauma or spasm	Otitis media	Tracheal dilatation*
	Paroxysmal coughing*	
Pneumothorax	Pneumonia*	
Recurrent laryngeal nerve injury	Sepsis	
	Sinusitis	
Spinal cord injuries	Subcutaneous or medi- astinal emphysema	
Subcutaneous or medi- astinal emphysema	Subglottic edema	
Thyroid injury	Tracheal injury and di- latation*	
	Tracheoesophageal fis- tula*	
	Tracheal malacia*	

*Common to both endotracheal and tracheostomy tubes.

The upper airway generally is suctioned with clean technique using a large-bore tube, called a Yankauer pharyngeal suction tip, or with a standard suction catheter. Conversely, the lower airway is suctioned with a small catheter and aseptic technique. When the lower and upper airways are suctioned with the same catheter, the lower airway is always suctioned before the upper airway. The procedures for upper airway and tracheal suctioning are given in the boxes on pp. 314 and 315.

The main indication for suctioning the upper airway is gurgling or excessive drooling from the mouth. Lower airway suctioning is performed for large airway crackles, wheezes, or gurgles. Suctioning is not effective when adventitious breath sounds are assessed in the lung periphery. Because suctioning is associated with numerous complications, it is never a routine procedure; it is performed only when clinically indicated. The techniques for oral/nasal pharyngeal suctioning and tracheal suctioning are highlighted in the boxes on pp. 314 and 315.

Suctioning of the upper airway

1. Assemble the equipment and supplies needed. Choose an appropriate-size suction catheter. Table 14-1, p. 292 contains a guide for choosing the proper size. The suction pressure is set as low as possible to minimize mucosal injury from high negative pressure. Most sources recommend setting the vacuum at 80 to 100 mm Hg. Some sources allow up to 150 mm Hg. Full vacuum (that is, suction pressures above 300 mm Hg) are never recommended for suctioning the airway.

2. Explain the procedure to the patient, and encourage the use of deep breathing. This elicits cooperation and helps to allay anxiety. The patient is positioned supine or in semi-Fowler position with the head in a neutral position, as indicated, to facilitate ventilation, oxygenation, and suctioning and to prevent strain on the nurse.

3. Place a towel or drape over the patient to minimize contamination with secretions.

4. Wash hands to decrease transmission of microorganisms.

5. Put on a pair of gloves; using two gloves minimizes the transmission of organisms among patient, nurse, and environment.

6. Suction a small amount of water through the catheter to check proper functioning of equipment and to lubricate the catheter. If using a standard suction catheter, lubricate the catheter with a small amount of water-soluble jelly, especially for nasal suctioning.

7. If using a Yankauer tip, it is inserted and gently moved around both sides of the mouth and over the tongue to remove oral secretions. When performing suctioning with a standard suction catheter, insert the catheter gently into the naris. (A nasal pharyngeal airway may be inserted first.) Whenever possible, choose the side without polyps or obstruction from a deviated septum. Following the floor of the nose, insert the catheter medially and inferiorly, about 6 to 8 cm in the adult, to reach the posterior pharynx.

8. Apply intermittent suction only on withdrawal of the catheter. Do not apply suction on insertion. Mucosal injury is greater when suction is applied continuously and when advancing the catheter.

9. If the opposite naris is congested, suction as above and then suction the mouth with the same suction catheter. Oral secretions are suctioned to reduce the risk of aspiration.

10. The catheter can be rinsed with water between passes to clear the tubing of mucus. Excessive mucus in the tubing decreases the efficiency of the suction machine, especially portable ones.

11. The Yankauer tip catheter is frequently reused for up to 24 hours and then discarded. The standard suction catheter is coiled around the hand. The glove is pulled off inside out around the catheter to contain contamination and then discarded in an appropriate receptacle.

12. The suction tubing is rinsed with water or with a disinfectant according to institution policy.

13. Chart the intervention, including quantity, color, consistency, and odor of secretions and the effect on the patient.

Suctioning of the trachea

1. (Follow steps 1 through 4 for upper airway suctioning.) If the patient is not intubated, the neck is hyperextended or a towel roll is placed between the shoulder blades to ease the catheter's entry into the trachea.
2. Put on gloves. The glove on the dominant hand is sterile and touches only sterile supplies; the glove on the opposite hand is either sterile or clean, but it does not touch sterile supplies.
3. Test the equipment by suctioning a small amount of sterile water or saline through the catheter.
4. If suctioning through the nose, lubricate the tip of the catheter with a small amount of water-soluble jelly. Excessive jelly eventually dries in the patient's airway and may cause obstruction.
5. Depending on institution policy, hyperinflate the patient. Some patients also require hyperoxygenation.
6. a. With a patient who has not been intubated or who does not have a tracheostomy, insert the catheter through the most patent naris or nasal airway. Mask oxygen usually is pulled away slightly or removed; leave the nasal cannula in place, or pull it out slightly. Having the patient stick out his tongue facilitates entry into the trachea and prevents the tongue from obstructing the posterior pharynx.
   b. With a patient who has been intubated or who has a tracheostomy, open the cap on the swivel adapter or remove the oxygen source (for example, a t-tube or tracheostomy collar).
7. a. Quickly insert the suction catheter during inspiration until the patient coughs or resistance is felt. In patients who are not intubated, the catheter must be inserted during inspiration, because the epiglottis is open only during inspiration. Coughing frequently is a sign that the catheter is at the carina.
   b. If there is difficulty entering the trachea in a patient who has not been intubated, the suction catheter is inserted much like a nasal endotracheal tube. Disconnect the suction catheter from the connecting tubing. Listen at the vent of the catheter while inserting it. As long as air flow is heard, the catheter is moving in the proper direction. When air flow ceases, the catheter usually has entered the esophagus. Assess the patient to be sure he is breathing.
8. Pull the catheter back about 1 cm before applying suction to minimize trauma to tracheal mucosa.
9. a. Intermittently apply suction while removing the suction catheter. Suction is applied for 10 to 15 seconds or less to minimize complications. Whenever possible, rotate the catheter while pulling it out. This is not possible with closed-system in-line suction catheters.
   b. If the patient develops distress, the suction catheter may be left in place temporarily and oxygen administered through the catheter by connecting oxygen to the catheter instead of suction. This patient may benefit from hyperoxygenation before subsequent suctioning. In some instances the catheter itself causes the problem by either obstructing or irritating the airway and must be removed.
   c. If the catheter is difficult to place in the trachea, do not remove it completely between the two passes. Leave it in place, and apply oxygen as above, if indicated. Instruct the patient to try not to talk or cough excessively to avoid injuring the vocal cords.
10. Replace the cap on the swivel adapter or oxygen source, and allow the patient to recover for at least 1 minute. The patient often is hyperinflated, hyperoxygenated, or both during this period.
11. The catheter is inserted a second time as indicated by assessment. Between passes the catheter is rinsed with sterile water or saline. Care is taken not to contaminate the catheter while waiting for the patient to recover.
12. After the lower airway has been suctioned, the nurse may use the same catheter to suction the nose, mouth, and pharynx. Once the catheter has been used in the nose and mouth, it is not reinserted into the trachea.
13. (Follow steps 10-13 for upper airway suctioning.) Rinse the catheter with water or saline. Some institutions also use a disinfectant rinse.

The primary complication of suctioning is hypoxemia. Not only secretions but also oxygen and air are suctioned from the airway. As air is removed, atelectasis develops from excessive negative pressure. At first the atelectasis involves a small area and is called microatelectasis. Repeated unnecessary suctioning causes localized and then generalized atelectasis. A secondary complication usually caused by hypoxemia is dysrhythmia. The dysrhythmias, such as bradycardia, tachycardia, premature ventricular systole, or asystole, are potentially life threatening.

Another complication of suctioning is varying degrees of mucosal trauma. Continuous suction causes the tip of the catheter to adhere to tracheal mucosa. As the catheter is withdrawn, ciliated epithelium is drawn into the catheter, leaving a denuded area. Loss of ciliated cells impairs adequate functioning of the mucociliary escalator and predisposes the patient to retention of mucus and infection. In some instances the injured area is hemorrhagic. It may continue to bleed, especially in patients with altered hemostasis. Although most patients demonstrate blood-streaked mucus, a few develop frank hemoptysis from suctioning. When nasotracheal suctioning is performed repeatedly, nasal mucosa are also injured. The mucosa may become denuded of epithelial cells, edematous, or hemorrhagic. Using a nasal pharyngeal airway prevents excessive injury to nasal mucosa.

With patients who have not been intubated, repeated introduction of the suction catheter through the upper respiratory tract, such as nasotracheal suctioning, introduces oral bacteria into the lower respiratory tract. In intubated patients, the lower respiratory tract is colonized with hospital bacteria within 48 hours. Aerosolized bacteria enter the lungs through the ventilator circuit, and oral bacteria follow the exterior of the endotracheal tube into the lower airway. Once colonized, the lower respiratory tract is susceptible to bacterial invasion and infection.

Some patients develop paroxysmal coughing from stimulation of the lower respiratory tract with a suction catheter. Bronchospasm is frequently initiated. When paroxysmal coughing is a problem, using inhaled bronchodilators, limiting the frequency and depth of suctioning, and instilling a small amount of dilute (1%) lidocaine in nonallergic patients may minimize complications.

In patients with severe hypertension (especially hypertensive crisis) and increased intracranial pressure, suctioning is particularly hazardous. Suctioning and coughing markedly increase systemic or intracranial pressure, which is sustained for several minutes to hours after suctioning. In the case of systemic hypertension, the patient may have an intracranial hemorrhage. Repeated passes of the suction catheter, especially more than two times, in a patient with increased intracranial pressure is often associated with a sustained increase in the baseline pressure. There also is the risk of herniation with suctioning in patients with increased intracranial pressure. When suctioning is limited to prevent increases in intracranial pressure, the risk of mucus retention and resultant atelectasis and pneumonia increases. Knowing when and when not to suction a patient with increased intracranial pressure is difficult and requires accurate assessment.

The anatomy of the lungs favors right lung suctioning (just as with intubation). The angle of the left lung is sharper, making it more difficult for the suction catheter to enter. Blindly passing a standard suction catheter into the lower airway, the nurse has a one in three chance of entering the left lung.

Use of a coudé suction catheter increases the chance of entering the left or the right lung selectively, especially in an intubated patient. A catheter designed to selectively enter the left lung (Broncitrac "L") currently is being researched. It is much more expensive than a standard or coudé suction catheter and requires the use of a standard suction catheter to remove secretions from the right lung. When left lung collapse from mucus retention is a problem, use of a specialized catheter is necessary and is cost effective when compared with bronchoscopy. Failure to remove secretions adequately from the lower airway can result in mucus plugging and collapse of one or more lobes.

BRONCHOSCOPY

Bronchoscopy is a procedure performed by pulmonologists, intensivists, and surgeons. A bronchoscope is a small flexible tube containing fiberoptics. (There is also a rigid bronchoscope used exclusively in the operating room; this discussion is directed toward flexible bronchoscopy.) When the bronchoscope is connected to a special light source, the physician can see the inside of the nose, larynx, trachea, or larger airways. The physician guides the bronchoscope into the entrances of the lobes and segments. The diameter of the bronchoscope varies from about 3 to 6 mm, depending on the manufacturer and the model. The physician can clear only the larger airways of secretions because of the size of the bronchoscope. It is used primarily to diagnose suspected tumors or hemoptysis but may be used to clear the larger airways when suctioning is ineffective. When the bronchoscope is used to augment suctioning, the physician selectively suctions the entrance to each lobe or segment. As previously stated, chest physical therapy is just as effective as bronchoscopy, especially when combined with suctioning.

To prepare the patient for bronchoscopy, begin by withholding food and oral fluids for at least 3 to 6 hours, depending on the patient and the physician. After the procedure the patient's gag reflex is impaired, and food and oral fluids are withheld for at least 2 hours or until the gag reflex returns. In fluid- or dehydration-sensitive patients, intravenous fluids are necessary during this period. Depending on the physician's preferences, bronchoscopy is performed under local or general anesthesia. When local anesthesia is used, especially in the intensive care unit, the nurse sometimes is required to assist the physician. A brief review of the procedure and possible specimens follows. After the bronchoscopy, many patients complain of an irritated throat. Room-temperature or warm fluids are soothing.

The patient is generally positioned supine in the bed or on a fluoroscopy table, although a few physicians perform the procedure with the patient upright. Most physicians administer a preoperative medication consisting of a sedative and an anticholinergic agent to dry oral secretions, but bronchoscopy can be performed without systemic medication. A topical anesthetic, such as lidocaine (1% to 10%), is sprayed into the pharynx with a mask or hand-held nebulizer. Some physicians ask the patient first to gargle with the anesthetic solution. The physician tests the numbness of the gag reflex by touching a tongue blade against the posterior pharynx. When the gag reflex is sufficiently diminished, the physician anesthetizes the nasal passage. Viscous lidocaine is often used in addition to the nebulized solution. The bronchoscope is lubricated, usually with viscous lidocaine or Cetacaine, and inserted into the most patent naris. When nasal mucosa are edematous, the naris is sprayed with a nasal decongestant plus antihistamine, such as Afrin, or co-caine, a potent vasoconstrictor and anesthetic. When positioned above the epiglottis, anesthetic is administered through the bronchoscope to anesthetize the vocal cords. Additional topical anesthesia is sometimes necessary as the bronchoscope is repositioned in the airway.

Various specimens are obtained with the bronchoscope. The first speci-mens are called bronchial washings. They are the secretions suctioned through the bronchoscope as the physician passes through the upper airway and throughout the lower airway. Bronchial washings are usually sent for culture (routine and fungal) and cytological tests, as indicated. Some physi-cians do not send bronchial washings for culture, because the specimen is contaminated with upper airway flora.

When the physician wants cultures of fungi, viruses, or bacteria exclusive to the lower airway, a protected brush catheter is used or bronchoalveolar lavage is performed. A protected brush catheter is sometimes called a Bartlett brush, after its inventor. The protected brush catheter is a sterile brush en-closed in a double-lumen catheter with a wax plug at the distal end. After the catheter has been positioned, the plug is expelled and the brush is extended. The physician moves the brush up and down along the mucosa. Before re-moval the brush is pulled back into its sheath. Once withdrawn the brush is pushed out of its sheath and cut off with sterile scissors into saline or a cul-ture medium such as thioglycolate or phosphate-buffered saline. Quantitative cultures often are performed with a protected brush catheter.

Bronchoalveolar lavage is a technique used to study alveolar cells and to identify alveolar invasion by bacteria. The bronchoscope is wedged in a bron-chus; then 1-5 aliquots of 30 to 50 ml of sterile, nonbacteriostatic normal saline is instilled and immediately withdrawn. Usually about 50% to 75% of each aliquot is withdrawn. The remaining fluid either is suctioned by the bronchoscope after the wedge is broken or is reabsorbed. Bronchoalveolar la-vage fluid is usually sent for culture, cell counts, or cytological tests.

Some cultures do not require the use of a protected brush; a standard cy-tological brush is used to obtain the specimen. These tests include cultures for viruses, chlamydia, *Legionella* species, and acid-fast bacteria. Viral and chlamydial cultures are placed in special culture media and are usually grown by a special laboratory. *Legionella* organisms and acid-fast bacteria are trans-ported to the laboratory in a dry, sterile specimen cup.

To diagnose a tumor, endobronchial or transbronchial biopsies are taken. When an endobronchial tumor is seen, the physician inserts a biopsy forceps through the bronchoscope and removes a tiny piece of the tumor for analysis. Sometimes the physician sees narrowing of the airway or widening of the ca-rina. In these instances a tumor is suspected, and the area is biopsied. When the main carina is involved, fluid is sometimes aspirated from the area with a Wang needle. Frequently the physician sees no obvious tumor, but an abnor-mality is present on the chest x-ray film. The physician then performs a trans-bronchial biopsy. Using fluoroscopy, the physician directs the biopsy forceps to the suspected area.

The complications associated with bronchoscopy depend on the proce-dure. The most common complication is bronchospasm, which sometimes re-quires the administration of inhaled or systemic bronchodilators. The risk of bleeding is ever-present, and greater when brushes or biopsies are taken. Bronchoscopy therefore usually is performed only when coagulation studies are normal. Patients can develop cardiac dysrhythmias even though supplemental oxygen is administered throughout the procedure. Many patients develop a low-grade fever in the 24 hours after the procedure, and a few patients develop pneumonitis. Pneumothorax, a major risk of bronchoscopy, can occur when biopsies are obtained.

THORACENTESIS

Thoracentesis is insertion of a needle into the pleural space to evacuate fluid or, in rare cases, air (for example, with a small, simple pneumothorax, the physician may choose to evacuate air manually). Thoracentesis usually is performed to obtain a sample of pleural fluid for diagnosis or to relieve dyspnea and discomfort in patients with reaccumulating pleural effusions. Thoracentesis frequently precedes insertion of a chest tube for pleural effusions. Ideally the patient is sitting upright on the edge of the bed and leaning forward on a bedside table. This allows the fluid to drain to the base of the lung, enhancing fluid removal. Alternately, the patient is positioned recumbent or side lying with the affected lung dependent.

While the nurse helps the patient maintain proper position, the physician percusses the diaphragm and fluid level. The area is infiltrated with a local anesthetic and cleaned with an antibacterial solution. A spinal needle attached to a three-way stopcock or a through-the-needle catheter is inserted into the pleural space just above the diaphragm. Specimens are withdrawn, and the remaining fluid is drawn into a vacuum bottle. The needle or catheter is withdrawn, and a dressing is applied to the site. Because the incidence of pneumothorax is high, a chest x-ray film is taken after the procedure.

Complications associated with thoracentesis vary from minor to major. The primary major complication is pneumothorax. Other complications include reexpansion pulmonary edema, infection of the pleural space, pain, persistent cough, dry taps (not obtaining fluid), traumatic taps (obtaining bloody fluid), puncture of the liver or spleen, and subcutaneous fluid collections.

CHEST TUBES

Chest tubes are inserted for three reasons: to remove air, to facilitate drainage of fluids, and to prevent air or fluid from reentering the chest. The chest tube is connected to a drainage system that works on the principle that fluids, being heavier, sink, and air, being lighter, rises.

A chest tube is a flexible plastic tube that is inserted by a physician or by specially trained personnel to drain air or fluid or both from the pleural cavity (pleural chest tube) or from the mediastinal space (mediastinal chest tube). The tube may be angled or straight and may be made of vinyl, silastic, or latex nonthrombogenic material. Most chest tubes used are straight. The length and diameter of a chest tube varies with the size. A pediatric chest tube is shorter and narrower than an adult chest tube. The average pediatric chest tube is a few millimeters wide, whereas the average adult tube is about 1 cm wide and 51 cm (20 inches) long. Chest tubes usually are ordered by their French (FR) size. When air alone needs to be evacuated in an adult, a size 32 FR or smaller is used. Fluid evacuation is optimized in an adult when a size 28 FR or larger tube is inserted.

The box on p. 320 lists common indications for insertion of a chest tube. A pneumothorax is caused when either the parietal or visceral pleura is interrupted, and air enters the pleural space. Air in the pleural space is positive

---

Indications for chest tubes

Air (pneumothorax or pneumomediastinum)

    Barotrauma (mechanical ventilation)
    Bronchopleural fistula
    Iatrogenic causes (central line insertion, pleural biopsy)
    Spontaneous alveolar rupture
    Surgical thoracotomy (lung, cardiac, or spine)
    Tension pneumothorax with mediastinal shift
    Traumatic causes (blunt chest trauma, rib fracture, sucking chest wound)

Fluid

    Cardiac tamponade
    Chylothorax (fatty pleural effusion)
    Empyema (infected pleural fluid)
    Hemothorax (bloody pleural fluid)
    Pericardial effusion
    Pleural effusion
    Surgical thoracotomy (blood and debris)
    Tension effusion or hemothorax (pleural effusion with mediastinal shift)

---

and causes the lung to recoil. Insertion of a chest tube reestablishes normal intrathoracic pressures. In rare cases a pneumothorax progresses to a tension pneumothorax. When this occurs, the lung collapses entirely and increased pressure in the pleural space pushes the mediastinum to the opposite side. Venous return is impaired, and cardiac output is decreased. The patient develops cardiopulmonary arrest and dies unless treatment is begun quickly. Before a chest tube is inserted, an 18-gauge needle is inserted into the second or third intercostal space anteriorly to relieve the pressure.

Air enters the mediastinal space *(pneumomediastinum)* as a result of alveolar rupture near the hilum. Pneumomediastinum is common after blunt chest trauma and barotrauma from mechanical ventilation with high levels of PEEP. Frequently some air remains in the mediastinum immediately after cardiac surgery; it is rapidly evacuated.

Fluid accumulates in the pleural space as a result of fluid overload, chest cancer, trauma, or surgery. Fluid accumulating in the pleural space compresses lung tissue, causing atelectasis.

Fluid in the pericardial sac is called a *pericardial effusion*. When excessive, pericardial fluid causes *cardiac tamponade,* which can be life threatening. The absolute volume of fluid in the pericardial sac often is not as important as how fast the fluid accumulates. In susceptible patients, an increase of 25 ml of pericardial fluid induces cardiac tamponade. Other patients are not symptomatic until 100 ml or more of pericardial fluid accumulates. When a pericardial effusion accumulates very slowly, the patient may have 1 to 2 L of fluid in the pericardial sac before tamponade develops. Cardiac tamponade limits contraction of the heart and is associated with hypotension, jugular venous distention, and elevated central venous pressure. The chest x-ray film shows an enlarged cardiac silhouette.

Each chest tube has one large hole at the end and several small holes for drainage. More holes mean less chance of occlusion by tissue or clots. A radiopaque line extends the entire length of the chest tube with breaks over the holes. This line helps the physician determine correct chest tube position on the chest x-ray film. The last break is within the rib cage in a properly positioned pleural chest tube. If the last break is outside the rib cage, air can enter, producing a pneumothorax. The physician also can identify kinks in the chest tube and can note when the chest tube has been inserted too far.

The term *thoracotomy* refers to an incision in the chest wall that can be 1 cm to several inches in length. When a tube is inserted through a small incision in an otherwise closed chest, the term *thoracostomy* is used. A chest tube is positioned to enhance drainage. Because air rises and fluid is pulled down by gravity, chest tubes to drain air and fluid are positioned differently. A pleural chest tube to evacuate air usually is inserted in the second or third intercostal space at the midclavicular line; a pleural chest tube to drain fluid is inserted in the fourth, fifth, or sixth intercostal space at the anterior axillary or midaxillary line. More lateral placement is uncomfortable to lie on. Other sites are sometimes chosen and the tube directed anteriorly to evacuate air and posteriorly to drain fluid. During an intraoperative procedure chest tubes are positioned under direct visualization and may exit at a different point. Mediastinal chest tubes usually exit anteriorly on either side of the sternum.

The physician usually orders an analgesic, a sedative, or both before inserting a chest tube. The procedure for inserting a chest tube needs to be as sterile as possible, even when inserted outside of the hospital during an emergency. The area is cleaned with an antibacterial agent and then infiltrated with a local anesthetic, such as lidocaine (1% to 2% with or without epinephrine). An incision is made in the skin, and the chest tube is inserted. Depending on the situation, the physician inserts a metal trocar with the chest tube attached. Alternately, and more commonly, forceps are used to bluntly dissect intercostal muscles, requiring manual insertion and direction of a chest tube.

The chest tube immediately is connected to a water-sealed drainage unit (see following section) or placed directly underwater (such as in a bottle of sterile water or normal saline). The chest tube is sutured into place, and a sterile occlusive dressing is applied. Petrolatum-impregnated gauze is commonly used to prevent air from entering the chest, but its use is under scrutiny, since skin maceration may occur with prolonged use. Care is taken to ensure that the gauze dressing is occlusive and that all connections are tight and securely taped or banded. When taping connections in a spiral, be sure to allow visibility of the connection. Finally, the chest tube is anchored to the trunk, apart from the dressing, to prevent tension on it. A chest x-ray film is taken to verify the position and removal of air or fluid.

Drainage systems

A variety of drainage systems are available for use with chest tubes, including one-bottle systems, two-bottle systems, three-bottle systems, and four-bottle systems (Fig. 14-5). Commercial drainage systems are patterned after one of these types. Understanding the function of single- and multiple-bottle systems allows the nurse to apply this knowledge to commercial systems.

One-bottle system. A one-bottle system ideally is used to evacuate a pneumothorax. Because of its design, a one-bottle system is not used for fluid

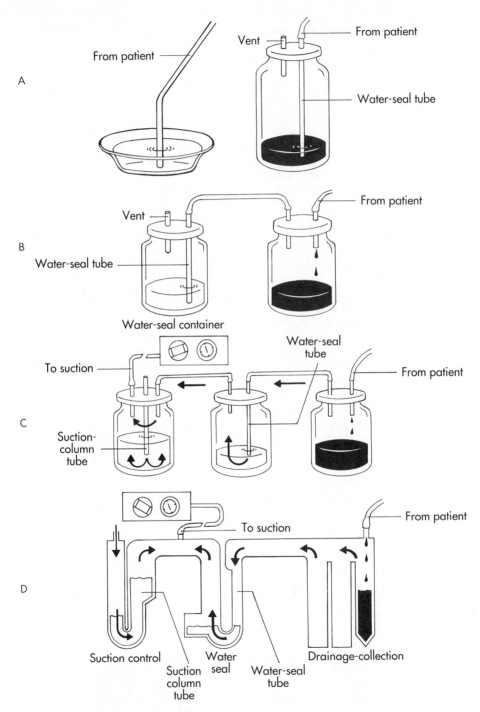

Fig. 14-5. Chest drainage systems. **A,** One-bottle type. **B,** Two-bottle type. **C,** Three-bottle type. **D,** Commercial type.

drainage. The bottle functions both as the water seal and the collection chamber. A one-bottle system has a long tube submerged in water and a short tube that vents to the atmosphere. To obtain a water seal, sterile water is poured aseptically into the bottle before the bottle is connected to the chest tube. The drainage tube is immersed under 2 cm of water for an effective seal. When intrathoracic pressure exceeds the water seal level (that is, 2 cm of water), excessive air or fluid in the pleural space is pushed out. An effective water seal isolates the pleural space from entry of air. Air is allowed to leave the pleural space but not to return. If the water seal is lost by evaporation or by tipping the bottle and exposing the end of the tube to air, negative intrapleural pressure pulls air into the patient's chest. The result of losing the water seal is a pneumothorax.

One problem with the one-bottle system is accumulation of fluid in the bottle. Raising the depth of the water seal, either with sterile water or with drainage from the patient's chest, increases the work of breathing and increases the amount of positive pressure necessary to evacuate air from the chest. Fluid drainage is impaired as the fluid column rises.

The one-bottle system usually is left open to air, although it may be connected to a suction source. When suction is needed, a vacuum regulator is connected to the short vent tubing and set to the vacuum ordered by the physician.

The water seal tube is useful for assessing proper functioning of the chest tube. In a spontaneously breathing patient, fluid in the water seal is drawn up during inhalation in response to negative intrapleural pressure. With exhalation, intrapleural pressure is more positive and pushes fluid down. In a patient receiving positive pressure mechanical ventilation, fluid in the water seal tube moves directly opposite (that is, down on inhalation and up on exhalation). The term *tidaling* is used when up and down movement of the fluid column accompanies respiratory movements. Tidaling indicates that the chest tube is in contact with the pleural space. Lack of tidaling is associated with an obstructed tube. The tube may lie against pleura surfaces or contain clots.

Bubbling of air through the tube and into the water indicates an air leak, except when vented mediastinal chest tubes are used. Bubbling in the water seal chamber is expected, and its absence indicates an abnormality, such as occlusion or kinking, with vented mediastinal chest tubes. When the chest tube is properly positioned and the connections are secure, the air leak is coming from the pleural space. Occasionally the chest tube needs additional sutures to prevent air from entering the pleural space around the chest tube. This is assessed by applying pressure over the chest tube insertion site. If the bubbling stops with pressure over the chest tube, the physician is notified.

Less often the leak is not a result of loose sutures or an actual air leak in the lung. The nurse is careful to assess for leaks in the system by momentarily (1 to 3 seconds) clamping the chest tube at the insertion site and observing for bubbling in the water seal chamber. (Note: A chest tube is never clamped for more than 10 to 15 seconds and then only when changing the bottle, since a tension pneumothorax may occur.) If a leak is still present, it is in the system. To locate the leak in the system, the nurse successively places a clamp just below each connection and assesses for leaks. When the leak stops, that connection is loose. In rare instances there may be a crack in the commercial drainage unit, necessitating replacement.

Two-bottle system. A two-bottle system is used when there is fluid drainage with or without an air leak. In the two-bottle system, the first bottle contains two short tubes and is essentially a fluid trap. The second bottle contains a long water seal tube and a short air vent or suction tube. The long tube connects the first and second bottles and is the water seal. (The second bottle of a two-bottle system looks like a one-bottle system, except that it is connected to the first bottle instead of to the patient.) The advantage of a two-bottle system is that the work of breathing is not increased as the drainage rises. Air leaks are assessed in the second bottle as air bubbles through the long tube. When necessary, suction is applied through the short tube in the second bottle.

Three-bottle system. The three-bottle system is used to evacuate any volume of fluid or air with controlled suction. A three bottle system is a two-bottle system with the addition of a third bottle to control suction. The suction-control bottle contains a long tube and two short tubes. One short tube connects bottles two and three. The second short tube is connected to an external suction source at a pressure that causes gentle, continuous bubbling in bottle three. Vigorous bubbling is not necessary and enhances fluid evaporation. The long tube is submerged in water and vented to the atmosphere. *Suction is limited to the depth that the long tube is submerged in water, regardless of the amount of suction applied by the external suction source.* If 20-cm suction is needed, the long tube is submerged 20 cm. Evaporation of water occurs as a result of bubbling in bottle three, thus decreasing the amount of effective suction. Therefore the water level is assessed frequently and replenished as needed. To revert a three-bottle system to water seal, the suction source or suction bottle must be disconnected to allow venting to the atmosphere. When suction is discontinued, a three-bottle system essentially becomes a two-bottle system.

Four-bottle system. A four-bottle system is rarely used. It contains a second water seal bottle connected to the fluid drainage bottle (bottle no. 1). Bottle four contains a long tube submerged 2 cm in water and a short tube vented to the atmosphere. With a four-bottle system, bottle one contains three short tubes. One short tube is connected to the chest tube for drainage, a second is connected to the water seal bottle, and the third is connected to bottle four. The fourth bottle acts as a safety valve to vent excessive positive pressure in the event the suction vent is obstructed or disconnected.

Commercial systems. One of the most popular commercial chest drainage units is the Pleurevac (Deknatel) (Fig. 14-5, *D*). It is essentially a three-bottle system. Chambers in commercial units often are color coded. In the Pleurevac, for example, the fluid collection chamber is white, the water seal chamber is red, and the suction control chamber is blue. Depending on the manufacturer and the model, commercial chest drainage units may contain added features. Most units have a positive pressure release valve to vent excessive positive pressure; a few have manual release buttons to vent excessive negative pressure, such as from suctioning. Newer models of chest drainage are instituting waterless suction control chambers. With these units, when decreasing the amount of suction, pressure applied against the pleura remains at the previous higher level unless manually vented. These units are also more susceptible to vacuum fluctuations from wall sources.

Fluid collection chambers vary among commercial models. Some commercial units allow independent measurement of drainage from two chest tubes. A Y-connector is not necessary to join the tubes, and the physician can decide independently when to remove each tube. In most units the fluid collection chamber is calibrated to allow accurate measurement of volumes as small as 0.5 to 1 ml, especially in an infant model. To achieve this accuracy, the fluid collection chamber is divided into several connected chambers. Chest drainage flows into the first chamber. When drainage exceeds this volume, fluid flows into the next area, much like water over a dam. When the unit is tipped, fluid moves between fluid collection chambers, making accurate measurement more difficult. The amount of drainage from the chambers is added to obtain the total volume. Autotransfusion frequently is available with commercial units. The autotransfusion system connects to the drainage tubing and essentially becomes the first chamber. When autotransfusion is no longer needed, the unit becomes a standard chest drainage system.

Commercial units have other features that are useful in patient care. Some units gauge the amount of air leak with a meter in the water seal chamber. Most commercial units are free standing, and some contain self-sealing ports to aspirate drainage or water from the water seal or suction control chambers. Unfortunately, drainage aspirated from the fluid collection chamber is not always the most current. For culturing fluid from a chest tube that has been in place for an extended period, more accurate, current drainage is obtained from the drainage tubing. Since most drainage tubing is self-sealing latex, the chest tube does not have to be opened to obtain a fluid sample.

Nursing care of patients with chest tubes

Nursing care of patients with chest tubes requires frequent assessment and special care during other nursing activities, such as turning the patient. Nursing care begins with establishing baseline vital signs, assessing pulmonary and cardiac status, and determining the patient's pain level, as well as encouraging deep-breathing and coughing exercises to enhance air and fluid evacuation from the pleural space. The nurse particularly observes for subcutaneous emphysema and splinting with pain. The nurse is careful to provide adequate analgesics as needed and to splint the patient's chest tube site and thoracotomy incisions during deep-breathing exercises. (Note: A special thoracotomy pillow, called a lung pillow, and a special mediastinotomy pillow, called the heart pillow, are available from Shumsky. These pillows are designed to conform to the patient's anatomy for splinting; they are the proper firmness to splint an incision adequately. They also contain anatomical drawings suitable for preoperative teaching.) Administration of pain medication is necessary but may be detrimental if excessive. Patients do not breathe deeply when in pain or when heavily medicated.

After assessing the patient, the nurse checks the chest tube and drainage tubing. The nurse maintains an occlusive dressing (adhesive or waterproof tape adheres the best). Paper tape is not occlusive and does not provide an adequately secure dressing or connection. A loose dressing allows air or bacteria to enter the pleural cavity. If the dressing is saturated or soiled, it is reinforced or changed according to institution policy. A wet dressing is an ideal medium for bacterial growth. If the patient's skin is irritated, a protective barrier such as Duoderm or Stomahesive is applied to the skin before taping.

The next step in assessment is to examine the connection of the chest tube to the drainage unit. A straight-line connector is preferred to a tapered connector. The connection is securely taped or banded. The nurse continues to assess the tubing for kinks or clots while draining fluid in the tubing into the fluid collection system. The tubing is coiled on the bed and drains directly into the collection bottle without dependent loops. When dependent loops are present, drainage of air and fluid is impeded.

With proper care most chest tubes drain fluid adequately. The nurse augments drainage by lifting the tubing off the bed, encouraging its movement toward the fluid collection chamber. Sometimes chest drainage is thick and slow to move. Clots may form on the walls of the chest tube or drainage tubing. Quickly squeezing and releasing the tubing loosens these clots in most instances. When clots cannot be loosened from the walls of the chest tube, the physician may insert a suction or Fogarty catheter into the chest tube and suction or pull out clots. Sometimes the chest tube is replaced. When clots obstruct the tubing to the fluid drainage system, the unit is replaced.

Controversy exists over the practices of milking and stripping, terms often confused or used interchangeably. Generally, milking is safer than stripping. Milking involves holding the tube firmly in one hand while the other hand, sliding *toward* the patient, compresses the tube. This forces clots in the tube back into the chest for gradual reabsorption. A procedure that some nurses refer to as milking involves squeezing, twisting, or rolling the tube over a clamp or between the fingers to break up clots for drainage into the fluid collection chamber.

Stripping is used primarily to maintain patency of mediastinal chest tubes with fresh bleeding in the early postoperative period. The nurse stabilizes and occludes the chest tube at the insertion site with one hand. The thumb and forefinger of the other hand, lubricated with water-soluble jelly, quickly stretch the tubing *away from* the chest. The hand on the chest tube releases first, immediately followed by the stripping hand, creating higher suction within the chest. Commercial chest tube strippers are available. Negative pressures in excess of 200 to 400 mm Hg can be generated with stripping. If not performed cautiously, fragile tissue, delicate sutures, and blood vessels can be sucked into the chest tube. Excessive bleeding may occur with chest tube stripping.

After assessing the drainage tubing, the nurse stoops to assess the drainage system at eye level. Drainage level is usually marked on a piece of tape or directly on the unit. Most commercial units have an opaque area for drawing a line and indicating the date and time of assessment. The nurse observes the amount of drainage since the last assessment. When a chest tube is first placed, assessments are made at least hourly. The interval is increased to every other hour and then every 4 hours until the chest tube is removed.

The nurse assesses the color (bright, dark; red, yellow, brown) and consistency (serous, viscous, clots) of the drainage and compares it with those in previous reports. In the immediate postoperative period, the drainage often is dark red, fresh blood. A change in color to bright red indicates fresh bleeding. Over several hours to days, postoperative chest drainage becomes more serous. Chest drainage from a pleural effusion is characteristically serous or milky (chylothorax). Infected pleural fluid often is purulent green to brown, depending on the organism, and frequently odorous. New onset of odor indicates a possible infection.

The nurse observes the chest drainage unit for proper functioning. The water seal level is assessed for tidaling with inhalation and exhalation. Recall that tidaling is absent in patients with obstructed tubes and is also diminished in patients receiving PEEP. If tidaling is absent with the application of suction, *momentarily* disconnect the suction to assess tidaling. Excessive tidaling is sometimes present with atelectasis or increased secretions.

When observing the water seal chamber, the nurse assesses for air leak. If an air leak is present, the nurse notes how it is associated with inspiration and expiration. In a mechanically ventilated patient, the air leak usually follows delivery of a breath. Bubbling from a pneumothorax usually occurs only during exhalation. Some patients demonstrate an air leak only when coughing (higher intrapleural pressure). When a bronchopleural fistula is present, the leak often occurs throughout the breathing cycle. A continuous air leak also occurs when there is an air leak in the system. (Location of a leak is discussed in the section on the single-bottle drainage system.)

The nurse finally assesses the suction control bottle or chamber. When using bottles, the tube is submerged under the ordered level of water. Evaporated water is replaced to ensure that adequate suction is being applied to the chest. Excessive water is removed with a suction catheter or syringe and extension tubing. Gentle bubbling should be present in the suction control chamber. Vigorous bubbling requires adjustment of the suction regulator to a lower level. The absence of bubbling indicates that inadequate suction may be applied to the pleural space. When suction is not being used, the nurse assesses that the suction control chamber is not connected to suction and is vented to the atmosphere.

Care is taken when turning the patient, helping the patient into the chair, or ambulating the patient to maintain patency of the chest tube and chest drainage unit. The nurse moves the tubings into position before moving the patient. If the chest tube and connections are securely taped, the tube should not inadvertently become disconnected. However, this sometimes may happen. If the tubing has fallen on the floor or is contaminated, it is not reconnected to the chest tube. The nurse immediately inserts the chest tube into a container of sterile water or saline, such as is used to fill the suction control chamber, to provide water seal while preparing a sterile chest drainage system. An infection introduced by reconnecting a contaminated tubing is expensive. Before connecting the chest tube to a new unit, some institutions require cleaning the end with an antibacterial or alcohol swab.

Special chest tubes

One special chest tube is designed to reexpand the lung after a simple pneumothorax, such as occurs with placement of a central venous catheter. This small pneumothorax catheter (the first was a Cook catheter, although other manufacturers produce a similar catheter) is inserted percutaneously, like an intravenous catheter (see Fig. 11-3). It usually is connected to a Heimlich valve, which allows air and fluid to drain out but prevents air from entering the chest. If drainage is excessive, the catheter is connected to a vented drainage bag or glove. When air is released through the valve, a squawking sound is heard. A sterile dressing is sometimes loosely taped over the end of the tube to catch drainage. Care is taken to prevent occlusion of the tip of the Heimlich valve, which may impair evacuation of air from the pleural space.

The decision to remove a chest tube is based on the amount of air and fluid drainage. If no air leak has been observed in the water seal chamber for 24 hours or longer, the chest tube usually is removed. Some physicians leave a chest tube in place during the entire period a patient is receiving positive pressure mechanical ventilation. A daily total of 100 ml or less of fluid usually indicates it is time for the chest tube to be removed. Fluid drainage over 100 ml per day is difficult for some patients to reabsorb. Excessive pleural fluid may require pleurodesis (discussed later in this chapter). With patients who have had cardiac surgery, the chest tube usually is removed in 2 to 3 days. After lung resection surgery, a chest tube is needed for about 1 week.

Chest tubes usually are removed by physicians or specially trained nurses. The patient is medicated with an analgesic, suction is discontinued, and the tape is removed from the patient's chest, exposing the sutures. The patient is asked to take a deep breath. At the peak of inspiration, when the lung is maximally inflated, the chest tube is quickly pulled out. Some physicians suture the opening. If purse-string sutures were used, they are closed as the tube is removed. If not, an occlusive dressing is applied to the site. It is common practice to apply petrolatum-impregnated gauze over an incision that was not sutured. The occlusive dressing is removed if the patient develops respiratory distress indicative of a pneumothorax. When two chest tubes are joined by a Y-connector, either or both are removed. If both are to be removed, the second chest tube is clamped while the first is being removed.

If a chest tube is placed for empyema, it is left in place until the infection resolves. Because of the fibrin clotting associated with an empyema, some physicians routinely irrigate the pleural space to enhance drainage of empyema fluid. In some cases an empyema tube is removed slowly, about 1 cm per week. This tube usually is removed from water seal and the drainage bottle and cut off at the skin. A large safety pin is inserted crosswise to prevent inward migration.

PLEURODESIS

Pleurodesis, which is also called pleurosclerotherapy, is used to prevent recurrence of a pneumothorax or pleural effusion, especially those caused by cancer. Pleurodesis is the instillation of an irritating substance into the pleural space. The most common substances used for pleurodesis are tetracycline (20 mg/kg), talc, kaolin, or nitrogen mustard. Once inserted, the irritant causes a local reaction that encourages adherence of the parietal and visceral pleura. A successful procedure prevents recurrent pneumothorax and reaccumulation of pleural fluid.

To initiate pleurodesis, the physician first inserts a chest tube, which is allowed to drain for one or more days, until the air leak or fluid drainage is minimal. Instead of removing the chest tube, the physician instills the irritant, suspended in about 50 ml of sterile normal saline, into the chest tube. The physician may first instill 20 ml of 1% or 2% lidocaine, since pleurodesis is painful. The patient also is given intramuscular or intravenous analgesics before the procedure. After all of the irritant has been instilled in the patient's chest, a 20- to 50-ml bolus of air is inserted and the chest tube is clamped. The patient is rolled from side-to-back-to-side-to-front in Trendelenburg and reverse Trendelenburg position to coat thoroughly all areas of the pleura. The patient's position is changed every 15 to 30 minutes for 1 to 2 hours. At the end of this time, the chest tube clamp is removed, allowing drainage. Suction usually is applied to enhance drainage. Brown (old bloody) drainage usually flows immediately from the tube. When pleurodesis has been performed successfully, drainage ceases in a day or two and the chest tube is removed.

CONCLUSION

This chapter has discussed invasive techniques, excluding mechanical ventilation, for improving oxygenation and ventilation. Many topics were presented, because there are numerous ways to improve gas exchange, depending on the problem. Although the physician usually initiates the treatment, it is the nurse who subsequently cares for the patient and the equipment. Competently caring for a patient with an endotracheal tube, tracheostomy tube, or chest tube is a challenge. By understanding the care of a patient who has been intubated or one with a chest tube, the nurse makes better clinical decisions and possibly prevents a complication.

BIBLIOGRAPHY

Ackerman MH: The use of bolus normal saline instillations in artificial airways: is it useful or necessary? *Heart Lung* 14(5):505-506, 1985.

Allan D: Patients with an endotracheal tube or tracheostomy, *Nursing Times* 80(13):36-38, 1984.

Amborn SA: Clinical signs associated with the amount of tracheobronchial secretions, *Nurs Res* 25(2):121-126, 1976.

Barnes CA, Kirchhoff KT: Minimizing hypoxemia due to endotracheal suctioning: a review of the literature, *Heart Lung* 15(2):164-176, 1986.

Birdsall C: What suction pressure should I use? *Am J Nurs* 85(6):866, 1985.

Blodgett D: *Manual of respiratory care procedures*, Philadelphia, 1980, JB Lippincott.

Bostick JA, Wendelgass ST: Normal saline instillation as part of the suctioning procedure: effects on Pao$_2$ and amount of secretions, *Heart Lung* 16(5):532-537, 1987.

Brook I: Microbiological studies of tracheostomy site wounds, *Eur J Respir Dis* 71(5):380-383, 1987.

Brown I: Trach care: take care—infection on the prowl, *Nursing 82* 12(5):45-49, 1982.

Burden N: Preparing for medical emergencies in the ambulatory setting, *Curr Rev Post Anesth Care Nurs* 9(17):134, 1987.

Burton GC, Hodgkin JE: *Respiratory care: a guide to clinical practice,* ed 2, Philadelphia, 1984, JB Lippincott.

Carroll P: Safe suctioning, *Nursing 89* 19(9):48-51, 1989.

Carroll PF: The ins and outs of chest drainage systems, *Nursing 86* 16(12):26-34, 1986.

Connor PA: When and how do you use a Heimlich flutter valve? *AJN* 87(3):288-290, 1987.

Cooper KL, Burns K, Torsiello P: How do you use a double-lumen endobronchial tube? *Am J Nurs* 89(11):1503-1506, 1989.

Cosenza JJ, Norton LC: Secretion clearance: state of the art from a nursing perspective, *Crit Care Nurse* 6(4):23-39, 1986.

Craven DE, Driks MR: Nosocomial pneumonia in the intubated patient, *Semin Respir Infect* 2(1):20-33, 1987.

Crow S, Carroll PF: Changing the suction catheter each time you enter a tracheostomy: necessity or waste? *Nursing Life* 5(3):44-45, 1985.

Dennison RD: Managing the patient with upper airway obstruction, *Nursing 87* 17(10):34-42, 1987.

Duncan CR, Erickson RS: Pressures associated with chest tube stripping, *Heart Lung* 11(2):166-171, 1982.

Duncan CR, Erickson RS, Weigel RM: Effect of chest tube management on drainage after cardiac surgery, *Heart Lung* 16(1):1-9, 1987.

Dunleap E: Safe and easy ways to secure breathing tubes, *RN* 50(8):26-27, 1987.

Erickson RS: Chest tubes: they're really not that complicated, *Nursing 81* 11(5):34-43, 1981.

Erickson RS: Mastering the ins and outs of chest drainage, part 1, *Nursing 89* 19(5):37-44, 1989.

Erickson, RS: Mastering the ins and outs of chest drainage, part 2, *Nursing 89* 19(6):46-50, 1989.

Farley J: Myths and facts about chest tubes, *Nursing 88* 18(6):16, 1988.

Fluck RR: Suctioning: intermittent or continuous? *Respir Care* 30(10):839, 1985.

Fuchs PL: Streamlining your suctioning techniques, part 1: nasotracheal suctioning. *Nursing 84* 14(5):55-61, 1984.

Fuchs PL: Streamlining your suctioning techniques, part 2: endotracheal suctioning, *Nursing 84* 14(6):46-51, 1984.

Fuchs PL: Streamlining your suctioning techniques, part 3: tracheostomy suctioning, *Nursing 84* 14(7):39-43, 1984.

Gatch G, Myre L, Black RE: Foreign body aspiration in children: causes, diagnosis, and prevention, *AORN J* 46(5):850-861, 1987.

Goodwin BA: Pediatric resuscitation, *Crit Care Nurse Quart* 10(4):69-79, 1988.

Guzzetta CE, Dossey BM: *Cardiovascular nursing: body-mind tapestry*, St Louis, 1984, Mosby–Year Book.

Harper R: *A guide to respiratory care: physiology and clinical applications*, Philadelphia, 1982, JB Lippincott.

Heffner JE: Airway management in the critically ill patient, *Crit Care Clin* 6(3):533-550, 1990.

Heffner JE, Miller KS, Sahn SA: Tracheostomy in the intensive care unit, part 1: indications, technique, management, *Chest* 90(2):269-274, 1986.

Heffner JE, Miller KS, Sahn SA: Tracheostomy in the intensive care unit, part 2: complications, *Chest* 90(3):430-436, 1986.

Heimlich HJ: A life-saving maneuver to prevent choking, *JAMA* 234(4):398-401, 1975.

Helling TS, Gyles NR, Eisenstein CL, Soracco CA: Complications following blunt and penetrating injuries in 216 victims of chest trauma requiring tube thoracostomy, *J Trauma* 29(10):1367-1370, 1989.

Hewitt JB, Janssen WR: A management strategy for malignancy-induced pleural effusions: long-term thoracostomy drainage, *Oncol Nurs Forum* 14(5):17-22, 1987.

Jung RC, Gottlieb LS: Comparison of tracheobronchial suction catheters in humans: visualization by fiberoptic bronchoscopy, *Chest* 69(2):179-181, 1979.

Kaufman J, Hardy-Ribakow D: What parents need to know about trach care, *RN* 51(10):99-104, 1988.

Knauss PJ: Chest tube stripping: is it necessary? *Focus Crit Care* 12(6):41-43, 1985.

Linden BE, Aguilar EA, Allen SJ: Sinusitis in the nasotracheally intubated patient, *Arch Otolaryngol Head Neck Surg* 114(8):860-861, 1988.

Lockhart JS, Griffin C: Occluded trach tube, *Nursing 87* 17(4):33, 1987.

Mapp CS: Trach care: are you aware of all the dangers? *Nursing 88* 18(7):34-43, 1988.

Martin DA, Redland AR: Legal and ethical issues in resuscitation and withholding of treatment, *Crit Care Nurse Quart* 10(4):1-8, 1988.

McPherson SP: *Respiratory therapy equipment*, St Louis, 1985, Mosby–Year Book.

Middaugh RE, Middaugh DJ, Menk EJ: Current considerations in respiratory and acid-base management during cardiopulmonary resuscitation, *Crit Care Nurse Quart* 10(4):25-33, 1988.

Miracle VA, Allnutt DR: How to perform basic airway management, *Nursing 90* 20(4):55-60, 1990.

Netter F: *The CIBA collection of medical illustrations*, vol 7, *Respiratory system*, New York, 1979, CIBA Pharmaceutical Co.

Noll ML, Hix CD, Scott G: Closed tracheal suction systems: effectiveness and nursing implications, *AACN Clin Issues Crit Care Nurs* 1(2):318-328, 1990.

Norton LC, Conforti CG: The effects of body position on oxygenation, *Heart Lung* 14(1):45-52, 1985.

O'Flaherty D, Adams AP: The end-tidal carbon dioxide detector: assessment of a new method to distinguish esophageal from tracheal intubation, *Anaesthesia* 45(8):653-655, 1990.

Palau D, Jones S: Test your skill at trouble shooting tubes, *RN* 49(10):43-45, 1986.

Pons PT: Esophageal obturator airway, *Emerg Med Clin North Am* 6(4):693-698, 1988.

Rathler MC, McNamara M: Teaching families to give trach care at home, *Nursing 82* 12(6):70-71, 1982.

Riegel B, Forshee T: A review and critique of the literature on preoxygenation for endotracheal suctioning, *Heart Lung* 14(5):507-518, 1985.

Rosequist CC: Current standards and guidelines for cardiopulmonary resuscitation and emergency cardiac care, *Heart Lung* 16(4):408-418, 1987.

Rudy E, Baun M, Stone K, et al: The relationship between endotracheal suctioning and changes in intracranial pressure: a review of the literature, *Heart Lung* 15(5):488-494, 1986.

Runton N, Zazal GH: The decannulation process in children, *J Pediatr Nurs* 4(5):370-374, 1989.

Shapiro B, Harrison R, et al: *Clinical applications of respiratory care*, ed 3, Chicago, 1985, Mosby–Year Book.

Shoemaker WC, Thompson WL, Holbrook PR: *The Society of Critical Care Medicine Textbook of Critical Care*, Philadelphia, 1984, WB Saunders.

Snowberger P: Decreasing endotracheal damage due to excessive cuff pressures, *Dimens Crit Care Nurs* 5(3):136-143, 1986.

Standards and guidelines for cardiopulmonary resuscitation (CPR) and emergency cardiac care, *Heart Lung* 16:408, 1987.

Stone KS: Ventilator versus manual resuscitation bag as the method for delivering hyperoxygenation before endotracheal suctioning, *AACN Clin Issues Crit Care* 1(2):289-299, 1990.

Villeneuve MJ, Hodnett ED: Cerebrovascular status and Trendelenburg position in severe head injury, *Axone* 11(3):64-67, 1990.

Visintine RE, Baick CH: Ruptured stomach after Heimlich maneuver, *JAMA* 234(4):415, 1975.

Wade JF: *Comprehensive respiratory care: physiology and technique*, ed 3, St Louis, 1982, Mosby–Year Book.

Willens J, Copel L: Performing CPR on adults, *Nursing 89* 19(1):34-43, 1989.

Willens JS, Copel LC: Performing CPR on infants, *Nursing 89* 19(3):47-53, 1989.

Willens JS, Copel LC: Performing CPR on children, *Nursing 89* 19(2):57-64, 1989.

Wilson EB, Malley N: Discharge planning for the patient with a new tracheostomy, *Crit Care Nurse* 10(7):73-79, 1990.

C H·A·P·T·E·R — *15*

Methods of Mechanical Ventilation

Objectives

- *Examine methods of noninvasive and invasive mechanical ventilation.*
- *Describe the procedure for cardiopulmonary resuscitation.*
- *List the indications for and complications of nasal and mask continuous positive airway pressure (CPAP).*
- *Differentiate the modes of positive-pressure mechanical ventilation.*
- *Identify complications of mechanical ventilation.*
- *Discuss different ventilator settings.*
- *State which settings to change based on arterial blood gas analysis.*
- *Explain techniques to wean a patient from mechanical ventilation.*
- *Discuss signs of failure to wean.*
- *Discuss jet ventilation.*

NONINVASIVE MECHANICAL VENTILATION

The decision to ventilate a patient does not always require intubation; there are several types of noninvasive mechanical ventilation. In general, these noninvasive methods are used in the home and not in the critical care setting, although they are also used in the intensive care unit. This section discusses negative-pressure ventilation and nasal and oral positive-pressure mechanical ventilation. A subsequent section examines types of invasive mechanical ventilation.

Negative-pressure ventilation

Negative-pressure ventilation is the natural form of ventilation. In a spontaneously breathing patient, subatmospheric pressure is created by increasing the volume in the chest; this is accomplished through contraction of the diaphragm and intercostal muscles. This negative pressure draws air into the patient's lungs. When the inspiratory muscles relax, the chest wall recoils to its natural relaxed state and exhalation is passive. Negative-pressure ventilators imitate spontaneous natural ventilation.

There are several different types of negative-pressure ventilators, all of which work on the same theory. Negative pressure is applied to the patient's chest, creating a vacuum. The chest wall subsequently is pulled out. As the chest wall expands, negative intrathoracic pressure is created and air is sucked into the patient's lungs. When the vacuum is released, the chest wall recoils, allowing exhalation.

Negative-pressure ventilators were used extensively in the post-polio era. They fell out of favor as positive-pressure ventilators were developed and improved. Studies are in progress to identify more clinical uses for noninvasive negative-pressure ventilators. Patients with chronic obstructive pulmonary disease (COPD) are the focus of most study in this area. Negative-pressure ventilators currently in use are the iron lung, chest cuirass, poncho wrap, and pneumobelt. Another type of negative-pressure ventilation is the rocking bed.

The *iron lung*, or body tank ventilator, is the most effective—and most limiting—negative-pressure ventilator. The first iron lung was invented by Drinker and Shaw in 1928. The iron lung is an airtight cylinder that encloses the patient from his neck to his feet. Foam rubber placed around the neck prevents air leaks. The iron lung is used mainly for patients with normal airways who cannot maintain adequate ventilation. A neonatal Isolette negative-pressure ventilator works similarly to an iron lung.

The iron lung surrounds the patient's body with subatmospheric pressure. The pressure in the patient's lungs is atmospheric, since the head and upper airway are exposed to the environment. The pressure difference between the mouth and chest wall causes a gradient that expands the chest and pulls air into the patient's chest. A diaphragm at the patient's feet moves in and out to create negative pressure. In early models, a manual pump was continuously compressed and released by care givers. Someone was always awake to operate the pump. Current models use electricity to power the diaphragm.

Patients in iron lungs require total care. Some patients can breathe on their own for minutes to hours a day out of the iron lung, although most patients require continuous support. Most iron lungs are stationary, but portable models are available. Immobility and its resultant problems are a prime concern with patients in an iron lung. In addition, because the abdominal wall is also subject to negative pressure, abdominal pooling of blood can occur, decreasing venous return and cardiac output.

Drinker collaborated with Collins in the late 1930s to produce a portable iron lung, of sorts, that would eliminate the problem of abdominal pooling of blood. The result is a *chest cuirass,* commonly referred to as the turtle shell. It is much more portable than the iron lung.

With the cuirass, a dome-shaped, rigid shell covers the anterior and lateral chest wall, giving the appearance of a turtle shell. With the cuirass, subatmospheric pressure is exerted only on the chest wall by an electric pump that works similarly to a vacuum cleaner. The physician determines the therapeutic level of negative pressure by assessing tidal volumes and arterial blood gases while the patient is ventilated by the cuirass. The maximum amount of negative pressure exerted depends on the fit of the cuirass. When the fit allows air to be pulled in around the rim, less pressure is applied to the chest.

Chest cuirasses come in many sizes to accommodate tall, short, thin, and obese pediatric and adult patients. Looser fits generate less pressure and less ventilation than snug fits. Foam on the rim cushions the skin from abrasion and enhances the seal. Additional foam padding is applied to improve the seal in a looser fitting cuirass. A plaster mold of the patient's chest is used to make a custom chest cuirass when a standard model does not fit, such as in cases of severe kyphoscoliosis. Manufacturing a custom-molded chest cuirass takes several weeks.

Although the chest cuirass is more portable than the iron lung, the patient is still tied to a short leash. The electric pump is noisy and has no alarms.

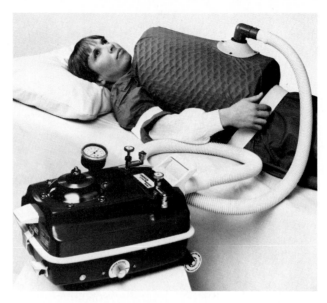

Fig. 15-1. Patient wearing a poncho wrap negative-pressure ventilator. (Courtesy of JH Emerson Co, Cambridge, Mass.)

Patients generally cannot rely on the chest cuirass for complete ventilatory support. The chest cuirass usually is used for patients who need nocturnal ventilation for hypoventilation syndromes or weak respiratory muscles.

The *poncho wrap* is a form of chest cuirass (Fig. 15-1). With the poncho wrap, the patient wears a metal cage similar to a turtle shell. A large poncho covers the cage and encases the entire thorax from the hips to the neck, including the arms. A drawstring closes securely around the neck, and elastic or Velcro bands encase the wrists and hips to prevent air leaks. The poncho wrap is connected to an electric pump that, like a vacuum cleaner, pulls air from within the poncho, creating a vacuum and expanding the lungs. Preventing leaks is a problem with this type of ventilator. The poncho wrap is considered easier to use in acute conditions, because it does not require the special sizing concerns of a chest cuirass. The poncho wrap may be used instead of custom molding a chest cuirass.

The *pneumobelt* is the least invasive and often the least effective negative-pressure ventilator. It consists of an inflatable rubber bladder or diaphragm held in place by a binder or straps. When the bladder is inflated with air, the abdominal contents are compressed, pushing the diaphragm up and allowing or gently forcing exhalation. As air is released from the bladder, the abdominal contents resume their normal position, allowing the diaphragm to descend. Negative pressure is created when the diaphragm moves downward; inspiration results. Because of its design, the pneumobelt is less effective and therefore not used in obese or very thin individuals.

The *rocking bed* is similar to the pneumobelt in that it uses intraabdominal pressure to augment ventilation. The rocking bed gently rocks the patient from head to toe instead of the customary side to side. As the patient is tipped on his head, the abdominal contents push up against the diaphragm, encouraging exhalation. As the head elevates, the abdominal contents move down, allowing the diaphragm to descend; the patient inhales.

With all of the negative-pressure ventilators, effectiveness initially is assessed by the patient's inability to speak during inspiration. If the patient can speak during what is supposed to be inspiration, the pressure is not great enough to cause adequate inspiration. Phonation occurs only during exhalation of air over the vocal cords, just as in normal people. The ultimate assessment of effectiveness is normal arterial blood gases.

Negative-pressure ventilators have several advantages and disadvantages. The main advantage is preservation of physiological ventilation and intrathoracic pressure changes. Cardiac output is preserved, because venous return is normal (in direct contrast to impeded venous return with positive-pressure ventilation). In addition, the patient does not have to be intubated and predisposed to infection from an artificial airway. Some patients being converted to negative-pressure ventilation from positive-pressure ventilation, as well as patients with ineffective airway clearance who require suctioning, may need an artificial airway temporarily. A tracheostomy makes fitting a chest cuirass and poncho wrap difficult.

The primary disadvantages of negative-pressure ventilation are pain, formation of pressure sores, and limited communication because of the tight seal required for effective ventilation. Early in the period of adjustment to negative-pressure ventilation, particularly to the chest cuirass, bruising develops on the lateral chest. Skin care is essential. Applying tincture of benzoin and transparent dressings helps prevent skin breakdown. Patient care also is affected by complications of immobility, especially with the iron lung. Patients who require supplemental oxygen must have the oxygen supplied separately. A nasal cannula commonly is used, although some patients need a mask. When high concentrations of oxygen are needed, the patient usually requires intubation and positive-pressure ventilation. In addition, with negative-pressure ventilation, precise minute volumes are unknown. Because ventilation is pressure based, changes in compliance because of bronchospasm, fluid, or secretions result in delivery of decreased volumes.

Positive-pressure ventilation

The simplest and often the first kind of noninvasive mechanical ventilation used is artificial or mouth-to-mouth respiration performed during cardiopulmonary resuscitation. This blowing of air into the mouth is positive-pressure ventilation. A mechanical ventilator performs the same function when attached to a special mask or mouthpiece instead of an endotracheal tube. Emergency resuscitation is followed by mask positive-pressure ventilation.

Emergency resuscitation. Cessation of breathing (respiratory arrest) or heart beat (cardiac arrest) requires immediate intervention by the nurse. Failure to restore pulse and respirations results in cyanosis in 1 minute and permanent organ damage in just 4 to 5 minutes. Cardiac arrest frequently is caused by myocardial infarction, although it also is caused by hemorrhage, pericardial tamponade, pulmonary embolism, and valvular heart disease. Respiratory arrest usually follows cardiac arrest within minutes. It also may be the primary event, following blockage of the upper or lower airway by secretions or a foreign body. Respiratory arrest also occurs in drug overdose, cerebrovascular accident, near drowning, and electrocution. Since cardiac arrest usually follows respiratory arrest within minutes, the nurse needs to

---

Cardiopulmonary resuscitation (CPR)

1. Evaluate responsiveness
   - Shake or tap the patient to arouse him
   - Shout, "Are you OK?"
2. Call for help, or call a code
   - 911 or 0 or special hospital code
3. Establish *Airway*
   - Head-tilt/chin-lift maneuver
   - Jaw-thrust maneuver
   - Mouth sweep to remove debris
   - Oral or nasal airway
4. Restore *Breathing*
   - Assess for air movement by looking at chest, listening for or feeling air movement from nose and mouth
   - Mouth-to-mouth ventilation
   - Mouth-to-nose ventilation
   - Mouth-to-stoma ventilation
   - Ambu ventilation
   - Oral or nasal intubation
   - Mechanical ventilation
5. Restore *Circulation*
   - External cardiac compressions
   - Defibrillation

---

know how to restore both pulse and respirations.

In performing emergency cardiopulmonary resuscitation (CPR), the nurse remembers ABC: airway, breathing, and circulation; this is the order for cardiopulmonary resuscitation. The box above lists actions to take when the nurse suspects a patient has had a cardiopulmonary arrest.

Certification in basic cardiopulmonary life support, through the American Heart Association or the American Red Cross, assures basic competency in performing CPR. Families of patients at risk for cardiopulmonary arrest are certified for basic life support, which includes techniques of cardiopulmonary resuscitation. Parents of high-risk infants, or children and families of cardiac patients or patients with a home mechanical ventilator commonly achieve basic certification. For nurses working with critically ill patients, certification in advanced cardiopulmonary life support (ACLS) often is desired and sometimes is required by the institution. ACLS includes protocols for administering medication, intubation procedures, defibrillation techniques, and other invasive measures to restore cardiopulmonary function. The information in this section is not meant to certify the nurse to perform CPR, but to serve as an adjunct.

Obtaining a patent airway is the first step in CPR. To obtain a patent airway, the nurse first properly positions the patient by placing him supine and tilting the head backward (unless this is contraindicated because of neck, back, or facial injuries). A backboard is placed under the thorax for performing external chest compressions. To relieve upper airway obstruction from the tongue and palate, the neck ideally is hyperextended using the head-tilt/chin-lift maneuver. When hyperextension cannot be used, the nurse uses a jaw-thrust method.

To perform the *head-tilt/chin-lift* maneuver, the nurse pushes firmly backward on the forehead with the palm of one hand while using the other hand to grasp and lift the bony part of the jaw near the chin. Pulling up on the jaw while pushing back on the forehead hyperextends the neck. A small towel roll under the shoulders enhances extension. This procedure is not used in patients with cervical spine injuries.

The *jaw-thrust* maneuver, also called jutting the jaw, is performed by grasping the corners of the lower jaw with both hands and lifting. Some nurses prefer to place a thumb in the mouth and pull the jaw forward. The patient's mouth usually falls open when the head is tilted back or the jaw thrust out.

An oral airway sometimes is inserted, when available, to prevent the tongue from obstructing the airway. If particulates are noted in the mouth, they are removed by sweeping the mouth with the first two fingers. A hooking motion starting at one cheek and continuing around the base of the tongue to the other cheek removes most particulates or foreign bodies. Oral pharyngeal suctioning frequently is necessary. Care is taken to avoid pushing the foreign body deeper into the airway. In cases of foreign body aspiration, an abdominal thrust maneuver is performed to dislodge the foreign body.

Positioning the patient and the head should take the nurse about 10 to 15 seconds. After the airway has been opened, the nurse listens for air movement. In some instances relieving airway obstruction restores breathing, and supplemental oxygen is temporarily applied by mask. In other instances artificial ventilation is needed.

Depending on the patient and the skill of the care giver or nurse, a variety of techniques can be used when no medical facilities are available. In this situation, mouth-to-mouth, mouth-to-nose, or mouth-to-stoma resuscitation is initiated. The nurse delivers two slow, full breaths into the patient's lungs and then briefly assesses for return of spontaneous ventilations. Each breath is delivered over 1 to 1½ seconds. In health care institutions, an air-bag-mask unit, also called an ambu, is used to restore breathing. Intubation is performed when skilled personnel are available. If breathing is not restored, artificial ventilations continue. For adults, ventilations are performed every 5 seconds or 12 times a minute. Children are ventilated more rapidly, every 3 seconds or 20 times a minute. The airway again is assessed for particulates or a foreign body if there is resistance to manual ventilations (assuming neck position is correct).

After establishing a patent airway and restoring breathing, circulation must be restored, if absent. To evaluate circulation the nurse assesses the carotid pulse for about 5 seconds. If this pulse is absent, external cardiac compressions are begun. Proper hand position is important to prevent further injury to the patient. Properly positioned hands are located 2 cm or 2 fingerbreadths above the xiphoid process directly over the sternum. In adults, the nurse compresses the sternum about 2 inches; in infants and children, the depth is 1 to 1½ inches. Compressions occur at a rate of 80 to 100 per minute in adults and children and 100 to 200 per minute in infants. Since the patient in cardiac arrest does not breathe, ventilations are administered after every five external chest compressions. Some patients require defibrillation for dysrhythmias.

Continuous positive airway pressure (CPAP). Although some systems provide only positive pressure during expiration (called expiratory positive airway pressure [EPAP] or spontaneous positive end-expiratory pressure [sPEEP]), this discussion is limited to the more common CPAP. EPAP is less effective in increasing functional residual capacity. It has the advantage (also a disadvantage) of requiring lower flow rates, which result in less air swallowing and abdominal distention.

Nasal CPAP (see Fig. 10-5) was first used by an anesthesiologist approximately 80 years ago. Over 50 years ago it began to be used to treat hypoxemia secondary to pulmonary edema and pneumonia and to allow flying at high altitudes. Twenty years ago, CPAP was rediscovered in the treatment of infant respiratory distress syndrome, adult respiratory distress syndrome (ARDS), and exertional dyspnea in COPD. Now it commonly is used in patients with obstructive sleep apnea to keep the airway from collapsing during sleep. Nasal or mask CPAP may be used to avoid endotracheal reintubation after extubation. It also has been used in other instances to avoid intubation or as a treatment for acute respiratory failure, pulmonary contusion, flail chest, cardiogenic pulmonary edema, ARDS, pulmonary embolism, bronchiolitis, fat emboli, pneumonitis, viral pneumonia, and asthma.

With CPAP, the patient breathes spontaneously at an elevated baseline (above atmospheric) pressure. Pressures ranging from 2.5 to 15 cwp are delivered through one of several types of devices, one of which is a threshold resister valve. This pressure not only distends oral pharyngeal tissue, but also keeps alveoli from collapsing. The end result is an increase in functional residual capacity. Improvement in arterial oxygen tension (Pao_2) usually is accompanied by decreases in intrapulmonary shunting, the work of breathing, and oxygen consumption.

Either continuous-flow or demand-valve gas delivery systems are available for administering CPAP. Continuous-flow CPAP is more common. With this system, high-flow gas is continuously directed from a bag reservoir or pump into the mask (or artificial airway). Air flow is not controlled by a valve in the continuous-flow CPAP system. The air is always available to the patient. With a demand-valve CPAP system, the patient opens a valve to receive air flow. The flow control opens in response to a drop in airway pressure, usually 1 cwp. Inhalation usually opens the valve, but it also may be opened by a leak in the system. Some patients have difficulty opening the valve, especially when applied through the Bennett MA-2 and some Bear ventilators.

Many companies manufacture nasal and face masks for CPAP. Face mask CPAP usually is limited to closely monitored patients in a hospital. CPAP also is used for intubated patients as a weaning mode when atelectasis prevents use of a T tube. Face mask therapy usually is continuous, whereas nasal CPAP is intermittent. Nasal CPAP is used extensively in the home. The nasal masks come in a variety of sizes to accommodate broad and narrow noses, as well as long and short noses. A fitting guide is available to help in selecting the proper mask. The masks are transparent, lightweight, and have a soft, pliable seal around the rim. The mask used in nasal CPAP is secured by elastic straps that go around the patient's head. A tight seal is best but not essential as long as the system pressure is maintained. Open mouths do not preserve pressure. Since some patients have difficulty keeping their mouths closed, a chin strap often is necessary.

Potential complications of CPAP

Aerophagia
Aspiration
Retention of carbon dioxide
Decrease in cardiac output
Discomfort
Disruption of tracheal or esophageal anastomosis
Erythema
Irritation of facial skin
Gastric distention
Hypoventilation
Intolerance
Pneumocephalus
Pressure sores
Pulmonary barotrauma

Various complications arise with CPAP, and these are summarized in the box above. The most common complication of nasal masks is irritation of the face and nasal bridge. Some patients develop erythema where the mask touches the skin or pressure sores across the bridge of the nose. A foam pad or small adhesive bandage can be used to cushion the nose and prevents irritation. A few patients cannot tolerate the positive-pressure sensation. Compared with the risks of intubation or permanent tracheostomy, most patients gradually develop a tolerance of the pressure sensation and other discomforts. The best way to minimize these problems is to increase the interval of nasal CPAP slowly over several days until the prescribed number of hours is reached.

The incidence of these and other complications is small. Hypoventilation is the most critical complication of nasal CPAP and usually occurs at high levels of CPAP. Overdistention of normal alveoli can increase the ratio of dead space to tidal volume. Carbon dioxide retention can lead to hypercapnia. Fatigue, weakness, oversedation, and lethargy also lead to hypoventilation.

Swallowing air is a potential complication of nasal CPAP but is more common in mask CPAP. Continued aerophagia results in gastric distention. Patients with aerophagia belch frequently. Emesis and possible aspiration of gastric contents are a hazard. When a full face mask rather than a nasal mask is used, the risk of emesis and aspiration is great, especially in a patient with an altered level of consciousness. A nasogastric or orogastric tube can be inserted to decompress the stomach in hospitalized patients.

Because inhaled air is under positive pressure, there is the risk of barotrauma. It is believed that the risk of pulmonary barotrauma is reduced because the patient is breathing spontaneously. It is possible that fresh sutures in the upper or lower airway or in the esophagus could be disrupted. If basilar skull fractures are present, air can enter the cranium (pneumocephalus). Positive-pressure breathing also is associated with a decrease in cardiac output from decreased venous return secondary to increased intrathoracic pressure. In patients with hypovolemia, the increase in intrathoracic pressure is magnified and can result in hypotension.

INVASIVE MECHANICAL VENTILATION

Invasive mechanical ventilation is instituted when the patient cannot maintain adequate ventilation (hypercapnia with acidemia), oxygenation (hypoxemia), or both with noninvasive measures. The following discussion is limited to mechanical ventilation with a positive-pressure mechanical ventilator through an artificial airway such as an endotracheal tube or tracheostomy tube.

A positive-pressure mechanical ventilator is a device that forces air into the lungs and allows the patient to exhale passively. A ventilator is classified as one of the types: time cycled, pressure cycled, or volume cycled. (Since time-cycled mechanical ventilation is rarely used in hospitalized adults, it is not discussed at length.) A time-cycled mechanical ventilator delivers air to the patient for a preset length of time (inspiration). The patient exhales passively. Volume, pressure, and flow depend on the ventilator and the patient.

A pressure-cycled mechanical ventilator (also called a pressure-limited ventilator) is used primarily in infants and for treatments with intermittent positive pressure breathing (IPPB). A newer form of pressure-cycled ventilation, called *pressure support,* currently is being used to wean patients from mechanical ventilation. The physician determines pressure, flow, and frequency. Volume is determined by these variables in combination with lung compliance. With a pressure-cycled mechanical ventilator, the breath is delivered until a preset pressure is reached. The physician usually sets the pressure based on the tidal volumes achieved at various levels of pressure. Lung volumes are intermittently or continuously monitored with a spirometer and remain in a given range as long as lung compliance is stable. As lung compliance decreases (that is, as the lungs become stiffer), lung volumes decrease. Pressure-cycled mechanical ventilators are not effective in ventilating patients with stiff lungs (including pneumonia or ARDS) or who have changing lung compliance and airway resistance.

Volume-cycled mechanical ventilators are commonly used both in the hospital and at home. A volume-cycled ventilator delivers a constant preset volume of gas to the patient regardless of airway resistance and compliance. (*Note:* The ventilator has a safety valve and an alarm that prevent delivering a full breath under excessive pressure.) The physician determines volume, flow, and frequency. The pressure required to deliver the ventilator breaths depends on lung compliance. When lung compliance is normal, the pressure is relatively low, about 30 cwp or less. As compliance decreases, the pressure required to deliver the breath increases. Most ventilators used in the hospital can deliver volume at pressures up to about 120 cwp, making them suitable for critically ill patients with altered lung mechanics.

When a breath is delivered by a volume-cycled ventilator, a small amount of the breath is lost within the ventilator and circuit. In most patients, the amount is a negligible 3 to 4 ml/cwp and depends on the type of ventilator circuit and the amount of pressure required to deliver the breath. In patients requiring high pressures to deliver the volume, the amount of tidal volume lost is greater. For instance, in the patient with normal ventilating pressures (20 cwp at a tidal volume of 700 ml) the amount of displaced tidal volume is 20×3 to 4, or 60 to 80 ml. The amount of air reaching the patient's lungs is actually $700 - 60$ to 80, or 620 to 640 ml. If lung compliance decreases in the same patient (such as occurs with pneumonia or ARDS), the ventilating pressure increases, perhaps to 60 cwp. Instead of losing 60 to 80 ml of tidal volume, the patient now loses 60 × 3 to 4, or 180 to 240 ml. Effective tidal volume is reduced to 460 to 520 ml. The additional loss of volume can contribute to atelectasis. It is not unusual for the physician to adjust the tidal volume or rate to increase the patient's effective minute ventilation. It is important to remember that increasing the tidal volume can also raise the ventilating pressure, and thus reduce tidal volume.

Modes of ventilation

Volume-cycled ventilators can deliver one or more modes of ventilation. The traditional modes of ventilation are controlled mandatory ventilation (CMV), assist control (AC), intermittent mandatory ventilation (IMV), or synchronous IMV (SIMV). Newer modes of mechanical ventilation are pressure-support ventilation (PSV), asynchronous lung ventilation (ALV), independent lung ventilation (ILV) or differential lung ventilation (DLV), inverse ratio ventilation (IRV), airway pressure release ventilation (APRV), proportional assist ventilation (PAV), and mandatory minute ventilation (MMV) or augmented minute ventilation (AMV). (A discussion of jet ventilation, which requires a special mechanical ventilator and nursing care, follows the section on weaning.) Documentation of theory, indications, and effectiveness are scant on most of the newer modes of mechanical ventilation and are not discussed in detail. The definitions for each of these modes is presented in Table 15-1 on pp. 342-343.

Controlled ventilation (CMV) was widely used before the development of assist controlled (AC) and intermittent mandatory ventilation (IMV). With CMV, the sensitivity control is off. On most ventilators, CMV is converted to AC by adjusting the sensitivity to allow the patient to initiate a breath. A disadvantage of AC over CMV is that the patient can hyperventilate with AC, because the patient determines frequency. In most instances the hyperventilation is controlled by lowering the tidal volume or sedating the patient (as long as the backup rate and volume are adequate).

IMV is a widely used mode of mechanical ventilation and weaning. Unlike with AC, using IMV usually is not associated with hyperventilation and resultant alkalemia. The patient routinely requires less sedation. A disadvantage of IMV is that most ventilators are configured to deliver the breaths after opening of a demand valve. The demand valve differs on each ventilator; some require more work to open the valve. Continuous-flow IMV is associated with less work of breathing but requires more time and expense to set up and maintain.

Pressure-support ventilation (PSV) frequently is used with IMV to decrease the work of breathing. When properly applied, PSV increases the volume of spontaneous breaths, allowing the respiratory muscles to work without developing fatigue. PSV helps the patient overcome resistance and compliance problems and is more comfortable than other modes of mechanical ventilation. In most patients a pressure-support level of 20 cwp provides adequate assistance to overcome the work of breathing and prevent muscle fatigue.

Ventilator settings. To implement traditional modes of ventilation, the nurse must understand the various possible settings. These include tidal and sigh volumes; low, high, and sigh pressure limits; rate; concentration of inspired oxygen (FiO_2); positive end-expiratory pressure (PEEP); peak flow; inspiration to expiration ratio (I:E), and sensitivity. In the critically ill patient, *tidal volume* usually is set at 10 to 15 ml per kilogram of lean body weight, but this value can be altered based on the patient's condition, arterial blood gases, and readiness to wean. In the average 70-kg adult, the tidal volume is set at 600 to 900 ml. In adults the tidal volume usually ranges from 500 to 1000 ml.

Sigh volume is set to deliver a breath that is 15 to 20 ml/kg, or about one and a half times the patient's tidal volume. The sigh is delivered at regular intervals or is triggered manually, such as for suctioning. Sighs usually are used only in the controlled (CMV) or assist controlled (AC) modes of ventilation to prevent atelectasis. With many other modes of ventilation the patient can generate a spontaneous sigh.

A certain pressure is required to deliver a tidal volume or sigh volume breath with a volume-cycled ventilator. This pressure, read on the pressure manometer, is called *peak ventilating pressure*. Ideally it is measured by means of a probe near the airway (proximal airway pressure) rather than by a machine system pressure reading. To prevent breaths from being delivered to the patient with excessive force, a high-pressure alarm limit is set, usually 10 cwp higher than normal peak ventilating pressure. The sigh pressure alarm limit is set 10 cwp higher than the pressure required to deliver a sigh breath. When the pressure exceeds the set high limit, excess volume is vented and not delivered to the patient. If the high-pressure alarm limit is set too high or is not set, the patient may develop barotrauma or other problems.

The peak ventilating pressure is also useful in setting the low-pressure alarm limit. This usually is set 10 cwp below the normal peak ventilating pressure. When the ventilator fails to achieve the minimum low pressure, an alarm is sounded. Depending on the situation, when the low-pressure alarm sounds, the patient is breathing shallowly or there is a leak in the circuit. The low-pressure alarm may also indicate improved lung mechanics.

The *rate* or frequency of breathing is set to meet the patient's minimum requirements, usually 10 to 16 breaths per minute. When the rate is meant to supplement the patient's own breathing, such as AC or intermittent mandatory ventilation (IMV), a backup rate of about 75% is used, depending on the patient's condition. The rate is lower in patients being weaned from mechanical ventilation.

The physician determines the appropriate mode, rate, and frequency based on the arterial carbon dioxide tension (Pa_{CO_2}) and pH from the arterial blood gases. In general, the minute ventilation is decreased to increase the Pa_{CO_2} and decrease the pH (hyperventilation); the minute ventilation is increased for hypoventilation (that is, decreased pH and increased Pa_{CO_2}). (See Table 15-2).

The Fi_{O_2} is directly set on some ventilators. On others the oxygen is blended externally to achieve the proper mix. In some situations, especially continuous-flow IMV, both the ventilator dial and the oxygen blender are adjusted to achieve the ordered flow. Some microprocessor-controlled ventilators allow for temporary increases in the Fi_{O_2} to 100%. The interval usually is 2 minutes and allows for oxygenation before or after suctioning without the worry of returning the dial or dials to previously ordered settings.

The physician determines the amount of oxygen. In critically ill patients, 100% oxygen frequently is administered when the patient first begins using the ventilator. Based on the arterial blood gases, the physician calculates an arterial/alveolar ratio (a/A O_2) at the current Fi_{O_2} and predicts the Fi_{O_2} to achieve an arterial oxygen tension (Pa_{O_2}) between 60 to 100 mm Hg and an arterial oxygen saturation (Sa_{O_2}) of 90% or higher (see Chapter 9 for review of a/A$_{O_2}$). Alternately, the physician orders a given Fi_{O_2} and increases or de-

Table 15-1. Modes of mechanical ventilation

Mode	Definition	Indications
Controlled ventilation (CMV)	Patient receives a preset volume and preset frequency and cannot generate spontaneous breaths. Ventilator is not set to sense patient efforts. Minute ventilation is determined by physician.	Apnea, surgery, respiratory muscle paralysis, sedation, drug overdose, status epilepticus, tetany
Assist controlled (AC)	Patient receives a preset volume and a minimum frequency. Ventilator sensitivity is set to deliver preset volume for spontaneous breathing efforts. Total frequency and minute ventilation are determined by patient.	All; used in most institutions when patient is first intubated
Intermittent mandatory ventilation (IMV) or synchronous intermittent mandatory ventilation (SIMV)	Patient receives a preset volume and preset frequency. Between ventilator breaths the patient breathes spontaneous volume and frequency. With IMV, the ventilator delivers a ventilator breath at any time in the patient's respiratory cycle and may cause overinflation. SIMV spaces ventilator breaths between patient breaths to prevent overinflation or stacking. IMV is delivered from a continuous-flow gas source or a demand valve. The latter is associated with increased work of breathing in most ventilators.	All; used as a weaning mode or to decrease alkalemia from hyperventilation caused by patient overbreathing with AC
Pressure-support ventilation (PSV)	Patient determines inspiratory flow rate, inspiratory time, and frequency. Ventilator delivers a preset positive pressure to overcome compliance and resistance problems that aid in decreasing the work of breathing. PSV is available only on the newer microprocessor-controlled ventilators.	High resistance, low compliance, possibly weaning, long-term mechanical ventilation, especially when combined with IMV or SIMV

Method	Description	Indication
Independent lung ventilation (ILV)	Each lung is independently ventilated. A special double-lumen endotracheal tube (Bronchocath or Carlens), which isolates each lung from the other, is necessary for ILV. ILV usually requires sedation and special suctioning techniques through the smaller lumens. Higher levels of oxygen and PEEP are applied to the diseased lung, preventing injury to the normal lung.	Unilateral lung disease such as lung contusion, pneumonia, hemoptysis, bronchopleural fistula
Airway pressure release ventilation (APRV)	Patient receives continuous positive airway pressure (CPAP) ventilation, except that during exhalation a valve opens, allowing the pressure to release to a lower or ambient pressure. The physician determines the CPAP level, the frequency of pressure releases, the level of CPAP during the release, and the duration of the pressure release or expiration.	Unknown; inadequate alveolar ventilation, possibly ARDS with air-flow obstruction
Inverse ratio ventilation (IRV)	Patient has a prolonged inspiratory phase. The inspiration to expiration ratio (I:E) is 1+:1. All breaths are ventilator controlled, requiring patient sedation or paralysis.	ARDS with refractory hypoxemia
Proportional assist ventilation (PAV)	Ventilator changes airway pressure based on inspired volume or flow or both to decrease the work of breathing.	Unclear; not useful for apnea
Mandatory minute ventilation (MMV) or augmented minute ventilation (AMV)	Patient breathes spontaneously. If the patient's minute ventilation falls below a preset level, the ventilator delivers breath(s) at a preset volume until reaching the minimum minute ventilation.	Possibly weaning or respiratory muscle fatigue

Table 15-2. Ventilator settings based on arterial blood gases

Action desired	Assist controlled ventilation (AC)	Intermittent mandatory ventilation (IMV)
Decrease arterial oxygen saturation (Pa_{O_2})	Decrease Fi_{O_2}	Decrease Fi_{O_2}
Decrease arterial oxygen saturation (Sa_{O_2})	Decrease PEEP	Decrease PEEP
Increase Pa_{O_2}	Increase Fi_{O_2}	Increase Fi_{O_2}
Increase Sa_{O_2}	Increase PEEP	Increase PEEP
	Correct alkalemia	Correct alkalemia
	Administer blood if hemoglobin is under 12-15 g/dl	Administer blood if hemoglobin is under 12-15 g/dl
	Increase cardiac output	Increase cardiac output
	Correct hypophosphatemia	Correct hypophosphatemia
Decrease Pa_{CO_2}	Increase rate	Increase rate
Increase pH	Increase tidal volume	Increase tidal volume
		Change to AC
Increase Pa_{CO_2}	Decrease tidal volume	Decrease rate
Decrease pH	Sedate patient*	Decrease tidal volume
	Increase dead space	Increase dead space
	Change to IMV	

*Decreasing the rate has no effect on overall minute ventilation with AC, since the patient controls the rate. Sedating the patient frequently decreases the rate.

creases it in increments of 10% to 20% until the desired Pa_{O_2} and Sa_{O_2} are obtained. Most patients require about 30% to 40% Fi_{O_2} for adequate oxygenation.

When a patient is difficult to oxygenate, other measures to improve oxygen transport and delivery are necessary. These measures are based on knowledge of the oxyhemoglobin curve and factors that improve oxygen delivery. Nursing interventions include administering blood to increase hemoglobin and the oxygen-carrying capacity; administering vasopressors, vasodilators, or other cardiac unloading agents to improve cardiac output; and reducing oxygen consumption through sedation, therapeutic paralysis, or hypothermia. Alkalemia and hypophosphatemia also impair oxygen transport and delivery and require correction.

PEEP is set directly on most ventilators. With some ventilators a knob is turned while observing the pressure manometer until it indicates the proper amount of positive pressure. On other ventilators the amount of PEEP is set digitally and observed on the pressure manometer. Some physicians believe that all patients need PEEP; others do not hold this view. Physicians who advocate using PEEP use the term physiological PEEP and usually are referring to 2.5 to 5 cwp PEEP. In patients having difficulty oxygenating, PEEP usually is added when the Fi_{O_2} is 50% or greater to decrease the risk of oxygen toxicity. Depending on the institution and the physician, the patient is started on 2.5 to 5 cwp PEEP. The level of PEEP usually is increased in 2.5-cwp increments. The physician uses arterial blood gases and compliance measurements to determine optimal levels of PEEP.

Peak flow or inspiratory flow rate, is the speed with which the gas is pushed into the patient's lungs. It is controlled by a calibrated dial or entered digitally. Peak flow rates range from 20 to 120 LPM, although most patients require 40 to 60 LPM. In patients with obstructive lung diseases, who require longer exhalation times, the peak flow is increased. Peak flow also is increased as the patient's frequency or rate increases. The faster or higher the peak flow, the shorter the time for inhalation; the slower or lower the peak flow, the longer the time for inhalation. (Peak flow thus affects the I:E ratio.) When the peak flow is too slow to deliver the minute ventilation, a ratio light or alarm is activated.

The *inspiratory to expiratory ratio* is set on some ventilators. Usually set in seconds, a normal inspiratory time is about ½ to 1½ seconds. Some ventilators require setting of the I:E ratio. Normal I:E is 1:2 but is increased to 1:3 to 1:5 when a prolonged exhalation is needed. A longer expiratory time is associated with increased alveolar emptying. With inverse ratio ventilation (IRV), the I:E is reversed, prolonging inhalation. Many ventilators cannot have a longer inspiratory time than expiratory time.

Sensitivity is set on some older ventilators that are not controlled by a microprocessor. In newer ventilators, sensitivity is built into the mode control. When sensitivity is manually adjusted for assist controlled ventilation (AC), the nurse increases the sensitivity until the patient pulls the needle on the pressure manometer to about −2 cwp. When the ventilator is more sensitive (for example, the needle is pulled to −1 cwp), the ventilator is prone to self-cycle. Decreasing sensitivity below −2 cwp requires the patient to generate more negative pressure to deliver a breath and increases the work of breathing.

Other settings available on various ventilators include different wave forms or ways to deliver the breath (for example, sine, square, accelerating, or decelerating). Most ventilators contain an inspiratory pause or hold, which usually is used to assess static compliance but also may be useful in preventing or treating atelectasis. Some ventilators require digital entry of the amount of desired pressure support or calculation of compliance when a compliance compensation factor for the circuit is inserted.

Complications of mechanical ventilation

Although mechanical ventilation often is used to treat life-threatening conditions, some of the complications of mechanical ventilation are also life threatening. The most common complications are listed in the box on p. 346. Not discussed, but certainly present, are the patient's anxiety and inability to communicate effectively.

The most common complications of mechanical ventilation usually occur while the ventilator is being adjusted to meet the patient's metabolic needs. Hypoventilation or hyperventilation are the most common initial problems in ventilator management. Based on analysis of arterial blood gases, the physician adjusts the patient's rate, volume, or mode to correct the resulting acidemia or alkalemia. Respiratory alkalosis often is considered the more dangerous of the two, because it impairs cerebral perfusion and predisposes the patient to cardiac dysrhythmias. Respiratory alkalosis also is a common cause of inability to wean the patient from mechanical ventilation. Some clinicians believe that using intermittent mandatory ventilation (IMV) prevents or more readily corrects respiratory alkalosis, but this has not been proven in the literature.

Complications of mechanical ventilation

Alveolar hypoventilation
Alveolar hyperventilation
Atelectasis
Barotrauma (pneumothorax, pneumomediastinum, subcutaneous emphysema)
Bronchopleural fistula
Decreased cardiac output
Gastric distention
Gastrointestinal bleeding
Hypotension
Ileus
Increased intracranial pressure
Malnutrition
Pneumonia
Positive fluid balance
Ventilator malfunction

Atelectasis develops for several reasons in mechanically ventilated patients. A patient may receive tidal volumes that are too low, although this is unusual. The more common causes of atelectasis are inefficient or inadequate removal of secretions and loss or inactivation of surfactant. Intubation of a main stem bronchus, usually the right, leads to atelectasis in the opposite lung. Pneumonia may follow atelectasis.

Nosocomial (hospital-acquired) pneumonia is common in mechanically ventilated patients. The incidence varies among institutions and patient groups. Clinicians realize that patients are colonized with hospital bacteria within about 48 hours of intubation, as evidenced by culture of respiratory secretions. Colonization does not imply infection; it often is difficult to decide if the patient is merely colonized or truly infected based on positive culture data. In fairly healthy patients, colonization does not progress to infection. As the patient's clinical condition declines, the likelihood of nosocomial pneumonia increases. Recent studies suggest that use of histamine type 2 gastric acid blockers or antacids increases nosocomial pneumonia. In addition, hypotension is believed to allow transient release of enteric pathogens into systemic circulation for transport to the lung and other susceptible body areas.

The most important means of preventing nosocomial pneumonia are hand washing and using aseptic technique when suctioning or manipulating the ventilator circuit. Many hospitals pay less than $1 for a standard suction catheter; the cost of a nosocomial pneumonia exceeds $1000. Using an inadvertently contaminated suction catheter is not cost effective. Using in-line suction catheters may reduce the incidence of nosocomial pneumonia.

The term *barotrauma* collectively refers to any positive-pressure injury to the lung. In most instances overdistention of alveoli is the cause. Thus very large tidal volumes or high levels of PEEP usually are involved. High peak (and mean) ventilating pressures usually are seen in patients with barotrauma injuries and lead to alveolar rupture. Sometimes the lung is punctured during insertion of a central venous catheter in a mechanically ventilated patient. The incidence of pleural or lung puncture varies with the skill of the person inserting the catheter, ventilator settings, and the patient's status. The most life-threatening consequence of barotrauma is development of a pneumothorax, which prevents lung expansion, worsening oxygenation and ultimately ventilation. With positive-pressure breathing, a simple pneumothorax can progress to a tension pneumothorax and cardiopulmonary arrest. Air also can dissect into the mediastinum (pneumomediastinum) or peritoneum (pneumoperitoneum).

Bronchopleural fistula, often referred to as BPF, is a persistent air leak following spontaneous alveolar rupture or traumatic puncture. A chest tube must be inserted to evacuate pleural air, but this may increase the pressure gradient and prolong the leak when suction is applied. Healing of a bronchopleural fistula takes time. Measures reported to reduce these fistulas include avoiding PEEP, minimizing positive-pressure breaths (pressure support or IMV is useful), decreasing tidal volume, reducing inspiratory time, and decreasing the amount of chest wall suction.

The primary mechanism for decreased cardiac output is an increase in mean intrathoracic pressure from positive rather than negative pressure (spontaneous) breathing. Venous return into the right heart is impaired, especially when PEEP is applied. A second cause of decreased cardiac output is increased pulmonary vascular resistance secondary to positive-pressure breathing. Increased pulmonary vascular resistance impedes right ventricular outflow and thus cardiac output. The use of low lung volumes (hypoxic pulmonary vasoconstriction or extraalveolar vessel collapse) or high levels of PEEP (compression of capillaries) may increase pulmonary vascular resistance. When the intravascular fluid volume is inadequate, the effects of positive-pressure ventilation on cardiac output are more easily observed. Hypotension usually is the first sign of decreased cardiac output. Some patients develop hypotension when they first begin using the CMV or AC mode of ventilation; this condition frequently responds to a fluid challenge.

Gastric distention, ileus, or gastrointestinal bleeding may be seen in mechanically ventilated patients. The role of mechanical ventilation in the development of these problems is unclear. In a newly intubated patient, air swallowed during artificial or ambu breathing accounts for some gastric distention. In other patients, gastric distention may be caused by air leaking around the cuff. Instead of being released through the upper airway, the air passes through the lower esophageal sphincter into the stomach. Gastrointestinal bleeding seen in mechanically ventilated patients ranges from guaiac-positive nasogastric drainage or stools to overt bleeding. The incidence of guaiac-positive stools is fairly high. Some estimate that one fourth of ventilated patients develop them. Most patients do not have gross gastrointestinal bleeding that requires a blood transfusion. The development of one or more gastrointestinal complications, coupled with the inability to eat normally (as in intubated patients and many tracheostomy patients), leads to malnutrition. Many of the complications in mechanically ventilated patients, especially pneumonia, are affected by malnutrition.

Positive-pressure ventilation increases intracranial pressure (ICP) by impairing cerebral blood flow. The effects of positive-pressure breathing on increased intracranial pressure are enhanced when PEEP is applied. Cerebral perfusion pressure is affected by either increased jugular pressure or decreased cardiac output. (Cerebral perfusion pressure is calculated by subtracting ICP from the mean arterial blood pressure.)

The cause of positive fluid balance in the mechanically ventilated patient is not well known. It is known that positive-pressure ventilation is associated with release of antidiuretic hormone (ADH). Secretion of ADH encourages the kidneys to retain water and salt, and consequently, body water is increased. Some patients receiving mechanical ventilation develop decreased renal blood flow and other forms of renal insufficiency. The mechanisms of this and the relationship to mechanical ventilation are unclear.

The final preventable complication of mechanical ventilation is ventilator malfunction. The range of problems with mechanical ventilators varies. The worst possibility is total ventilator failure, or failure to cycle. A fairly common problem is accumulation of water in the ventilator circuit, which increases airway resistance and may cause inadvertent increases in PEEP. For this reason water routinely is drained from the circuit at least every 2 hours or an in-line trap is used. Water is never drained back into the cascade, since infection could develop. Other problems include failure to deliver set tidal volume, failure of high- or low-pressure alarms, inadequate humidification, low FIO_2, and overheating inspired air. Frequent ventilator *and patient* assessments prevent or rapidly correct problems.

Weaning

Weaning is the process of removing the patient from mechanical ventilation. Extubation or decannulation follows weaning in many instances, but neither is actually a part of weaning from mechanical ventilation. Weaning and extubation or decannulation are two separate processes that should not be confused. The patient may still receive humidity, oxygen, and suctioning through the endotracheal or tracheostomy tube. For most patients, weaning is simple and quick. Remember, most patients are weaned from mechanical ventilation (and rapidly extubated) in the operating room or postanesthesia recovery room.

Weaning is an art combined with science that requires accurate and frequent assessment of the patient. Readiness to wean from mechanical ventilation is suggested by assessment of several criteria or parameters. Ventilation, oxygenation, and other factors are guidelines to be used in determining readiness to wean (Table 15-3). No single parameter successfully predicts ability to wean from mechanical ventilation. Meeting most of the criteria usually indicates readiness to wean; however, some weanable patients meet few criteria, and some nonweanable patients meet many criteria.

Several equally important factors are involved in weaning a patient from mechanical ventilation. The first is that the patient must be medically stable. The reason that the patient required mechanical ventilation must be resolved (for example, infection or sepsis has been treated, surgery has been completed, blood pressure has stabilized). The patient may receive intravenous vasopressors or intraaortic balloon counterpulsation and still be medically stable. In reality, some patients cannot be weaned without cardiac support, which is removed later.

Adequate nutrition is essential to weaning from mechanical ventilation. Although most patients can tolerate 2 to 3 days without nutrition other than intravenous glucose, they cannot tolerate prolonged periods without protein and with minimal calories. (Recall that there are less than 200 calories and no protein in 1000 ml of D_5W). Protein-calorie malnutrition results. The body catabolizes muscle, including the diaphragm and other respiratory muscles, to meet its metabolic needs. Malnutrition predisposes the patient to nosocomial pneumonia, reduces the ventilatory response to hypoxia, and de-

Table 15-3. Guidelines for readiness to wean (weaning parameters)

Ventilation criteria	pH 7.35-7.45
	Pa_{CO_2} normal for patient
Dead space/tidal volume	$(V_D/V_T) < 0.6$
	Vital capacity > 10-15 ml/kg
	Tidal volume (spontaneous) > 5 ml/kg
	Minute ventilation 5-10 LPM
	Negative Inspiratory Force (NIF) > -20 cwp
	Maximum voluntary ventilation > 2 times resting minute ventilation
	Respiratory rate ≤ 35
Oxygenation criteria	$Fi_{O_2} \leq 40\%$
	PEEP ≤ 5 cwp
	$Pa_{O_2} \geq 60$ mm Hg
	$Sa_{O_2} \geq 90\%$
	$(A\text{-}a)O_2 < 350$ mm Hg on 100% Fi_{O_2}
	$a/A_{O_2} > 0.2$
Shunt fraction	$Q_S/Q_T \leq 20\%$
(Q_S/Q_T)	$Pa_{O_2}/Fi_{O_2} > 200$ mm Hg
Other criteria	Medically stable
	Psychologically ready
	Optimal muscle strength
	Method for adequate communication
	Albumin > 2 mg/dl
	Phosphate 2.5-4.5 mg/dl
	Potassium 3.5-5.5 mEq/L
	Calcium 8.5-10.5 mg/dl
	Magnesium 1.5-2.5 mEq/L
	Euthyroid
	Hemoglobin > 12 g/dl

creases respiratory muscle strength and endurance. It does not matter whether the patient's protein and calories are ingested through oral feedings, a gastrointestinal feeding tube, intravenous routes, or a combination of these. Most adult patients require about 2000 calories daily for weaning; more calories are needed if the patient has an infection or extensive healing in progress. The dietitian (using an equation or indirect calorimetry) calculates the patient's calorie needs, including protein, and suggests methods for achieving the goal. Patients with excessively low albumin and protein stores require repletion before weaning is attempted.

Along with adequate nutrition, the patient must have an adequate metabolic state. The most important minerals are phosphorus, calcium, potassium, and magnesium. Trace elements are also important. Endocrine abnormalities, such as hypothyroidism, affect the drive to breathe, whereas metabolic abnormalities, including hypophosphatemia, hypocalcemia, hypokalemia, and hypomagnesemia, adversely affect the muscles' ability to contract forcefully. The minerals and thyroid hormone must be repleted before initiating weaning.

The patient's overall muscle strength is important in removing a patient successfully from mechanical ventilation. The diaphragm and abdominal muscles are used in normal breathing, as well as for coughing. Patients who use accessory muscles or have abnormal breathing patterns may have pro-longed weaning or may be unable to be weaned. It also is important to maintain strength of arm and leg muscles. Patients should sit in the chair at least twice daily and sometimes more often in difficult to wean patients. Sitting in the chair facilitates diaphragmatic excursion, since the abdominal contents are not pushing up against the diaphragm. Patients who do poorly at weaning in the bed often excel while in the chair. Some patients are strong enough to ambulate with assistance from an ambu or a portable ventilator.

Finally, the patient must be psychologically ready for weaning and must be able to communicate his feelings adequately. Patients receiving mechanical ventilator support psychologically adjust in several phases: preoccupation with survival; denial of threat to life accompanied by fantasy to be free of the mechanical ventilator; depression, with gradual accommodation to reality; and active participation in rehabilitative care. Patients may go through one or more stages at different intervals of hospitalization and rehabilitation. In the survival phase, the patient allows nurses and machines to assume responsibility for body functions, although feelings of anxiety, helplessness, and dependency are present. Some patients enter the denial and fantasy phase expressing ambivalence about the lifesaving mechanical ventilator that has them on a "short leash." The patient fears not only that he is dependent on the mechanical ventilator, but also that he will die if it is removed suddenly. A third phase is very common in chronically ventilated patients. The patient is unsure whether he is going to live, wean from mechanical ventilation, or die. Depression sets in as the patient realizes the reality of the situation. Some patients realistically or unrealistically assess the gravity of their situation and request no further resuscitation for acute life-threatening events. Counseling is necessary to help the patient make appropriate decisions, since the patient has trouble dealing with today and may not be able to "see tomorrow." The final, most productive phase has a fully cooperative patient striving to get better and go home.

To help the patient cope with mechanical ventilation, the nurse initiates several interventions. In the preoperative period, the patient learns about possible continued intubation and mechanical ventilation. This is particularly true of cardiac and throat surgery patients. The patient is told of the inability to speak because of the tube; unless contraindicated (laryngectomy), the patient is informed that he will regain speech when the tube is removed or changed to fenestrated tracheostomy tube or talking tracheostomy tube. Daily, or more frequently, the patient is informed of progress with his condition, including that he requires less support from the ventilator. Patients who have been mechanically ventilated for some time become anxious when suddenly one day the physician or nurse announces that the ventilator will be discontinued. This anxiety can be eased if the patient is informed of his improving ventilatory and oxygenation status. Some patients feel less dyspneic when a bedside fan blows air toward them during a weaning trial.

In patients who are difficult to wean, the nurse coordinates a patient care conference, which helps focus the patient care team. All individuals involved in the patient's care attend; sometimes the patient attends as well (usually at not the first, but at subsequent conferences). When possible, the same nurse (primary nurse) or group of nurses cares for the patient, because patients trust a familiar, caring nurse. A familiar nurse also is more astute in picking up small changes in the patient's condition and knows his habits, routines, and family members. A schedule of activities and goals is developed (such as that shown in the boxes below for a fictitious patient named John Wittman). The schedules includes all of the patient's activities, as well as periods of rest. Activities are spaced, and the patient knows who or what to expect. Small, measurable goals are developed, such as "walks 10 steps by Friday 6/10" or "sits up in chair for 30 min t.i.d." The schedule and goals are posted on the wall or door in the patient's room, because the patient must be able to see them.

Schedule for John Wittman

7 AM	Bronchodilators Chest physical therapy (PT) in bed
8 AM	Breakfast Bath
9 AM	Up in chair Physical therapy exercises
10 AM	Free
11 AM	Bronchodilators Chest PT in bed
12 noon	Lunch
1 PM	Speech or occupational therapy
2 PM	Ambulate, then chair
3:30 PM	Bronchodilators Chest PT in bed
4-6 PM	Free Dinner in chair
9 PM	Bronchodilators Chest PT in bed Bed for night
12 midnight-6 AM	Sleep with minimal disturbance

Goals for John Wittman

Goal	M	T	W	Th	F	Sa	Su
Sit in chair three times daily	●	●	2	2	●		
Drink three cans of Ensure daily	●	2	2	●	2		
Walk to door	●	–	–	–	–	–	–
Walk 10 feet	●	–	–	–	–	–	–
Walk 12 feet	–	●	●	–	–	–	–
Walk 14 feet	–	–	–	●	●		
Comb hair and wash face	●	●	●	●	●		
Shave	×	●	–	●	●		
Perform assisted bath	–	–	●	×	●		

–, not applicable; ×, did not do; ●, successful.

The initial step in weaning a patient from mechanical ventilation is to lower the oxygenation support. First, the physician usually decreases the Fio_2 to 40% or less to reduce the hazard of oxygen toxicity, although some physicians wean the Fio_2 to 50%. If the patient is subsequently extubated, it often is difficult to oxygenate the patient when the Fio_2 is greater than 50%. After the Fio_2 has been weaned, the PEEP is weaned to 5 cwp or less. When barotrauma is a problem, the physician may choose to wean the PEEP to a lower value before weaning the Fio_2. Decreasing the Fio_2 and PEEP may take minutes or hours to days or weeks to accomplish. At this point the patient is ready to be weaned from the ventilatory aspects of mechanical ventilation, assuming that the pH and $Paco_2$ have been maintained in a normal range. After that, the patient is ready to be weaned from complete ventilatory support.

There is no one right way to wean the patient from ventilation aspects, although different plans have their proponents. The three primary means are abrupt removal, the traditional method (also called Brigg's or T piece trials) and the IMV method. The latest technique for weaning patients uses pressure support with IMV. Most patients can be weaned using either IMV or AC. The exception is patients who have increased work of breathing when opening the demand valve on the mechanical ventilator. Either a continuous-flow IMV or AC–T piece trial aids in weaning these susceptible patients. The most important point is to apply only one method of weaning consistently.

The abrupt method of weaning from mechanical ventilation is fairly self-explanatory. The patient is abruptly removed from the ventilator. This occurs after anesthesia has worn off and in many postoperative cardiac patients. In most instances the ventilator circuit provides supplemental oxygen without rate or volume while the clinician observes the patient's breathing. Alternately, the patient is placed on a limited T piece (or T tube) trial. Occasionally arterial blood gases are assessed, but usually not.

The traditional method of weaning uses the AC (or, less commonly, the IMV) mode of mechanical ventilation. Weaning parameters are assessed to determine readiness to wean before initiating a trial. The ventilator provides most (at least 75%) or all of the patient's minute ventilation when he is using the ventilator. Some report greater success in hard-to-wean patients when the tidal volume during rest periods is physiological (that is, about 5 ml/kg). At intervals the patient is removed from the ventilator and placed on a T piece (analogous to a tight-fitting mask for the endotracheal or tracheostomy tube) or tracheostomy collar with supplemental oxygen (Fig. 15-2). This is a separate system from the ventilator and increases patient cost. Most patients receive an Fio_2 that is 10% higher on the T piece than that supplied by the ventilator. When patients have problems with atelectasis, the physician may order CPAP trials (a rate of 0 and designated amount of PEEP given through the mechanical ventilator), instead of T tube trials.

The patient spontaneously breathes at his own rate and depth of breathing. The T piece trial may be as short as a few minutes or as long as several hours. The first trial usually lasts 5 minutes, and the physician or nurse is in constant attendance. When a tube 7 cm or smaller in diameter is used in the adult, T piece trials are limited because of the increased work of breathing through the small-diameter tube. Deflating the cuff increases airway size and may decrease the work of breathing.

If the patient is doing well, the physician may extubate him. Alternately, at

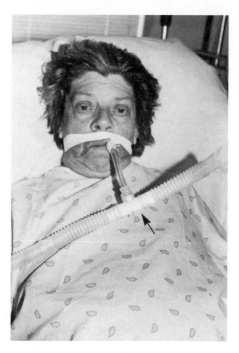

Fig. 15-2. T piece for weaning.

the end of the trial, the patient is returned to the mechanical ventilator to rest. Additional trials are scheduled throughout the day but stop at bedtime. The patient is allowed to sleep using the mechanical ventilator for full ventilatory support. When the patient is breathing on the T piece throughout the day, the trial extends throughout the night. The patient may remain intubated for airway protection and removal of secretions even after the need for mechanical ventilation no longer exists.

With IMV weaning, the patient continues to use the ventilator. Several methods are used for IMV weaning. One method involves decreasing the ventilator rate by one or two breaths per minute every hour, as tolerated by the patient, until zero is reached. The rate is turned up to a resting level if the patient tires and at night. On subsequent mornings the IMV rate is decreased to the previous day's lowest level. The physician further decreases the rate, as tolerated by the patient.

In some institutions IMV weaning is accomplished by decreasing the rate by one or two breaths per minute every *day*, and the ventilator is not turned to a resting level at night. The patient continually assumes the work of breathing, and the level of work is increased daily.

Some differentiate traditional and IMV weaning with the analogy of training for a marathon. With AC–T piece weaning, the patient runs (breathes) a little farther (longer) each time (trial) until able to run (breathe) 26 miles (24 hours). There are rest periods between periods of intense exercise. With IMV weaning, the patient runs (breathes) until the goal of 26 miles (24 hours) is reached. Each time the rate is decreased, the patient runs a little faster (assumes more work of breathing).

Many of the new microprocessor-controlled ventilators contain pressure support for supplemental ventilation or weaning. PSV weaning involves components of both traditional and IMV weaning. PSV weaning is like traditional AC–T piece weaning in that the patient breathes spontaneously. When weaning with PSV, the physician slowly decreases the amount of pressure support, similar to decreasing the rate in IMV. The amount of pressure support usually is decreased in increments of 1 to 5 cwp, as tolerated by the patient. When the level of PSV reaches 5 cwp, the patient is said to be weaned. The physician may try a T piece trial or may extubate the patient. The superiority of PSV over any other method has not been demonstrated.

The physician usually writes orders to initiate weaning with some of the specifics, particularly the length of the trial, left to the nurse. Ideally weaning attempts begin in the early morning and conclude in the evening. In the morning the patient is more rested and better able to cope with weaning. As the day wears on and into night, the patient tends to tire physically and emotionally.

The nurse is careful to optimize the patient's airway before beginning any weaning trial. This includes administering a bronchodilator, followed by chest physical therapy and suctioning. When possible the nurse sits the patient upright in the chair. Although the patient can sit up in the bed, the chair is preferred because positioning and maintaining good position in the bed is difficult. The nurse initiates the weaning trial while attempting to keep other major physical activities (and skeletal muscle oxygen consumption) to a minimum. For instance, the physical therapist should not require active exercises during early weaning trials. As the patient's weaning interval increases, these activities are included.

During the weaning trial the nurse assesses the patient frequently. In some instances, when alarms are not used (such as with T piece or CPAP trials), the nurse assesses the patient continuously. The patient's condition, including vital signs, are assessed at least every 10 minutes for 30 minutes during the first weaning trial. Most institutions then require assessments every 30 minutes times 2, followed by hourly assessments times 2 and then assessments every 2 hours. A little shortness of breath, discomfort, or fatigue is seen in many patients. The patient is suctioned as needed. In patients with marginal secretion clearance and tenuous ability to wean, initiating 1 to 5 minutes of ambu bagging every 2 hours aids in secretion removal and provides a rest period for the patient. Signs of failure or impending failure to wean are given in the box on p. 355.

The earliest signs of failing to wean usually are decrease in the spontaneous tidal volume and increase in the respiratory rate. The patient frequently develops abnormal patterns of breathing or apnea (see Chapter 5). The patient becomes confused, disoriented, or lethargic. If oxygenation is a problem, angina, cyanosis, or dysrhythmias occur. If any of these problems develop, the nurse obtains an arterial blood gas and, without waiting for the results, returns the patient to resting ventilator settings, as ordered by the physician. In some instances (for example, life-threatening conditions or inability to rapidly obtain an arterial blood gas), the patient is returned to the ventilator without obtaining arterial blood gases. When arterial blood gases are not drawn, however, it often is impossible to tell if the problem was secondary to inadequate ventilation or oxygenation. When the results of the arterial blood gas tests are available, the nurse analyzes them in conjunction with the pa-

---

Signs of failure with weaning trial

Accessory muscle use, respiratory alternans, or paradoxical breathing development
Agitation
Angina
Cyanosis
Decrease in tidal volume 100 ml per breath or less than 3-5 ml/kg
Dysrhythmias
Heart rate: >120 beats per minute, *or* increases or decreases 10 beats per minute
Lethargy
Mental confusion
pH <7.30
Pao_2 <55 mm Hg
Respiratory rate: <8, >35, or increases 10 breaths above baseline
Sao_2 <90%
Systolic blood pressure: decreases or increases 20 mm Hg

Table 15-4. Assessing the patient's progress in weaning trials

Date/time	8/11 9 AM	10 PM	8/12 12 noon	10 PM
Ventilator	Bird			
Fio_2/PEEP	40/5	40/5	40/5	
Tidal volume (V_T)	700	700	700	
Ventilator rate/total rate	10/10	10/12	10/10	
Mode	AC	AC	AC	
Spontaneous	T tube			
Fio_2	40	40	40	40
V_T	200	150	250	200
Vital capacity (VC)	600	450	700	600
Rate	30	40	25	30
Interval	1 hour	2 hour	2 hour	2 hour
Comments	dyspnea	mucus plug	OK	tired
pH/$Paco_2$/Pao_2	7.35/44/68	7.28/52/64	7.40/40/80	7.35/45/75

tient's clinical condition at the time the arterial blood gases were drawn.

During and usually at the end of the weaning trial or day, the nurse or respiratory therapist assesses the patient's weaning parameters and vital signs. When these are compared with earlier values, the nurse learns more about the patient's condition and muscle strength. A flow sheet, such as the one in Table 15-4, helps in observing the patient's progress.

Jet ventilation

A jet ventilator is a special type of volume ventilator used to deliver high-frequency ventilation. It delivers very small tidal volumes at very high rates and is subdivided into the most common high-frequency jet ventilation (HFJV), the less common high-frequency positive-pressure ventilation (HF-PPV), and the least common high-frequency oscillator (HFO). The character-

Table 15-5. Types of high-frequency ventilators

	Rate/minute	Volume	I:E
High-frequency jet ventilation (HFJV)	100-600	2-5 ml/kg	1:2-8
High-frequency positive-pressure ventilation (HFPPV)	60-120	3-5 ml/kg	1:0.3
High-frequency oscillator (HFO)	60-3600	1-3 ml/kg	1:?

istics of the various types are summarized in Table 15-5. In some instances the tidal volume is equal to or less than anatomical dead space, and rates exceed 100 to 150 breaths per minute. The usual range for high-frequency jet ventilation is 100 to 400 breaths per minute. Some special types of high-frequency ventilators are called oscillators. With high-frequency oscillation, up to 3600 breaths per minute are generated.

There is debate as to exactly how jet ventilators transport gas, making the physiology difficult to understand. Two processes, convection and diffusion, are involved in delivering gas to the alveoli. Of the various types of convective flow, streaming is the most prevalent in the small airways. With convective streaming, the faster-moving inspired gas flows toward the alveoli in the center of the airways, whereas the slower-moving expiratory gas travels in the periphery of the airway. Another form of convection, seen in both large and small airways, is augmented dispersion, in which turbulence creates swirling of gases. Some think of this as waves of air, similar to ocean waves, flowing in and out of the lung. Both laminar and lateral flow of gas occur with augmented dispersion to facilitate mixing. Once in the alveoli, gas transport occurs by diffusion.

The theoretical basis for using HFJV is to decrease mean airway pressures and minimize the risk of barotrauma. Therefore the main uses of HFJV are in ventilating patients with bronchopleural fistulas and in patients undergoing laryngoscopy, bronchoscopy, or upper airway surgery. Although many use HFJV in patients with ARDS, there appears to be no advantage, based on available research, to support its benefit over conventional ventilation.

HFJV is delivered through a 2-mm metal or plastic cannula or tube that acts as a gas injector or Venturi to entrain atmospheric air. An endotracheal tube has been designed to deliver HFJV (Fig. 15-3). It has two ports in addition to the pilot balloon. One port is for infusion of saline to humidify the gas, and the other is for delivering the gas or monitoring airway pressures. Many institutions jet the gas through a specially designed adapter that fits over the end of the endotracheal tube rather than replacing the endotracheal tube in a critically ill patient.

The ventilator settings for HFJV differ from conventional ventilation, and it is difficult to adequately humidify the inspired gas. The physician determines the rate, the driving pressure, and the I:E ratio. The adjustment of ventilator settings is unconventional in HFJV. The guidelines for adjusting the settings based on arterial blood gas values are summarized in Table 15-6.

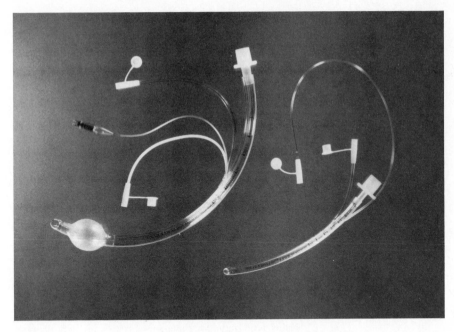

Fig. 15-3. Jet ventilator endotracheal tube (note the additional tube ports). Left: adult; Right: pediatric. (Courtesy of Mallinckrodt Medical, Inc. St. Louis)

Table 15-6. Guidelines for adjusting a jet ventilator

To decrease Pa_{CO_2}	Increase driving pressure
	Increase inspiratory time
	Decrease respiratory rate
To increase Pa_{CO_2}	Decrease driving pressure
	Decrease inspiratory time
	Increase respiratory rate
To increase Pa_{O_2}	Increase Fi_{O_2}
	Increase PEEP
	Increase inspiratory time
To decrease Pa_{O_2}	Decrease Fi_{O_2}
	Decrease PEEP
	Decrease inspiratory time

The humidification problem is reduced by continuously infusing half-normal to normal saline into the airway. The rate of infusion varies; in adults, the rate is approximately 20 ml/hour, depending on the secretions. More or less saline is administered for thick or thin secretions, respectively. Suctioning also can be a problem because of the need to remove the jet infuser. If the jet is left on, it "flies" about and may injure the patient or nurse. Most nurses temporarily place the jet ventilator on standby when suctioning or have an assistant hold the jet infuser.

CONCLUSION

This chapter has introduced the concepts of noninvasive and invasive mechanical ventilation, which are lifesaving or life-sustaining measures. It is easy for the nurse to become overwhelmed by the technical aspects of mechanical ventilation, but as she becomes more knowledgeable about caring for patients using various types of ventilators, patient care improves. This discussion of different types of ventilators, including the jet ventilator, modes of ventilation, and complications of mechanical ventilation, as well as methods of changing ventilator settings and weaning the patient from mechanical ventilation, gives the nurse a theoretical basis for caring for a patient using mechanical ventilation. This knowledge, combined with experience, prepares the nurse to assess the patient's condition rapidly and to implement appropriate interventions, such as notifying the physician to adjust ventilator settings, returning a patient to the mechanical ventilator during a weaning trial, or encouraging the patient to continue with the weaning trial a little longer.

BIBLIOGRAPHY

Aldrich TK: The patient at risk of ventilator dependency, *Eur Respir J* 7:645s-650s, 1989.

Aldrich TK, Karpel JP, Uhrlass RM, et al: Weaning from mechanical ventilation: adjunctive use of inspiratory muscle resistive training, *Crit Care Med* 17(2):143-147, 1989.

Bach JR, Alba AS: Management of chronic alveolar hypoventilation by nasal ventilation, *Chest* 97(1):52-57, 1990.

Benotti PN, Bistrian B: Metabolic and nutritional aspects of weaning from mechanical ventilation, *Crit Care Med* 17(2):181-185, 1989.

Blaufuss JA, Wallace CJ: Two negative pressure ventilators: current clinical applications and nursing care, *Crit Care Nur Q* 9(4):14-30, 1987.

Bolgiano CS, Saah ML: Measurement of bedside ventilatory parameters, *Crit Care Nurse* 10(1):60-66, 1990.

Branson RD, Hurst JM, DeHaven CB: Mask CPAP: state of the art, *Respir Care* 30(10):846-857, 1985.

Brochard L, Harf A, Loring H, Lemaire F: Inspiratory pressure support prevents diaphragmatic fatigue during weaning from mechanical ventilation, *Am Rev Respir Dis* 139(2):513-521, 1989.

Burns SM: Advances in ventilator therapy: high-frequency, pressure support and nocturnal nasal positive pressure ventilation, *Focus Crit Care* 17(3):227-237, 1990.

Burton GC, Hodgkin JE: *Respiratory care: a guide to clinical practice*, ed 2, Philadelphia, 1984, JB Lippincott.

Byra C: High-frequency ventilation, *Crit Care Nurse* 5(6):42-47, 1985.

Carlon GC, Griffin JP: Clinical experience with high-frequency jet ventilation, *Curr Rev Respir Ther* 5(11):87-92, 1983.

Carroll PF: Caring for ventilator patients, *Nursing 86* 16(2):34-40, 1986.

Chatburn RL: More on estimating appropriate pressure support levels, *Respir Care* 30(10):925, 1985.

Clark K: Psychosocial aspects of prolonged ventilator dependency, *Respir Care* 31(4):329-333, 1986.

Curgian LM, Sparapani M: The chest cuirass and related nursing management, *Rehabil Nurs* 11(4):17-19, 1986.

Duncan AW, Oh TE, Hillman DR: PEEP and CPAP *Anaesth Intensive Care* 14(3):236-250, 1986.

Fiastro JF, Habib MP, Quan SF: Pressure support compensation for inspiratory work due to endotracheal tubes and demand continuous positive airway pressure, *Chest* 93(3):499-505, 1988.

Foltz BD, Benumof JL: Mechanisms of hypoxemia and hypercapnia in the perioperative period, *Crit Care Clin* 3(2):269-286, 1987.

Fromme LR, Kaplow R: High-frequency jet ventilation, *Am J Nurs* 84(11):1380-1383, 1984.

Garner W, Downs JB, Stock MC, Rasanen J: Airway pressure release ventilation (APRV): a human trial, *Chest* 94(4):779-781, 1988.

Geisman LK: Advances in weaning from mechanical ventilation, *Crit Care Nurs Clin North Am* 1(4):697-705, 1989.

Grossbach I: Trouble-shooting ventilator- and patient-related problems. I., *Crit Care Nurse* 6(4):58-70, 1986.

Grossbach I: Trouble-shooting ventilator- and patient-related problems. II., *Crit Care Nurse* 6(5):64-79, 1986.

Grossbach-Landis I: Weaning from mechanical ventilation, *Crit Care Update* 10(3):7-27, 1983.

Hagarty E: Weaning your COPD patient from the ventilator, *RN* 47(7):36-40, 1984.

Harper R: *A guide to respiratory care: physiology and clinical applications,* Philadelphia, 1982, JB Lippincott.

Henneman EA: Effect of nursing contact on the stress response of patients being weaned from mechanical ventilation, *Heart Lung* 18(5):483-489, 1989.

Henning R: Clinical applications of mechanical ventilation, *Anaesth Intensive Care* 14(3):267-280, 1986.

Holliday JE, Hyers TM: The reduction of weaning time from mechanical ventilation using tidal volume and relaxation biofeedback, *Am Rev Respir Dis* 141(5 pt1):1214-1220, 1990.

Hurst JM, Branson RD, Davis K: High-frequency percussive ventilation in the management of elevated intracranial pressure, *J Trauma* 28(9):1363-1367, 1988.

Javaheri S, Kazemi H: Metabolic alkalosis and hypoventilation in humans, *Am Rev Respir Dis* 136(4):1011-1016, 1987.

Kacmarek RM: The role of pressure support ventilation in reducing work of breathing, *Respir Care* 33(2):99-120, 1988.

Kaplow R, Fromme LR: Nursing care plan for the patient receiving high-frequency jet ventilation, *Crit Care Nurse* 5(1):25-27, 1985.

Kemper M, Weissman C, Askanazi J, et al: Metabolic and respiratory changes during weaning from mechanical ventilation, *Chest* 92(6):979-983, 1987.

Kerby GR, Mayer LS, Pingleton SK: Nocturnal positive pressure ventilation via nasal mask, *Am Rev Respir Dis* 135(3):738-740, 1987.

Levy RD, Bradley TD, Newman SL, et al: Negative pressure ventilation: effects on ventilation during sleep in normal subject, *Chest* 95(1):95-99, 1989.

Mammel MC, Boros SJ: Airway damage and mechanical ventilation: a review and commentary, *Pediatr Pulmonol* 3(6):443-447, 1987.

Mayo JM, Hammer JB: A nurse's guide to mechanical ventilation, *RN* 50(8):18-24, 1987.

McPherson SP: *Respiratory therapy equipment,* St Louis, 1985, Mosby—Year Book.

Millman RP, Kipp GJ, Beadles SC, Braman SS: A home monitoring system for nasal CPAP, *Chest* 93(4):730-733, 1988.

Nett LM, Morganroth ML, Petty TL: Weaning from the ventilator: protocols that work, *Am J Nurs* 87(9):1173-7, 1987.

Nett LM, Morganroth ML, Petty TL: Weaning from the ventilator: in specific clinical situations, *Am J Nurs* 87(9):1178-1180, 1987.

Nett LM, Morganroth ML, Petty TL: Weaning from the ventilator: weaning the unweanable, *Am J Nurs* 97(9):1181-1184, 1987.

Netter F: *The CIBA collection of medical illustrations,* vol 7, *Respiratory system,* New York, 1979, CIBA Pharmaceutical Co.

Norton LC, Neureuter A: Weaning the long-term ventilator-dependent patient: common problems and management, *Crit Care Nurse* 9(1):42-52, 1989.

Norton LC, Chulay M, Tyler M, et al: Common problems and state of the art in nursing care of the mechanically ventilated patient, *Am Rev Respir Dis* 138(4):1055-1056, 1988.

Nugent KM: The importance of position in achieving optimal gas exchange in the patient with unilateral lung disease, *IM* 7(3):170, 1986.

Pierson DJ: Weaning from mechanical ventilation in acute respiratory failure: concepts, indications, and techniques, *Respir Care* 28(5):646-662, 1983.

Pierson DJ: Complications associated with mechanical ventilation, *Crit Care Clin* 6(3):711-724, 1990.

Ploysongsang Y, Rashkin MC, Ranganathan VH: Serial physiologic studies of a chronic obstructive pulmonary disease patient in acute respiratory failure: clues for weaning? *Respiration* 57(2):122-126, 1990.

Popovich J: PEEP: maximizing the benefits without hampering the heart, *J of Respir Dis* p. 33, March, 1986.

Rouby JJ, Viars P: Clinical use of high-frequency ventilation, *Acta Anaesthesiol Scand Suppl* 90:134-139, 1989.

Samodelov LF, Falke KJ: Total inspiratory work with modern demand valve devices compared to continuous flow CPAP, *Intensive Care Med* 14(6):632-639, 1988.

Sassoon CS, Mahutte CK, Light RW: Ventilator modes: old and new, *Crit Care Clin* 6(3):605-634, 1990.

Sassoon CS, Giron AE, Ely EA, Light RW: Inspiratory work of breathing on flow-by and demand-flow continuous positive airway pressure, *Crit Care Med* 17(11):1108-1114, 1989.

Shapiro B, Harrison R, et al: *Clinical applications of respiratory care,* ed 3, Chicago, 1985, Mosby—Year Book.

Shapiro SH, Macklem PT, Gray-Donald K, et al: A randomized clinical trial of negative pressure ventilation in severe chronic obstructive pulmonary disease: design and methods, *J Clin Epidemiol* 44(6):483-496, 1991.

Shoemaker WC, Thompson WL, Holbrook PR: *The Society of Critical Care Medicine textbook of critical care,* Philadelphia, 1984, WB Saunders.

Stone AM, Bone RC: Successful weaning from mechanical ventilation: strategies to avoid failure, *Postgrad Med* 86(5):315-319, 1989.

Swinamer DL, Fedoruk LM, Jones RL, et al: Energy expenditure associated with CPAP and T piece spontaneous ventilatory trials. Changes following prolonged mechanical ventilation. *Chest* 96(4):867-872, 1989.

Tobin MJ, Yang K: Weaning from mechanical ventilation, *Crit Care Clin* 6(3):725-747, 1990.

Tomlinson JR, Miller KS, Lorch DG, et al: A prospective comparison of IMV and T piece weaning from mechanical ventilation, *Chest* 96(2):348-352, 1989.

Villar J, Winston B, Slutsky AS: Nonconventional techniques of ventilatory support, *Crit Care Clin* 6(3):579-603, 1990.

Wade JF: *Comprehensive respiratory care: physiology and technique,* ed 3, St Louis, 1982, Mosby–Year Book.

Wissing DR, Romero MD, George RB: Comparing the newer modes of mechanical ventilation: a guide to design advances and specific clinical applications, *J Crit Ill* p. 41, March, 1987.

Witta K: New techniques for weaning difficult patients from mechanical ventilation, *AACN Clinical Issues in Critical Care Nursing* 1(2):260-266, 1990.

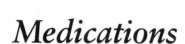

C H · A · P · T · E · R 16

Medications

*O*bjectives:

- Differentiate the types and actions of bronchodilators.
- Identify the actions and side effects of antibiotics and steroids.
- Discuss the use of antitussives, decongestants, antihistamines, expectorants, diuretics, and mucolytics in patients with pulmonary dysfunction.
- Evaluate criteria for proper use of an inhaler.
- Give the preferred order of administration when several types of inhalers are used.
- Discuss the types and use of vaccines in pulmonary disease.

Medications are an important component of the treatment of pulmonary disease. Drug regimens include both those prescribed by a physician and over-the-counter medications. This chapter discusses the different classes of medications used to treat pulmonary diseases. Bronchodilators are emphasized because they are commonly prescribed. Other classes of medications reviewed are antibiotics, antitussives, diuretics, mucolytics, decongestants, mast cell stabilizers, expectorants, and steroids.

BRONCHODILATORS

Bronchodilators are some of the most important medications used to improve or treat symptoms of pulmonary disease.* Frequently pulmonary disease is manifested by impaired expiratory air flow caused by bronchoconstriction or mucus. A bronchodilator decreases spasm of the muscles lining the airways and facilitates expectoration of mucus by enlarging the diameter of the airway. The three groups of bronchodilators discussed in this section are beta adrenergic agonists, anticholinergic agents, and methylxanthines.

The diameter of the airway can be reduced by one or more mechanisms. A common cause is smooth muscle contraction. Inflammation or edema can cause swelling of the airway mucosa, decreasing the diameter of the airway. Excessive secretion of mucus from goblet cells and mucous glands impairs the flow of air through the airways. Bronchodilators and other medications are aimed at correcting one or more of these problems.

---

*Although steroids and mast cell stabilizers are classed as bronchodilators, they are discussed separately.

Smooth muscle contraction is affected by intracellular concentrations of messengers. The ratio of these messenger chemical compounds (cyclic 3′,5′-adenosine monophosphate [cAMP] in the sympathetic nervous system and cyclic 3′,5′-guanosine monophosphate [cGMP] in the parasympathetic nervous system) enhances or inhibits bronchodilation. Increased levels of cAMP or decreased levels of cGMP promote bronchodilation (decrease muscle tone), whereas decreased levels of cAMP and increased levels of cGMP induce bronchoconstriction (increase muscle tone). Production of cAMP is desirable, since it promotes bronchodilation. Several stimuli promote cAMP. The intracellular enzyme adenylate cyclase, formerly adenyl cyclase, is a catalyst for converting adenosine triphosphate (ATP) to cAMP. Similarly, inhibiting the intracellular enzyme phosphodiesterase prevents the rapid breakdown of cAMP (a kind of increase in cAMP). Major bronchodilators enhance the production of cAMP either by stimulating production of adenylate cyclase or by inhibiting phosphodiesterase.

The muscles of the airway are affected by both the parasympathetic and sympathetic nervous systems through the transmitters acetylcholine, epinephrine, and norepinephrine. Acetylcholine is released by cholinergic fibers. The primary cholinergic fiber is the vagus nerve, which, when stimulated, causes bronchospasm and excessive secretion of mucus. Epinephrine and norepinephrine are catecholamines, the transmitters of the sympathetic nervous system. Epinephrine and norepinephrine are also classified as adrenergic agents, sympathomimetic agents, or adrenoreceptor stimulators by various sources.

The adrenergic agents are subgrouped according to the receptors they stimulate. The main groups are alpha and beta receptors. Alpha receptors are located in smooth muscle and exocrine glands. Alpha receptors primarily have cardiac effects, resulting in increased blood pressure. Stimulation of alpha receptors results in increased bronchomotor tone (bronchoconstriction), release of anaphylactic mediators, and increased bronchial secretions. Beta receptors increase cAMP through the action of adenylate cyclase and are further subclassed as beta-1 or beta-2 receptors.

Beta-1 receptors are not found in the lungs. The primary effect of stimulation of these receptors is an increase in the rate and force of heart contraction, which increases heart rate and blood pressure and could cause dysrhythmias. Beta-2 receptors are located in the lungs and in other skeletal muscles and tissues. Stimulation of beta-2 receptors causes bronchodilation; inhibition of these receptors (for example, with cardiac beta blockers such as propanolol) causes bronchoconstriction in patients with hyperreactive airways. Unfortunately, stimulation of the beta-2 receptors also causes stimulation of the nervous system, resulting in nervousness, insomnia, and tremors. The beta-2 adrenergic bronchodilators include catecholamines (epinephrine, isoproterenol, isoetharine), resorcinols (metaproterenol, terbutaline), and saligenins (albuterol). The catecholamines have a short half-life, making them frequently unsuitable for long-term administration but very useful for acute bronchospasm. The resorcinols and saligenins have a longer half-life, making them more useful as long-term medications.

Adrenergic agonists

Adrenergic agonists are available for inhalation or oral ingestion (Table 16-1). Only epinephrine and terbutaline are manufactured in a subcutaneous form. Because of its cardiac side effects, epinephrine usually is not adminis-

Table 16-1. Bronchodilators

Drug	Dosage	Onset/duration of action	Alpha/beta-1/beta-2 effects*	Trade names
Adrenergic agonists				
Albuterol	Nebulizer: 0.5 ml q 4-6 hr Metered-dose inhaler (MDI): 2 puffs q 4-6 hr Rotacaps: 1 q 4-6 hr Tablet: 2-4 mg q 6-8 hr Syrup: (2 mg/5 ml) 5-10 ml q 6-8 hr	1-30 minutes/4-6 hr	0/1-2/4	Proventil, Ventolin
Epinephrine	Subcutaneous route (1:1000): 0.1-0.5 ml q 30 minutes up to 1 ml, then q 4-6 hr Nebulizer (racemic epinephrine): 0.3-1 ml q 2-4 hr MDI: 1-2 puffs q 4-6 hr	1-5 minutes/1-2 hr	2-3/3-4/2-3	Adrenalin, Primatene Mist, Asthmahaler, Vaponefrin, Micronefrin
Isoetharine	Nebulizer (1%): 0.25-1 ml q 3-6 hr MDI: 1-2 puffs q 3-6 hr	1-5 minutes/2-3 hr	0/1-2/3	Bronkosol, Bronkometer
Metaproterenol	Nebulizer (5%): 0.2-0.3 ml q 3-6 hr MDI: 2-3 puffs q 3-6 hr Tablet: 10-20 mg q 6-8 hr Syrup: (10 mg/5 ml) 5-10 ml q 6-8 hr	1-30 minutes/4 hr	0/2-3/2-3	Alupent
Terbutaline	Subcutaneous route (1 mg/ml): 0.25 ml q 15-30 minutes up to 0.5 ml, then q 4 hr MDI: 1-2 puffs q 4-6 hr Tablet: 2.5-5 mg q 8 hr	1-30 minutes/2-8 hr	0/1-2/3-4	Brethine, Bricanyl, Brethaire
Anticholinergic agents				
Atropine	Nebulizer: 0.025-0.075 mg/kg up to 2.5 mg q 4-6 hr	15-30 minutes/3-5 hr	—	Atropine
Ipratropium	Nebulizer (0.025%): 1-2 ml q 4-6 hr MDI: 2-4 puffs q 4-6 hr	3-30 minutes/3-6 hr	—	Atrovent

*Scale: 1, least action to 4, most action.

tered to patients over 40 to 50 years of age unless it is certain that the patient does not have coronary artery disease. However, it is important to note that over-the-counter inhalers such as Primatene Mist contain epinephrine and are used by patients of all ages. Patients who have been using Primatene Mist often feel that prescription beta adrenergic inhalers are ineffective because they do not get the sympathetic "rush" and tachycardia felt with epinephrine. When the inhaler is used more often than recommended, the bronchospasm may become refractory. Terbutaline is also used to inhibit uterine muscle contractions in pregnant women with premature labor.

The onset of action of adrenergic agonists varies from 1 minute to about 15 minutes and is sustained for 1 to 6 hours, depending on the preparation and beta-2 selectivity (see Table 16-1). Epinephrine has a quick onset of action and a relatively short duration of action, which necessitates frequent dosing. Onset of action is slower in oral preparations.

The best adrenergic bronchodilator is the most selective (beta-2) for bronchodilation because there is optimal bronchodilation with fewer side effects. Therefore the newer beta adrenergic agonists, such as albuterol, are preferred. Side effects depend on the amount of alpha and beta potencies, as well as the route. More frequent and more severe side effects are seen with subcutaneous administration followed by oral ingestion (also systemic) and then inhaled dosing. Compared with inhaled forms, oral preparations have more systemic side effects and do not have a significantly longer duration of action; therefore the preferred means of administration is inhalation. Side effects are few with beta-2 selective albuterol, metaproterenol, and inhaled terbutaline. Common side effects of the bronchodilators are listed in the box below; the most common side effects are transient tachycardia and mild tremor, which resolve within a few minutes.

Common side effects of bronchodilators

Adrenergic agonists	Anticholinergic agents
Dizziness	Blurred vision*
Dysrhythmias	Cough
Headaches	Difficulty voiding*
Hypertension	Dizziness
Hypokalemia	Dry mouth
Insomnia	Dysphagia*
Nausea	Dysrhythmias*
Pallor	Gastrointestinal discomfort
Palpitations	Glaucoma exacerbation*
Sweating	Headaches
Tachycardia	Mental changes*
Tremors	Nausea
	Nervousness
	Throat discomfort
	Urinary retention*

*Seen primarily with atropine.

Anticholinergic agents

Anticholinergic bronchodilators act by blocking the cholinergic response from parasympathetic stimulation. Intracellular levels of cGMP decline when the cholinergic response is blocked. Recall that methacholine is used to induce bronchospasm (a cholinergic response) in pulmonary function testing to diagnose asthma. The main anticholinergic medications are atropine and ipratropium (see Table 16-1).

Atropine (brand name is the same), which is derived from belladonna, is a very potent anticholinergic medication used primarily to treat bradycardia by blocking vagal tone. It also causes dilated and paralyzed pupils; reduces respiratory, oral, and nasal secretions; decreases bladder and gastrointestinal spasm (causing urinary retention, ileus, and gastroparesis); and decreases sweating. Ipratropium (Atrovent) is a relatively new anticholinergic agent that has fewer side effects than atropine. Ipratropium does not affect ocular pressure unless mistakenly sprayed into the eye. It is more convenient and less expensive to use than atropine, and resistance is not a problem, as it is with the adrenergic bronchodilators.

Methylxanthines

Theophylline and its main salt, aminophylline, are the most commonly used methylxanthine medications. Caffeine, which is found in coffee, tea, cola, and cocoa, is a naturally occurring xanthine. Methylxanthines cause bronchodilation by inhibiting phosphodiesterase and increasing levels of cAMP. These medications have other pulmonary effects as well. Methylxanthines stimulate breathing, enhance ciliary function, inhibit the release of histamine, vasodilate pulmonary vessels and decrease pulmonary hypertension, and improve diaphragmatic contractility. In addition to their pulmonary effects, methylxanthines vasodilate coronary artery blood vessels, vasoconstrict cerebral blood vessels, promote diuresis, stimulate central nervous system and skeletal muscles, and increase secretion of gastric acid.

The effects of theophylline are directly related to its level in the blood. A blood level of 10 to 20 μg/dl is considered therapeutic, although patients often show improvement in pulmonary function with subtherapeutic levels. The American Thoracic Society recommends 8 μg/dl as a normal lower limit of theophylline. Physicians generally try to keep the level on the low side of normal to minimize side effects. This also gives them a margin for increasing the dose safely during an exacerbation. A blood level above 20 μg/dl is considered toxic. The frequency and severity of side effects increase as the level increases. The box on p. 366 lists the side effects of theophylline.

Aminophylline is 75% to 85% less active than theophylline. Activity varies with the amount of theophylline in a given preparation. Products contain 48% to 100% active theophylline. When changing a patient from intravenous aminophylline to oral theophylline, the physician calculates the amount of aminophylline administered to the patient over 24 hours. The aminophylline dosage is reduced by about 75% to 85% to determine the correct theophylline dose. For instance, a patient is admitted to the hospital with an acute exacerbation of asthma. The physician begins intravenous aminophylline. After 2 or 3 days the patient is better and ready to take oral medications. The patient currently receives 1000 mg of aminophylline over a 24-hour period. The suggested theophylline dosage is 750 to 850 mg. If the theophylline drug is to be taken twice a day, the patient is given about 400

Side effects of theophylline

Abdominal pain	Nausea
Anorexia	Nervousness
Dehydration (secondary	Palpitations
to diuresis)	Premature ventricular beats
Diarrhea	Seizures
Dysrhythmias	Tachycardia
Flushing	Tachypnea
Headaches	Tremors
Insomnia	Ventricular tachycardia
Irritability	Vomiting
Muscle twitching	

---

mg per dose; if the drug is to be taken four times a day, the dose is 200 mg. Blood levels must be determined to arrive at the correct dosage of a theophylline medication. The dosage is increased or decreased based on the theophylline level.

Theophylline is rapidly absorbed in the gastrointestinal tract or intravenously. Roughly 90% of the drug is metabolized in the liver and excreted in the urine in an inactive form. The remaining 10% is excreted unchanged in the urine. Theophylline clearance is altered by age, diet, smoking history, cardiac and liver functions, and other medications. Elderly people require lower dosages, whereas children frequently require higher dosages because of their metabolic rate. Metabolism of theophylline is more constant when the doses are evenly spaced over a 24-hour period. Each dose is taken with the same amount and type of food (protein or carbohydrate).

People who smoke generally require higher dosages than those who don't. The half-life of theophylline in an nonsmoker averages 7 to 9 hours; in a person who smokes, the half-life is about 4 to 5 hours. If the individual quits smoking, the dosage frequently must be adjusted. Impaired hepatic and cardiac function slow the utilization of theophylline, often requiring a lower dose. Sometimes one of the signs of impaired cardiac function or congestive heart failure is an increasing level of theophylline.

A variety of medications alter theophylline clearance. The most common ones are erythromycin antibiotics and cimetidine. The box below lists the causes of increased and decreased blood levels. Because of its absorption

---

Factors affecting theophylline blood level

Increases blood level	Decreases blood level
Allopurinol	Charcoal ingestion
Cimetidine	Cigarette smoking
Ciprofloxacin	Isoproterenol
Congestive heart failure	Phenobarbital
Erythromycin	Phenytoin
Liver disease	Rifampin
Oral contraceptives	
Shock	

---

characteristics and potential side effects, theophylline is not used in patients with any of the following: unstable blood pressure, gastrointestinal bleeding, hepatic failure, hyperthyroidism, nausea, a history of seizures, tachyrhythmias, extreme tremulousness, peptic ulcer, or vomiting.

When a patient is admitted to the hospital in acute respiratory distress from an exacerbation of pulmonary disease, intravenous aminophylline frequently is initiated. The loading dose is approximately 6 mg/kg (5 mg/kg if theophylline is used), although the range varies from 4 to 9 mg/kg. If the patient has recently taken a dose of theophylline, a lower loading dose is chosen. (The physician may do a finger stick theophylline test to aid in decision making. The existing serum level is subtracted from the desired level, and the result is multiplied by 0.5 to obtain the loading dose.) Patients with congestive heart failure, liver disease, or cor pulmonale frequently receive doses as low as 0.2 mg/kg. A common loading dose is 200 to 500 mg of aminophylline administered over 30 minutes. An intravenous infusion of aminophylline is started after the loading dose has been administered. The maintenance dosage is determined by theophylline blood levels. If the level is low, the rate of infusion is increased; if it is high, the infusion is slowed or stopped for 1 hour or longer.

When the bronchospasm has resolved, the patient is switched to an oral preparation. Oral preparations are available in three forms: rapid release or plain preparation (most elixirs, some sprinkles, and some pills), slow release (timed-release capsules or tablets with sustained action over 8 to 12 hours), or once a day (sustained action over 24 hours). Most patients who need daily therapy take slow-release or once-a-day preparations. Patients with intermittent bronchospasm (primarily asthma), who use an inhaler as first-line therapy, supplement with rapid-release preparations when symptoms are not relieved with the inhaler. When switching a patient from intravenous to oral therapy, the intravenous theophylline is continued for about 2 hours after administration of the oral theophylline. The goal is to allow oral absorption to near peak concentrations before discontinuing intravenous therapy. Table 16-2 lists peak plasma concentration times of various types of theophylline.

Theophylline toxicity. Theophylline toxicity can occur at any time, often without warning. When the patient complains of unusual nausea, vomiting, headache, increased tremors, irritability or confusion, theophylline toxicity is considered. The blood level is determined, and treatment is initiated. Treatment depends on the patient's symptoms and the serum theophylline level. If the level is just above the normal range (that is, 20 to 25 μg/ml or mg/dl) one or two doses are withheld, in most cases. When theophylline is restarted, the dosage is decreased by about 25%. (If heart failure is the cause of the theophylline toxicity, it must be treated simultaneously. Theophylline toxicity can be avoided by choosing alternative antibiotics or by adjusting the theophylline dose when prescribing antibiotics that alter the theophylline level.)

If the theophylline level is higher than 25 μg/ml or if severe side effects are present, additional measures are necessary. A level above 30 μg/ml is considered a medical emergency. In an alert patient, initial treatment is to induce vomiting with syrup of ipecac, if vomiting has not already begun and if the patient recently has taken a dose of theophylline. The patient must be able to protect his airway from aspiration when vomiting is induced. Initial treatment is followed by administration of activated charcoal (30 to 60 g) orally or by nasogastric tube. Some physicians also order a cathartic, such as citrate

Table 16-2. Peak plasma concentration times of various types of theophylline

Product	Dosage*	Peak concentration	Brand names
Intravenous solution	Aminophylline: (6 mg/kg in 50 ml D_5W or normal saline (NS) load, then 0.5-1 mg/kg/hr) Theophylline: (5 mg/kg in 50 ml D_5W or NS load, then 0.4-0.9 mg/kg/hr)	20-30 minutes	Aminophylline, Theophylline
Once-a-day preparation	5-10 mg/kg, usually taken after dinner in patients who awaken frequently at night, because peak concentration then occurs at night; dose may also be taken in the morning. May be given q 12 hr in some patients who are rapid metabolizers	4-13 hr	Theo-24, Uniphyl
Slow-release tablet or capsule	5-10 mg/kg/day in two or three divided doses q 8-12 hr	3-7 hr	Constant-T, Respbid, Slo-Phyllin gyrocaps, Theo-Dur, Theolair-SR
Rapid release or Plain preparation	5-10 mg/kg/day in four to six divided doses q 4-6 hr	30 minutes-3 hr	Elixophylline, Slo-Phyllin, Theolair, Theophyl chewable tablets

*Dosage is titrated to maintain the theophylline blood level at 10 to 20 μg/ml.

of magnesia. If the blood level is above 50 to 60 μg/ml, charcoal hemoperfusion or hemodialysis is begun immediately in addition to gastric charcoal.

ANTIBIOTICS

Antibiotics are prescribed with some regularity for pulmonary patients. Infections in the lung stimulate production of mucus, which is not well tolerated by some patients, especially those with limited respiratory reserve. Sinusitis also exacerbates pulmonary disease in some patients. When the patient develops an infection, normal ventilation-perfusion relationships are altered. The patient may develop acute oxygenation or ventilation failure or both. In patients with marginal lung function, intubation and mechanical ventilation frequently are necessary. Rapid institution of antibiotics reduces mucus and improves arterial blood gases. It is important to remind the patient to increase fluid intake to thin mucus when an infection is present.

Antibiotics work by binding to the bacteria cell and inhibiting growth (bacteriostatic) or killing the bacteria (bacteriocidal). Treatment is ideally directed by cultures. The most commonly prescribed antibiotics are ampicillin, amoxicillin, tetracycline, and sulfa drugs (Septra). Erythromycin is avoided because of its effect on theophylline. When erythromycin is prescribed, the theophylline dosage is adjusted.

It is fairly common practice for a physician to prescribe antibiotics for a viral infection in pulmonary patients with limited reserve. Since the patient's immunity is altered, he is more susceptible to secondary bacterial invasion. The physician may give the patient a prescription of antibiotics to keep at home. The patient initiates antibiotics when he has signs and symptoms of an infection. These signs include increased sputum, cough, or fatigue; change in the color or thickness of sputum; and fever, chills, or night sweats. If the patient's condition does not improve or worsens within 3 days, he should call the physician. Some patients with chronic suppurative conditions, such as bronchiectasis, may take antibiotics for 7 to 10 days a month to suppress infection. There is always the risk of resistance or superinfection when antibiotics are used frequently.

The main side effect of antibiotics is gastrointestinal distress. The patient may complain of nausea or loose stools, and some patients have abdominal cramps.

Antiviral agents sometimes are used to treat the herpes simplex, influenza A, varicella zoster, and respiratory syncytial viruses. Some of these drugs are amantadine (Amantadine HCL), acyclovir (Zovirax), interferon (Intron A, Alferon N), ribavirin (Virazole) and rimantadine HCL.

Some physicians use aerosolized antibiotics to reduce lung bacteria in patients with chronic suppurative conditions such as cystic fibrosis or bronchiectasis. Aminoglycosides, such as gentamicin or tobramycin, are the most commonly used. These medications are nebulized like a bronchodilator. Some patients complain of increased coughing with nebulized antibiotics. The advantage of nebulizing antibiotics is that systemic adverse effects, such as renal failure, are reduced or eliminated.

A fairly new inhaled antibiotic is pentamidine (NebuPent), which is used to treat *Pneumocystis carinii* infection, an opportunistic infection in immunosuppressed patients. Pentamidine is administered through a special nebulizer device.

ANTITUSSIVES

The use of antitussives is controversial among pulmonary physicians. An antitussive is used to suppress an ineffective cough but never an effective cough, with few exceptions. One example of an ineffective cough is a dry, hacking, nonproductive cough. Antitussives are not given when secretions retained in the airways are not coughed out. The patient may require increased fluids, expectorants, or chest physical therapy to improve cough effectiveness. However, if a patient cannot get enough rest because of excessive coughing, an antitussive sometimes is prescribed.

There are various types of antitussive agents. In the critical care area, coughing is suppressed with the use of topical anesthetics such as lidocaine. The lidocaine is injected either through an endotracheal tube or transtracheally with a needle.

Systemic cough preparations are narcotic or nonnarcotic. The best narcotic cough suppressant is codeine (preferred) or morphine. The use of narcotics is limited because they cause respiratory depression. Narcotic cough medications also have adverse effects such as dry mouth, impaired mucociliary clearance, and bronchospasm from histamine release. Patients often develop constipation when using narcotic preparations.

Nonnarcotic cough preparations are available over the counter or by prescription. Many contain dextromethorphan or benzonatate. The nurse evaluates for correct use of over-the-counter antitussives. A common nonnarcotic prescription antitussive is Tessalon Perles.

DIURETICS

Diuretics are used when fluid overload is present. They are commonly used with congestive heart failure or cor pulmonale. The most common diuretics are furosemide (Lasix) and acetazolamide (Diamox). Recall that theophylline also has diuretic side effects. The patient receiving diuretic therapy usually needs dietary potassium supplements to prevent hypokalemia. The diet is assessed for adequate potassium intake, especially when supplemental potassium has not been prescribed. Serum potassium levels are assessed routinely.

MUCOLYTICS AND EXPECTORANTS

Mucolytic agents enhance mobilization and removal of secretions from the airway. The most important mucolytic agent is water. Adequate hydration is essential for easier expectoration of mucus, since sputum is composed of mucoproteins, water, electrolytes, and cellular debris. However, care is taken to not overhydrate the patient. Overhydration can, in effect, cause the patient to drown in his own secretions when fluid clearance is impaired (for example, some patients with congestive heart failure or renal failure can develop pulmonary edema). When a patient is dehydrated, secretions are thicker and more difficult to expectorate. Similarly, when sputum is infected, it contains more cellular debris, as well as deoxyribonucleic acid (DNA) from neutrophils and bacteria. The DNA and cellular debris thicken the sputum and change the color from clear or white to yellow, brown, or green.

Many clinicians recommend at least 2000 to 4000 ml of fluids daily. (A fluid is liquid at room temperature.) Fluids include water, juice, milk, and soft drinks, in addition to soup, pudding, gelatin, protein supplement drinks, and ice cream. At least four to eight 8-oz. glasses of water are needed daily in addition to other fluids. Undernourished or low-weight patients should choose high-calorie fluids, whereas overweight patients should select low-calorie fluids. The physician is consulted about fluid restrictions for patients with impaired cardiac and renal function.

When secretion removal is difficult despite adequate hydration, the patient may need pharmacological therapy. Expectorants are available in both inhaled and systemic form. The most common inhaled expectorant is acetylcysteine, sometimes better known as Mucomyst. However, acetylcysteine is an irritant that may also cause bronchospasm and inhibit ciliary function. Acetylcysteine often is preceded by or combined with a bronchodilator to prevent bronchospasm. When acetylcysteine is given, the patient develops bronchorrhea and coughing is stimulated. The drug has a rotten egg (sulfurlike) odor and an unpleasant taste that patients dislike. A 20% solution of acetylcysteine usually is diluted with an equal amount of normal saline or sodium bicarbonate to make a 10% solution, which is equally effective.

Oral expectorants include potassium iodide and guaifenesin. A saturated solution of potassium iodide (SSKI), available only by prescription, has been used for many years as an expectorant. It activates the submucosal bronchial glands to produce more watery secretions. SSKI may also have a direct mucolytic effect by breaking the protein bonds in mucus. Some evidence suggests that SSKI stimulates ciliary function and may have an antiinflammatory effect. SSKI usually is prescribed as 5 to 20 drops in a glass of water three or four times a day. Unfortunately, many patients complain of the metallic taste left by SSKI, and some develop acne or parotid swelling. Because thyroid function may be affected by long-term use of SSKI, thyroid function should be assessed within 2 months of beginning treatment and then at least yearly.

Many over-the-counter cough and cold preparations contain guaifenesin, formerly called glyceryl guaiacolate. Guaifenesin acts by vagal stimulation and by direct stimulation of the bronchial glands. The usual dosage is 100 to 400 mg four to six times daily, although some physicians prescribe up to 1200 mg of guaifenesin (the long-acting form, such as Humibid) twice daily. Common side effects of guaifenesin, if overused include nausea, vomiting, and drowsiness. Expectorants, including guaifenesin, should be used intermittently.

Iodinated glycerol (Organidin) is classified as a mucolytic expectorant. The usual dosage is two tablets four times daily with a glass of liquid.

DECONGESTANTS AND ANTIHISTAMINES

Decongestants and antihistamines are used to treat upper airway congestion. A decongestant vasoconstricts localized blood vessels. The reduced blood flow (decreased hydrostatic pressure) prevents fluid exudation into the tissues, decreasing edema. Decongestants are used only on a limited basis. Most physicians recommend limiting use to 3- to 7-day intervals. Prolonged use may result in rebound congestion when the drug is discontinued. If this occurs, the patient develops increased congestion.

Both over-the-counter and prescription decongestants are used. The most common over-the-counter preparation is pseudoephedrine (Sudafed, Actifed) (30 to 60 mg four times daily). It is available in many preparations, as well as alone. The patient should consult the physician before taking any over-the-counter medication containing a decongestant and should notify the physician if symptoms do not improve within a few days. The physician usually orders a prescription decongestant, such as Tavist-D.

Antihistamines are used to control the symptoms of sneezing, rhinitis, and itchy, watery eyes (that is, cold or allergy symptoms). Antihistamines are used consistently by some physicians and rarely by others. The patient should talk with his physician about appropriate use of antihistamines, since many of these drugs cause drowsiness. Newer prescription antihistamines, such as terfenadine (Seldane) or astemizole (Hismanal), do not cause drowsiness.

MAST CELL STABILIZERS

Cromolyn sodium or disodium cromoglycate (Aarane, Intal), a mast cell stabilizer, is used by some patients with asthma. Cromolyn is not a direct bronchodilator but has bronchodilatory effects by preventing the bronchospasm seen in asthma, including exercise-induced asthma. It is a prophylactic agent and is not used for acute bronchospasm. After deposition in the lung, cromolyn is absorbed into the blood and excreted within 4 hours into the urine and bile. Cromolyn presumably works by preventing the antigen-antibody response of the mast cells and may prevent calcium from entering the cell. Histamine release is diminished or obliterated. Intal is the only cromolyn sodium drug currently marketed in the United States, although other similar mast cell stabilizers are under investigation and may be released soon.

Intal is available in capsule form for inhalation, as a liquid for nebulization, and as a metered-dose inhaler (MDI). The dosage for Intal usually is one capsule, one nebulizer ampule, or two puffs, respectively, one to four times daily. The powder is administered in a special turbo inhaler called a Spinhaler. Cromolyn may be taken continuously or for only a few weeks to months of the year when allergy symptoms peak. Although some patients notice a positive effect within a few days, many do not see an effect for about 6 weeks. If the patient does not improve symptomatically or objectively (pulmonary function tests) within 4 weeks, the dosage is increased. After 6 to 8 weeks without improvement, the drug is discontinued.

The side effects of Intal are few and usually mild. In rare cases the patient develops a skin rash. Patients who use Intal may complain of hoarseness, irritated throat, cough, and bronchospasm. For this reason Intal often is preceded by administration of a bronchodilator.

CORTICOSTEROIDS

Corticosteroids, specifically glucocorticoids, are used to treat a wide variety of acute and chronic pulmonary diseases (see box below). Steroids have antiinflammatory and bronchodilatory effects, among others. The antinflammatory effects include preventing the release of lysosomal enzymes in delayed hypersensitivity reactions, decreasing circulating lymphocytes, eosinophils, and tissue mast cells, and inhibiting histamine and other mediators. Steroids produce bronchodilatory effects by increasing cAMP and lowering the stimulation threshold for beta-2 receptors. Steroids also improve circulatory function and heart contraction and enhance the patient's general sense of wellbeing. In sarcoidosis, the serum levels of angiotensin-converting enzyme are reduced through steroid therapy.

Steroids may be given intravenously (in the hospitalized patient), orally, or via an MDI. The dosage depends on the steroid preparation and the patient's response. The primary intravenous steroids are hydrocortisone (Solu-Cortef), a short acting agent, and methylprednisolone (Solu-Medrol), an intermediate-acting agent (preferred). The infusion may be given continuously or intermittently (every 4 to 8 hours). After the acute bronchospasm or inflammation has resolved (as demonstrated through control of wheezing or improvement in pulmonary function tests), the patient is given oral steroids.

Pulmonary Diseases treated with steroids

Active collagen-vascular diseases
Allergic bronchopulmonary aspergillosis (ABPA)
Asthma and status asthmaticus
Cancer
Chronic bronchitis
Chronic obstructive pulmonary disease (COPD)
Hypersensitivity pneumonitis
Idiopathic pulmonary fibrosis
Pneumoconioses
Sarcoidosis
Tracheitis

Prednisone is the most common oral steroid used. It is intermediate acting. The acute dosage is 1 mg per kilogram of lean body weight per day, which is about 60 mg in most patients. The entire dose may be taken in the morning, or the dose may be divided and taken in the morning after breakfast and in the evening after dinner. Depending on the clinical situation, the patient continues this high dosage for days to weeks. The usual quick burst of steroids in acute asthma is taken for about 2 weeks. In sarcoidosis, the treatment may last 6 months. A few patients need continuous steroid therapy but at a fairly low dosage.

A tapering regimen for a typical short burst of steroids is 60 mg daily for 2 days, 50 mg for 2 days, 40 mg for 2 days, 20 mg for 2 days, 15 mg for 2 days, 10 mg for 2 days, and 5 mg for 2 days; then drug is discontinued. When steroid use is prolonged, the patient is tapered from 60 mg/day to 20 mg/day over the course of 2 to 4 weeks. The final tapering is much slower. Dosages are decreased at weekly, monthly, or even less frequent intervals. Some patients take 5 to 15 mg a day indefinitely. When continuous steroids are needed, some physicians prefer to use alternate-day dosing to minimize adrenal and pituitary suppression and to reduce systemic side effects. With this regimen, the patient takes 5 to 20 mg every other day. On alternate days, the dosage is 0 or at least less than the previous day. For instance, the patient who usually takes 20 mg daily may, on alternate-day dosing, take 20 mg one day and 10 mg the next, or 20 mg one day and 0 the next. Sometimes the dosage on the "take it" day is increased to further reduce the dosage on the off day.

It is important to reduce the dosage of oral steroids or discontinue them because of their side effects. In an effort to do this, the physician may prescribe inhaled steroids with oral steroids, although inhaled steroids can also be used alone. Inhaled steroids have fewer systemic side effects than oral steroids and are used to wean patients from oral steroids, as well as to prevent their use. Depending on the preparation, inhaled steroids are administered two to four times daily. The normal dosage for most inhaled steroids is two to four puffs every 6 to 12 hours, not to exceed 2000 µg a day. Although a usual daily dosage is 24 puffs, some patients require 40 puffs daily. Common inhaled steroids include beclomethasone (Vanceril, Beclovent), flunisolide (Aerobid), and triamcinolone (Azmacort).

Prolonged use of oral steroid can give rise to many side effects. In most instances risk is related to dosage; the higher the dosage and the longer the use of oral steroids, the greater the chance of side effects. Common side effects are listed in the box on p. 374.

Immunological suppression with steroids is important in caring for patients who are prone to develop infections. Steroids lessen or mask the symptoms of infection, making identification difficult. For instance, patients on steroids do not mount traditional fevers to infection. They also do not develop positive responses to skin testing, including the purified protein derivative (PPD) test for tuberculosis. In addition, when patients with unknown tuberculosis are treated with steroids, the tuberculosis may be reactivated.

Osteoporosis is a serious side effect of chronic steroid use. Leaching of calcium from the bones increases the incidence of pathological fractures. Some patients develop compression fractures of the spine from coughing or stepping down a little harder than usual. The pain from these fractures limits breathing. In postmenopausal women, estrogen replacement is initiated to help prevent osteoporosis. Calcium supplementation is controversial but usu-

---

Common side effects of steroids

Oral form
Cataracts
Cushing syndrome (moonlike
    facial swelling, central obe-
    sity with hump over back
    and neck, stretch marks
    over limbs and trunk, acne,
    hirsutism)
Dependency
Euphoria
Fragile skin and capillaries
Gastrointestinal upset
Gastrointestinal bleeding
Growth retardation (children)
Hyperglycemia
Impaired immunological sta-
    tus
Impaired wound healing
Increased appetite
Insomnia
Myopathy
Nervousness
Osteoporosis
Personality changes
Psychoses
Thrush
Weight gain

Inhaled form
Irritated throat
Oral fungal infections (for ex-
    ample, candidiasis)
Thrush

---

ally recommended.

Hyperglycemia may occur with use of oral steroids. It is more common in patients with a familial history of diabetes. The patient may be able to control the serum glucose with diet, although insulin sometimes is required.

A cushingoid effect is very common in patients on prolonged steroid therapy. The patient develops a moonlike or round face. Truncal obesity and a hump on the back and shoulders occur from increased fat deposits. Weight control is essential to prevent obesity. Patients taking steroids must be cautioned that they probably will have an increased appetite. Patients taking prolonged oral steroid supplementation complain of weakened muscles in the upper arms and thighs. Truncal obesity makes the arms and legs look smaller, and there may be muscle wasting as well. Bruising resulting from fragile capillaries and skin is common with even slight injuries that the patient does not remember.

Gastrointestinal distress also is common in patients taking steroids. The most frequent complaints are nausea, cramping, and diarrhea. Gastrointestinal bleeding does occur and can be prevented with antacids or H_2 blockers such as cimetidine (Tagamet) or ranitidine (Zantac). (Remember that cimetidine alters the theophylline level.) Most patients say that symptoms can be lessened by taking the prednisone on a full stomach.

Steroids also have numerous emotional effects. Patients have an artificial sense of well-being that makes effectiveness difficult to interpret. Objective measures, such as pulmonary function tests, must be used to determine effectiveness, since the physician may not be able to rely on the patient's interpretation of effect. Patients often have mood swings, and depression and apathy are fairly common after the drug has been discontinued.

Inhaled steroid preparations have two major advantages over oral forms: systemic absorption is minimal, and the side effects are few. Minimal systemic absorption and lower dosage are presumed to be reason for reduced number of side effects. Many patients complain of an irritated throat, a problem that can be diminished by using a spacer. A spacer is an extension device that allows the MDI to be activated at least 4 cm from the mouth, thus reducing the aerosol impaction in the back of the throat. Candidiasis, identified by white patches or white coating in the mouth, usually occurs because the patient did not rinse his mouth after each use of the MDI. (A spacer also reduces the incidence of candidiasis.) When rinsing the mouth, the patient must be sure to spit the mouth rinse out. Swallowing the rinse may result in fungal infections of the esophagus. A mouthwash high in alcohol (such as Listerine or Cepacol) may prevent thrush but is contraindicated in patients with dry mouth, such as with cancer. When an oral fungal infection occurs, the treatment usually is simple. The patient may use Nystatin swish and swallow or clotrimazole lozenges (Mycelex Troches) four times daily. If treatment is started early, systemic problems are few. If oral fungal infections are not treated, the patient may develop systemic infections that require 6 weeks of intravenous amphotericin B.

METHODS OF ADMINISTRATION

Beta adrenergic, anticholinergic, steroid, and mast cell stabilizer medications are prescribed as nebulizers or inhalers. Most patients use an inhaler. The nebulizer is reserved for patients who cannot use inhalers or who do not obtain relief of bronchospasm with inhalers. Most children under 5 years of age use a nebulizer with a mask or sometimes a mouthpiece. The child is switched to an inhaler when he is old enough to comprehend and follow directions and has sufficient skill to take the medication. Among adults, patients with advanced obstructive airway disease often use a nebulizer to control bronchospasm. Sometimes chronic steroid use can be avoided by using a nebulizer. In addition, patients who cannot adequately coordinate activating an inhaler and breathing, even with a spacer, usually need a nebulizer to get the medication into their lungs.

A variety of different machines are available for nebulizing medications. In the hospital, oxygen or air is forced through a jet nebulizer. At home, most patients, especially those dependent on a ventilator, use an air compressor with a jet nebulizer cup to deliver nebulized medications (Fig. 16-1). The most common nebulizer in use in the home is the Pulmo-aide. Ultrasonic nebulizers also are available, such as the Pulmosonic or Microstat. Some nebulizers are powered only by electricity, whereas others have battery packs or plug into the lighter receptacle in a car.

When a nebulizer is used in the home, it is essential to teach the patient how to clean and disinfect it adequately. The nebulizer cup is rinsed under running water after each use. The cup is cleaned with soap and water at least daily. It is placed between two paper towels to dry and stored in a loosely closed (not zippered or twist tied) plastic bag. Depending on the patient's condition and the environment, the cup is disinfected at least weekly.

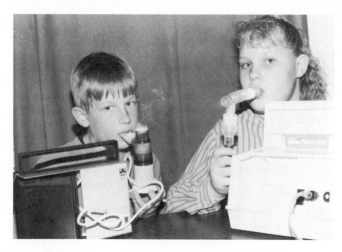

Fig. 16-1. Some patients must use nebulizers for inhaled bronchodilators.

Nebulizer medication generally is more expensive than inhaler medication. Beta adrenergic bronchodilators are available in multidose bottles. They (and mast cell stabilizer medications) also are available in single-use bottles, snap-tip glass vials, or plastic snap-top tubes, depending on the manufacturer. In addition, nebulizers cost several hundred dollars, depending on the model and features. Most insurance companies pay 80% of the cost of the equipment, and the patient is responsible for the remaining 20%. Health maintenance organizations (HMOs) cover the cost of the equipment only if durable medical equipment is covered under the plan. Medicare currently does not allow its members to purchase nebulizers; the patient rents the machine indefinitely. The advantage of rental is that the patient is not responsible for maintenance or repairs.

Inhalers

There are three types of inhalers: metered-dose inhaler (MDI), turbo or spin inhaler (cromolyn or Intal), and rotacaps (Ventolin). The most common is the metered-dose inhaler. Beta adrenergic, anticholinergic, steroid, and mast cell stabilizer medications are available in an MDI.

The MDI is a simple device, but it often is difficult to use correctly. Proper use requires precise timing of five steps: (1) shaking the MDI, (2) positioning it correctly, (3) activating the inhaler, (4) exhaling completely and then slowly inhaling, and (5) breath holding. The inhaler must be well shaken to mix the medication with the propellant; failure to shake the MDI results in incorrect dosing.

Current research suggests that the best technique is to activate the inhaler at least 4 cm from a wide open mouth. This is in direct contrast to product literature and techniques taught 15 years ago. Commercials on television for over-the-counter inhalers do not show the open mouth technique. If a patient cannot hold the MDI in front of the mouth, a spacer is needed. Table 16-3 presents a teaching aid for using an inhaler correctly.

Activating the MDI is the next step. Most patients place the thumb on the underside of the MDI and one or two fingers on top of it. However, some

Table 16-3. Technique for using an inhaler

Action	Rationale
1. Shake the inhaler 15 to 20 times.	1. To mix the medication with the propellant.
2. Hold the inhaler about four fingers in front of your mouth. Aim the inhaler directly into the mouth, not toward the eyes, cheeks, or chin. If a spacer is used, the MDI is placed in it. The spacer is placed directly in the mouth.	2. To allow the medication to become a vapor to inhale. If the MDI is placed in the mouth, the medication will hit the back of the throat before becoming a vapor, which the patient wants to inhale. (Holding the inhaler in front of the patient and activating it shows the patient that the most spray or vapor develops about 6 to 10 inches from the mouthpiece. Be sure that the path of the vapor is across the patient's line of vision and not into the patient's or the nurse's face.)
3. Exhale completely (to functional residual capacity).	3. To allow the medication to come into the lungs with the first air breathed in. The medication is not wasted in dead space ventilation.
4. Open your mouth wide (drop your jaw) and activate the MDI.	4. To draw air in behind the medication. The mouth serves as a reservoir for the medication to vaporize. Be sure that the patient does not breathe in before activating the MDI.
5. Breathe in slowly and deeply to total lung capacity over 5 or 6 seconds.	5. To prevent premature deposition of medication by breathing in too fast and to deposit the medication deep in the airways.
6. Close your mouth and hold your breath for 10 seconds.	6. To allow the medication to deposit on the airways. Not holding the breath or exhaling too rapidly blows the medication out into the air. Be sure the patient does not exhale through the nose or mouth.
7. Wait at least 1 to 5 minutes and repeat the process for each additional puff ordered.	7. To allow the medication to begin to work, so subsequent puffs go deeper and are more effective.

patients need both thumbs and two to four fingers to activate the MDI. Patients with arthritis or hand weakness have difficulty activating an MDI. A product called VentEase helps arthritic patients activate the MDI. However, VentEase is made for tall inhalers; a wedge must be placed in the top of the VentEase when short inhalers (such as Alupent and Atrovent) are used for the device to work. Some patients have difficulty directing the MDI at the open mouth, especially when dyspneic, anxious, or tremulous.

The next step, slow inhalation, first requires complete exhalation. Then the patient inhales to total lung capacity (TLC) slowly over 5 or 6 seconds. Inhalation begins at functional residual capacity (FRC) after the MDI has been activated. Many patients do not exhale to FRC before activating the inhaler, or they do not breathe to TLC after activating it. The InspirEase and Aero-Chamber spacers cue the patient who is inhaling too fast with a whistle.

The final step for correct MDI use is breath holding. The literature suggests a 10-second breath holding maneuver. Holding the breath allows the medication to deposit in the lungs. This is very difficult in dyspneic or anxious patients. If the patient cannot hold his breath or exhales prematurely,

---

MDI order when several drugs are taken

1 Beta adrenergic drug
2 Anticholinergic drug
3 Mast cell stabilizer
4 Steroid

---

less of the medication is deposited in the lungs. Inability to hold the breath may be resolved with the use of the InspirEase spacer. If this spacer is not helpful, a nebulizer is necessary.

The order in which inhalers are used is based on principles of action (see box above). The MDI with the quickest onset of action is used first to relieve bronchospasm and enhance deposition of subsequent puffs. For this reason beta adrenergic inhalers are used first. They are followed by the slower acting anticholinergic inhalers. Some patients cough when using anticholinergic inhalers, which is another reason to bronchodilate with beta adrenergic inhalers first. The third drug is the mast cell stabilizer, which requires preadministration of a bronchodilator in many patients. The last drug inhaled is the steroid. Maximum bronchodilation should precede use of a steroid inhaler. After using a steroid inhaler, the patient should rinse his mouth. With some patients rinsing the mouth also is recommended after using beta adrenergic and anticholinergic inhalers to reduce systemic absorption.

Spacers for inhalers

Recall that a spacer is an extension device that allows the MDI to be activated at least 4 cm from the mouth, thus reducing the aerosol impaction in the back of the throat. More of the medication usually gets to the airways. Only about 10% to 20% of the medication from an MDI without a spacer reaches the lung, whereas with a spacer up to 53% enters the lungs, maximizing bronchodilation. Some patients require less frequent doses of medication when using a spacer. In addition, side effects, such as oral candidiasis, are reduced because of decreased systemic absorption. Patients complain less of "bad taste" and throat irritation when using a spacer.

Many types of spacers are available. A simple, inexpensive model is the cardboard tube from a toilet paper, paper towel, or wrapping paper roll that is cut to a length of 3 to 6 inches. A more durable version is a piece of plastic respiratory therapy tubing used for aerosols or ventilator circuits. The mouthpiece of the inhaler is placed at one end, and the other end is placed in the mouth. Care must be taken to direct the inhaler toward the mouth in a straight line.

The primary commercial spacers are the AeroChamber and the InspirEase (Fig. 16-2). A commercial spacer costs about $20 to $25. Some spacers, such as the InspirEase, require bag changes at an additional yearly cost of less than $25.

The AeroChamber is a 145 ml round tube (about two times larger in diameter than respiratory therapy tubing) with a hole for attaching the MDI mouthpiece at the distal end. The proximal end has a one-way valve, and the distal end has a whistle to indicate too rapid inhalation. The patient places the AeroChamber in the mouth and activates the MDI. The patient then con-

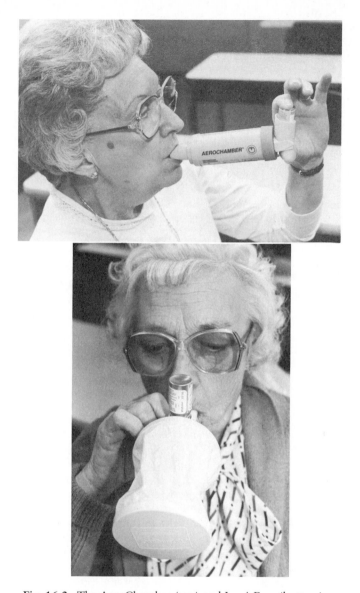

Fig. 16-2. The AeroChamber (top) and InspirEase (bottom) are examples of commercial spacers.

tinues as if no spacer were used. One advantage of the AeroChamber is that the patient can also use the VentEase to activate the MDI if arthritis or hand weakness is a problem.

The InspirEase is composed of a mouthpiece (formerly two mouthpieces in two shades of blue) and a 700 ml collapsible blue plastic bag. The mouthpiece has two extension pins that fit into holes in the plastic bag. Once seated, the mouthpiece is rotated about one-quarter turn to fit securely. The patient places the MDI canister *without its mouthpiece* into the mouthpiece of the InspirEase. The technique for using the InspirEase is presented in Table

Table 16-4. Use of a metered-dose inhaler with InspirEase

1. Attach the mouthpiece to the bag if not already done.	1. Prepares InspirEase.
2. Shake the MDI and place the MDI canister in mouthpiece. (Note: can also place MDI cannister in mouthpiece and then shake.)	2. Mixes medication with propellant.
3. Place the mouthpiece in the mouth, and exhale completely to FRC into the bag.	3. Allows the medication to come into the lungs with the first air breathed in.
4. Activate the MDI. Inhale slowly and deeply. The bag will collapse against the mouthpiece.	4. Prevents premature deposition of medication by breathing in too fast and helps deposit the medication deep in the airways. If the patient breathes in too fast, a whistle is heard.
5. Hold breath for as long as possible, and exhale into the bag; the bag will expand.	5. Allows the medication to deposit on the airways. Not holding the breath or exhaling too rapidly blows the medication out into the air. The patient exhales dead space air into the bag. Medication in the exhaled air is blown into the bag.
6. Breathe in again from the bag without compressing the MDI.	6. Medication blown into the bag from the previous exhalation is rebreathed.
7. Remove InspirEase, and exhale.	7. All done with first puff.
8. Wait 1 to 5 minutes, and repeat for each additional puff.	8. Allows the medication to begin to work so that subsequent puffs go deeper and are more effective.

16-4. The InspirEase whistles when the inspiratory flow rate exceeds 0.3 L per second. In addition, if the patient cannot hold his breath or breathe deeply, he exhales into the bag. Medication from dead space areas enters the bag, to be rebreathed on a subsequent breath. Thus the patient can receive more of the medication consistently. The patient's level of dyspnea, anxiety, or tremulousness has less effect on delivery of the medication. The bag of the InspirEase is changed when it becomes cracked or soiled. Some patients change the bag monthly, others change it three or four times a year.

Some inhalers have built-in spacers. One such MDI is the steroid Azmacort. Unfortunately, each time the patient gets a refill on the medication, he pays for a new spacer. The advantage of receiving a new spacer with each refill is that cleanliness, a concern with some patients, is guaranteed at regular intervals.

Care of a metered-dose inhaler

The mouthpiece of the MDI or spacer is washed in warm, soapy water at least daily. If the patient has an infection, the mouthpiece is washed after each use.

It is important for the patient to know how much medication remains in the MDI. Most inhalers last about 3 to 4 weeks if two puffs are taken four times daily. (Most inhalers contain 200 puffs.) The patient can estimate how much medication remains by dropping the inhaler into a bowl of water (Fig. 16-3). If the MDI lies on the bottom of the bowl, it is full. If it stands on the bottom of the bowl, it is about three fourths full. As the MDI nears half full, it rises to the surface. When the MDI is one quarter full, it turns partly on its side on the surface of the water. An inhaler that lies on top of the water is empty.

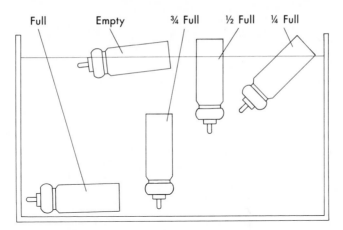

Full   Empty   ¾ Full   ½ Full   ¼ Full

Fig. 16-3. The amount of medication remaining in a metered-dose inhaler is assessed by dropping the canister into a bowl of water. The patient should obtain a refil when the inhaler rises to the surface and begins to tip over. (From Beare P, Myers J: *Principles and practice of adult health nursing,* St Louis, 1990, Mosby–Year Book.)

VACCINES

Most physicians recommend the pneumococcal pneumonia and flu vaccines for patients with chronic pulmonary diseases on the ground that the patient cannot tolerate a major respiratory tract infection. Individuals living with a patient who is at risk may also need vaccination. Many institutions recommend that either or both of these vaccines be administered to health care workers. Similarly, nursing homes or extended care facilities may choose to administer vaccines to health care workers and residents. The influenza vaccine is safe for pregnant women.

The current recommendation for the pneumococcal pneumonia vaccine is one injection in a lifetime, since recent studies suggest that antibody titers are still present 5 years after administration. (It is a misnomer to call this vaccine a pneumonia vaccine, since all types of pneumococcal infection, including otitis media, are affected. In addition, the vaccine does not prevent all types of pneumonia. However, most clinicians still call it the pneumonia vaccine.) A booster is not recommended, and vaccination may not be suggested in patients who have had recent pneumococcal pneumonia or other infection (because of preexisting pneumococcal antibodies).

Different pneumonia preparations are available, including Pneumovax and Pnu-Imune 23 (Lederle). The preparations contain protection for up to 23 of the most prevalent types of pneumococci. However, the vaccine is effective only against the named types of pneumococci. About 25 µg of each type is given in the 0.5 ml dose. Some pneumococcal vaccines are not recommended for children under 2 years of age; others are administered as early as 3 months of age. The vaccine is given subcutaneously or intramuscularly.

The major adverse reactions with most pneumococcal vaccines is localized soreness at the injection site for about 3 days. Some patients develop low-grade fever and mild myalgia for about 24 hours. Anaphylaxis is rare, as are high fever and marked swelling at the site.

The influenza vaccine, commonly called the flu shot, is given annually. Flu-zone (Squibb) is a trivalent influenza vaccine prepared from chicken embryos infected with a specific type of influenza virus. The virus is inactivated, concentrated, and highly purified and therefore cannot cause influenza. The influenza vaccine is effective against two type A strains and one type B strain of influenza. It is made for administration in a particular influenza year, such as the 1991-92 formula. Consecutive years may contain one or more of the same strains.

Before administration, the nurse assesses for allergy to egg or egg products and for signs of active infection. Flu vaccine is not administered during an acute infection. The flu vaccine vial or syringe is shaken well. It is administered to individuals over 6 months of age into the muscle. The dosage for children under 3 years is 0.25 ml, and for individuals over age 3, 0.5 ml. The deltoid muscle commonly is used in the adult; the anterolateral thigh is used in children. The ideal time to administer the flu vaccine is in the fall, before December, when influenza activity sharply increases. Antibody response is altered in immunosuppressed patients. The influenza vaccine is reported to inhibit the clearance of warfarin, theophylline, phenytoin, and aminopyrine but most patients have no adverse clinical effects.

The major side effects of the influenza vaccine are fever, malaise, and myalgia, especially in patients who have not taken the flu vaccine previously. These symptoms usually appear in 6 to 12 hours and last for 1 or 2 days.

CONCLUSION

The nurse needs to know about the various medications used with pulmonary patients to understand proper administration. This chapter has reviewed the basic actions of medications, listed common dosages, and discussed common side effects. With this knowledge, the nurse can properly administer a variety of medications to the patient. In addition, the nurse can identify areas in which patient education is needed and thus can teach the patient such skills as proper use of an inhaler or how to recognize the signs and symptoms of an infection.

BIBLIOGRAPHY

Alberts WM, Corrigan KC: Corticosteroid therapy for chronic obstructive pulmonary disease: is it worth the risks? *Postgrad Med* 81(5):131-134, 1987.

Anthonisen NR, Manfreda J, Warren CP, et al: Antibiotic therapy in exacerbations of chronic obstructive pulmonary disease, *Ann Intern Med* 106(2):196-204, 1987.

Anthonisen NR, Wright EC: Response to inhaled bronchodilators in COPD, *Chest* 91(5 suppl):36s-39s, 1987.

Armitage JM, Williams SJ: Inhaler technique in the elderly, *Age & Aging* 17(4):275-278, 1988.

Bâ M, Spier S, Lapierre G, Lamarre A: Wet nebulizer versus spacer and metered-dose inhaler via tidal breathing, *J Asthma* 26(6):355-358, 1989.

Benton G, Thomas RC, Nickerson BG, et al: Experience with a metered-dose inhaler with a spacer in the pediatric emergency department, *Am J Dis Child* 143(6):678-681, 1989.

Berry RB, Shinto RA, Wong FH, et al: Nebulizer versus spacer for bronchodilator delivery in patients hospitalized for acute exacerbations of COPD, *Chest* 96(6):1241-1246, 1989.

Brim S: Aerosol therapy: a nurse's guide, *Home Healthc Nurse* 6(6):37-41, 1989.

Brim S: A quick guide for home use of inhalant medications, *Pediatr Nurs* 15(1):87-88, 94, 1989.

Brown DH, Kasuya A, Leikin JB: Endotracheal drug administration in the critical care setting, *J Emerg Med* 5(5):407-414, 1987.

Burton GC, Hodgkin JE: *Respiratory care: a guide to clinical practice*, ed 2, Philadelphia, 1984, JB Lippincott.

Chapman KR, Wanner A: Controversies in pulmonary medicine: patients with COPD should be started initially on anticholinergic bronchodilators, *Am Rev Respir Dis* 138(4):1074-1075, 1988.

Chervinsky P: Concomitant bronchodilator therapy and ipratropium bromide: a clinical review, *Am J Med* 81(suppl 5A):67-73, 1986.

Coady TJ, Stewart CJ, Davies HJ: Synchronization of bronchodilator release, *Practitioner* 217(1298):273-275, 1976.

Crompton G: Problems patients have using pressurized aerosol inhalers, *Euro J of Respir Dis* suppl 119:101-104, 1982.

Crompton GK: The adult patient's difficulties with inhalers, *Lung* (168 suppl):658-662, 1990.

DeBlaquiere P, Christensen DB, Carter WB, Martin TR: Use and abuse of metered-dose inhalers by patients with chronic lung disease: a controlled, randomized trial of two instruction methods, *Am Rev Respir Dis* 140(4):910-916, 1989.

Dipalma JR: Beta$_2$ agonists for acute asthma, *Am Fam Physician* 31(5):184-187, 1985.

Dolovich M, Ruffin RE, Roberts R, Newhouse MT: Optimal delivery of aerosols from metered-dose inhalers, *Chest* 80(suppl 6):911-915, 1981.

Emerman CL, Devlin C, Connors AF: Risk of toxicity in patients with elevated theophylline levels, *Ann Emerg Med* 19(6):643-648, 1990.

Epstein SW, Parsons JE, Corey PN, et al: A comparison of three means of pressurized aerosol inhaler use, *Am Rev Respir Dis* 128(2):253-255, 1983.

Foster WM, Bergofsky EH: Airway mucous membrane: effects of beta-adrenergic and anticholinergic stimulation, *Am J Med* 81(suppl 5A):28-35, 1986.

Foxworth JW, Reisz GR, Knudson SM, et al: Theophylline and diaphragmatic contractility: investigation of a dose-response relationship, *Am Rev Respir Dis* 138(6):1532-1534, 1988.

Fuller HD, Dolovitch MB, Posmituck G, et al: Pressurized aerosol versus jet aerosol delivery to mechanically ventilated patients: comparison of dose to the lungs, *Am Rev Respir Dis* 141(2):440-4, 1990.

Gold WM: Cholinergic pharmacology in asthma. In Austen KF, Lichtenstein LM, eds: *Asthma*, New York, 1973, Academic Press.

Greenbaum R: Down the tube, *Anaesthesia* 42(9):927-928, 1987.

Grieco MH, Larsen K, Petraco AJ: In vivo comparison of triamcinolone and beclomethasone inhalation delivery systems, *Ann Allergy* 45(4):231-234, 1980.

Gross NJ: The use of anticholinergic agents in the treatment of airways disease, *Clin Chest Med* 9(4):591-598, 1988.

Gross NJ: Anticholinergic agents in COPD, *Chest* 91(suppl 5):52s-57s, 1987.

Hahn K: Slow teaching the COPD patient, *Nursing 87* 17(4):34-42, 1987.

Horsley MG, Bailie GR: Risk factors for inadequate use of pressurized aerosol inhalers, *J Clin Pharm Ther* 13(2):139-143, 1988.

Huchon G: Aerosol deposition in the alveolar space, *Lung* 168(suppl):672-676, 1990.

Jenne JW: Theophylline as a bronchodilator in COPD and its combination with inhaled beta-adrenergic drugs, *Chest* 92(suppl 1):7s-14s, 1987.

Jones MD, Yeager H: Inhaler and spacer use in obstructive airway diseases, *Am Fam Physician* 42(4):1007-1013, 1990.

Kelling JS, Strohl KP, Smith RL, Altose M: Physician knowledge in the use of canister nebulizers, *Chest* 83(4):612-614, 1983.

Kirilloff LH, Tibbals SC: Drugs for asthma: a complete guide, Am J Nurs 83(1):55-61, 1983.

Konig P: Spacer devices used with metered-dose inhalers: breakthrough or gimmick? *Chest* 88(2):276, 1988.

Larsson S, Svedmyr N: Bronchodilating effect and side effects of beta 2-adrenoceptor stimulants by different modes of administration (tablets, metered aerosol, and combination thereof), a study with salbutamol in asthmatics, *Am Rev Respir Dis* 116(5):861-869, 1977.

Lazarus SC: Rational therapy of acute asthma, *Ann Allergy* 63(6 part 2):585-590, 1989.

Lee H, Evans HE: Aerosol inhalation teaching device, *J Pediatr* 110(2):249-252, 1987.

Leech JA, Gervais A, Ruben FL: Efficacy of pneumococcal vaccine in severe chronic obstructive pulmonary disease, *Can Med Assoc J* 136(4):361-365, 1987.

Mahler DA: The role of theophylline in the treatment of dyspnea in COPD, *Chest* 92(suppl 1):2s-6s, 1987.

Mallol J, Barrueto L, Girardi G, Toro O: Bronchodilator effects of fenoterol and ipratropium bromide in infants with acute wheezing: use of MDI with a spacer device, *Pediatr Pulmonol* 3(5):352-356, 1987.

Matthay RA: Favorable cardiovascular effects of theophylline in COPD, *Chest* 92(suppl 1):22s-26s, 1987.

McFadden ER: Clinical use of beta adrenergic agonists, *J Allergy Clin Immunol* 76(2 pt 2):352-356, 1985.

Middleton E: A rational approach to asthma therapy, *Postgrad Med* 67(3):107-116, 1980.

Morgan EJ, Petty TL: Summary of the National Mucolytic Study, *Chest* 97(suppl 2):24s-27s, 1990.

Netter F: *The CIBA collection of medical illustrations*, vol 7, *Respiratory system*, New York, 1979, CIBA Pharmaceutical Co.

Newhouse M, Dolovich M: Aerosol therapy: nebulizer versus metered-dose inhaler, *Chest* 91(6):799-800, 1987.

Newman SP, Clark AR, Talaee N, Clarke SW: Pressurized aerosol deposition in the human lung with and without an "open" spacer device, *Thorax* 44(9):706-710, 1989.

Newman SP, Clark SW: The proper use of metered-dose inhalers, *Chest* 86(3):343-344, 1984.

Noseda A, Yernault JC: Sympathomimetics in acute severe asthma: inhaled or parenteral, nebulizer or spacer? *Eur Respir J* 2(4):377-382, 1989.

O'Callaghan C, Milner AD, Swarbrick A: Spacer device with face mask attachment for giving bronchodilators to infants with asthma, *BMJ* 298(6667):160-161, 1989.

Pauwels R: The effects of theophylline on airway inflammation, *Chest* 92(suppl 1):32s-37s, 1987.

Petty TL: Drug strategies for airflow obstruction, *Am J Nurs* 87(2):180-184, 1987.

Petty TL: Future trends in the management of asthma and chronic obstructive pulmonary disease, *Am J Med* 79(6A):38-42, 1985.

Physicians' Desk Reference, 1990 edition, Oradell, NJ, Medical Economics.

Salzman GA, Pyszczynski DR: Oropharyngeal candidiasis in patients treated with beclomethasone dipropionate delivered by metered-dose inhaler alone and with Aerochamber, *J Allergy Clin Immunol* 81(2):424-428, 1988.

Seifert CF, Hamilton SF: Incorrect instructions for use of metered-dose inhalers, *Am J Hosp Pharm* 45(1):75-76, 1988.

Sennhauser FH, Sly PD: Pressure flow characteristics of the valve in spacer devices, *Arch Dis Child* 64(9):1305-1307, 1989.

Shim C, Williams MH: The adequacy of inhalation of aerosol from canister nebulizers, *Am J Med* 69(6):891-894, 1980.

Stoller JK: Systemic corticosteroids in stable chronic obstructive pulmonary disease: do they work? *Chest* 91(2):155-156, 1987.

Storms WW, Bodman SF, Nathan RA, et al: Use of ipratropium bromide in asthma: results of a multi-clinic study, *Am J Med* 81(suppl 5A):61-66, 1986.

Summer W, Elston R, Tharpe L, et al: Aerosol bronchodilator delivery methods: relative impact on pulmonary function and cost of respiratory care, *Arch Intern Med* 149(3):618-623, 1989.

Tal A, Paul M, Weitzman S: Proper use of metered-dose inhalers: the role of the primary care physician, *Isr J Med Sci* 23(3):168-170, 1987.

Teo J, Kwang LW, Yip WC: An inexpensive spacer for use with metered-dose bronchodilators in young asthmatic children, *Pediatr Pulmonol* 5(4):244-246, 1988.

Wade JF: Comprehensive respiratory care: physiology and technique, ed 3, St Louis, 1982, Mosby–Year Book.

Wanner A, Sackner MA: *Pulmonary diseases: mechanisms of altered structure and function,* Boston, 1983, Little, Brown.

Wiest PM, Flanigan T, Salata RA, et al: Serious infectious complications of corticosteroid therapy for COPD, *Chest* 95(6):1180-1184, 1989.

Ziment I: Pharmacologic therapy of obstructive airway disease, *Clin Chest Med* 11(3):461-486, 1990.

Ziment I, Niewoehner DE: Controversies in pulmonary medicine: aminophylline should be administered for all exacerbations of COPD, *Am Rev Respir Dis* 138(4):1070, 1988.

Home Care of Patients with Respiratory Dysfunction

Unit 5 focuses on what happens when the patient with a respiratory disorder is sent home. The discussion encompasses home oxygen therapy (Chapter 17), home mechanical ventilation (Chapter 18), and pulmonary rehabilitation (Chapter 19). Patients with pulmonary dysfunction frequently still need the benefits of hospital technology at home, such as supplemental oxygen or a mechanical ventilator; this causes anxiety for the patient and his family and disrupts the pattern of home life. It is important for the nurse to understand the patient's needs; she also must know about the equipment required and must be able to teach the patient and family members how to use it. In some instances the nurse may need to choose a supplier for oxygen and equipment for the mechanical ventilator; guidelines for performing this task are presented. Patients with obstructive and restrictive lung diseases frequently need pulmonary rehabilitation upon discharge. Many of the concepts of pulmonary rehabilitation, especially energy conservation techniques, are applicable to all patients with pulmonary dysfunction. Pulmonary rehabilitation may be a formal procedure, as in a hospital-based program, or an informal one, as in home education and exercise. Because reimbursement is low and ultimately the patient must become independent in a home exercise program, the nurse often teaches concepts of pulmonary rehabilitation. A teaching plan and patient education guides are included in Chapter 19.

C·H·A·P·T·E·R *17*

Home Oxygen Therapy

Oxygen therapy has been used in hospitals for over a century, but long-term oxygen therapy in the home has been available only for about 20 or 30 years. Research has demonstrated the benefit of administering oxygen in the home for chronic hypoxemia. (The systemic effects of chronic hypoxemia are shown in the box on p. 387.) Both morbidity and mortality are decreased when appropriate patients have oxygen therapy at home. Using oxygen at home used to be cumbersome, hazardous, and difficult. However, many improvements have been made in home oxygen delivery over the past few years. This chapter reviews the indications for home oxygen therapy, as well as patient assessment, and discusses the types of oxygen delivery devices available in the home. Because home oxygen therapy is one of the most expensive medications prescribed, costs and reimbursement issues are also discussed. Finally, this chapter reviews how to choose an appropriate oxygen vendor.

INDICATIONS FOR HOME OXYGEN THERAPY

A classic study in home oxygen therapy was the NOTT (nocturnal oxygen therapy trial), funded by the National Institutes of Health (NIH). The study was a multi center trial involving patients with severe chronic obstructive pulmonary disease (COPD). All patients had an FEV_1 (forced expiratory volume in 1 second) below 600 ml and a resting arterial oxygen tension (Pao_2) below 55 mmHg (or 60 mm Hg with evidence of tissue hypoxia, including polycythemia, cor pulmonale, or electrocardiographical evidence of right ventricular hypertrophy). The 203 patients were randomly assigned to either 12-hour nocturnal oxygen therapy or 24-hour continuous oxygen therapy. The patients were followed for 2 years. Results indicated that the nocturnal group averaged about 12 hours of oxygen daily, whereas the continuous group used oxygen about 17 to 18 hours daily. The group with continuous oxygen therapy showed an improved survival rate and fewer complications, including hospitalizations. A similar British study confirmed these findings.

In the hospital oxygen is freely administered to patients with either hypoxemia or the potential for hypoxemia. Home oxygen therapy is initiated with several goals in view: to relieve hypoxemia; to reverse the signs, symptoms, and physiological abnormalities resulting from tissue hypoxia; and to improve the patient's general physical condition, including activity and exercise tolerance and cognitive functioning. An additional goal is to improve survival; in other words, to decrease mortality from chronic hypoxemia.

The need for home oxygen therapy was recognized in the late 1960s, when improved physical functioning was identified in patients who received home

386

Effects of Hypoxemia

Pulmonary system	Cardiac system	Neurological system	Renal system
Constricts pulmonary blood vessels	Causes right ventricular hypertrophy	Decreases mentation	Decreases blood flow in severe hypoxemia
Elevates mean pulmonary artery pressure	Increases heart rate	Decreases coordination and reaction time	Stimulates erythropoietin to increase red blood cell production and causes polycythemia
Causes cor pulmonale	Increases initially, but ultimately decreases cardiac output	Decreases visual acuity	
		Dilates cerebral vessels and causes transient ischemic attacks	
		Causes sleeplessness and restlessness	

---

oxygen therapy. Over the next 10 to 15 years, researchers found that patients treated with oxygen at home were hospitalized less often. They also noted that patients lived longer with long-term oxygen administration in the home. As study of patients receiving home oxygen continued, it was noted that the patient's cognitive and mental functioning improved significantly. Patients demonstrated improved intelligence, motor coordination, memory, and visual coordination. They also became more independent. Polycythemia and pulmonary hypertension, side effects of chronic hypoxemia, are reversible with administration of oxygen for at least 15 hours daily.

Assessment

Oxygen use in the home is not limited to patients with pulmonary disease; some patients with primary cardiac disease are also candidates. Home oxygen is used in any patient who has a PaO_2 of 55 mm Hg or less or an arterial oxygen saturation (SaO_2) of 88% or less on room air at rest, during sleep, or with exertion. Oxygen is prescribed when other methods of improving gas exchange are inadequate, such as optimal treatment of bronchospasm, pneumonia, and heart failure, as well as cessation of smoking. In patients with marginal gas exchange (PaO_2, 56 to 59 mm Hg or SaO_2, 89%), oxygen is prescribed with evidence of tissue hypoxia, such as cor pulmonale, pulmonary hypertension, erythrocytosis, increasing exertion-induced hypoxemia, impaired mentation, or central nervous system dysfunction. These guidelines are based on criteria used in the home oxygen research trials. They are also the guidelines used for reimbursement of home oxygen therapy by third-party payers.

Assessment of the need for home oxygen therapy is not based on a single measurement of oxygen (PaO_2 or SaO_2). Several measurements taken days or weeks apart, when the patient is not acutely ill, determine need. The primary method to determine the need for home oxygen is an arterial blood gas (ABG) analysis. The specimen is drawn *at rest* after the patient has been breathing room air (21%) oxygen for at least 20 to 30 minutes. If the patient's condition deteriorates before this interval elapses, an ABG specimen is drawn and oxygen is administered. The patient's oxygen level is reassessed after the oxygen has been administered to determine the adequacy of the treatment. The goal of oxygen therapy depends on the physician, although most physicians aim for a PaO_2 of approximately 70 mm Hg or an SaO_2 of about 90% to 92%.

Even when the patient's oxygenation is adequate with room air at rest, it may still be abnormal during sleep or exertion. One of two methods is used to determine *sleep-induced* oxygen desaturation. The patient may undergo complete polysomnography (a sleep study), or he may just sleep with a pulse oximeter secured in place. (A paper recorder or the ability to transfer information from the oximeter into a computer base is essential.) The polysomnograph or oximeter records changes in oxygen saturation and pulse as the patient sleeps. If the Sao_2 decreases during sleep, oxygen supplementation during sleep is necessary.

Some patients may have adequate oxygenation at rest and during sleep but desaturate with exertion. To assess *exertion-induced* oxygen desaturation, an exercise evaluation is performed. (Recall that the normal response to exercise is an increase in oxygenation.) The best assessment of exertion-induced desaturation occurs in a formal exercise laboratory. A physician assesses cardiac function (and may also collect exhaled gases) as the patient walks on a treadmill or rides a bicycle. The patient's blood pressure, heart rate, and often pulse oximetry or serial ABG are monitored at various speeds and inclines (tensions) of walking (or biking). The physician adjusts the amount of oxygen to the amount of exercise that the patient can perform. Low levels of exertion may require slightly less oxygen than regular exercise. The alternative to this is ambulating the patient in the hall with a portable pulse oximeter in place. An ABG specimen may be drawn to assess acid-base status at the end of the walk.

A typical oxygen prescription includes a liter flow for rest, exercise, and sleep. In some patients these are the same. In many patients, the liter flow varies. In addition, the means of delivering the oxygen may include an oxygen-conserving device for patients with high requirements. Continuous use, if indicated, is noted on the prescription, which also states the number of hours for daily use when less than 24 hours. Many years ago the designation *prn* (meaning "as needed") was used in prescribing oxygen; this is no longer acceptable. A prn interval is not considered reimbursable by third-party payers. (It makes sense if one considers that a physician would not order amiodarone or theophylline prn, so why oxygen?)

TYPES OF HOME OXYGEN

Three types of oxygen systems are available for home use: compressed oxygen cylinders, liquid oxygen, and oxygen concentrators. Detailed information about each system is available from oxygen suppliers or manufacturers. Table 17-1 differentiates liquid, compressed gas, and concentrator oxygen.

Compressed gas cylinders

Compressed oxygen gas cylinders have been available for over a century, since 1888. They are very safe when used properly. Before pressurized cabins were developed, pilots used compressed oxygen to fly safely at higher altitudes. Compressed gas cylinders are also used by firefighters entering burning buildings. (Recall that oxygen is *combustible,* meaning that it will support a fire; it is not *flammable,* meaning that it does not ignite.)

Compressed gas cylinders store gaseous oxygen under high pressure (about 2200 psi). Oxygen is delivered through a regulator/flowmeter that accurately gauges the oxygen liter flow. (Patients usually buy a regulator/flowmeter for

Table 17-1. Home oxygen systems

	Compressed gas cylinders	Liquid oxygen systems	Concentrator
Primary use	Intermittent therapy, such as for exercise or sleep only	High liter flows and active patients	Moderate liter flows and patients with limited mobility inside or outside the home
Advantages	100% oxygen; relatively inexpensive; no loss of gas during storage; relatively portable; delivers up to 15 LPM	100% oxygen; conveniently portable; portable units can be refilled at home; delivers up to 6 LPM	Fixed monthly cost; minimal interruption of household by supplier; no refills of "main tank"; most units deliver up to 4 or 5 LPM
Disadvantages	Bulky; possibly unsightly; needs frequent refilling with continuous use	Usually weekly delivery required for refill; evaporates if not used; potential for frostbite at connections and if spilled	Oxygen concentration decreases as liter flow increases (usually 85% to 90%); requires power supply; increases electric bill $15 to $20 a month; requires second system for portability (usually gas cylinders)

less than $200 rather than renting one indefinitely; the purchase pays for itself within a year.) Compressed oxygen usually is stored in green steel or aluminum cylinders, whereas air is stored in yellow tanks and carbon dioxide in grey ones.

The cylinders are available in various sizes and volumes. Those most often used in the home are C (240 L), D (360 L), E (625 L), M (3030 L), G (5300 L), and H (6000 L). C and D cylinders are portable units; G and H cylinders are stationary units. At 2 LPM a D cylinder lasts about 3 hours. Other tanks and their approximate hours are: C cylinder (2 hours), E cylinder (5 hours), M cylinder (25 hours), G cylinder (44 hours), and H cylinder (50 hours). Obviously, compressed gas cylinders do not hold very much oxygen. If a patient requires continuous oxygen at 2 LPM, either several tanks are needed in the home or the supplier must make daily visits. Two or more large tanks usually are connected or banked together in the home. Because of transportation costs for the supplier, a patient uses compressed gas cylinders for outside activities and a concentrator for stationary home needs.

The advantage of compressed gas cylinders is that the gas may be stored when not in use without loss of oxygen. The tanks are relatively portable and can be carried over the shoulder in a backpack-type device (D cylinder weighs about 10 to 13 pounds) or pushed in a cart (E cylinder weighs about 17 to 19 pounds). Some patients have difficulty lifting the E cylinder up curbs or steps and into cars or buses. Much smaller, lighter tanks (for example, C cylinder [7 pounds] and Mada [5 to 7 pounds]) are sometimes used and filled from the large stationary tanks (Fig. 17-1). Few patients

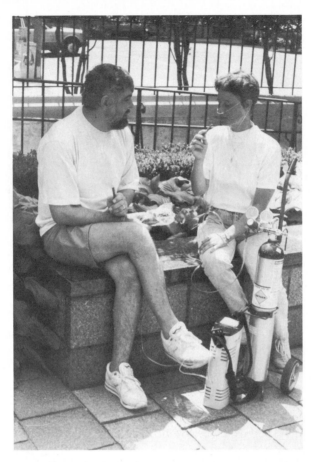

Fig. 17-1. Size and appearance comparison of portable oxygen systems. Left: Portable liquid oxygen system. Right: "E" tank.

transfill compressed gas oxygen tanks. Most patients learn to change the regulator/flowmeter between portable C, D, or E tanks. Aluminum cylinders weigh less than steel ones.

All compressed gas cylinders are bulky and somewhat ugly. There is no hiding that the patient is using oxygen. Many patients complain of having the green tanks in their home. A threat from having compressed gas cylinders in the home is the potential for the regulator/flowmeter to become dislodged from the cylinder, usually from the cylinder falling. If this happens, the cylinder shoots around the room like a torpedo, destroying property and possibly injuring someone. The chances of this happening are very slim if the tanks are properly stored or secured. Larger tanks are secured in large floor rings to prevent tipping. Smaller units are secured in upright position in metal cages. The portable unit is secured in a wheeled device. The regulator/flowmeter assembly can be protected with a wire cage.

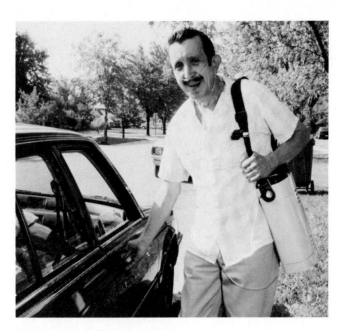

Fig. 17-2. Portable liquid oxygen contains more oxygen in the same space compared with compressed gas oxygen. Patients can be away from the main oxygen system for up to 8 hours at 2 LPM. (From Beare P, Myers J: *Principles and practice of adult health nursing,* St Louis, 1990, Mosby–Year Book.)

Liquid oxygen

Oxygen liquefies when cooled to about −183° F and occupies 1/860 the space of the gas. Liquid oxygen is stored in a Thermos–type container at about −300° F under low pressure (that is, about 22 psi). As the air exits the tank, it warms and vaporizes. Liquid oxygen is supplied in most hospitals and institutions. Home systems, of which there are about six manufacturers, are available for use in many areas. In some cases the availability of a liquid system is limited by the supplier or the patient's location.

The main advantage of liquid oxygen is increased portability in a lightweight tank. There are roughly two sizes of the stationary tanks (20 and 30 liquid liters or 17,200 and 25,800 gaseous liters, respectively) and two sizes of the portable tanks (about 0.5 and 1 liter). The large stationary unit is used as the primary oxygen source and for refilling the portable unit. The large unit lasts about 5 to 8 days at 2 LPM, depending on the size of the large reservoir and how many times the small portable unit is used. At 2 LPM, the small portable tanks last about 4 to 8 hours, depending on size (Fig. 17-2). They weigh about 7.5 to 10 pounds and are either carried over the shoulder or back, in the hand, or wheeled in a cart. To efficiently use oxygen, once the portable unit is filled, it is used until empty because the large reservoir is more efficient at cooling than the portable. Care is taken to prevent the portable liquid oxygen tank from tipping, since this creates increased pressure inside the tank and venting of oxygen to the atmosphere.

One disadvantage is that liquid oxygen evaporates at a very slow rate, making it impractical for intermittent users. A large home liquid oxygen tank will evaporate in about 1 month if not used at all. A second disadvantage is that the supplier must refill the tank about weekly or biweekly. High-flow oxygen users (3 LPM and above) may need two large tanks to make once-weekly filling possible. Most oxygen suppliers place the liquid oxygen patient on a route with a standard filling day every week. This may be inconvenient, since the patient must remain home to await filling.

A potential problem with liquid oxygen is frostbite burns from spilling. Frost forms on the connection between the large reservoir and the portable tank. Patients must use care when filling and removing the portable tank to prevent frostbite. In addition, if the humidity is high, the portable and large reservoir may be temporarily frozen together. The portable unit usually is filled about 30 minutes before its intended use in case this happens. The connection thaws fairly rapidly at room temperature.

Oxygen concentrator

The oxygen concentrator is an electrically powered device that filters oxygen from room air for immediate use by passing room air through molecular sieves to remove carbon dioxide, nitrogen, and water. Several manufacturers make concentrators; one manufacturer makes a suitcase—type model, although most concentrators are the size of a nightstand.

The main advantage of an oxygen concentrator is that the cost of the oxygen is stable. The supplier usually checks the equipment monthly to clean filters and assess oxygen percentage, although some patients clean both internal and external filters themselves. The concentrator provides a limitless supply of oxygen as long as power is supplied to the unit. In areas with frequent power outages or in rural areas, a generator often is needed to supply the power. (An alarm sounds when power is interrupted.) All homes with a concentrator have at least one E size compressed gas cylinder or larger in reserve for use during a power failure. In the winter, the extra heat generated by the concentrator often is a blessing; however, in the summer it becomes a disadvantage.

The main disadvantage of the concentrator is that it does not provide 100% oxygen. As the liter flow increases, the Fio_2 decreases. When the patient is prescribed 3 to 4 LPM of oxygen, the patient's oxygen level must be rechecked on the concentrator to assure adequate oxygenation. Other disadvantages include the need for a second system that is portable. Although the concentrator, which weighs 25 to 50 pounds, is portable (it can be moved from room to room or carried outside the home), it must have a power source. A compressed gas system usually is used for portability. The noisy hum from older concentrators is both annoying and comforting. Some patients complain about the increase in the electrical bill, an expense not covered by insurance. The increase usually is about $15 to $20, depending on the geographical location.

Regardless of which system is used, the main tank is kept in a centrally located position. In most cases the living room or the bedroom is chosen. The patient is given a 50-foot length of oxygen supply tubing attached to an oxygen cannula. Connections are avoided whenever possible because of the potential for leaks. Care is taken to avoid tripping on the oxygen supply tubing throughout the day and night. If the patient must be up in the dark, night lights are necessary to see and avoid the tubing. When pets are in the home, additional care is needed to prevent them from chewing on the tubing.

Compliance can be a problem with patients who need oxygen. The patient feels dependent on a machine that has a short leash, 6 to 50 feet. Some patients fear that they will become addicted to the oxygen. It helps to remind the patient that everyone is addicted to oxygen and no one can live without it. Some people just need a little more, just as some people need additional medications to make the heart beat regular. Reminding the patient that oxygen is a medication is also helpful. It is important to suggest that oxygen is like any other tool, such as glasses or a hearing aid. It takes time to become accustomed to using such aids, but after a while a person can't do without them. Oxygen is meant to improve the quality of life, not impair it. The nurse also reviews the systemic hazards of low oxygen (see Table 17-1) and the benefits of adequate oxygen. The nurse also may recommend use of a different nasal cannula (for example, clear versus green tubing or smaller prongs) or an oxygen-conserving system. Oxygen can be administered through a cannula mounted on special eyeglasses (Oxyframes, Oxyspecs). The choice of frames is limited but may meet a patient's emotional needs.

When oxygen is first prescribed, many patients feel uncomfortable using it outside the home. They worry that people will avoid them, and have a fear of combustion. Then there is the myth that oxygen will explode; it will not explode, but it will support fire. Some people who use oxygen mistakenly believe that they cannot live in the same home as a person who smokes. In fact this is desirable, but for a different reason; it is unhealthy to live with a smoker. Second-hand smoke is very dangerous. A patient using oxygen can be in the same room with a smoker as long as the smoker is about 5 to 10 feet away from the oxygen source. A patient who uses oxygen cannot smoke with the oxygen on; severe facial and airway burns can result. Remember that oxygen supports a fire; it will make a fire, including a cigarette, burn hotter and faster.

With regard to traveling outside the home, the oxygen user is concerned about how he looks. Some nasal cannula are very noticeable. The color green stands out on all skin colors, whereas a clear nasal cannula is not as noticeable. Similarly, green tanks are obvious, and brown plastic cases are less so.

People often are rude. They stare, and parents hush small children who inquire about the "funny thing on his face" or the "green tank in a cart." The patient is taught to respond to inquiring looks with answers such as, "Yes, this is oxygen." When appropriate, it may help to say that smoking caused the problem. Perhaps the patient can provide impetus for the questioner to avoid or quit smoking.

OXYGEN-CONSERVING DEVICES

Some patients receive inadequate oxygenation with a standard nasal cannula or require a device to enhance oxygen time on a portable unit. Others wish to decrease the cost of oxygen. The apparatuses for accomplishing these ends are called oxygen-conserving devices, and there are several kinds.

One of the simplest models is the oxygen reservoir cannula. Oxymizer and Oxymizer pendant (Chad Therapeutics) are two types of oxygen reservoir cannulas that use a membrane to deliver or reserve oxygen flow (Fig. 17-3). The Oxymizer contains a moustache-like reservoir just under the nose; its counterpart, the Oxymizer pendant, contains a disc-shaped pendant on the chest. The Oxymizer stores oxygen in the reservoir during exhalation and delivers it during inhalation. Most oxygen cannulas vent the oxygen to the at-

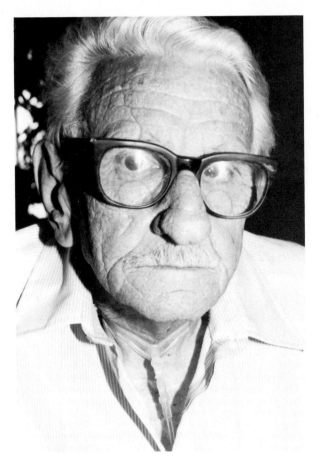

Fig. 17-3. Transtracheal oxygen delivers oxygen directly into the trachea and often allows the patient to use lower liter flows. The external catheter can be hidden under clothing.

mosphere during exhalation. Using the reservoir cannula increases the size of the anatomical reservoir to deliver more oxygen. In patients who receive relatively low flows of oxygen, less oxygen is needed. Patients who are inadequately oxygenated on high flows of oxygen may be better oxygenated. The Oxymizer has a respiratory rate limitation of about 30 per minute.

When the Oxymizer cannula is insufficient to improve oxygenation, the physician and patient may jointly choose insertion of a transtracheal catheter. Oxygenation is enhanced, as is aesthetic value, since there is no visible oxygen cannula. The catheter exits from under the shirt at the waistline and is attached with a small alligator-type clip to prevent accidental removal. Some patients are more compliant with this device. There is also less nasal or upper lip irritation.

There are at least three types of transtracheal catheters currently marketed. They have undergone many changes in the past 5 to 10 years to produce a reliable product. (*Note:* The first transtracheal catheter was an intravenous intracath inserted backwards into a pediatric tracheostomy tube. The tubing cracked, and there were problems with fluid and secretion buildup on the inside of the tracheostomy tube.) Two similar current models are the Micro-trach (Ballard Medical Products) and Scoop (Transtracheal Associates) They are one-piece polyethylene catheters.

There are two types of Scoop catheters. One contains a hole just at the end of the catheter, similar to the Microtrach, and the other contains several small holes (much like a nasogastric tube) in addition to the end hole. The catheter is inserted under local anesthesia much as with the Seldinger technique for a central venous catheter, only the goal is insertion into the trachea instead of into a blood vessel.

The third type of transtracheal catheter, the ITOC (Cook), is similar to a Hickman catheter for chronic intravenous access. The ITOC is placed under local or general anesthesia. The catheter is tunneled under the skin from the lower edge of the ribs up to the trachea. The trachea is surgically visualized, and the catheter is inserted. Two fiber cuffs help hold the surgically sutured catheter in place. The tracheotomy site is sutured closed.

The care of the three transtracheal catheters differs somewhat. All of them are flushed one or more times daily with a 5- to 10-ml bolus of normal saline. The site is cleaned with soap and water. With the ITOC, care is similar to that for a Hickman catheter. A transparent dressing is needed at the site. In some instances the Scoop catheter is removed, cleaned, and reinserted by the patient. The technique usually is performed without a wire guide, although a wire guide may be used in some cases. There is always the possibility that the patient may be unable to recannulate the tracheostomy hole, necessitating a visit to the emergency room or physician. The patient receives a new Micro-trach or Scoop catheter every 1 or 3 months, respectively, as directed by the manufacturer and the physician.

When a patient first receives a transtracheal catheter, he may notice more coughing. The cough occurs because of tracheal irritation from the new catheter and subsides in a few days. A cough medication frequently is used for the first week to prevent dislodgement of the catheter. Later, the cough sometimes produces a brown mucus ball that forms on the end of the catheter. The ball usually appears just after the catheter has been cleaned. The patient should notify the physician if the site appears abnormal (reddened or swollen) or has a purulent discharge. Antibiotics are needed to treat the infection. In the case of the ITOC, if infection is observed, the catheter may need to be removed to prevent septicemia.

Other types of oxygen-conserving devices are available that are noninvasive and worn externally. The most common device is a pulse-dose demand oxygen device. The two main pulse-dose demand oxygen devices are the Oxymatic (Chad Therapeutics) and the Pulsair oxygen system ($Cryo_2$ systems). A sensor detects inspiration and delivers oxygen to the patient. With exhalation, oxygen flow ceases. An audible click is heard in some models. In most models air can be heard (a whoosh sound) during inhalation. These devices have a rate limitation of about 30 to 35 breaths per minute and require nasal inspiration. The devices generally do not work well in mouth breathers. The Oxymatic can be used on either a liquid oxygen tank or a compressed gas cylinder, whereas the Pulsair is an entire liquid oxygen system.

REIMBURSEMENT CRITERIA

"How much will it cost?" is a common question from patients who are just starting treatment with oxygen. The answer depends on the type of health

Table 17-2. Approximate cost of oxygen

	1 LPM	2 LPM	3 LPM
Commercial			
Liquid oxygen*	System rental up to $200 monthly, plus up to additional $300 in oxygen	System rental same, plus up to additional $600 in oxygen	System rental same, plus up to additional $800 in oxygen
Oxygen concentrator	Up to $500	Up to $500	Up to $500
Compressed gas tanks $21 per D/E tank	10 hr/tank	5 hr/tank	3 hr/tank
Patient cost at 20% (4%)	Up to $100 ($20) monthly	Up to $160 ($32) monthly	Up to $200 ($40) monthly
Medicare†			
Medicare allowable	Pays 50% of allowable for flows under 1 LPM; 100% of allowable for flows between 1 and 4 LPM; and 150% of allowable for flows over 4 LPM in approved patients		
Midwest area	About $250, plus $70 for portable model and $40-$50 for rental of cylinder regulator	About $250, plus $70 for portable model and $40-$50 for rental of cylinder regulator	About $250, plus $70 for portable model and $40-$50 for rental of cylinder regulator
Patient cost without/ with secondary coverage	About $56/$12 monthly	About $56/$12 monthly	About $56/$12 monthly

*Based on oxygen fill per week (35 pounds at 1 LPM, 65 pounds at 2 LPM, and 90 pounds at 3 LPM) at an oxygen cost of $1 to $2.25 per pound.
†Subject to change.

care coverage the patient has. Most commercial third-party payers and state medical aid programs pay 80% of the cost. A few plans have 100% coverage, but these are rare. Some HMOs do not cover oxygen or any other durable medical equipment such as wheelchairs or hospital beds. Medicare pays at a special rate, called Medicare allowable, determined by the government (Health Care Finance Association).

The Medicare allowable varies by geographical region, and it changes as dictated by the government. Medicare pays 80% of the Medicare allowable; the patient or secondary insurance pays the remaining 20%. A secondary insurance to commercial insurance or Medicare usually pays 80% of the remaining 20%. This leaves the patient with about 20% of the original 20% of the total cost of oxygen, or 4%, as a monthly bill. Even 4% of the cost of oxygen is too much for some patients.

Many reputable oxygen suppliers accept the insurer's payment as full payment if the patient shows financial need. Payment plans for the remaining 4% are negotiable. Rather than forgo the oxygen, patients are encouraged to discuss financial problems and options with the supplier. Table 17-2 lists the approximate cost of oxygen in the Midwest in late 1990.

CHOOSING A VENDOR

Choosing which oxygen supplier the patient will use is not the purview of the nurse in many institutions. A social worker, respiratory therapist, or home health care agency makes the choice. In some instances the institution is its own home equipment supplier. It is essential to develop a good relationship with one or more suppliers. Patient care is enhanced by effective two-way communication. If the patient's needs change, either notifies the other. For instance, on a routine visit to the home, the home oxygen supplier may note that the patient is more dyspneic or cyanotic; he notifies the referral source, nurse, or physician for potential change in the oxygen prescription. Or, after a visit to the physician's office, the patient's oxygen prescription may change, necessitating a call to the oxygen supplier.

When the nurse is in charge of choosing the supplier, several factors must be considered, including the supplier's location, the education and training of its staff, the equipment and service available, and the cost. The supplier should be located within 100 miles of the patient's home. A location farther away than this compromises care if the equipment should malfunction. Although interruption of oxygen may not be as important as with a ventilator, the patient needs service within a reasonable period. Travel time in good weather should not exceed about 1½ to 2 hours. Remember that travel time is increased in rainy or icy weather. The patient must have sufficient backup supplies to last until service personnel arrive.

Many durable medical equipment suppliers employ respiratory therapists or nurses to educate patients about the equipment and to provide follow-up assessments. Each patient receiving oxygen is commonly seen at 1 to 3 month intervals to assess the adequacy of therapy. A brief report indicates the patient's status and compliance with therapy. The personnel who deliver and refill oxygen equipment usually are not medically trained. They frequently are good-natured truck drivers who interact well with patients and have a working understanding of the equipment. These delivery personnel often clue the respiratory therapist or nurse about potential problems, such as if the patient is using less or more oxygen.

The equipment provided by the oxygen supplier varies. Some companies are full-service suppliers, offering compressed gas cylinders, liquid oxygen systems, and oxygen concentrators. Other suppliers, such as the corner drugstore, do not carry liquid oxygen because of the expense and maintenance. Similarly, some do not carry mechanical ventilators, apnea monitors, or other very specialized equipment. It is important that the patient receive all equipment from one supplier; then there is just one person to call in case of problems and one bill. Also, there is less interruption of the patient's home life by suppliers.

The cost of equipment varies by geographical region, and the patient can do nothing about this cost. However, cost also varies by supplier within a region. It is important to compare cost and service among suppliers. It often is cheaper for the patient to haul compressed gas cylinders directly to a company that fills the cylinders and then home, if he can. Such companies usually are open only 8 AM to 5 PM Monday through Friday; the patient is on his own after these hours. With an oxygen supplier, the patient usually can receive refills 24 hours a day, 7 days a week in an emergency. The supplier also takes responsibility for care and maintenance of the equipment.

CONCLUSION

Great advances have been made in home oxygen therapy in the past 20 years. Patient's lives are enhanced with the use of home oxygen. It is very scary, however, to begin using oxygen at home. A lot of myths, such as oxygen blowing up, need to be dispelled. The types of oxygen delivery devices are numerous. Knowledge of the various devices helps the nurse to help the patient make appropriate decisions when a change of therapy is necessary.

BIBLIOGRAPHY

Anderson KL: Long-term oxygen therapy: indications and guidelines for use, *Home Healthc Nurse* 7(3):40-47, 1989.

Bolgiano CS, Bunting K, Schoenberger MM: Administering oxygen therapy: what you need to know, *Nursing 90* 20(6):47-51, 1990.

Christopher KL, Spofford BT, Petrun MD, et al: A program for transtracheal oxygen delivery: assessment of safety and efficacy, *Ann Intern Med* 107(6):802-808, 1987.

Foss MA: Oxygen therapy, *Professional Nurse* 5(4):188-190, 1990.

Georgopoulos D, Anthonisen NR: Continuous oxygen therapy for the chronically hypoxemic patient, *Ann Rev Med* 41:223-230, 1990.

Hahn K: Tips for giving oxygen therapy, *Nursing 90* 20(2):70, 1990.

Heimlich HJ: Oxygen delivery for ambulatory patients: how the Micro-Trach increases mobility, *Postgrad Med* 84(6):68-73, 77-79, 1988.

Hoffman LA, Johnson JT, Wesmiller SW, et al: Transtracheal delivery of oxygen: efficiency and safety for long-term continuous therapy, *Annals of Otology, Rhinology & Laryngology* 100(2):108-115, 1991.

Massey LW, Hussey JD, Albert RK: Inaccurate oxygen delivery in some portable liquid oxygen devices, *Am Rev Respir Dis* 137(1):204-205, 1988.

McPherson SP: *Respiratory therapy equipment*, St Louis, 1985, Mosby–Year Book.

Mims BC: The risks of oxygen therapy, *RN* 50(7):20-26, 1987.

Moore-Gillon J: Oxygen-conserving delivery devices, *Respir Med* 83(4):263-264, 1989.

Moore-Gillon J: The role of oxygen saving devices in patients with chronic hypoxemia, *Lung* 168 suppl:814-815, 1990.

Netter F: *The CIBA collection of medical illustrations*, vol 7, *Respiratory system*, New York, 1979, CIBA Pharmaceutical Co.

Nocturnal Oxygen Therapy Trial Group: Continuous or nocturnal oxygen therapy in hypoxemic chronic obstructive lung disease: a clinical trial, *Ann Intern Med* 93(3):391-398, 1980.

Petty TL: Practical tips on prescribing home oxygen therapy, *Postgrad Med* 84(6):83-85, 88-90, 1988.

Pierson DJ: Pulse oximetry versus arterial blood gas specimens in long-term oxygen therapy, *Lung* 168 suppl:782-788, 1990.

Shigeoka JW, Bonekat HW: The current status of oxygen-conserving devices, *Respir Care* 30(10):833-836, 1985.

Tiep BL, Lewis MI: Oxygen conservation and oxygen-conserving devices in chronic lung disease: a review, *Chest* 92(2):263-272, 1987.

Tiep BL: Long-term home oxygen therapy, *Clin Chest Med* 11(3):505-521, 1990.

Tiep BL, Christopher KL, Spofford BT, et al: Pulsed nasal and transtracheal oxygen delivery, *Chest* 97(2):364-368, 1990.

Wade JF: *Comprehensive respiratory care: physiology and technique*, ed 3, St Louis, 1982, Mosby–Year Book.

Wesmiller SW, Hoffman LA, Sciurba FC, et al: Exercise tolerance during nasal cannula and transtracheal oxygen delivery, *Am Rev Respir Dis* 141(3):789-791, 1990.

Young LY, Creighton DE, Sauve RS: The needs of families of infants discharged home with continuous oxygen therapy, *J Obstet Gynecol Neonatal Nurs* 17(3):187-193, 1988.

C H·A·P·T·E·R ─────── *18*

Home Mechanical Ventilation

*O*bjectives:

- Identify common diseases that require home mechanical ventilation.
- Evaluate a patient's readiness to be discharged home.
- Discuss the function of each member of the patient care conference.
- Assess the home preparedness for caring for a mechanically ventilated patient.
- Develop a teaching plan for the home ventilator patient.
- Identify problem solving discharge techniques which increase the likelihood of success.

In the midtwentieth century, patients with neuromuscular diseases, such as polio, were sent home in iron lungs. In the 1970s, patients were discharged with positive-pressure mechanical ventilation. The goals of home mechanical ventilation are to reduce mortality and extend life span, to improve physical and emotional functioning, to improve the quality of life or the quality of death, and to improve cost effectiveness. This chapter discusses sending a patient home with positive-pressure mechanical ventilation. Much of the same information can be applied to the much easier negative-pressure mechanical ventilators.

ASSESSING THE PATIENT

The typical candidate for home mechanical ventilation is medically stable. In most instances the patient does not need intravenous fluids except for intermittent parenteral antibiotic therapy. The patient may receive enteral feedings or may feed himself. Thus the only reason the patient remains hospitalized is the need for mechanical ventilation to normalize arterial blood gases. Many diseases or disorders create a need for home mechanical ventilation; these are summarized in the box on p. 400. Note that the cause of hypoventilation may originate in the nervous system (neuromuscular disorders), in the thorax or around the lung (restrictive disorders), or in the lung parenchyma or airways (obstructive disorders).

The physician usually initiates a referral for home mechanical ventilation, although in many instances it is the nurse who observes that a patient is a potential candidate. The physician determines that the patient cannot be weaned from mechanical ventilation. This determination is made after several

---

Diseases requiring home mechanical ventilation

Neuromuscular disorders	Obstructive disorders	Restrictive disorders
Amyotrophic lateral sclerosis	Bronchiectasis	Congestive heart failure
Arnold-Chiari malformation	Bronchiolitis obliterans	Fibrothorax
Guillain-Barré syndrome	Bronchopulmonary dysplasia	Hyaline membrane disease
Multiple sclerosis	Chronic bronchitis and emphy-	Interstitial pulmonary fibrosis
Muscular dystrophy	sema (COPD)	Kyphoscoliosis
Myasthenia gravis	Cystic fibrosis	Obesity
Ondine's curse	Obstructive airway disease	Sarcoidosis
Polymyositis	Sleep apnea syndrome	
Spinal cord injuries above and		
sometimes below the fourth		
cervical vertebra		
Surgical injury to the phrenic		
nerve		

---

unsuccessful weaning attempts. In rare instances, based on the history and physical examination, the physician may make this determination when the patient is intubated. The physician uses arterial blood gas analysis, pulmonary function tests or weaning parameters, acid-base status, nutritional status, chest x-ray films, functional ability, growth charts in infants and children, and endurance tests to determine whether a patient is unable to wean from mechanical ventilation. Some institutions have specific criteria for discharge.

The physician is responsible for providing continuing care for the patient at home or for locating a physician to assume the care. This is a 24-hour, 7 day-a-week responsibility and not to be taken lightly. Most problems can be handled over the telephone, but often the physician must be available for a home visit. Transportation to the hospital or physician's office is expensive, since an ambulance frequently is required. The physician relies on home health nurses to assess the patient accurately.

Patient care conference

Once the physician has determined that a patient cannot be weaned from mechanical ventilation, a patient care conference is held to determine the patient's suitability for being sent home. This is a multidisciplinary conference; all health care workers involved in the patient's care are invited. A typical conference includes the following professionals, as well as others: physician, nurse, social worker, respiratory therapist, speech therapist, occupational therapist, dietitian, and chaplain. Each discusses the patient's or family's needs and capabilities with regard to ongoing care. As a unit, the team decides if the patient has the resources to go home with a mechanical ventilator.

The physician highlights essential treatment and medications and discusses the patient's overall condition. The nurse lists the patient care problems and needed interventions such as suctioning, tracheostomy care, decubitus care, dressings, feedings, medications, and incontinence. One very important topic covered by the nurse is family support. This includes which family members have visited and how often. If family members who live in the vicinity of the hospital have not visited regularly during the patient's hospitalization, it is unlikely that they will be available to learn to care for the patient at home. Lack of family support is the biggest cause of placement in an institution instead of discharge home.

For example, a long-term ventilator patient was eligible by medical and nursing standards to go home with a mechanical ventilator. The family was approached about the possibility and wanted to take the patient home. At the patient care conference, the nurses noted that the family had visited less than every 7 to 10 days of a hospitalization that lasted several months. The team felt that the family's commitment was questionable based on previous behavior. But they discussed discharge planning options with the family in a multidisciplinary conference, and the family decided to take the patient home. Several institutional sessions, including some late evening ones, were scheduled at the family's convenience. The family rarely came as scheduled and did not notify the team to make other arrangements. The patient ultimately was discharged to an extended care facility. The family visited the patient at the new facility twice in 8 weeks.

The social worker identifies the patient's and family's financial and emotional resources. This includes finances, job status, community support, and respite care, among other factors. The respiratory therapist notes current ventilator settings and tells how they potentially can be met in the home. For instance, pressure support ventilation is not available in the home for continuous ventilation through a tracheostomy. The respiratory therapist recommends a home mechanical ventilator to meet the patient's needs.

Communication devices and the potential for swallowing food and fluids without aspiration are discussed by the speech therapist. The occupational and physical therapists review the patient's functional and cognitive limitations. Adaptive equipment is the specialty of the occupational therapist. These therapists also identify the patient's mobility needs and fine and gross motor skills. The therapists (or nurse) are involved later in teaching the caregivers about transfers between the bed and chair, positioning in the bed or chair, ambulation, eating, and other activities of daily living.

The dietitian discusses the patient's caloric and protein needs, taking into account wound healing, work of breathing, and other stresses. Nutrition is critical to maintaining quality of life (for example, muscle strength, wound healing, prevention of pressure sores, and resistance to infection). The dietitian identifies the best method of assuring adequate caloric intake, such as enteral tube feedings via bolus or continuous drip, oral feedings, or a combination.

When a patient is deemed suitable for discharge home with mechanical ventilation, another patient conference is held. Sometimes the two patient care conference are combined. All members of the previous patient care conference often attend, in addition to the home health nursing agency, the patient's caregivers, and the supplier for durable medical equipment. The goal of the second conference is to familiarize the family with the work involved in caring for a mechanically ventilated patient and to begin development of a teaching plan. At this conference it is essential to determine the patient's postdischarge code status. If the patient is to be resuscitated, the caregivers need to learn cardiopulmonary resuscitation.

The nurse explains what a typical day and night are like for the patient, including all treatments or therapies. It is important to stress that care extends into the night with most patients, even though an attempt is made to simplify the patient's nocturnal needs. The family is given a realistic idea of the care involved. It is important to assess adequate numbers of caregivers. Since one nurse is not responsible for 24-hour coverage, 7 days a week, it is ludicrous to expect the same of one family member. An unwritten rule of thumb is to train three or four caregivers. The care often is divided among two primary and one or two supportive caregivers after discharge. It is easy for caregivers to underestimate the amount of care required and become exhausted. When the patient comes home, caregivers learn the fatigue of being on call at all hours. Most caregivers work in shifts of 8 to 12 hours, just as nurses do, or a 16-hour and an 8-hour shift. This helps prevent sleep deprivation and illness in the caregivers. The nurse reminds caregivers that if they become ill, often no one is available to care for the patient adequately; thus the caregiver must take care of himself, too. If available, respite care or other support helps families remain vital.

Alternately, care is sometimes provided by an outside nursing agency. Few insurance agencies, including Medicare, pay for continuous nursing (that is, 24-hour care or shifts of nursing coverage). However, most insurance companies, including Medicare, reimburse for intermittent nursing visits lasting about an hour. In the beginning the visits are daily. They decrease to four or five times weekly, then two to three times weekly, and finally weekly. Weekly visits continue for one or two months as needed, but they are decreased to bimonthly and then monthly. Most of the time the visits remain monthly, if only to change the tracheostomy tube. The number and duration of nursing visits usually can be negotiated with the third-party payer, if a cost savings is demonstrable.

Several other items are discussed as part of the patient's care at this second conference, including medications, nutrition, mobility, elimination, communication, equipment and supplies, and finances. The goal is to begin compiling a list of skills to teach the patient and family and a list of equipment and supplies to order for the home.

The medication list is reduced to essential treatments. It is not unusual for several medications to be discontinued when a patient is prepared to be sent home. It is essential to minimize the number of medications to improve compliance and to reduce the potential for errors in the home. Also, fewer medications mean fewer side effects and complications from medications.

The typical home medication list may include a bronchodilator (inhaled, systemic, or both), a diuretic and potassium supplement, a cardiotonic agent such as digoxin, a sleeping or antianxiety medication, and an antipyretic medication. In some cases the patient requires injections, such as insulin, which the caregivers must learn to give. Current intravenous and some injectable medications may need to be administered orally or by means of enteral feeding tube. Liquids are preferred to crushing pills, which may clog the feeding tube if not administered properly. Antiulcer agents, anticoagulants, and parenteral antibiotics often are discontinued. An attempt is made to administer medications only between 6 or 8 AM and 10 PM. The hospital schedule is converted to a home schedule, with medications spaced over 16 hours rather than 24 hours. (Remember the goal is to try to provide a normal life for patient and caregivers.)

The patient's method of receiving nutrition (about 2000 to 2500 calories) and fluids is analyzed. A permanent enteral feeding tube is necessary in patients who have significant upper airway aspiration or who cannot consume an adequate number of calories or fluids orally. A gastric or small bowel feeding tube is percutaneously or surgically inserted at least 1 week before discharge.

Each type of tube has advantages and disadvantages. With a gastric feeding tube, feedings are the intermittent bolus type. This allows for a fairly normal feeding routine and usually little night interruption. However, a gastric tube carries the risk of reflux and aspiration in some patients. With a small-bowel feeding tube, the patient has minimal risk of aspiration from gastric reflux. Feedings are given by means of continuous infusion to minimize diarrhea and enhance absorption. Sometimes the family may need to fill the feeding bag during the night, and a feeding pump and associated supplies are needed. Caregivers also learn to clean and reuse the feeding bag properly to prevent bacterial contamination and reduce cost. The bag is cleaned daily and changed at weekly intervals or more often. In this era of use-and-toss disposable supplies, it is difficult for some nurses to remember the importance of cleaning and reusing supplies to minimize cost.

At the conference, the family is given a realistic idea of the patient's mobility. In the hospital, the nurse often asks families to step out of the room when the patient is being helped into the chair or turned in bed to preserve the patient's privacy. Some patients require minimal assistance, but others need two to four assistants to help them get into the chair. In the home there are rarely this many people around. With patients who need the most help, a Hoyer lift often is needed to get the patient in and out of bed. The physical therapist usually teaches skills related to getting out of and into the bed, whereas the nurse discusses mobility in bed, such as turning and positioning. However, either the nurse or the physical therapist could provide this education.

The patient's elimination needs also are discussed, including his bowel and bladder routines. Some patients are continent and ask for the bedpan or commode; others are incontinent of bladder, bowel, or both. An enema or suppository is needed with particular patients, although many have diarrhea. The need to keep the skin clean of excretions to prevent skin breakdown is stressed. If the patient already has skin breakdown, the care of the decubitus is reviewed. Sometimes it is difficult for sons of mothers and daughters of fathers to provide personal hygiene, including perineal washing, intermittent catheterization, and enemas.

The adequacy and methods of patient-family communication on a long-term basis are examined. The speech therapist can discuss the various types of communication devices. Some are sophisticated, computer-assisted devices that actually talk for the patient. They frequently are very expensive but necessary in some patients. Other devices include an electrolarynx or writing board. Ideally the patient tolerates the cuff down on the tracheostomy tube and has spontaneous speech. A Passy Muir valve facilitates speech when placed in the exhalation tubing before the exhalation valve. Some patients who need a cuffed tracheostomy tube mouth understandable words. Others require assistive devices such as a talking tracheostomy tube. Remember that a fenestrated tube is used only when the patient is not receiving continuous ventilation.

In most cases home care requires a multitude of equipment and supplies. Adequate storage space near the patient is essential. Typical equipment includes a ventilator with cascade (and possibly a back-up ventilator) (Fig. 18-

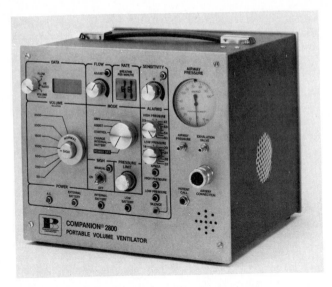

Fig. 18-1. Mechancial ventilators used in the home are small and relatively portable. (From Weilitz P: Pocket guide to respiratory care, St Louis, 1991, Mosby–Year Book.)

1), manual resuscitation bag, compressor for bronchodilator treatments, suction machine, feeding pump, alternating pressure pad for pressure reduction, Hoyer lift, bedside commode, geriatric chair or wheelchair, hospital bed, and oxygen concentrator.

The list of supplies is also lengthy. Supplies to last at least 1 month are kept in the home. Patients usually need oxygen and ventilator circuit tubing, nebulizer cups and tubing, tracheostomy dressings, suction catheters, normal saline lavage, normal saline or water for rinsing suction catheters, cotton-tipped swabs, tracheostomy ties, and feeding tube supplies, including several cases of tube feeding.

The final area discussed at the patient care conference is finances. The patient's insurance program already has been investigated. The patient and family are told what is covered and how much they are responsible for paying. It is not unusual for the total bill for equipment and supplies to be about $2,000 a month. Medications up to several hundred dollars a month and electricity to operate the equipment (about $50 a month) are additional and may not be covered by insurance. Some insurance plans cover 80% of the total cost, whereas others cover only 80% of the equipment and none of the cost of supplies. It is important to streamline care within financial constraints. For instance, the family may use paper towels or washcloths instead of tracheostomy dressings; suction catheters frequently are used for at least 24 hours before cleaning or disposal.

Nursing care is the most expensive component of a home ventilator patient. In 1991 in the Midwest, the cost of nursing assistance was $20 to $50 an hour, depending on the level of skill needed. Some caregivers require minimal assistance; others need extensive help. The cost ranges from about $1,000 a month for six 1-hour visits a week to $7,000 to $10,000 a month for daily nocturnal coverage alone, to $30,000 a month for continuous nursing care. The latter often is not fiscally effective for the insurance agency but may improve the patient's quality of life.

Contrary to popular belief, finances are not the main factor that prevents ventilator patients from being sent home—lack of family involvement is. Other sources of financial assistance can be arranged. The social services department seeks alternative sources of funding if finances are limited.

After the important issues have been discussed, the caregivers are approached about willingness to proceed. It is important to stress that the decision not be made hastily. Ideally, the patient care conference is not the caregivers' first exposure to the idea of home mechanical ventilation. The caregivers also must not be made to feel bad or inadequate if they choose not to take the patient home with a mechanical ventilator. In some cases the patient is sent to an intermediate facility to regain strength before discharge home. If the caregivers choose to initiate home mechanical ventilation, they commit a block of time to learning necessary skills. It takes a minimum of 2 to 4 hours daily for 2 to 3 weeks to prepare the caregivers adequately.

The team determines if the home situation is safe and adequate for support of the patient and caregivers. After the patient and caregivers are accepted for home mechanical ventilation, two activities occur simultaneously: assessment of the home and development of a teaching plan.

ASSESSING THE HOME

Immediately after the staff finds that a patient is ready to be sent home with a mechanical ventilator, the home is assessed. Just as with the patient and family, numerous assessments are made of the home. The home assessment usually is performed by the ventilator supplier or durable medical equipment (DME) vendor. Early assessment is necessary to allow time for changes or additions to be made.

The first area assessed in the home is accessibility. Where is the home located? In the city, an address usually is easy to locate, because houses are numbered and streets are paved. In rural areas, the vendor relies on accurate directions to locate the home. House numbers often are unavailable. Upon arriving at the site, the vendor notes how easy it is to get to the home. The home must be easily located day and night in all types of weather. Are the roads narrow and winding or hazardous? Is the road or driveway paved, gravel, or dirt? A stretcher or wheelchair is difficult to maneuver on rocks or in mud. Is the home in a floodplain from creeks or rivers? Patients may not be sent home to houses in floodplains because of the hazard of maintaining electrical equipment or transporting the patient from the home. The vendor assesses the home's entrance. Are there several stairs, forming an obstacle? A ramp is built as needed for accessibility with mobile patients.

The vendor assesses the allocation of space inside the home. This entails several areas, including the patient's room. The patient's room ideally is located near water, waste disposal, food preparation, and emergency exits. It is essential that the patient's room hold all necessary equipment and supplies. A nearby room or closet stores extra supplies. For these reasons the patient often is not located in the back bedroom or up winding stairs in a second story bedroom. The vendor assesses the width of stairs, hallways, and doors for accessibility of wheelchairs, geriatric chairs, walkers, and stretchers. The patient ideally is located near the family entertainment area. In some homes the family converts the dining room or living room into the patient's bedroom. This is both good and bad. The patient is near the family, but family life is greatly interrupted and the patient's privacy is diminished. A private room is a better choice for all concerned whenever possible.

Adequate electrical supply must be verified well before discharge. A 20-A room service usually is adequate to supply power to all electrical equipment. In some older homes a 10- to 15-A service is available and needs to be upgraded. (Circuit breakers are more convenient than fuses but not essential.) Many older homes also have only one or two double outlets in each room, for a total of two to four plug-ins. Most patients with positive-pressure mechanical ventilation require six or more outlets for equipment alone (ventilator, cascade, suction machine, oxygen concentrator, sometimes an electric bed, alternating pressure pad, nebulizer or compressor, bed side lamp, fan). In some instances the number of outlets can be increased by using a power strip for items not in continuous use, such as the nebulizer and suction machine. It is unsafe to overload any circuit and to draw extension cords from another room. Although adding one or two outlets is expensive, it is safer and improves the resale value of the house.

Water is necessary for hydration and for cleaning equipment and supplies. In some rural homes water comes from a well. It is important to have the water tested for purity. If the water is contaminated with unsafe levels of microorganisms, it is treated before the patient is sent home. Alternately, the water is boiled for at least 10 minutes to kill the bacteria. In addition, high levels of a few minerals may damage equipment with prolonged use. Sometimes bottled water is necessary.

The vendor verifies emergency services to the patient's home. He identifies the electric company for source of power. In gas-heated homes, the gas company also is named. It is essential for the electric company to be notified of the patient's need for life-support equipment. In the event of a power outage, the area is given priority for repairs. In addition, the electric company notifies the patient of planned power outages for maintenance and repair. (The patient uses a generator or ambu during power outage.) Other emergency services are similarly notified of the patient's condition. These include the fire department, nearest hospital emergency department, ambulance company, police department, water department, gas company, and highway department (snow removal and road maintenance). The patient, the vendor, the hospital, or the physician must notify each emergency service by *certified* letter of the patient's status. When the patient no longer requires the priority status (death or weaning), the emergency services are notified. Some companies send yearly renewals for priority listing to the physician.

The final area of assessment for the patient's home care is to identify community resources. These vary among communities. The most important community resources are respite care and caregiver support. Few areas offer respite care. If several families in the area have cared for ventilator patients, they may be able to trade services. Clergy are essential to the support of the patient and caregivers. Local or state politicians may also be helpful in identifying funding or changing laws. Some communities have various economic resources for patients. These local organizations may pay for partial or total rent or purchase of particular items. Sometimes equipment is loaned, such as from some offices of the American Lung Association, which accepts equipment donations.

DEVELOPING A TEACHING PLAN

The primary nurse, or perhaps a nurse specialist or home care nurse, is responsible for developing the teaching plan. At the patient care conference, all facets of the patient's care are discussed. Ideally, good notes are taken, making development of the teaching plan easier. The nurse identifies problems, develops nursing diagnoses, and establishes a measurable patient goal. Table 18-1 lists common nursing diagnoses and related interventions to teach.

Using principles of education and common sense, the teaching plan is developed. Simple skills are taught first, followed by more complex skills. The caregivers' ability to assimilate information and to demonstrate their understanding limits the rapidity of instruction. Each day previously learned skills are reviewed by the nurse and demonstrated by caregivers. Caregivers need to return demonstrate each skill at least three times independently; then the skill is deemed learned and needs further review only if a problem is observed with the caregivers performing it. A checklist such as that shown in Table 18-2 is used for each caregiver. Dates are inserted or changed as needed. Most caregivers require about 2 to 3 weeks or more of instruction before the patient is sent home.

Table 18-1. Typical problems with home care patients

Problems	Nursing diagnoses	Interventions
Patient unable to perform activities of daily living unassisted or with minimal assistance	Self-care deficit	Bathing; bed making; range of motion, flexibility, and strengthening exercises
Actual or potential skin breakdown	Potential for altered skin integrity	Bed and chair positioning; bed and chair transfers (Hoyer lift); pressure sore treatments or prevention; dressings
Patient losing weight, unable to eat orally or aspirates	Inadequate nutrition	Specialized feeding techniques; tube feedings; protein supplements
Inadequate or nonproductive cough or thick sputum	Ineffective airway clearance	Tracheostomy care; augmented cough; hydration; suctioning; chest physical therapy; nebulized bronchodilators; mobility
Limited participation in self-care; decreased appetite; inability to sleep	Depression	Patient participation; transfer to floor from intensive care unit
Abnormal arterial blood gases, impaired patient function, including mentation and exercise	Impaired gas exchange	Oxygen; mechanical ventilator; positive end-expiratory pressure (PEEP)

Table 18-2. Sample caregiver checklist
Patient Name__Joan Wittman__Caregiver Name__Marcia Wittman__

Date to instruct	Skill	Date done*	Return demonstration*		
			1	2	3
Day 1	Hygiene	3/13	3/14		
	bath	PD	TJ		
	shaving				
	mouth care				
	perineal care				
	hair washing				
Day 1	Dressings	3/13	3/14		
	tracheostomy	PD	TJ		
	feeding tube				
	pressure sores				
	other incisions or wounds				
Day 1-2	Enema	3/13	3/16		
		PD	TJ		
Day 1-3	Mobility	3/13	3/14		
	range-of-motion arms and legs	PD	TJ		
	positioning in bed				
	positioning in chair				
	bed-chair transfer				
	chair-bed transfers				
	application of splints				
Day 2-3	Medications				
	action and side effects				
Day 3-5	Tube feeding				
	type and volume				
	residuals (gastric tubes)				
	flushing				
	cleaning bag				
Day 5	Administering medications				
	Vital signs as needed				
Day 6	Tracheostomy care				
	stoma and outer cannula				
	ties				
	inner cannula				
	cuff inflation and deflation				
	changing tracheostomy tube				
Day 6	Secretion-enhancing maneuvers				
	chest physical therapy				
	augmented cough				
Day 6	Manual resuscitation bag				
	use				
	cleaning				
Day 6-7	Suctioning				
	lavaging				
	tracheostomy				
	oral and nasal techniques				
	signs of infection				

Table 18-2. Sample caregiver checklist—cont'd

Date to instruct	Skill	Date done*	Return demonstration*		
			1	2	3
Day 7	Ambulation				
Day 7	Cardiopulmonary resuscitation (CPR)				

Day 8-10	Ventilator
	  settings
	  troubleshooting alarms
	  draining water				

Day 8-10	Ventilator
	  circuit assembly and changing
	  cascade
	  cleaning and disinfecting
	  exhalation valve
	  portable battery hook-up				

Day 8-10	Oxygen				
Day 8-10	Nebulizer				

*Instructor's or reviewer's initials.

Simple skills, such as those learned in the first nursing clinical, are taught first. These include bathing and other hygiene measures, positioning in bed and chair, transferring between bed and chair, and vital signs, when needed. These simple skills help to get the caregivers familiar with the patient and lessen their fear of the hospital environment and equipment. All of these simple skills are learned and perfected within the first few days of eduction.

Other skills require more knowledge and a higher skill level. They are also more "invasive" and require manipulation of equipment. At this point, equipment to be used in the home (for example, the feeding pump, suction machine, nebulizer or compressor, and ventilator) is placed in the patient's room, if this has not been done already so caregivers are taught with actual equipment. Included in this group are administration of medications and tube feedings, tracheostomy care, airway care, and ventilator management.

Because they are simpler and often associated with fewer risks, tube feeding and medication administration are covered before airway care. The patient is given a 3 × 5 card for each medication listing the name, primary action in simple terms (water pill versus diuretic), dosage, and major side effects (limit to just a few) (see Fig. 19-2). The time the medication is to be administered is highlighted. Remember that hospital dosing times are not necessarily those recommended at home. Group the dosing times into 3 or 4 evenly spaced intervals to avoid nocturnal administration. It helps to think how the nurse would take the medication at home.

When planning to teach airway care, first teach noninvasive techniques and then invasive techniques. Recall what scares new nurses the most, and apply this to the family. For instance, cleaning the tracheostomy stoma and changing the ties is less frightening than removing the inner cannula and suctioning. Some tubes do not have an inner cannula; most physicians prefer using an inner cannula in home patients, even though they do not require one in hospitalized patients, because the inner cannula can be removed and cleaned, especially if the patient is not suctioned and airway obstruction occurs. Other patients do not have a cuff. If possible the patient is sent home without a cuff, which is prone to leaks and requires more frequent changes. In some instances a foam cuff, which requires minimal monitoring, is used.

Care of uncuffed tracheostomy tubes is simpler to teach and to learn. The tracheostomy tube is changed about once a month, according to the physician's orders. The tracheostomy tube is changed with the caregivers present a day or longer before discharge; some institutions require caregivers to change the tracheostomy tube before the patient is sent home.

Of all the airway skills, suctioning causes the most anxiety. Removing the inner cannula for cleaning and using a manual resuscitation bag help prepare the family for suctioning as they become familiar with the swivel adapter and ventilator circuit. The caregivers can practice suctioning by inserting the catheter into a soda bottle with water in the bottom only and a tracheostomy tube taped in the top. The caregivers apply suction to withdraw fluid; this helps to familiarize them with suction apparatus and general principles before suctioning the patient. The caregivers can practice holding their breath from a *normal inhalation, not a deep breath*, while inserting the suction catheter into the soda bottle and then removing it to simulate the patient's feelings. A general rule of thumb is to be in and out of the airway before the low pressure or apnea alarm sounds, about 15 to 20 seconds at most.

In the home, clean technique usually is implemented instead of the aseptic technique learned and practiced by nurses. The home has fewer pathogens than the hospital, and usually the caregivers are not in contact with several other patients. In many instances the same suction catheter is used for a 24-hour period before disposal. Some patients clean and reuse suction catheters for an indefinite period. Tap water or boiled water is used to rinse catheters. When clean technique is used, stress the importance of hand washing before suctioning and adequate rinsing of the catheter after suctioning. Well-rinsed suction catheters are stored between two clean, dry, paper towels after suctioning. They are never stored in a closed or zippered plastic bag, which promotes growth of bacteria. For clean technique to work, supplies must be kept clean. Otherwise clean technique becomes dirty technique, and the patient becomes infected.

The final area covered is care of the mechanical ventilator. This lesson usually is covered by a respiratory therapist from the vendor or hospital. The lesson includes administering oxygen and inhaled bronchodilators, changing and cleaning the ventilator circuit, and troubleshooting the ventilator alarms. Bagging the patient precedes care of the mechanical ventilator and usually is taught with suctioning. A handout on what to assess for each alarm is helpful and usually can be obtained from the vendor.

The caregivers should begin to assume care of the patient in the hospital immediately after learning a skill. When there, they practice learned skills on the patient. Each day a new skill or set of skills is added. If the caregivers practice daily, the job is less overwhelming, and hospital (institution) staff can assess areas of concentration and independence. As seen in Table 18-2, it takes at least 2 weeks to educate a family. Often a third week is needed to perfect skills before discharge.

IMPLEMENTING THE DISCHARGE

Implementing the discharge begins with the vendor bringing home equipment into the hospital for the caregiver to use. The patient is connected to the home ventilator, and settings are determined to provide adequate gas exchange. One or two days before discharge, the equipment is delivered to the patient's home.

When caregivers have learned all areas of the patient's care, they are brought into the hospital to provide total care for the patient for a period of 48 to 60 hours. This usually occurs from Friday evening to Monday morning. A sleeping cot or reclining chair is needed for the caregivers to rest. The caregivers determine among themselves how to arrange care schedules. Some prefer to divide the shifts into 8- or 12-hour segments. Doing this before discharge helps caregivers realize complete responsibility for the patient's care and think about how they will arrange care at home. The nursing staff assesses the caregivers' adequacy of skills and care. They provide assistance and education as needed, but the caregivers are responsible for the patient's care. The role of the nursing staff is primarily supervisory and supportive. This is a very stressful time for the family. They need to prove themselves capable of caring for the patient, and many learn what a sleepless night is like.

After the caregivers have provided total care for the patient and have been deemed capable, the discharge date is confirmed. In many cases the tentative date was set weeks before and depended on the caregivers' learning many skills. The date may have been adjusted several times to allow the caregivers to demonstrate competence. Tuesday or Wednesday is the preferred day for discharge. If problems arise, they are easier to solve in the middle of the week than during the weekend; nursing agency staffing also is better. The social services department arranges for a life-support ambulance to transport the patient home on the scheduled date. The discharge time varies but usually is around 10 AM. Again, problems are easier to solve during the day than at night.

On the day of discharge the respiratory therapist accompanies the patient home. The vendor may remain with the caregivers for 4 to 6 hours, arranging equipment and supplies and providing final instructions. The vendor usually is present the first time the caregivers change the ventilator circuit. Most vendors make daily visits for 1 to 2 weeks until they and the caregivers are assured of the caregivers' competence. Vendor visits slowly decrease to three or four times weekly, to weekly, and finally to monthly.

In some instances the patient is weaned from mechanical ventilation in the home. Weaning at home occurs much more slowly than in the hospital with most mechanically ventilated patients. One ventilator setting change a week or a month is the norm in many patients. The exception is the patient with a reversible neuromuscular disorder, such as Guillain-Barré's disease, who rapidly regains function over a short period; these patients are weaned more rapidly. The physician dictates weaning guidelines, which are implemented by the nurse and the caregivers.

ALTERNATIVES

Many patients cannot go home with a mechanical ventilator, for numerous reasons. The patient may have too much cardiopulmonary instability, require a higher nursing skill level than can be provided at home, have inadequate family support, or have no financial support. These patients often are placed in extended care facilities. However, in many localities there are few to no extended-care ventilator beds available, except for the wealthy, who can afford private care facilities. Waiting lists for Medicare or medical assistance beds in nonprivate facilities extend several months. Patients remain in the hospital until a facility is located or the patient dies. In many instances the facility is not located near family and may be several hours' drive away.

CONCLUSION

Care of a ventilator-dependent patient is a rewarding challenge. It is even more challenging to prepare lay caregivers to take a patient home with a mechanical ventilator. A successful discharge requires a multidisciplinary approach and a committed nursing staff. The discharge process begins with a patient care conference. Those involved in the patient care conference are the physician, nurse, social worker, respiratory therapist, speech therapist, occupational therapist, dietitian, caregivers, patient, chaplain, durable medical equipment supplier, and home health nursing agency. At the patient care conference, patient and family needs are reviewed. The nurse develops and coordinates the teaching plan, which is executed over a period of several weeks. Each member of the multidisciplinary team has an essential role in teaching the caregivers. The home is assessed, and equipment delivered before the patient is discharged. The durable medical equipment vendor assumes responsibility for establishing the patient and equipment in the home. Home health nurses help the caregivers make the transition from hospital to home. These nurses assess the patient and continue to teach the caregivers. Once home, some patients are weaned, and others receive continuous mechanical ventilation.

BIBLIOGRAPHY

Dettenmeier PA: Planning for successful home mechanical ventilation, *AACN Clin Issues Crit Care* 1(2):267-279, 1990.

Dettenmeier PA, Jackson NC: Chronic hypoventilation syndrome: treatment with noninvasive mechanical ventilation, *AACN Clin Issues Crit Care Nurs* 2(3):415-431, 1991.

Goldberg AI, Frownfelter D: The ventilator-assisted individuals study, *Chest* 98(2): 428-433, 1990.

Goldberg AI, Noah Z, Fleming M, et al: Quality of care for life-supported children who require prolonged mechanical ventilation at home, *QRB* 13(3):81-88, 1987.

Haynes N, Raine SF, Rushing P: Discharging ICU ventilator-dependent patients to home health care, *Crit Care Nurse* 10(7):39-41, 1990.

Make BJ: Mechanical ventilation in the home, *Crit Care Clin* 6(3):785-796, 1990.

Martinez M, Mitchell A: Home planning and discharge for the ventilator-dependent patient: a case study, *Crit Care Nurse* 9(7):79-82, 1989.

McCabe MK: Ventilator patient care: a team approach, *Nurs Manag* 21(9):128a-b, 1990.

Robinson S: Discharge planning for the homeward-bound ventilator dependent client: a case study, *Axon* 11(4):77-80, 1990.

Storm DS, Baumgartner RG: Achieving self-care in the ventilator-dependent patient: a critical analysis of a case study, *Int J Nurs Stud* 24(2):95-106, 1987.

Thompson CL, Richmond M: Teaching home care for ventilator-dependent patients: the patient's perception, *Heart Lung* 19(1):79-83, 1990.

Whitford KM: Health care needs of ventilator-dependent children, *Pediatr Nurs* 14(3): 216-219, 1988.

C·H·A·P·T·E·R ——— *19*——

Pulmonary Rehabilitation

*O*bjectives:

- Describe the role of dyspnea in muscle deconditioning.
- Identify components of an exercise prescription.
- Develop a patient education program for pulmonary rehabilitation.
- Describe techniques of energy conservation.
- Discuss the types of exercises for pulmonary rehabilitation.
- Identify stress reduction techniques.
- Describe techniques that would help a patient to quit smoking.

Pulmonary rehabilitation is designed to return the patient to his fullest physical and emotional potential by controlling symptoms or disease and promoting or maintaining health. Pulmonary rehabilitation itself involves many activities and a variety of pulmonary patients. One of the many benefits of pulmonary rehabilitation is improved self-care, which results from increased muscle strength and endurance, improved central and peripheral oxygen transport, and improved activities of daily living. In patients with a history of chronic pulmonary disease, the number of hospitalizations decreases significantly, often by half. The length of stay in the hospital also is decreased. Less time is lost from work, school, and leisure activities. Further, as exercise tolerance increases, the patient's attitude and sense of well-being also improves (Brashea and Rhodes, 1978).

Pulmonary rehabilitation programs are multidisciplinary; they involve at least a physician, nurse, and respiratory therapist. Additional personnel may include physical therapist, speech therapist, occupational therapist, nutritionist, social worker and counselor, and exercise specialists. Some programs also use pharmacists and vocational counselors. The multidisciplinary team develops a pulmonary rehabilitation program that involves the patient's and family's education, life-style changes, and exercise training. Although the components are similar, programs vary for inpatients and outpatients, as well as with the type of lung disease.

In pulmonary rehabilitation programs, patient education is a formal program with established lectures or momentary bedside education. All members of the multidisciplinary team contribute to the educational program. To avoid unnecessary overlap and gaps in the educational content, the health care professionals must collaborate on the teaching plan and communicate

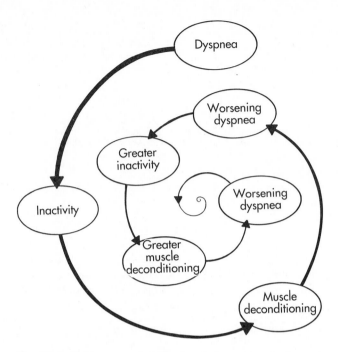

Fig. 19-1. Pulmonary rehabilitation helps to break the cycle of dyspnea, inactivity, and deconditioning.

with one another about the patient's progress. Some overlap is necessary, however, to reinforce learning. For instance, the nurse, respiratory therapist, stress counselor, and exercise therapist all teach breathing control as they work with the patient. Care is taken to avoid teaching the patient conflicting information from various sources.

For many reasons patients with chronic pulmonary diseases often are caught in a vicious cycle that impairs their ability to perform physical tasks. Dyspnea leads to inactivity; inactivity promotes muscle deconditioning. Deconditioned muscles waste energy and increase shortness of breath (Fig. 19-1). The shortness of breath or dyspnea that occurs with chronic pulmonary disease often initiates the cycle early in the course of the disease. Exercise training in pulmonary rehabilitation helps to break the cycle initiated by dyspnea, inactivity, and muscle deconditioning.

Pulmonary rehabilitation usually is an integral part of chronic care, but it is equally important in acute care. Both outpatients and inpatients need pulmonary rehabilitation. Patients being mechanically ventilated need education and exercise. Deep-breathing and coughing exercises in patients with pneumonia or who have had surgery are a form of acute care pulmonary rehabilitation. To improve lung compliance, the patient with chronic obstructive pulmonary disease (COPD) learns to do pursed-lip and diaphragmatic breathing, inhaling and exhaling slowly and deeply, whereas patients with interstitial lung disease learn to breathe shallower and faster. This chapter is designed to review the basic components of pulmonary rehabilitation. The chapter focuses on outpatients with chronic pulmonary disease. The chapter includes several illustrated boxes, called "Patient education guides," that are written in language most patients will be able to understand. The nurse is encouraged to copy these patient education guides for distribution.

ASSESSMENT
Candidates for pulmonary rehabilitation

In observing the patients enrolled in formal exercise training pulmonary rehabilitation programs, the nurse notes that most participants have *severe* obstructive or restrictive pulmonary disease. These patients derive both educational and exercise benefit, but they may have benefited more from earlier enrollment in a program, since physical ability in severe disease usually is very limited. Patients who benefit most from pulmonary rehabilitation programs have an FEV_1 (forced expiratory volume in 1 second) above 1 L or between 30% and 70% of predicted. Pulmonary rehabilitation ideally begins with the diagnosis of pulmonary disease; that is, before severe disability occurs. Recall that the first sign of pulmonary disease often is dyspnea.

The diagnosis of COPD, emphysema, chronic bronchitis, cystic fibrosis, interstitial pulmonary fibrosis, asthma, acute respiratory failure, or recurring pneumonia is a clue that the patient may require pulmonary rehabilitation. A patient who has had thoracic surgery also may need pulmonary rehabilitation. In hospitalized patients, the physician, nurse, or therapist may recommend pulmonary rehabilitation. Education and training begin in the intensive care unit and continue through acute care on the floor and discharge home. (Alternately, education begins in the physician's office and continues in the community.) Since an acutely ill patient has limited ability to learn or exercise, the program often is simplified. The inpatient program often involves a slide or tape program or a series of lectures interspersed with physical therapy. In some instances the patient is referred to another facility or specialized center for pulmonary rehabilitation after discharge.

Outpatient pulmonary rehabilitation exercise training programs usually are developed and implemented by hospitals, especially those focused on teaching or community service. Criteria vary for admission to such programs, but most limit admittance to *motivated* patients with evidence of dysfunction by pulmonary function testing who are interested in self-care and who are felt to be able to improve their physical condition. Patients with unstable or disabling nonpulmonary disease, such as ischemic heart disease, usually are excluded. Lack of motivation is a reason for failure in a pulmonary rehabilitation program and often results in exclusion from the program. Motivation frequently is assessed by willingness to quit smoking, which worsens pulmonary function. Patients sometimes are required to quit smoking before or shortly after entering a pulmonary rehabilitation program. The patient's interest in breaking the smoking habit is vital to success. Use of supplemental oxygen does not exclude a patient from an exercise program; however, most patients do not require oxygen if enrolled early in the disease process.

In some programs participants are segregated by diagnosis, (for example, asthmatics in one group, patients with COPD in another) or by the severity of the disease; this is done because the rehabilitation needs of the various subgroups vary. For example, asthmatics often are younger than other patients with obstructive lung diseases, and their exercise programs are more vigorous. In addition, patients with cardiac dysfunction usually are separated from those with pulmonary dysfunction, because they have different educational and exercise needs.

Exercise

Objective tests are performed before a patient enrolls in a pulmonary rehabilitation exercise program to determine the patient's physical condition and ability before rehabilitation is begun. The patient also undergoes a complete history (including allergies, smoking, chest pain, myocardial infarction, sputum characteristics, and tuberculosis exposure and skin test status) and physical examination. The physician analyzes the results of various tests including a complete blood count, electrolytes, alpha-1 antitrypsin, thyroid panel, electrocardiogram, resting arterial blood gases, and pulmonary function tests. If the patient meets enrollment criteria, he usually performs a physician-directed pulmonary exercise test with frequent blood pressure checks, serial exhaled gases, serial arterial blood gases (usually by means of an indwelling arterial line, which also measures blood pressure), continuous pulse oximetry, and continuous electrocardiography to assess exercise capacity. Some physicians insert a pulmonary artery catheter to measure pulmonary artery pressure, cardiac output, and venous oxygenation.

Exercise tests enable the physician to measure the patient's exercise tolerance objectively in relation to present physiological status. The exercise test differentiates pulmonary from cardiac limitations, as well as muscle deconditioning. The patient must have coordinated motor skills and be able to follow directions to be eligible to undergo an exercise test or to participate in a formal exercise program. The main problems in exercising a patient with pulmonary disease are hypoxemia, hypertension, abnormal right heart function, and air trapping.

An exercise test can be performed on a bicycle or a treadmill. When a treadmill is used, the physician controls the speed and grade (incline) to determine the patient's level of fatigue. The various protocols for exercise testing implemented by the physician include the Naughton, modified Naughton, and Low Performance Protocol.

Most patients with pulmonary dysfunction are walked on the treadmill at a speed of about 1 to 1½ mph, whereas cardiac patients frequently can walk much faster. The incline begins on a flat level and is increased every 1 to 2 minutes by 2% to 4%. Increasing the incline is analogous to walking uphill and rapidly fatigues most patients. Just before increasing either the speed or the incline and at the patient's exercise limit (the end of the test), the physician samples exhaled gases and arterial blood gases. Oxygen is added or increased to meet the patient's demands. The test ends when serious electrocardiographic or cardiac changes occur, when the patient feels symptom limited (he is unable to walk any longer because of either dyspnea or muscle fatigue), or when the patient has reached a preselected, age-determined heart rate (see box on p. 417).

The purpose of exercise testing is to determine a safe level of exercise and the need for supplemental oxygen. The patient usually is given a training heart rate range based on the test. The exercise prescription usually specifies (1) method or mode of exercise (walking, biking, inspiratory muscle trainer, treadmill, arm ergometer, 6- or 12-minute walk), (2) intensity (miles per hour, distance, or time to a given maximum heart rate) (3) frequency (times per day or week), and (4) duration (usually minutes or miles). Upper extremity exercises are also used in a pulmonary exercise training program and are discussed later in the chapter.

Criteria for terminating an exercise test

General

Symptoms force patient to quit

Heart rate

70% to 85% of the following figure: 220 − patient's age (determined by physician)

Blood pressure

Significant decrease in systolic blood pressure
20 mm Hg increase in diastolic blood pressure
50 to 100 mm Hg increase in systolic blood pressure

Cardiac dysrhythmia

Ventricular or supraventricular beats greater than 6/min
Atrial or ventricular paroxysmal tachycardia
New T wave inversion of 3 mm Hg or more
New ST segment elevation or depression of 2 mm Hg or more

Signs of insufficient peripheral oxygenation and ventilation

Clammy skin
Cyanosis
Dizziness
Lack of coordination
Mental confusion
Muscle cramps
Nausea
Pallor
Severe dyspnea

Once enrolled in a pulmonary rehabilitation training program, the patient's progress is measured subjectively and objectively. The patient makes the subjective assessments. For example, he may report that he can perform activities of daily living with less shortness of breath. He also may be able to perform activities that he previously was unable to do.

Objective assessment of the patient usually includes a simple measurement of exercise tolerance or a formal exercise test. The simplest test of exercise tolerance is a 6- or 12-minute walk. The distance a patient walks in the specified time (either 6 or 12 minutes) is recorded at the beginning of a program and at intervals (usually every 2 or 3 months) thereafter. A formal exercise test is needed occasionally to assess oxygen requirements for exercise. In most programs, this is done every 12 to 18 months unless the patient's condition dictates an earlier need. Subsequent formal exercise retesting often is less extensive than the initial test.

Education

Several techniques can be used to identify the educational needs of a particular patient. The patient may complete a multiple choice questionnaire about the disease and treatments. The nurse discusses the answers with the patient and uses this discussion to reinforce the patient's knowledge about the treatment plan. One direct way to assess patient knowledge is to ask the patient about his understanding of a particular topic, such as, "Why are cilia important?" "Tell me what you know about asthma," "Show me how you use your inhaler," "Demonstrate pursed-lip and diaphragmatic breathing," or "What activities are hard for you to perform because of shortness of breath?" (See interviewing techniques in Chapter 4.) Observation of skills is essential for evaluating the patient's ability to perform the task (for example, use of a metered-dose inhaler). The nurse uses this assessment to begin developing an individualized educational plan.

An educational program should be tailored to the patient's and family's needs. The components of the educational plan can include anatomy, physiology, pathophysiology, medications, exercise, and energy conservation. Additional topics are developed and presented if the patient needs them. Some patients require intensive education in one or more areas. The most common problem requiring education is taking medications, particularly metered-dose inhalers.

The nurse also plans according the patient's age and style of learning (visual or auditory, group or individual). Consideration of the patient's preferred method of learning enhances learning and can even improve the rehabilitation process. Handouts are a helpful adjunct to teaching and can be kept for reviewing at home and sharing with family and friends. Pamphlets are available from several organizations, such as the American Lung Association, the American Heart Association, and the American Cancer Society (free or for a nominal charge). The nurse reviews the pamphlet with the patient and his family; simply handing the patient a pamphlet does not constitute learning. Table 19-1 contains a list of typical pulmonary rehabilitation topics that the nurse should address.

Some nurses are surprised at how little patients know about normal body functioning. Keep in mind that many patients with chronic pulmonary disease are elderly and have not benefited from the science education of students in the past few decades. When discussing normal lung anatomy, nurses may find that using a diagram or lung model is very helpful. Literature from drug companies, respiratory aids, and agencies such as the American Lung Association contain helpful drawings to review with the patient. Many points should be emphasized in each of the major areas listed in Table 19-1. These points are briefly presented below.

Anatomy, physiology, and pathophysiology. Sometimes anatomy, physiology, and pathophysiology are combined in one lecture or session. An understanding of normal anatomy and physiology is necessary to understand changes with disease. In discussing normal lung anatomy and physiology, begin by tracing the path of air from the nose or mouth to the airway. Stress the roles of warming, filtering, and humidifying inhaled air. It helps to point out the location and function of the sinuses so that patients can understand why sinus infections have an impact on pulmonary secretions. When discussing airway structure, emphasize the size of the trachea and alveoli and how changes in size can affect breathing or breathlessness. In patients with bronchospasm, discuss the muscles lining the airways and how they are influenced by allergens or emotions. Patients with chronic pulmonary diseases need to know the location of the diaphragm, how it works, and how changes in abdominal contents can affect the diaphragmatic function. Patients who produce mucus need a basic understanding of the normal function of cilia and

Table 19-1. Pulmonary rehabilitation topics

Subject	Topics to discuss
Anatomy and physiology	Upper and lower airways, cilia, alveoli, gas exchange
Pathophysiology	Obstructive and restrictive diseases and special types of each for enrolled patients (for example, bronchiectasis, fibrosis)
Medications	Inhaled and systemic bronchodilators, steroids, antibiotics, decongestants, expectorants, diuretics, and so forth
Breathing exercises	Pursed-lip and diaphragmatic breathing, effective cough
Energy conservation techniques	Personal hygiene, stairs, cleaning, and cooking
Exercise	Warm up, cool down, flexibility, strengthening, and endurance exercises; training heart rate as appropriate
Oxygen	Need, types of oxygen delivery systems, oxygen-conserving devices
Stress reduction	Coping mechanisms, techniques for relief, meditation, relaxation exercises
Nutrition	General and specific (potassium, cholesterol, fats versus carbohydrates, fluid intake)
Sexual function	Causes of dysfunction, alternative techniques

how mucus is produced and eliminated from the lung. Stress that cilia are destroyed or paralyzed by smoking and thus cannot effectively clear mucus from the lungs.

Discussion of pathophysiology centers on the diseases of the patients in the program. Understanding the problems in each disease lays a foundation for treatments presented later. Asthmatics learn what triggers or exacerbates wheezing. Stress the difference between emphysema and bronchitis, because they often are confused. Emphysema involves distended or destroyed alveoli (recall Swiss cheese) and chronic bronchitis involves airways narrowed by edema, inflammation or secretions. Many patients have COPD, which is a combination disorder. It helps to explain that although patients with obstructive lung disease feel that they have trouble getting air in, the cause of much dyspnea actually is an inability to get air out of the lungs. Conversely, with patients who have interstitial lung disease, the nurse should stress the limitations in getting air in. It is important to differentiate reversible conditions (bronchospasm) from nonreversible ones (destroyed air sacs).

Medications. Often the patient does not completely understand the purpose of his medications. The physician prescribes the medication and tells him it will help his breathing. Some patients seek further information, but many do not, and consequently most patients use medications improperly. Doses are taken late or missed because the patient does not understand the pharmacology of the drug. Some medications are taken on a empty stomach and others with food. Patients commonly administer inhaled medications improperly, because they have not been taught how to do it correctly. Therefore education about medications is a necessary component of pulmonary rehabilitation.

There are many areas of focus when teaching about medications. First, it is important for the nurse to teach, in simple terms, the drug's primary therapeutic action, such as decreases muscle spasm or kills or stunts (bacteriostatic) bacteria. Stress that there usually is an adjustment period of about 1 month when using a new medication. The patient must know the name of the drug, the dosage, and the number of times per day it is to be taken. Finally, the patient learns about major side effects and the signs of toxicity or adverse events. (See Chapter 16.)

A handout is needed to teach effectively about medications. The nurse can give the patient a blank sheet of paper divided into five columns. As the nurse talks, the patient fills in the blanks. In the first column the patient writes the drug's name and in the second column, the dosage. The third column contains special instructions such as take with food or a full glass of water. The fourth column lists the frequency or times of day to take the medication. The fifth column has major side effects, adverse events, or signs of toxicity. At the bottom of the card, there may be times of day listed and the medications to take (Fig. 19-2). If the patient cannot complete the card, the nurse should fill in the blanks for him. In the clinic or physician's office, this is good nursing practice and often results in improved patient compliance with medications.

Breathing techniques. Pursed-lip and diaphragmatic breathing (PL-DB) are integral to the education of patients with obstructive lung disease but are not necessary with interstitial lung disease. PL-DB prevents or reduces collapse of small airways on exhalation, a problem in obstructive lung diseases. By improving the exhalation of air, they prevent or reduce air trapping and allow inhalation of more "fresh" air. Elimination of carbon dioxide is enhanced, and oxygen intake is improved. The patient inhales larger tidal volumes and reduces the respiratory rate to improve overall lung compliance. Wasted ventilation and use of accessory muscles are minimized.

PL-DB actually involves two techniques that are learned separately and then practiced together. Being able to perform PL-DB without thinking requires the patient to perform the technique repeatedly. Initially the patient practices pursed-lip breathing for 5 minutes every hour while awake and with exertional activities. Over time the breathing pattern becomes a habit and is performed unconsciously.

Pursed-lip breathing is the easier of the two techniques to learn and can be performed anywhere, anytime, and usually is overlooked by passersby. The patient purses his lips as if to whistle. The lips become a gate to control exhalation. When performing pursed-lip breathing, it is essential to exhale at least two to three times as long as to inhale. For instance, if it takes the patient 1 second to inhale, he should exhale for at least 2 to 3 seconds. The patient does not force or blow the air out, but holds it back for slow, controlled exhalation. Watch to make sure patients are not forcing the air out. (See also the patient education guide on breathing techniques on p. 423.)

Diaphragmatic breathing is more difficult to learn. Like pursed-lip breathing, diaphragmatic breathing can be performed anywhere without drawing attention to the patient. Recall that the diaphragm is the main muscle of inhalation. Using upper rib and other accessory muscles increases the work of breathing. An analogy for explaining the importance of diaphragm breathing is to tell the patient that he spends $1 each time a muscle of breathing is used. It is more cost effective to use the diaphragm and spend $1 for each breath than to use accessory muscles and spend $5 to $10.

First, teach the patient to locate the diaphragm by sniffing while holding the hand just under the breastbone and above the waist. As the patient sniffs in, the diaphragm "jumps" out. A paradoxical diaphragm goes in instead of out on inhalation. Second, the patient concentrates on making the diaphragm expand on inhalation and contract on exhalation. Most patients find it easier

Sample Medication Schedule

Medication schedule for _Robert Clark_				
Medicine (action)	Dosage	Special instruction	Frequency	Side effects
Atrovent (broncho dilator)	2 puffs 1-5 minutes apart	Use with spacer; take before meals and chest PT	every 4-6 hours	cough
theodur (broncho dilator)	300 mg	with food	2x daily	jitters, nausea Call physician if increased nausea or vomiting or if wheezing
Alupent (broncho dilator)	2 puffs 1-5 minutes apart	use before Atrovent and with spacer	every 4-6 hours	jitters, fast pulse or palpitations
Azmacort (steroid)	4 puffs 1-5 minutes apart	Use with spacer after Atrovent and rinse mouth	2x daily	oral yeast/fungal infections Call physician for sores or white plaques in mouth.

Fig. 19-2. Sample medication schedule.

Medication schedule for _Robert Clark_

Daily Schedule for Medications

_____

Times	Medications
7 am	Alupent Atrovent Azmacort with spacer
8 am	theodur
11 am	Alupent Atrovent with spacer
5 pm	Alupent Atrovent Azmacort with spacer
7 pm	theodur
10:30 pm	Alupent Atrovent with spacer

Fig. 19-2, cont'd.

Patient education guide
Breathing techniques

Pursed-lip breathing

Breathe in slowly through your nose; feel your lungs fill with air.
Purse your lips as if to whistle or kiss.
Breathe out *very* slowly through your pursed lips.
Use your lips as a gate to control air leaving the lungs.
It should take you at least two or three times as long to breathe out as
   to breathe in; for example, if it takes you 2 to 3 seconds to breathe
   in, breathe out for at least 4 to 6 seconds.

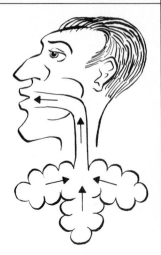

Diaphragmatic breathing

It often is easier to perform diaphragmatic breathing
   while sitting, because then your abdomen is not pushing
   up on your diaphragm.
Place one hand on your abdomen just above your waist
   and your other hand on your upper chest. While sniffing, feel your lower hand jump; this is your diaphragm.
Breathe in through your nose and feel your lower hand
   (diaphragm) push out. Your upper hand should not
   move.
Breathe out through pursed lips, and feel your lower hand
   (diaphragm) move in.

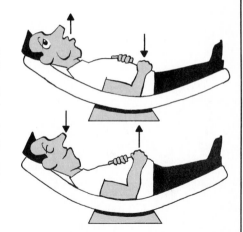

Lateral chest expansion

Place your hands on your lower ribs at your sides.
Breathe in through your nose, and concentrate on pushing
   your hands out.
Keep your shoulders still.
Breathe out, and feel your hands move in.

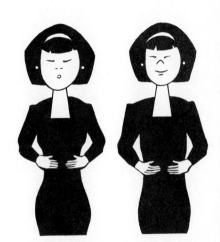

to practice diaphragmatic breathing in an upright or semiupright position, because abdominal contents are pulled down by gravity. This allows more efficient use of the diaphragm. As the patient gains experience in performing diaphragmatic breathing accurately, weight is added over the diaphragm. Some patients purchase special weights, and others use home products such as canned goods (dried rice or beans) or books of varying weights.

Some clinicians recommend locating the diaphragm laterally and performing a technique called lateral chest expansion. The patient places his hands over the lower lateral rib cage. The patient concentrates on expanding the area under the hands with inhalation. It is essential with both diaphragmatic breathing and lateral rib expansion to keep the upper rib cage and shoulders quiet during inhalation and exhalation. Using muscles other than the diaphragm increases the work of breathing.

Energy conservation. Once the techniques of pursed-lip and diaphragmatic breathing have been learned, they are applied to the areas of energy conservation and exercises. Energy conservation techniques help the patient perform activities of daily living, help decrease the dyspnea and fatigue associated with performing a task, and help improve the patient's self-confidence and independence. Positions for the patient to assume when short of breath are summarized in the patient education guide on p. 425.

A nurse, physician, or respiratory or physical therapist initiates a referral for energy conservation techniques training. An occupational therapist evaluates the need for energy conservation techniques and usually teaches them. The main educational points for energy conservation are to PACE ACTIVITIES and to EXHALE ON EXERTION. It is just as important not to rush during these activities (pacing) as it is to use other techniques that reduce the workload. Rest periods are interspersed with periods of activity or work.

Using the arms above the level of the shoulders involves a major expenditure of energy. Thus combing the hair, washing the face, and brushing the teeth may be difficult. Before washing or combing the hair, washing or shaving the face, or brushing the teeth, the patient makes sure that his airway is free of secretions and has maximal bronchodilation. Use of bronchodilators and chest physical therapy usually precedes these activities.

Hygiene. The nurse recommends ways the patient can improve his ability to perform activities of daily living. Suggestions for reducing energy expenditure include resting the elbows on the sink basin and sitting in a chair to perform upper body grooming. The patient inhales as he raises his arms and exhales (using pursed-lip and diaphragmatic breathing) while combing his hair, brushing his hair or teeth, and washing his face or hair. Some patients can complete one or two strokes of the hygiene activity, whereas others complete half of the face or hair as they exhale. The speed with which each activity is completed depends on the patient's condition. The patient frequently needs to repeat the breathing sequence several times until the task has been completed. Very breathless patients might consider changing their hair style to a simpler one (a short, straight cut or a minimal-maintenance perm), using an electric shaver, or perhaps allowing the beard to grow. Alternately, a barber or hairdresser can perform these activities of daily living.

Bathing is made easier by sitting on a stool with rubber-tipped legs and using a hand-held shower nozzle or spray attachment on the faucet. Sitting in the bathtub is restful, but it may be difficult to get out of a bathtub without assistance. Some patients' breathing is affected by being in a steamy bath-

Patient education guide
Positions to assume when short of breath

Stand with your heels about 1 foot from a wall; lean back, putting your back and head against the
  wall and your arms at your sides.
Alternatively, face the wall. Place one foot near the wall and one foot slightly back. Rest your fore-
  arms and head on the wall.
Sit, leaning slightly forward, and rest your elbows on your knees or on a table.
Lie on your side with your head and chest supported by two or three pillows.

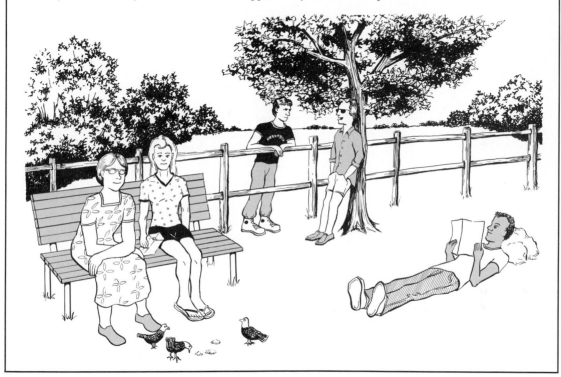

room; other patients need the additional humidity. With the former group,
leaving the door open allows steam to escape and reduces or eliminates the
feeling of suffocation from excessive humidity. Safety rails for entering and
exiting the shower and for sitting on and rising from the toilet seat are helpful. Swimming or using a whirlpool (hot tub) can eliminate some daily body
cleaning. After bathing, the patient must dry off. This, too, requires a fair
amount of energy. Many patients wrap up in a terry cloth robe to wrap up in
instead of towel drying. Others use three towels: one to sit on, one to wrap
around the shoulders, and one to put across the lap.

   Once dry, the patient dresses. It is more difficult to dress the lower body
than the upper body because of the excessive bending and pulling required.

Therefore the patient dresses from the bottom up, thus doing activities requiring greater energy expenditure first. Lower extremity dressing usually is performed while sitting. The patient puts on pants or skirt, socks, and shoes (slip-ons are preferred over shoes with laces) before standing. Upon standing, the patient pulls up the slacks or skirt. Permanent-press, lightweight, loose-fitting clothing with front closures makes dressing easier. In the summer, lightweight separates are recommended to allow body heat to dissipate. In winter, lightweight clothing is layered to conserve body heat. Heavy and tight-fitting garments usually are less comfortable and not recommended.

Walking and cleaning. Another basic activity of daily living is walking. Goals of walking distances for particular patients range from walking between rooms in the home to walking to the mailbox or shopping in a store. Some patients are very breathless when walking and require frequent, long rest periods to accomplish the goal. Energy conservation techniques can be applied to walking. The patient inhales while at a standstill and then walks a few steps as he exhales, using pursed-lip and diaphragmatic breathing. The patient stops, inhales, and walks as he exhales. Although the walk is somewhat halting at first, with practice the patient learns how to perform the walking-breathing sequence smoothly.

Shopping in a grocery store is easier than shopping in a mall. Unlike the mall, the grocery store has carts that can be used to support the patient; if the patient becomes fatigued, he can lean on the cart. Using a wheeled walker, pushing a wheelchair to sit in when tired, or riding in a motorized cart are ways to travel through malls without becoming exhausted. Many grocery and department stores now provide motorized carts for shopping.

One of the most strenuous of activities of daily living is climbing stairs. Energy conservation techniques for stair climbing are similar to those for walking. The patient inhales while standing on a step or landing and then climbs a few steps while exhaling. He rests on a step while inhaling and then climbs while exhaling. It usually takes the patient several breaths to climb a flight of stairs. However, using controlled-breathing techniques reduces the patient's breathlessness and prevents exhaustion. Descending the stairs requires less energy, because the patient does not have to pull his weight up; rather, he allows it to go down. Many patients practice the same breathing techniques when going down stairs.

The kitchen is an area of energy expenditure, since meal preparation and clean-up occur here. One of the patient's best defenses against excessive energy expenditure in the kitchen is a well-organized and well-stocked kitchen. Frequently used items such as dishes, canned goods, and staple supplies are placed at arm level, not on the top shelf or in a distant bottom cabinet. Lightweight plastic dishes are preferred to heavy china or ironstone. Electrical appliances are used in place of manual devices whenever possible, including a mixer, blender, electric knife, food processor, and dishwasher. Nonstick pans provide for easier clean-up and healthier eating. Sitting on a stool or chair and resting the arms on the counter to prepare meals (such as when cutting vegetables) or to wash dishes is an energy conserving technique. Letting dishes drip dry instead of hand drying them reduces energy expenditure and saves time.

Cleaning the house is another problem for many patients. Again, organization is the key. A wheeled cart with several shelves is useful for moving cleaning supplies such as dusters, polishes, wet cloths, and a pan of water with cleaning solution on the top. The patient pushes the cart around the room, using the cleaning supplies as needed. Items that need to be stored in another area are placed on lower shelves of the cart for later delivery. The patient pushes the cart to other rooms to deliver misplaced items.

Mopping floors and vacuuming requires the patient to use breathing exercises similar to those used in walking and climbing stairs (exhale on exertion). A self-wringing mop requires less energy. If a self-wringing mop is not used, the patient exhales while bending over to wring the mop and stands while inhaling. Bending over encourages exhalation by forcing air to leave the lungs. The patient mops while exhaling. At the end of the breath, the patient leans on the mop while inhaling and continues mopping during exhalation. Pacing is involved when the patient cleans one side or one fourth of the room at a time with rest periods in between. Similarly, the patient stands still while inhaling and pushes the vacuum during exhalation.

Other activities are condensed to reduce energy expenditure. For instance, when making the bed, the patient learns (as nurses do) to make one side first and then the other. The patient reduces trips upstairs or downstairs by using a basket to store supplies and then making one trip when the basket is full. The weight of the basket is important to the work of breathing, because a heavier basket requires more energy to carry. Some patients may need to carry two smaller, lighter loads instead of one very large heavy load.

Planning the daily and weekly calendar can also conserve energy. Periods of activity are interspersed with periods of rest, so that the patient is not exhausted early in the day. The activities requiring the most energy are scheduled early in the morning or after an afternoon nap, when the patient is rested. They are not scheduled immediately after a meal, when the blood supply is concentrated on digestion and the diaphragm is elevated by a full stomach. It is important for the patient to perform airway clearance techniques before performing activities requiring greater energy expenditure.

Activities requiring considerable energy (mowing the lawn) are spaced throughout the week. Some patients can perform such activities daily, whereas others must space the activities 1 or 2 days apart. For instance, many patients should not mow the lawn and go to a party on the same day. (By the way, a self-propelled lawn mower or hiring a neighbor to mow the lawn are energy conserving techniques. Although it is expensive to have someone else perform these activities, health is a concern, too.) Patients often are less tired if they separate house cleaning from shopping or laundry, because all of these activities expend great amounts of energy. The keys to energy conservation are to pace during the activity and to space energy-consuming activities. When appropriate, the patient uses pursed-lip and diaphragmatic breathing. For a summary of energy conservation techniques, see the Patient education guide on p. 428.

Exercise. Exercise is essential for strong muscles. It increases blood flow to muscles, the muscles' capacity to do work, endurance for longer exercise periods, and maximum oxygen uptake. In patients with lung disease, a pulmonary rehabilitation and exercise training program is individualized to the patient's level of physiological functioning, and it simulates normal daily activity, such as walking and stair climbing. Exercise is easy and inexpensive to implement in the home and requires minimal preparation time and supervision.

The main kinds of home exercise are walking, using a treadmill, bicycling,

Patient education guide
Energy conservation techniques

Breathing

Use pursed-lip and diaphragmatic breathing.
Remember to exhale on exertion.

Hygiene

Sit in a chair or stand and rest your arms on the
   sink when combing your hair, brushing your
   teeth, or washing your face.
In the bathtub, sit on a stool with rubber-tipped
   legs and use a hand-held shower or spray attachment.
Leave the bathroom door open if humidity both-
   ers you.
Install safety rails in the bathtub and over the toilet to assist in moving around safely.
Instead of drying off, wrap up in a terry cloth
   robe or sit on a towel, wrap a towel around
   your shoulders, and place a towel across your
   lap.

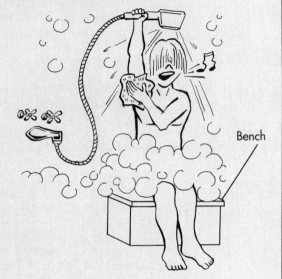

Bench

Clothing

Dress your lower body first, because bending over impairs breathing in.
Wear permanent-press, lightweight, loose-fitting clothing with front closures.
Layer lightweight clothing in winter rather than wearing heavyweight clothing.
Choose slip-on shoes instead of laced shoes, and clothing with snaps instead of buttons.
Wear clothing with elastic instead of fitted waists.

Walking

Breathe in through your nose. Walk a few steps while you breathe out through pursed lips.
Stop and breathe in through your nose.
Continue this pattern of breathing until you reach your destination.

Climbing stairs

Breathe in through your nose. Climb a few steps while you breathe out through pursed lips.
Stop as your breathe in through your nose; climb a few steps as you exhale.
Continue this pattern until you reach a landing or the top of the stairs.

Kitchen

Stock frequently used supplies at arm level.
Use lightweight plastic dishes (or aluminum pans) instead of heavy china or ironstone.
Use electrical appliances (mixer, blender, knife, food processor, dishwasher) in place of manual devices
   whenever possible.
Sit on a stool and rest your arms on the counter or table when preparing food or washing dishes.
Allow dishes to air dry rather than drying them by hand.
Cook larger portions and freeze or refrigerate some for later.

Housecleaning

The key is organization.

Push a wheeled cart with several shelves containing cleaning supplies (duster, polish, cleaning cloth, pan of water with cleaning solution) around and between rooms.

Place items needing to be stored in another area of the house on lower shelves.

Keep a box or basket at the top and bottom of stairs for placing items to be carried down and up, respectively. Make one trip when the box is full.

Completely clean one side or area of the room before moving to another area. Don't waste steps.

Finish making one side of the bed before starting the other side.

Use a self-wringing mop if possible. Breathe out while bending forward to mop, because bending forces air from the lungs. Breathe in while standing. Lean on the mop, if necessary.

Breathe in; while pushing vacuum, breathe out.

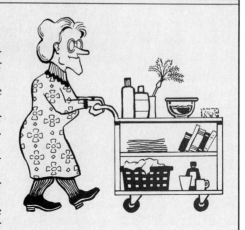

General

Schedule activities requiring lots of energy early in the day.

Perform chest therapy and take inhaled bronchodilators before heavy exertion.

Space activities requiring lots of energy, such as mowing the lawn, shopping, and vacuuming, throughout the week.

If possible, hire someone to perform tasks that cause excessive shortness of breath or fatigue.

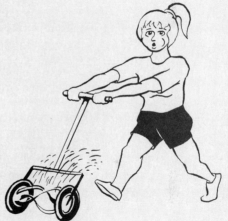

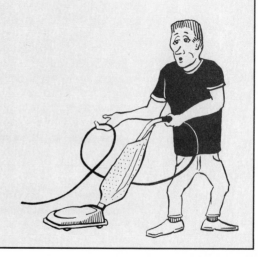

or climbing stairs. A few patients may use rowing or cross-country ski machines. Some physicians and exercise trainers do not recommend these machines or cycling because they do not simulate normal daily activity. Walking is inexpensive and can be done anywhere. Ideally the ground is level, and the surroundings are pleasant. Many local shopping malls open early to allow for year-round, climate-controlled walking, and some provide professional monitoring by nurses or other health professionals. In inclement weather, if the patient cannot walk outside or go to an enclosed walking area, he walks in his basement or elsewhere in the home.

Walking on a treadmill is convenient, since the patient never has to leave home. However, many inexpensive treadmills are unable to go slowly enough for patients with moderate pulmonary dysfunction; more expensive models capable of going 1 mph or less are needed. Some local health clubs may have suitable treadmills and provide necessary monitoring of a comprehensive training program. However, these programs often are expensive.

Bicycling is inexpensive and can be done in the home or outdoors. A stationary bicycle can exercise either the lower or both upper and lower extremities, depending on the model. A flywheel bicycle with adjustable tension, an odometer, and a tachometer is preferred for controlled biking. This allows the patient to assess objectively his level of activity and distance. Stair climbing is performed on portable or stationary stairs in the home.

Warm-up and cool-down exercises. A good exercise program always includes a warm-up and a cool-down period, which prepare the muscle for work and prevent injury. The muscles and joints become more flexible, and the heart slowly adapts to the increases and decreases in blood flow (cardiac output) during and after exercise, respectively. The patient monitors his pulse rate before warm-up exercises, as well as at the peak of exercise and 5 minutes after cool-down exercises. Exercise is adjusted to maintain the heart rate in the prescribed range. For some patients with moderate or severe pulmonary dysfunction, warm-up exercises are the only exercises performed in the beginning phase of exercise training. As the patient improves (as evidenced by less dyspnea or tachycardia with warm-up exercises), he progresses to walking or biking.

The patient also is careful to wait at least 1 hour after eating before exercising. Inhaled bronchodilators are taken at least 30 to 45 minutes before exercising (but less than 2 to 3 hours before, depending on the medication) for maximum bronchodilation. Ideally the patient exercises in the morning, when he is fully rested. Exercises are performed at least every other day for a recommended minimum of 20 to 30 minutes. Exercising fewer than three times a week limits the amount of muscle conditioning. Daily exercising is the most beneficial. Even on days when the patient doesn't feel like exercising, he should do it anyway but at a lower intensity.

Warm-up and cool-down exercises are performed for 5 to 10 minutes. These exercises focus on the arms and legs as separate and combined muscle groups and aid in relaxation. Arm exercises strengthen and recondition arm, shoulder, and upper chest muscles to improve breathing and to improve ability to perform activities of daily living requiring lifting. Leg exercises strengthen and recondition the quadriceps muscles, as well as the calf muscles. Together the activities improve strength, endurance, and coordination. Some patients use arm or ankle weights while performing the exercises to increase the workload. For the best training effect, exercises are performed continuously, rather than interspersed with rest periods. However, some patients need rest periods of about 1 minute between exercises. If the patient needs to recover for longer than 5 minutes, the activity is too strenuous, the number of repetitions must be reduced or the type of exercise changed. If the patient feels fatigued for more than an hour after exercise, the program needs to be adjusted. The Patient education guide on pp. 432-433 contains nine typical warm-up or cool-down exercises used in pulmonary rehabilitation exercise training.

Many other exercises for warm-up and cool-down activities can increase strength and flexibility. A physical therapist or exercise specialist can develop a program for the home. In addition, the American Lung Association has a two-part videotape that explains pursed-lip and diaphragmatic breathing and shows exercises performed sitting in or standing by a chair. The tape is geared to people with obstructive lung disease and is available for loan or purchase.

Oxygen. For the patient in pulmonary rehabilitation, many aspects are involved in learning to use oxygen (review Chapter 17). First, the patient learns why oxygen is needed. The potential risks of not using oxygen are explored, and organ damage is explained. Some patients are willing to use oxygen in the home but not outside the home. They are embarrassed and fear being noticed. Oxygen can also be burdensome, since many systems are heavy and restrict mobility. The analogy of remembering how long it takes to get used to wearing glasses or a hearing aid and how much better the patient feels with the device helps some patients wear oxygen. If the patient retains carbon dioxide, discuss the problems resulting from using too much oxygen; for example, worsening oxygenation from carbon dioxide retention (hypoventilation). Most patients benefit from learning about the three different forms of oxygen delivery systems and oxygen-conserving devices. If appropriate, the costs of the different systems are compared. Some patients learn about transtracheal oxygen devices.

Reducing stress. Stress is the physical and psychological response of our bodies to demands placed on us and to those we place on ourselves. Stress occurs every day. How we respond to stress depends on our perception of the stressor. Some stressors are negative, and others are positive. For instance, getting up early in the morning to go to work is stressful for some people, but there is a financial reward. Simple things such as dressing, cooking, or leaving the house become more stressful for patients who are dyspneic. The patient begins to worry hours or days in advance how he is going to manage, if he will become dyspneic, if he will run out of oxygen, and so forth.

Different levels of stress have different effects in the body. Mild stress heightens the body's ability to deliver more oxygen to tissues by increasing the heart rate, the rate and depth of breathing, and alertness. This often is called the "flight or fight" response. Excessive stress causes dryness of the mouth, irritability, dilated pupils, release of sugar by the liver, and urinary urgency. Some people break out in a "cold sweat."

Defense mechanisms aid in coping with an individual's response to stress. These defense mechanisms include denial (negating the presence of the stressor), conversion (expressing feelings through physical symptoms), displacement (redirecting emotions to a substitute), rationalization (making excuses), and sublimation (adopting socially acceptable alternatives to release tension). Defense mechanisms usually are helpful, but they can be harmful if taken to extremes. For example, some degree of denial (perhaps about the lung disease

---

Patient education guide
Warm-up and cool-down exercises

1. Sit on a kitchen chair with your feet flat on the floor and your back against the chair (or stand).
   Inhale as you bring your arms straight out in front of you at shoulder height. Do not lock your elbows, but keep your arms straight. (Alternately, the patient may elevate his arms to the side to form a "T.")
   Hold this position for a few seconds, if possible.
   Exhale as you slowly lower your arms to your lap or sides. Do not drop your arms quickly.
   Repeat five times. Increase by one repetition a day until you can do 20 repetitions.
2. Sit on a kitchen chair with your feet flat on the floor and your back against the chair (or stand).
   Inhale as you bring your arms up and touch your shoulders or the back of your neck. Keep elbows level with shoulders.
   Hold this position for a few seconds, if possible.
   Exhale as you slowly lower your arms.
   Repeat five times. Increase by one repetition a day until you can do 20 repetitions.
   The next two exercises are frequently called dowel rod exercises because the patient uses a rod or broomstick. They are performed while sitting or standing.
3. Sit on a kitchen chair with your feet flat on the floor and your back against the chair (or stand).
   Hold the rod in both hands on your lap.
   Inhale as you raise the rod above your head.
   Hold this position for a few seconds, if possible.
   Exhale as you slowly lower your arms.
   Repeat five times. Increase the repetitions by one each day until you can do 20 repetitions.
4. Sit on a kitchen chair with your feet flat on the floor and your back against the chair (or stand).
   Hold the rod in both hands on your lap.
   Inhale as you raise the rod above your head.
   Exhale as you lean to one side.
   Inhale as you return to the center.
   Exhale as you lean to the opposite side.
   Inhale as you return to the center.
   Exhale as you slowly lower your arms to your lap.
   Repeat five times. Increase the repetitions by one each day or every other day until you can do 20 repetitions.
5. Stand behind a straight-backed chair. Hold on lightly for support.
   Inhale as you slowly swing your leg out to the side; keep your back straight. (Alternately, raise the leg in front of you.)
   Hold this position for a few seconds, if possible.
   Exhale as you slowly draw your leg back. Do not drop your leg quickly.
   Repeat five times with each leg. Increase the repetitions by one each day or every other day until you can do 20 repetitions.
6. Stand beside a straight-backed chair. Hold on with one hand lightly for support.
   Squat.
   Place your hands on the floor for support, and extend one leg back to stretch the lower leg. Keep the lower back straight. The leg supporting the patient should be bent at the knee and should be perpendicular to the floor, usually balancing on the toes. The knee of the extended leg should not touch the ground, if possible. (Runner's stretch.)
   Return to squat position.
   Repeat with other leg. You may stand for a few moments in between leg stretches, if you need to.
7. Sit on a kitchen chair with your feet flat on the floor and your back against the chair (or stand next to chair).

Inhale as you raise both legs (or one leg) straight out in front of you at chair height. Do not lock your knees, but keep your legs straight.

Hold this position for a few seconds, if possible.

Exhale as you slowly lower your legs to the floor. Do not drop your legs quickly.

Repeat five times. Increase by one repetition a day until you can do 20 repetitions.

8. Inhale and exhale rhythmically as you march in place. The higher you lift your knees, the more energy is required.

    Try to march for 1 minute.

    Increase the duration of marching by 15 seconds every day until you can march for 1 to 2 minutes.

9. Lie down on a firm but comfortable surface with a small pillow under your head.

    Inhale.

    Exhale as you slowly draw your knee up to your chest.

    Hold this position for a few seconds, if possible.

    Inhale as you slowly lower your leg.

    Repeat five times with each leg. Increase repetitions by one each day until you can do 20 repetitions.

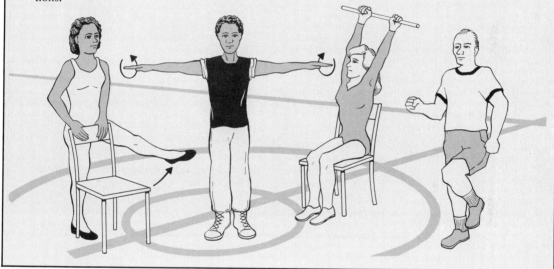

or death) is good if it prevents incapacitating depression, but denial should not prevent the normal process of adjusting to a problem. The nurse assesses which defense mechanisms the patient uses to cope with stress.

Stress reduction techniques are needed to conserve energy and to reduce oxygen consumption. The patient learns pursed-lip and diaphragmatic breathing, if indicated, to help control dyspnea. Other techniques include biofeedback, meditation, or listening to audiocassettes with relaxation techniques. Some patients benefit from using visualization or from watching videocassettes with restful pictures, music, and verbal cues. Pictures of a crowded elevator may create stress, whereas pictures of a vacation promote relaxation. Some patients use mind over matter or imagery to imagine themselves relaxing each body part. Different techniques are discussed and practiced to identify at least one that helps each patient. The nurse instructs the patient in autogenic phrases and guided relaxation, two techniques that promote relaxation (see Patient education guides on pp. 434-435).

Patient education guide
Autogenic phrases

(*Note:* After each phrase, breathe in and out slowly and deeply, as indicated. You may sit in a comfortable chair or lie on a restful surface and may need to adjust your position.)

I am closing my eyes. I feel quiet.

I am beginning to feel relaxed.

My feet feel heavy and relaxed.

My ankles, my knees, and my hips feel heavy, relaxed, and comfortable.

My stomach, chest, and back feel heavy, relaxed, and comfortable. They are quiet.

My neck, jaws, and forehead feel relaxed. They feel comfortable and smooth.

My whole body feels quiet, comfortable and relaxed. I am feeling relaxed.

My hands and arms (feet and legs) are heavy and warm. I am feeling quiet.

My whole body is relaxed and my hands (feet) are warm and relaxed.

My hands (feet) are warm. Warmth is flowing into my hands (feet).

I feel the warmth flowing down my arms (legs) into my hands (feet).

My hands and arms (feet and legs) are warm and relaxed.

My whole body feels quiet, comfortable, and relaxed.

My mind is quiet. I withdraw my thoughts from my surroundings, and I feel serene and still.

My thoughts are inward, and I am at ease.

Deep within my mind I can see that I am relaxed. I feel relaxed, comfortable, and still.

I am alert, but in a quiet, inward way.

My mind is calm and quiet.

I feel calm and quiet.

At the end of this quiet time, take a deep breath and repeat the following: I feel life and energy flowing through my feet, legs, stomach, and chest. I feel life and energy flowing through my hands, arms, shoulders, neck, and head. The energy makes me feel light and alive. As I stretch, I feel relaxed, alive, and full of energy.

Patient education guide
Guided relaxation

Sit in a comfortable chair with your hands resting in your lap, or lie on the floor with your hands at your sides.

Close your eyes.

Breathe in through your nose and out through your mouth. (For patients with obstructive lung disease, use "pursed lips" instead of "mouth.")

Breathe in through your nose and out through your mouth (pursed lips).

Feel your muscles start to loosen and relax.

Each time you breathe out, feel all the tight parts of your body start to get soft and relax.

Breathe in through your nose and out through your mouth (pursed lips).

Keep breathing slowly.

Think about your feet. Tighten your feet. Hold for a few seconds and relax. Feel the tightness leave your feet as you breathe out. Feel your feet getting heavy as you breathe out. Breathe in through your nose and out through your mouth (pursed lips).

Think about your legs. Tighten your legs. Hold for a few seconds and relax. Feel the tightness leave your legs as you breathe out. Feel your legs getting heavy each time you breathe out.

Think about your stomach. Tighten your stomach. Hold for a few seconds and relax. Feel the tightness leave your stomach as you breathe out. Feel your stomach getting heavy each time you breathe out.

Breathe in through your nose and out through your mouth (pursed lips).

Feel your relaxed feet, legs, and stomach. Let them stay that way.

Breathe in through your nose and out through your mouth (pursed lips). Think about your lower back. Feel the tightness leave your lower back as you breathe out. Feel your lower back getting heavy each time you breathe out.

Breathe in through your nose and out through your mouth (pursed lips). Think about your arms and shoulders. Tighten them. Hold for a few seconds and relax. Feel the tightness leave your arms and shoulders as you breathe out. Feel your arms and shoulders getting heavy each time you breathe out.

Feel the tightness in your neck and jaw. Relax your neck and jaw. Let the muscles become loose. Let any stiffness melt away.

Breathe in through your nose and out through your mouth (pursed lips). Think about your face, your cheeks, nose, eyes, and forehead. Tighten all the muscles in your face. Hold for a few seconds and relax. Roll your head gently in a circle. Feel the tightness leave your face as you breathe out. Feel your face getting relaxed as you breathe in through your nose and out through your mouth (pursed-lips).

Relax your mind. Think of a pleasant place such as the cool shade of green trees under blue skies. There is a gentle breeze against your face. You can hear the water flowing in a stream. Think of the quietest place you have ever been. Your whole body feels relaxed, quiet, and comfortable. Breathe in through your nose and out through your mouth (pursed lips). Experience how good relaxed feels.

Your whole body feels quiet, relaxed, and comfortable. Your breathing is easy. If you feel any tension, release it now.

Stay relaxed for a few minutes in your quiet place.

Slowly open your eyes. Gently and slowly stand up. Stretch your relaxed muscles.

Nutrition. Proper eating habits are another component of pulmonary education. Some patients require special dietary instruction, usually by a registered dietitian. (The nurse must be aware of the dietitian's lessons to provide reinforcement.) Individual education includes weight gain or reduction programs, and cholesterol- or salt-controlled diets. If group education is provided, topics may center around the role of cholesterol, potassium, calcium, or protein and carbohydrates in the diet.

Fluid intake or techniques to improve nutrition in dyspneic patients are addressed under the nutrition program. The patient learns ways to drink adequate fluids and meet caloric needs at the same time. Some patients may need low-calorie fluids, and others may need high-calorie fluids. Six small meals a day are preferable to three larger ones in dyspneic patients, because movement of the diaphragm is more restricted after larger meals. Some dyspneic patients tend to snack on convenience foods throughout the day instead of eating a balanced diet. It is much easier to eat a candy bar or a bag of chips than to prepare a nutritious snack. The dietitian can suggest simple, easy-to-prepare snacks. In addition, the candy bar may contribute to breathlessness, because the sugar (glucose) ultimately breaks down into carbon dioxide, which must be eliminated by the lungs. Most patients benefit from a high- or moderate-protein diet with moderate fat and carbohydrates. Patients with hypercapnia may benefit from a higher proportion of fat versus carbohydrate in the diet. In some patients with hypercapnia, the fat ratio is increased to 50% to 60% of calories other than protein.

Sexuality. There is more to sexuality than sexual intercourse, although it plays an important role. Sexuality is an important component of life, but one the patient rarely discusses. It is important that the nurse broach the subject with the patient, and she must be able to offer accurate and appropriate information or refer the patient to someone who can.

Patients frequently hint at problems with sexuality in speaking of "the sex we used to have." Some patients admit that they can no longer have sexual intercourse because of dyspnea. They also may suggest that intimacy has been impaired because of role changes. Some components of sexuality are discussed only in individual sessions, although many facets are appropriate for group discussion. In many instances a group discussion leads to private consultation with a nurse, physician, or sex therapist.

When discussing sexuality or sexual intercourse with a patient with lung disease, dyspnea plays an important role. The need to use oxygen alters some patient's or the partner's feelings of being sensual or sexual. Oxygen is a tubing to be dealt with during physical face contact, such as kissing. Some patients remove oxygen for these activities; however, removing the oxygen impairs function. Dyspnea also interferes with the patient's ability to have sexual intercourse. Alternate positions that require less energy are suggested. For many, a side-lying position is more comfortable than traditional positions. For others, having the woman assume the top position causes less dyspnea, especially if she is the one using oxygen. Patients may need to substitute other activities for sexual intercourse. The role of touching and holding and other ways to express deep feelings is discussed.

Techniques to help a patient quit smoking. Cigarette smoking causes premature death and is known to cause lung cancer and some head and neck cancers. It is responsible for many chronic pulmonary diseases and heart attacks, as well as stomach ulcers and bladder tumors. Smoking is associated with osteoporosis, miscarriage, and low-birth-weight babies, peripheral vascular disease, periodontal disease, and premature aging of the face. Smokers have less vitamin C in the body and altered vitamin B_{12} metabolism. Millions of Americans have quit smoking, millions want to quit smoking, and millions still smoke with no desire to quit. One of the obstacles to quitting smoking is the physiological nicotine addiction; there are also emotional and social factors.

What happens in the body when an individual smokes? Within a few seconds of lighting up and inhaling the cigarette smoke, the flavor of the cigarette stimulates the membranes of the lips, mouth, and throat. The smoke contains noxious gases such as acrolein, hydrocyanic acid, nitric oxide, nitrogen dioxide, acetone, ammonia, and carbon monoxide. Upon reaching the lungs, the smoke overwhelms the alveoli, depositing a residue of thousands of different chemicals, some of which are radioactive or cancer-causing chemicals. Tar is deposited in the large airways, where it alters ciliary function. The nicotine is rapidly absorbed into the blood stream. It reaches the brain and subsequently increases the heart rate by about 15 to 25 beats per minute; it also raises blood pressure 10 to 20 mm Hg.

People smoke for a variety of reasons. Most authorities agree that stimulation of senses and function, relaxation or pleasure enhancement, tension reduction, addiction, habit, and handling or rituals associated with smoking are common reasons for smoking cigarettes.

People also quit smoking for various reasons. The most common reasons are to become healthier, to set a good example, to improve aesthetic value (such as breath, stained fingers, or burn marks on clothing or furniture), to reduce expense, and to regain control from a bad habit. Smokers do not quit because someone else wants them to quit; they must quit for personal reasons or gain; that is, because they want to quit.

There are two ways to quit smoking—gradually or cold turkey, and many programs are available to help with the process. The various types of programs include self-help tapes and books, videocassettes or audiocassettes, and 6- to 8-week group or individual therapy sessions under the direction of a professionally trained leader. Most formal 6- to 8-week programs, such as those sponsored by the American Cancer Society or the American Lung Association, recommend that a person quit smoking abruptly. Gradually cutting down to one cigarette and naming the hour and the day of the last cigarette places great emphasis on the last cigarette. It is a moment to be savored and enjoyed. Many feel this enhances the need to return to smoking. Cold turkey or quitting abruptly relinquishes the power of the last cigarette; it is just one of many. When quitting smoking, all patients may experience craving for tobacco, irritability, anxiety, difficulty concentrating, restlessness, headache, drowsiness, and gastrointestinal disturbances.

Using a nicotine substitute such as Nicorette gum aids in diminishing the physiological cravings of nicotine withdrawal. The nicotine-containing gum is intermittently chewed to control the release of nicotine. The manufacturer recommends chewing until the mouth tingles or flavor is tasted, about 1 minute. The gum is then stored in the cheek or a plastic pill box until the feeling diminishes, about 1 to 2 minutes. It is chewed and stored repeatedly until the craving diminishes. Each piece is chewed in this fashion for about 30 to 60 minutes. Most patients chew 12 to 20 pieces of Nicorette gum a day and slowly reduce the number.

Smokers need to analyze when and why they smoke before quitting. Situations that stimulate the need to smoke need to be avoided or substituted for in the future. For instance, if the weekly management meeting, card game, or party is accompanied by smoking, it should be avoided for a while. If it can't be avoided, the individual needs to try alternative methods to provide distraction from smoking, such as a chewing behavior or humming. Delay lighting a cigarette as long as possible (for example, waiting 15 minutes or until the next hand). The craving usually diminishes by that time, and it may be easier not to light a cigarette. Imagination is important in quitting cigarettes. Some people place cigarette money in a fund and dream of what to buy in a week, month, or year. Others remember how bad they felt when smoking and how good not smoking feels.

While quitting cigarette smoking, the individual needs to occupy his hands and mouth with other activities such as chewing on toothpicks (especially flavored) or plastic straws, eating celery or carrots, increasing activity, taking a shower instead of smoking, and performing relaxation exercises. Many who are quitting smoking rely on a buddy to help them through the difficult times. Quitting smoking does not necessarily mean that the patient will gain weight, although excess weight usually is less harmful to health than cigarette smoking. Some people find themselves eating more food because it tastes better after quitting smoking. Keeping a food diary, chewing gum, and watching food choices aids in maintaining a normal weight.

The hardest period is the first 3 to 4 weeks; it gets easier for a while and then harder. People who have quit for 6 months or longer usually remain cigarette free. It is important to remember that only one cigarette can cause a patient to resume smoking. One cigarette quickly becomes one pack of cigarettes. Many people feel like a failure if they resume smoking after quitting for a time. Actually, most people quit several times before they really quit forever. A supportive environment is necessary to help the individual avoid resuming the habit.

Support group. A support group is an important component of pulmonary rehabilitation and involves patients with chronic lung diseases and their families or friends. Nurses, physical and respiratory therapists, physicians, dietitians, and counselors are resources for the members. Most support groups meet monthly for education and socialization. Patients share their experiences with one another and often have helpful suggestions on managing life with a chronic pulmonary disease. Peer pressure and peer support combine to improve compliance with the treatment regimen.

The support group meeting often has an educational focus. Members of the group may suggest topics or locate speakers under the guidance of a nurse or respiratory therapist. The topics may follow the general outline of topics presented in this chapter or expand into other areas. Many patients want to know about legal issues, such as wills or durable power of attorney. Others want more information about reimbursement issues, especially with Medicare, from a specially invited speaker. Other topics of interest frequently requested include heart disease, cancer diagnosis and therapy, updates on current therapy or research in chronic lung diseases, traveling with oxygen, and allergies. Instructive films or videotapes are sometimes shown. These can be obtained free of charge from drug companies, the American Lung Association, the American Heart Association, or the American Cancer Society, among others. In many locations the American Lung Association sponsors support groups for patients with lung diseases, especially asthma or COPD.

CONCLUSION

This chapter has reviewed concepts of comprehensive pulmonary rehabilitation, focusing primarily on the patient with obstructive airway disease. Exercise is a facet of care that frequently is overlooked, allowing debility to occur. Inactivity usually is the result of difficulty in breaking the vicious cycle of dyspnea, inactivity, and muscle wasting. Implementing an exercise program early promotes muscle strength and efficient use of oxygen. Various types of exercises to improve flexibility and muscle strength for the relatively inactive patient were presented. These exercises are performed sitting in a chair or standing beside it.

Other pulmonary rehabilitation topics that promote the patient's well-being have been discussed briefly to help the nurse identify and outline important concepts to share with individuals or groups of patients. These subjects included anatomy and physiology, pathophysiology, medications, breathing exercises, energy conservation techniques, oxygen, stress reduction, nutrition, and sexual function. Finally, techniques to help the patient quit smoking and support groups were reviewed so that the nurse may understand the problems associated with cigarette smoking and withdrawal and the need for peer support for patients with pulmonary diseases.

BIBLIOGRAPHY

Altose MD, Kendis C, Connors AF, DiMarco AF: Comparison of the effects of inspiratory muscle training and physical reconditioning on exercise capacity and dyspnea, *Am Rev Respir Dis* 133:A102, 1986.

Blackie SP and Pardy RL: Exercise testing in the assessment of pulmonary disease, *Clin Rev Allergy* 8(2-3):215-227, 1990.

Brashear RE, Rhodes ML: *Chronic obstructive lung disease: clinical treatment and management,* St Louis, 1978, Mosby–Year Book.

Brown S, Mann R: Breaking the cycle: control of breathlessness in chronic lung disease, *Professional Nurse* 5(6):325-326, 1990.

Burckhardt CS, Woods SL, Schultz AA, Ziebarth DM: Quality of life of adults with chronic illness: a psychometric study, *Res Nurs Health* 12:347-354, 1989.

Busch AJ, McClements JD: Effects of a supervised home exercise program on patients with severe chronic obstructive pulmonary disease, *Phys Ther* 68(4):469-474, 1988.

Carter R, Nicotra R, Clark L, et al: Exercise conditioning in the rehabilitation of patients with chronic obstructive pulmonary disease, *Arch Phys Med Rehabil* 69(2):118-122, 1988.

Cheong T, Magder S, Shapiro S, et al: Cardiac arrhythmias during exercise in severe chronic obstructive pulmonary disease, *Chest* 97(4):793-797, 1990.

Cox NJ, van Herwaarden CL, Folgering H, Binkhorst RA: Exercise and training in patients with chronic obstructive lung disease, *Sports Med* 6(3):180-192, 1988.

Foster S, Lopez D, Thomas HM: Pulmonary rehabilitation in COPD patients with elevated P_{CO_2}, *Am Rev Respir Dis* 138(6):1519-1523, 1988.

Foster S and Thomas H: Pulmonary rehabilitation in lung disease other than chronic obstructive pulmonary disease, *Am Rev Respir Dis* 141(3):601-604, 1990.

Gimenez M: Exercise training in patients with chronic airway obstruction, *Eur Respir J* 7(suppl):611s-617s, 1989.

Goldstein RS, McCullough C, Contreas MA: Approaches to rehabilitation of patients with ventilatory insufficiency, *Eur Respir J* 7(suppl):655s-659s, 1989.

Grassino A: Inspiratory muscle training in COPD patients, *Eur Respir J* 7(suppl):581s-586s, 1989.

Hahn K: Slow teaching the COPD patient, *Nursing 87* 17(4):34-42, 1987.

Hahn K: Sexuality and COPD, *Rehabil Nurs* 14(4):191-195, 1989.

Hahn K: Tips for giving oxygen therapy, *Nursing 90* 20(2):70, 1990.

Hasani A, Pavia D, Agnew J, et al: The effect of unproductive coughing/FET on regional mucus movement in the human lungs, *Respir Med* 85(suppl A):23-26, 1991.

Hodgekin JE: Pulmonary rehabilitation, *Clin Chest Med* 11(3):447-460, 1990.

Hoffman LA, Berg J, Rogers RM: Daily living with COPD: self-help skills to improve functional ability, *Postgrad Med* 86(6):153-154, 159-166, 1989.

Holle RH, Williams DV, Vandres JC, et al: Increased muscle efficiency and sustained benefits in an outpatient community hospital–based pulmonary rehabilitation program, *Chest* 94(6):1161-1168, 1988.

Hunter SM: Educating clients with COPD, *Home Healthc Nurse* 5(6):41-43, 1987.

Ingersoll GL: Respiratory muscle fatigue research: implications for clinical practice, *Appl Nurs Res* 2(1):6-15, 1989.

Kersten L: Changes in self-concept during pulmonary rehabilitation. I, *Heart Lung* 19(5 part 1):456-462, 1990.

Kersten L: Changes in self-concept during pulmonary rehabilitation. II, *Heart Lung* 19(5 part 1):463-470, 1990.

Kim MJ: Respiratory muscle training: implications for the patient, *Heart Lung* 13(4):333-340, 1984.

Lake FR, Henderson K, Briffe T, et al: Upper limb and lower limb exercise training in patients with chronic airflow obstruction, *Chest* 97(5):1077-1082, 1990.

Lareau S, Larson J: Ineffective breathing pattern related to airflow limitation, *Nurs Clin North Am* 22(1):179-191, 1987.

Larson JL, Kim MJ, Sharp JT, Larson DA: Inspiratory muscle training with a pressure threshold breathing device in patients with chronic obstructive pulmonary disease, *Am Rev Respir Dis* 138(3):689-696, 1988.

Make BJ, Paine R: Pulmonary rehabilitation for COPD patients, *Hosp Pract* 22(1A):26-27, 31-34, 1987.

Mall RW, Medeiros M: Objective evaluation of results of a pulmonary rehabilitation program in a community hospital, *Chest* 94(6):1156-1160, 1988.

Martin JG: Clinical intervention in chronic respiratory failure, *Chest* 97(3):105s-109s, 1990.

Mier A, Laroche C, Agnew J, et al: Tracheobronchial clearance in patients with bilateral diaphrammatic weakness, *Am Rev Respir Dis* 142(3):545-548, 1990.

Moody LE: Measurement of psychophysiologic response variables in chronic bronchitis and emphysema, *Appl Nurs Res* 3(1):36-38, 1990.

O'Ryan JA, Burns DG: *Pulmonary rehabilitation: from hospital to home,* Chicago, 1984, Mosby–Year Book.

Pardy RL, Reid WD, Belman MJ: Respiratory muscle training, *Clin Chest Med* 9(2):287-296, 1988.

Pavia D: The role of chest physiotherapy in mucus hypersecretion, *Lung* 168(suppl):614-621, 1990.

Pierson DJ: Home respiratory care in different countries, *Eur Respir J* 7(suppl):630s-636s, 1989.

Ries AL, Hawkins RW: Upper extremity exercise training in chronic obstructive pulmonary disease, *Chest* 93(4):688-692, 1988.

Rochester DF: Respiratory muscle function in health, *Heart Lung* 13(4):349-354, 1984.

Sweer L, Zwillich CW: Dyspnea in the patient with chronic obstructive pulmonary disease: etiology and management, *Clin Chest Med* 11(3):417-445, 1990.

Swerts PM, Kretzers LM, Terpstra-Lindeman E, et al: Exercise reconditioning in the rehabilitation of patients with chronic obstructive pulmonary disease: a short- and long-term analysis, *Arch Phys Med Rehabil* 71(8):570-573, 1990.

Toshima MT, Kaplan RM, and Ries AL: Experimental evaluation of rehabilitation in chronic obstructive pulmonary disease: short-term effects on exercise endurance and health status, *Health Psychol* 9(3):237-252, 1990.

Wasserman K, Sue DY, Casaburi R, Moricca RB: Selection criteria for exercise training in pulmonary rehabilitation, *Eur Respir J* 7(suppl):604s-610s, 1989.

Woods NF, Yates BC, Primomo J: Supporting families during chronic illness, *Image J Nurs Sch* 21(1):46-50, 1989.

Index

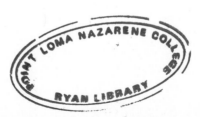

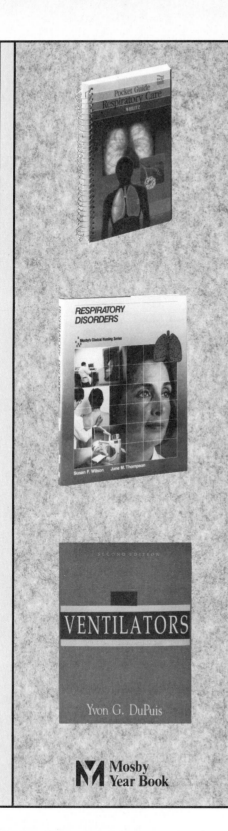